Veterinary Technician's Manual for
Small Animal Emergency and Critical Care

Veterinary Technician's Manual for
Small Animal Emergency
and Critical Care

Edited by

Christopher L. Norkus, BS, CVT, VTS (ECC), VTS (Anesthesia)
Ross University School of Veterinary Medicine
Basseterre, Saint Kitts, West Indies
Cummings School of Veterinary Medicine at Tufts University
North Grafton, Massachusetts

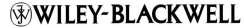

A John Wiley & Sons, Inc., Publication

This edition first published 2012 © 2012 by John Wiley & Sons, Ltd.

Wiley-Blackwell is an imprint of John Wiley & Sons, formed by the merger of Wiley's global Scientific, Technical and Medical business with Blackwell Publishing.

Registered office: John Wiley & Sons Ltd, The Atrium, Southern Gate, Chichester, West Sussex, PO19 8SQ, UK

Editorial offices: 2121 State Avenue, Ames, Iowa 50014-8300, USA
The Atrium, Southern Gate, Chichester, West Sussex, PO19 8SQ, UK
9600 Garsington Road, Oxford, OX4 2DQ, UK

For details of our global editorial offices, for customer services and for information about how to apply for permission to reuse the copyright material in this book please see our website at www.wiley.com/ wiley-blackwell.

Authorization to photocopy items for internal or personal use, or the internal or personal use of specific clients, is granted by Blackwell Publishing, provided that the base fee is paid directly to the Copyright Clearance Center, 222 Rosewood Drive, Danvers, MA 01923. For those organizations that have been granted a photocopy license by CCC, a separate system of payments has been arranged. The fee codes for users of the Transactional Reporting Service are ISBN-13: 978-0-8138-1057-7/2012.

Designations used by companies to distinguish their products are often claimed as trademarks. All brand names and product names used in this book are trade names, service marks, trademarks or registered trademarks of their respective owners. The publisher is not associated with any product or vendor mentioned in this book. This publication is designed to provide accurate and authoritative information in regard to the subject matter covered. It is sold on the understanding that the publisher is not engaged in rendering professional services. If professional advice or other expert assistance is required, the services of a competent professional should be sought.

Library of Congress Cataloging-in-Publication Data

Veterinary technician's manual for small animal emergency and critical care / edited by Christopher L. Norkus.
 p. ; cm.
 Includes bibliographical references and index.
 ISBN-13: 978-0-8138-1057-7 (pbk. : alk. paper)
 ISBN-10: 0-8138-1057-4 (pbk. : alk. paper) 1. Veterinary emergencies. I. Norkus, Christopher L.
 [DNLM: 1. Emergency Treatment–veterinary. 2. Pets. SF 778]
 SF778.V585 2011
 636.089'6025--dc23
                          2011021941

A catalogue record for this book is available from the British Library.

Set in 10/12 pt Sabon by Toppan Best-set Premedia Limited

Printed and bound in Malaysia by Vivar Printing Sdn Bhd

Disclaimer

1   2012

This book is dedicated to Charles P. Gandal, DVM

I "kept the faith" after all these years.

and

The Ross University School of Veterinary Medicine

Class of May 2011, "Pink for life."

Contents

Section 1: Initial Patient Management

Section 2: Specific Organ System Disorders

Section 3: Select Emergency/Critical Care Topics and Therapies

Companion website
This book is accompanied by a companion website: www.wiley.com/go/norkus

Contributors

Lori Baden Atkins, LVT, VTS (Emergency & Critical Care)
Veterinary Medical Teaching Hospital
Texas A&M University
College Station, TX

Amy N. Breton, CVT, VTS (Emergency & Critical Care)
Veterinary Emergency & Specialty Center of New England
Waltham, MA

Amy Campbell, CVT, VTS (Emergency & Critical Care)
Tufts Veterinary Emergency Treatment & Specialties
Walpole, MA

Mary Tefend Campbell, CVT, VTS (Emergency & Critical Care)
Carriage Hills Animal Hospital and Referral Center
Montgomery, AL

Jonathan A. Esmond, RVT, VTS (Emergency & Critical Care)
Advanced Critical Care & Internal Medicine
Tustin, CA;
Animal Emergency Clinic of the High Desert
Victorville, CA

Trish Farry, CVN, VTS (Emergency & Critical Care), VTS (Anesthesia), Cert IV (TAA)
School of Veterinary Science
The University of Queensland
Australia

Dana Heath, RVT, VTS (Emergency & Critical Care), VTS (Anesthesia)
Veterinary Medical Teaching Hospital
Texas A&M University
College Station, TX

Jennifer Keefe, CVT, VTS (Emergency & Critical Care), VTS (Anesthesia)
Angell Animal Medical Center
Boston, MA

David Liss, BA, RVT, VTS (Emergency & Critical Care)
Veterinary Specialists of the Valley
Woodland Hills, CA

Jaime Maher, CVT, VTS (Emergency & Critical Care)
Cummings School of Veterinary Medicine at Tufts University
North Grafton, MA

Christopher L. Norkus, BS, CVT, VTS
(Emergency & Critical Care), VTS
(Anesthesia)
Ross University School of Veterinary
Medicine
Basseterre, Saint Kitts, West Indies
Cummings School of Veterinary Medicine
at Tufts University
North Grafton, MA

Sally R. Powell, CVT, VTS (Emergency
& Critical Care)
MJR Veterinary Hospital at the
University of Pennsylvania
Philadelphia, PA

Angela Randels, CVT, VTS (Emergency
& Critical Care) VTS (Small Animal
Internal Medicine)
FIRST Regional Animal Hospital
Chandler, AZ

Jennifer K. Sager, BS, CVT, VTS
(Anesthesia), VTS (Emergency & Critical
Care)
University of Florida College of
Veterinary Medicine
Gainesville, FL

Lindan Spromberg, BS, LVT, VTS
(Emergency & Critical Care)
PIMA Medical Institute
Seattle WA

Andrea M. Steele, BSc, RVT, VTS
(Emergency & Critical Care)
Ontario Veterinary College Health
Sciences Centre
Guelph, Ontario, Canada

Kara B. Trent, CVT, VTS (Emergency &
Critical Care), VTS (Anesthesia)
VCA Veterinary Specialists of Northern
Colorado
Loveland, CO

Ann Elise Wortinger, BIS, LVT, VTS
(Emergency & Critical Care), VTS (Small
Animal Internal Medicine)
Sanford Brown College
Dearborn, MI.

Kimm Wuestenberg, CVT, VTS
(Emergency & Critical Care), VTS (Small
Animal Internal Medicine)
Phoenix, AZ

Preface

Let's face it. Our beloved household pets manage to get themselves into lots of trouble.

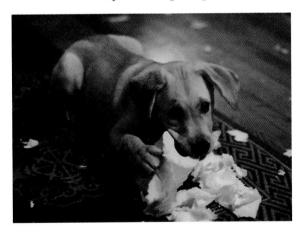

Essentially, our job in veterinary emergency and critical care medicine is to help get our animal friends out of harms' ways 24 hours a day, 7 days a week, and 365 days a year.

Veterinary Technician's Manual for Small Animal Emergency and Critical Care serves to provide veterinary paraprofessionals with a cutting edge reference as to the pathophysiology, epidemiology, signs, diagnosis, treatment, and general nursing techniques of the most common veterinary emergencies. The book has been organized into sections following that of the qualifying exam for the Academy of Veterinary Emergency & Critical Care Technicians (AVECCT) and may be a helpful aid for those preparing to write the exam. The end goal of this work, however, is to become a critical and respected resource which expands the knowledge base of veterinary paraprofessionals and, ultimately, results in better patient care and increased know-how when seconds count to save lives.

Christopher L. Norkus

Acknowledgment

A special thank you is necessary to my best friend Mark Holloway for his superior IT support in rescuing a majority of this book off of my dead laptop after I clumsily spilled soda on it.

C.L.N.

Veterinary Technician's Manual for
Small Animal Emergency and Critical Care

Section 1

Initial Patient Management

Triage and Initial Assessment of the Emergency Patient

Amy N. Breton

Introduction

One of the most important skills as a veterinary technician is the ability to be able to triage quickly and appropriately. Failure to triage appropriately may mean life or death for the patient.

Triage

The term triage comes from the French word that means "to sort" and was first used in World War I to sort and classify wounded soldiers based on the severity of their wounds (Grossman 2003). Emergency departments started using organized triage systems in the 1960s when hospitals began to see more patients than they had available resources for (Grossman 2003).

Telephone Triage

The initial triage may actually occur over the phone. Because the technicians cannot rely on their sense of touch, sight, and feel of the patient, technicians who are tasked to handle telephone calls should have strong clinical knowledge, excellent listening and communicating skills, and a sense of intuition (Grossman 2003).

A telephone triage log of the calls should be kept. Because it is a legal document, the log should be stored for several years depending on the state laws. It is important to note that several court cases have occurred involving a pet owner and a veterinary clinic because of the advice that was given over the phone. Remember that the recommendations you offer to the client can have legal ramifications, and it is important that you document the conversation to protect both yourself and the clinic.

Ideally, an organized system should be in place and all employees should follow the system (Grossman 2003). Each technician should ask the same initial questions of each

---

Box 1.1   Telephone Triage Questions

- Name, location, and telephone number of client
- Pet's name, age, sex, breed, and weight
- Pertinent medical history
- Current medications
- Current complaint
  - How is your pet breathing?
  - What is the color of the gums?
  - What is the level of consciousness (LOC)?
  - Current rectal temperature? (if able)
  - Is the pet able to stand/walk?

  Other questions may include the following:

- Is the pet eating? Is there vomiting, retching, or diarrhea?
- Is the abdomen distended or painful to the touch?
- Can the pet urinate? Are the urinations normal?
- Is there any bleeding? Where and how much?
- How much and when did the pet ingest the substance?
- How many and how long have the seizures been?
- Has there been any coughing?

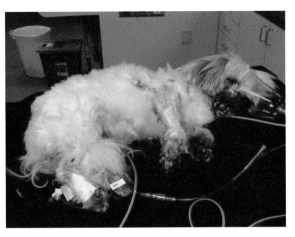

Figure 1.1   Cases brought to the emergency room, such as this dog hit by a car, must be triaged and examined quickly to address immediate life threats.

client that calls in order to ensure that each call is handled in a thorough manner. After the initial information is gathered, the questions may vary depending on what the presenting complaint is.

Each clinic may have a different policy on what advice can or cannot be given over the phone. No matter what the clinic's policy is, all owners should be instructed to come in with their pet no matter how insignificant the problem may appear. Because of owner error in interpreting their pet's condition, it is impossible to appropriately triage an animal over the phone. For example, owners frequently cannot tell if their pet is seizuring versus trembling out of fear. The safest suggestion is to always advise the owner to bring the pet into a veterinary hospital immediately. For legal purposes, it is important that the telephone triage log reflect this recommendation with each phone call. Any medical treatment suggested to clients over the phone must be documented in full in the telephone log.

Once you have suggested to the clients that they bring in their pet for a medical treatment, you should provide the owners with information about how to safely transport their pet to the clinic (Davis 2008). This may include placing pressure on a bleeding wound, putting a quick bandage on a bleeding area, keeping the animal immobile, or instructing the owner how to make a muzzle at home to ensure he/she is kept safe. Telephone triage is also important because it allows the medical team to prepare for the arrival of the patient at the hospital and to organize resources (Davis 2008). Intravenous fluids, catheters, oxygen, and crash cart supplies can be readied prior to the patient's arrival (Fig. 1.1).

Hospital Triage

Every patient that enters into the emergency room should be triaged by a veterinary technician within a minute of its arrival. It is better to assume every patient is critical than to allow a critical animal to wait for a triage while it is declining in health.

When triaging, it is important to be able to quickly assess each patient and to sort each into categories. All triage systems break down categories into either a three-, four-,

Table 1.1   Triage level acuity systems

3 Levels	Wait/Reassessment Time	Condition Examples
Resuscitative	Immediately	Cardiac arrest
Emergent	10–45 minutes	Fracture
Urgent	30 minutes–2 hours	Abscess

4 Levels	Wait/Reassessment Time	Condition Examples
Resuscitative	Immediately	Active seizures
Emergent	5–15 minutes	Serious laceration
Urgent	15–45 minutes	Eye injury
Nonurgent	1–2 hours	Constipation

5 Levels	Wait/Reassessment Time	Condition Examples
Resuscitation	Immediately	Severe respiratory distress
Emergent	5–15 minutes	Urinary obstruction
Urgent	15–45 minutes	Vomiting/diarrhea (no blood)
Semi-urgent	1–2 hours	Minor laceration
Routine	4 hours	Suture removal

Adapted from Grossman (2003), *Quick Reference to Triage.*

or five-tier system. While there is not a standard triaging system in veterinary medicine, most human medicine triage systems can be applied. In most human emergency departments in the United States, a triage acuity system is used to determine which patient can safely wait and which patient needs to be seen immediately (Hansen 2005).

In 2001, the Emergency Nurses Association of the United States was surveyed to ask what type of triage acuity scale was used by each hospital (Hansen 2005). An overwhelming 69% of the emergency departments used a three-level scale (Hansen 2005). Only two years later, another study was conducted and found that only 47% of emergency departments were using a three-level triage system, while there was an increase to 20% for those that used four-level and 20% that used five-level systems (Hansen 2005; see Table 1.1). The general consensus is that there is a trend toward four- and five-tier systems in hospitals. No matter what system is used, one thing is certain: the system should be organized and everyone at the clinic should use it.

In 1994, the animal trauma triage (ATT) scoring system was created (Table 1.2). The ATT scoring system is a way to classify and help predict the likelihood of a patient's survival after a traumatic incident (Wingfield and Raffe 2002). The system classified six different categories (perfusion, cardiac, respiratory, eye/muscle integument, skeletal, and

Table 1.2 The animal trauma triage scoring system

Grade	Perfusion	Cardiac	Respiratory	Eye/Muscle Integument	Skeletal	Neurological
0	Mucous membrane (MM) pink/moist Temp: >100°F Pulses strong or bounding	HR: K9: 60–140 F: 120–200 NSR	Normal respiratory rate	Abrasions, lacerations: only partial thickness Eyes: normal	Weight bearing on 3–4 limbs No fractures or joint laxity	Central: conscious and alert Only slightly dull Peripheral: normal
1	MM pale pink or hyperemic Temp: >100°F Pulses fair	HR: K9:140–180 F: 200–260 NSR or Ventricular premature complexes PCs (<20/minute)	Mild increased respiratory rate and effort Mild increase upper airway sounds	Abrasions, lacerations: full thickness but no deep tissue involvement Eye: corneal laceration/ulcer Orbit not perforated	Closed fracture Single joint laxity	Central: Conscious but dull, depressed Peripheral: Abnormal spinal reflexes with purposeful movement
2	MM pale Capillary refill time (CRT): 2–3 seconds Temp: <100°F	HR: K9:180+ F: 260+ Arrhythmias	Moderate increased respiratory effort with abdominal component Moderate increase upper airway sounds	Abrasions, lacerations: full thickness and deep tissue involvement Eye: corneal perforation, proptosis	Multiple grade 1 conditions Single long bone open fx Nonmandibular skull fx	Central: Unconscious, but responds to noxious stimuli Peripheral: Absent purposeful movement with intact nociception in two or more limbs Decrease anal and/or tail tone
3	MM gray, blue, or white Temp: >100°F No Femoral Pulses	HR: K9: <60 F: <120 Erratic arrhythmias	Marked respiratory effort or gasping Little to no detectable air passage	Abrasions, lacerations: full thickness and artery, nerve, or muscle involved Penetration to thoracic/abdominal cavity	Vertebral body fx/lux Except coccygeal Multiple open fx	Central: nonresponsive, refractory seizures Peripheral: absent nociception in two or more limbs

neurological) into a 0–3 scale system (Wingfield and Raffe 2002). The six scores are then added together with the highest possible score being 18 (Wingfield and Raffe 2002). The higher the score, the worse the prognosis. Ideally, the patient would have a score of 0, meaning that it is in perfect health. Each point increase from 0 resulted in a 2.3–2.6 decreased chance of survival.

Many times, clients become irate when other pets are seen before their own pet. It is imperative that clients are informed of how the emergency department functions to avoid confusion. Clients should be given an appropriate wait time and informed that if a more critical pet comes in, their wait time may be extended. Clients should be notified if wait times have changed. This task is often the responsibility of the triage technician. Being able to keep all clients happy in a waiting room is a skill that can take years to master.

Primary Assessment

The *primary assessment* will determine if the animal is having a true emergency and needs immediate treatment or if it is stable enough to wait. If the patient is deemed stable during the primary assessment, a more thorough secondary assessment will occur at another time depending on the amount of patients waiting to be seen in the waiting room. In many busy emergency rooms, the primary assessment may only include the collection of vital signs (pulse, temperature, respiratory rate/effort) and a brief owner history (chief complaint, current medications, and information from the referring veterinarian) (Table 1.3).

Table 1.3   Canine/feline normal and abnormal physical exam findings

Canine Normal	Canine Emergency Finding	Feline Normal	Feline Emergency Finding
Heart rate			
<30 lbs. 100–140 bpm 30–50 lbs. 80–120 bpm >50 lbs. 60–80 bpm	For any size dog: >160 bpm <60 bpm	140–200 bpm	<140 bpm >260 bpm
Respiration rate			
20–40 bpm	>50 bpm or any effort	20–40 bpm	>50 bpm or any effort
Mucous membrane			
Pink	Any color other than pink	Pink	Any color other than pink
Capillary refill			
<2 seconds	<1 second, >3 seconds	<2 seconds	<1 second, >3 seconds
Temperature			
100–102.9°F	<98°F, >105°F	100–102.9°F	<98°F, >105°F

The primary assessment should ideally begin with the triage interview (Grossman 2003). Since we cannot interview the pet itself, the triage interview should be directed toward the owner.

There may be a couple of circumstances that would prevent you from performing a triage interview. Treatment should be initiated on any pet that is considered a level-one triage acuity, also known as resuscitative. Examples of this would be cardiac arrest, active seizures, severe blunt trauma, anaphylaxis, uncontrolled hemorrhage, severe head trauma, open chest/abdominal wound, and any type of shock. Owners of these pets should be informed of the "why," "what," and "how much" in a clear and concise manner:

■ Why does their pet need immediate emergent treatment?
■ What treatment will be initiated?
■ A verbal rough estimate should be given of how much it will cost.

Many times, owners will not wish to proceed with treatment due to cost, age, or another underlying illness of the pet. The following depicts an example of a conversation when conducting a triage interview: "My name is Amanda. I would like your permission to start emergency treatment on Skipper because he is in shock and has a dangerously low heart rate. We will place an intravenous catheter, give him intravenous fluids, perform some initial blood work to try to get him more stable. This initial treatment will likely cost about $500–700. Is it okay if we start treatment immediately?" Many veterinary clinics will have the client sign a "quick estimate" which gives the clinic permission to start emergency treatment and shows a range of how much the client may spend.

Unless your patient is in need of resuscitative measures immediately, you will have ample time to conduct the triage interview and initial assessment on the pet. The triage interview should always begin with you introducing yourself and telling the client your title so they know who is handling their pet's care (Grossman 2003). Before even handling the animal you need to ask what the chief complaint is. This is imperative because if you fail to ask what the problem is and you reach for a femoral pulse, you may end up grabbing a leg that is broken. You should also politely ask if the pet will mind you touching it and if it is friendly. This question will hopefully prompt the client to tell if you the pet is aggressive or not.

While speaking to the client you should be observing the patient. It is important to use all your senses including sight, smell, hearing, touch, and intuition (Grossman 2003).

Assessing these systems should be done in a clear, conscious manner. The technique you develop for performing the primary assessment on a particular patient should be the same technique you use for each patient. While it is often "easier" to simply jump right to the area of complaint (like the broken leg), you cannot forget to examine the rest of the patient. If you have done your primary examination appropriately, you will have assessed the three major systems briefly: cardiovascular, respiratory, and central nervous systems (Hansen 2005).

Secondary Assessment

When time allows, a more detailed *secondary assessment* of the patient is performed by the attending veterinarian or technician. This is also the time when a more detailed client

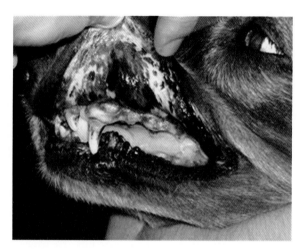

Figure 1.2 A dog with pale mucous membranes. Common causes include anemia and vasoconstriction. (Courtesy of Gareth Buckley DVM, DACVECC.)

interview is performed. This is often performed concurrently as treatment of the emergent patient is already underway.

To perform a full physical exam, you should start with the head and examine the patient's eyes, mouth, nose, and ears. The mucous membranes (MMs) and capillary refill time (CRT) should be obtained (Fig. 1.2). The submandibular lymph nodes should be palpated and any discharge or changes should be recorded.

As you proceed down the body, the forelimbs should be examined for any obvious injuries or nonsymmetry. You should auscultate the heart and feel a femoral or distal pulse at the same time. It is important you note that heart rate and pulse rate are the same. If they are not the same, this *pulse deficit* likely indicates some type of arrhythmia, such as ventricular premature contractions. You should auscultate the lungs in different fields. The abdomen should be examined and palpated. You should run your hands down the back of the patient and check the skin turgor of the patient. Lacerations, wounds, bruising, ectoparasites, and masses should all be noted (Fig. 1.3).

Once you get to the back of the patient, the tail should be lifted and the rectum should be examined. The popliteal and inguinal lymph nodes should be palpated. A temperature should be taken and pulses should be felt again. The hind legs should be examined and felt in a similar manner as the forelimbs. You should observe the patient's walking and its mannerisms when you are not touching it. Special attention should be paid to whether the patient appears mentally appropriate. This includes altered behavior, depression, head pressing, circling, and ataxia.

Cardiovascular

The most common conditions that can cause a change in cardiovascular status are hypovolemia, anemia, sepsis, or cardiac dysfuncion (Hughes 2005). It is important to be able to identify early indicators of failure in the cardiovascular system so that the patient does not decline further.

During a physical exam, MM color may be altered from a normal healthy pink to a muddy, grey, or pale color (Fig. 1.4). Any change in MM color is a life-threatening

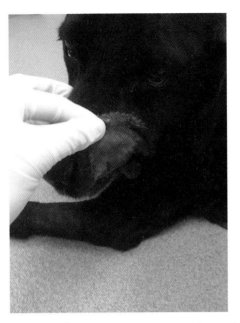

Figure 1.3 Hyperemic (red) mucous membranes may suggest a state of vasodilation such as would be seen with sepsis, systemic inflammatory response syndrome (SIRS), or anaphylaxis.

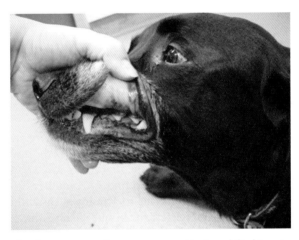

Figure 1.4 Icteric (jaundiced) mucous membranes correspond to hyperbilirubinemia and may suggest hemolysis, liver disease, bile duct obstruction, or feline sepsis.

emergency. CRT should always be under 2 seconds. During cardiovascular collapse, you may see an increase to 3 seconds or greater.

Heart rate may be either increased or decreased. Pulse strength may be either bounding or weak. Both the heart rate and pulse rate may be irregular or nonsynchronous. During auscultation, an arrhythmia or murmur may be detected. One of the key indicators in the early stage of shock is an elevated heart rate (Hughes 2005). Some patients may have an elevated heart rate due to excitement or anxiety, but the overall patient status must be assessed before this conclusion is made. A good example of this is a 3-year-old Labrador retriever who has high energy. On presentation, he appears very bright and alert.

His owners describe hematochezia. His physical exam is within normal limits, except that he has bounding pulses and a heart rate of 180 bpm. This dog is likely in the early stages of shock and is experiencing some cardiovascular collapse. Treatment should be initiated relatively soon.

There are numerous potential heart arrhythmias, and while some may not be life-threatening, until the patient receives a full cardiac workup, all arrhythmias should be considered potentially life-threatening. If during the physical exam a heart arrhythmia is auscultated, the patient should have an electrocardiogram (ECG) performed. An ECG strip should be performed for 5 minutes, and a strip should be recorded and placed in the patient's record. If the technician is not well-versed in interpreting heart arrhythmias, a veterinarian should be consulted to ensure that the patient is stable and can wait to be seen.

Respiratory

Any change in an animal's breathing is an emergency. Owners often mistake labored breathing as "panting" or shallow breathing as "sniffing." When performing a physical exam, it is important to step back and simply examine how the patient is breathing. Your sight will be the most important tool at determining if the patient is having difficulty breathing or not.

When observing a patient's breathing, there should not be an abdominal component when a patient is breathing normally. If there is abdominal effort, it should be noted if the chest and abdomen are moving together (synchronous) or opposite (asynchronous). Expiratory time and effort can also yield information. The normal inspiration:expiration (I:E) ratio is 1:2, meaning a patient exhales for twice as long as it inhales when breathing normally (Dodam 2002). Generally, increased expiration time can be a sign of lung pathology or intrathoracic problem, while an increased inspiration time can point to upper airway pathology or extrathoracic problem. Synchronous breathing is generally a sign that the abnormality is inside the lungs, while asynchronous breathing usually points to pleural space pathology (Mathews 2007).

MM color is also an important tool in determining respiratory function. Though not completely accurate (because lighting, anemia, or icterus hides the appearance of cyanotic membranes), any presence of cyanosis is an issue that needs to be addressed immediately. Severely anemic patients may mask the "blue" color of cyanosis because at least 5 g/dL of hemoglobin is required in order for patients to physically show the color blue. This is also true in patients that are extremely icteric or in severe shock. If the patient is severely white or jaundiced, it may mask the cyanosis.

If you have any question whether a patient is oxygenating well, oxygen supplementation should be given. Pulse oximetry may also be used to help. A pulse oximetry machine measures the oxygen saturation of hemoglobin (SpO_2), which is a very insensitive measure of oxygenation. Normally, animals should have a range of oxygen saturation from 98% to 100% on room air. The drawback to a pulse oximetry machine is that, at times, it is not very accurate. Patient movement, poor perfusion, hair, or any color other than pink MMs (icterus, cyanosis, and anemia) can cause the reading to be inaccurate. However, the pulse oximetry machine continues to be a fairly quick and easy test to use.

Since there are myriad reasons respiratory dysfunction may occur, it is possible that a patient suffering from only mild respiratory issues may have an extended wait time in the emergency room. If there is any question on the degree of respiratory dysfunction, the patient should be given oxygen supplementation until treatment and diagnostics can begin.

Central Nervous System

Upon initial presentation, the LOC should be assessed. There are many different methods to classify LOC. Depending on the text you read, there may be some minor changes to the LOC levels (Archer 2009).

An animal may be conscious but have abnormal mentation such as slow or inappropriate response to stimuli (Rivera 2003). When a patient presents to the clinic, it is important to simply observe the animal initially to see how mentally appropriate it is. You should observe the animal and ask yourself the following:

- Does the animal know where it is?
- Can it visually focus on its surroundings?
- Is the pet walking normally or is it ataxic?
- Are the pupils the same size and responsive to light?
- Are there any abnormal breathing patterns?
- Is there any seizure activity?
- Does the animal respond to painful stimuli?

It is important to note the patient's LOC upon presentation. Any patient that has a declining LOC presents an emergency case, and the overall prognosis of the patient worsens (Rivera 2003).

Complete History

As part of the secondary assessment, a more detailed complete history is obtained from the owners. During this interview, is it important to again remind clients of who you are and what treatment may have already been started on their pet. It is important then to confirm the correct signalment of the patient (e.g., age, sex, breed, spay/neuter status) and the owner's chief complaint as to why the pet was brought pet to the emergency room. It is important to ask about the progression of the complaint: Are things improving, getting worse, or staying the same? What interventions has the owner provided, if any (e.g., Has the pet been given aspirin)? Has the pet been seen by another veterinarian, and if so, what has been done? Has there been vomiting, diarrhea, melena, coughing, sneezing, changes to appetite, polyuria, polydipsia, or lethargy? What past medical history or surgical history does the pet have? Is it on any medication or supplement? Has the pet traveled recently? What is the pet normally fed with and how much? Is the pet's vaccination up-to-date, and if the pet is a cat, has the cat ever been tested for feline immunodeficiency virus (FIV) or feline leukemia virus (Felv)? These questions should be asked about every pet that comes into the hospital and should provide invaluable information to help in the treatment of the patient.

Unique Triages

The central nervous system, cardiovascular system, and respiratory system are the primary systems to initially evaluate because these systems determine whether the condition is a "life-threatening" emergency or not. However, there are some important other systems

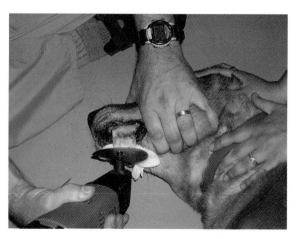

Figure 1.5   Marrow bones stuck on the lower jaw are a common example of an oral emergency. (Courtesy of Thomas Walker, DVM, DACVECC.)

that may not cause life-threatening emergencies but will certainly threaten the quality of life for the animal (Fig. 1.5).

Reproductive System

Certainly, the female herself may be stable, but there could be a reproductive emergency that jeopardizes the health of the unborn neonates. The following questions should be asked of the client:

- When is the pet due?
- Do you notice any discharge? What color? Is there any foul odor?
- How long has the mother been having contractions?
- How long in between puppies/kittens has it been?
- Do you see a puppy or kitten coming out? How long has it been there?
- Are you able to take a rectal temperature?

If a client comes in or calls because he/she is concerned about his/her pregnant pet, then the pet should receive a full workup.

When a reproductive emergency arrives at the clinic, ideally, all puppies/kittens that had already been born are brought to the clinic as well. This way they can be given right back to the mother to nurse when she is finally done delivering. Upon arrival, the neonates that have already been born should be removed from the mother and kept in a warm, clean area. This way the focus can be given only to the mother.

Even if the owners know how many puppies/kittens the mother is having, a lateral radiograph should still be taken to confirm how many more are expected. The radiograph will also be able to show if there is one puppy/kitten stuck in the birth canal. A radiograph should be taken immediately after the pet has been checked into the hospital. Sedation may be avoided since this may hinder the birthing process and may affect the puppies/kittens that have not yet been born.

Depending on the situation, drugs may be administered to help increase contractions, or the pet may be taken for a caesarian section. If a natural birth is going to be attempted, it is generally better to allow the pet to be with its owner(s) in a quiet room. Pets will try to stop delivering in places they are not comfortable, so making them as comfortable as possible is important. Reproductive emergencies are often time-consuming and utilize much of the staff.

Ocular Emergencies

While they may not be life-threatening, ocular emergencies are as important as any other emergency. There are some true ocular emergencies that, if left untreated, may result in permanent vision loss for a pet.

There are four true ocular emergencies: acute blindness, acute red or cloudy eye, acute painful eye, and anything dangling from the eye (Gilger 2006). It is imperative that these clients are told to come in immediately. As a rule of thumb, if an owner calls with concern regarding a pet's eye, it is best to have the patient come over to assess whether it is truly an emergency.

Upon arrival at the clinic, the pet should be triaged in a similar manner like all other pets. However, depending on the nature of the eye problem, the pet may need immediate treatment. An example would be if the eye is proptosed. While eye injuries are not life-threatening, they are very painful. Administering pain medications to the pet may allow you to perform a better ocular exam.

If there is any wait for the pet to be seen, it is imperative that the pet be given an Elizabethan collar so that the pet does not cause further injury to the eye.

Neurological Emergencies

Neurological emergencies require rapid assessment and quick treatment in order for the best prognosis to occur. The three most common neurological emergencies are acute spinal cord injury, acute brain injury, and tick paralysis (seen mainly in Australia) (Sturges 2006). Other neurological emergencies include all types of seizures.

Oftentimes, it is difficult to assess over the phone if a pet is just lame or if it is suffering from a more severe neurological issue. Many owners may describe generalized symptoms such as "whining, not wanting to walk, shaking, panting a lot, crying, yelping for no reason, or appearing stiff." This is one of the reasons that it is always best to have the owner bring the pet to the veterinary clinic so that the pet can be assessed appropriately.

If a neurological injury is suspected, you should advise the owner to minimize the pet's motion and to come to the clinic as soon as possible. Since oftentimes movement for the pet is painful, owners should be advised to use caution. For small dogs and cats, they should be placed in a carrier. For larger dogs, they may need assistance getting into the car. Owners can use a large blanket or a "necktie/panty hose" muzzle to place over their pet's head/mouth to avoid getting bitten.

Because of allodynia and hyperalgesia, it may be difficult sometimes to assess and localize the origin of where animals feel pain. These pets may become guarded, and simply touching their head may cause them to react.

While these animals should be triaged in the same manner as other pets, it may be impossible to work with them until they receive pain medications. Some veterinarians like to perform a quick neurological exam before the pet receives any medication. This is because the pet may be slightly sedated after medication, thus making exam findings difficult to interpret.

After your full physical exam, you will want to perform a brief neurological exam. This should start with the pet's LOC. Any change in its LOC is an emergency that needs immediate attention. You should also note whether or not the patient is "mentally appropriate." You should pay particular attention to the pet's eyes and whether the pupils are the same size, have normal reaction to light, and that the eyes do not have nystagmus or anisocoria. You should have the pet walk for you. If the pet is unable to walk, assistance may need to be given to the pet to get it to stand.

Once the pet is standing you should check for conscious proprioception (CP) deficit. Simply place the pet in a standing position, and take a paw and flex it so that the dorsal aspect of the paw is touching the ground. The animal should be able to recognize that it is not standing on the pad of its foot and will quickly "flip" its foot to the correct position. Any delay usually means the pet has a neurological deficit.

You should also check for deep pain with hemostats. You should pinch the bones on the toes on each foot of the animal. The pet should immediately withdraw its foot even with the littlest pressure. If the pet is delayed in responding or does not pull back at all, there is a neurological deficit.

While acute brain injury cases may be easier to label as an "emergency," acute spinal cord injuries may not. Owners of small dogs (dachshunds, miniature corgis) may arrive with these pets being carried and describe the injury as "must have hurt his foot." A good triage technician will remove the pet from the owner's arms and fully assess the pet for themselves. As a rule, any animal that shows any neurological deficit should have immediate treatment initiated. It is well documented that the prognosis of the neurological pet decreases dramatically the longer the pet had to wait before treatment.

Neonates and Special Species

While most small animals will be triaged in a similar manner, there are some special species that must be triaged using unique skills.

Neonates

Neonates are very delicate. Approximately 11%–34% of kittens and puppies will die within the first 12 weeks of their life (Fortney 2004). When a client calls with a medical emergency involving a neonate, it is important that instruction be given to the client on how to appropriately transport the neonate to the hospital.

Ideally, the sick neonate should be brought in separately. This is to minimize the risk of disease transmission and stress to the rest of the litter. The mother will generally become very stressed as well and may stop feeding the rest of the litter if brought to the hospital.

It is imperative that anyone transporting neonates be instructed on how to keep them warm during transport through the use of hot water bottles and warm blankets.

Thermoregulation is a severe problem in neonates. This is because of their lack of insulating fat (Fortney 2004). Shivering reflex and peripheral vasoconstriction responses are not fully developed for at least 1 week (Fortney 2004).

Upon entering the hospital, the neonate should be immediately addressed and placed into a warm environment. The owner should not be expected to be responsible for warming the neonate once in the hospital. A normal neonatal temperature is between 98 and 100°F. Rarely is overheating a problem, but certainly, electric blankets and heat lamps should be avoided because of the high risk of burns and overheating associated with them.

Dehydration and hypoglycemia are both great concerns for neonates. Even mild vomiting or diarrhea is considered an emergency in neonates because of how quickly they can become dehydrated. Hypoglycemia is particularly common in toy breed neonates (Fortney 2004). This is because neonates have an increased demand for glucose due to their low fat reserve (Fortney 2004). They also have poor liver and muscle glycogen reserves (Fortney 2004). A normal blood glucose is 90–140 mg/dL. Because hypoglycemia is so common, any neonate that presents into a veterinary clinic with signs of illness should immediately have a blood glucose performed.

Wildlife

Each state has its own regulations and laws pertaining to the handling of wildlife. It is important that each hospital becomes familiar with the laws. No matter where you are located you will, at some point, have someone bring wildlife into your veterinary clinic for treatment. Unless it is an endangered species, most state laws will allow for examination/assessment for rehabilitation, stabilization, or euthanasia. If the animal is deemed too sick/injured to be rehabilitated, then euthanasia should be performed unless it is an endangered species.

The United States Fish and Wildlife Service has a website that lists each state and the endangered species (www.ecos.fws.gov/tess_public/StateListing.do?state=all).

It is important that each hospital becomes familiar with what wildlife is endangered because it is illegal to euthanize without notifying the state first. These animals are generally treated no matter how severe the injury is in order to preserve the species.

If it is thought that the animal can be treated and rehabilitated, then the clinic may opt to start initial treatment and elect to transport to a facility with a wildlife rehabilitator. Unless the veterinary clinic has a licensed wildlife rehabilitator working, it is not recommended that a small animal hospital care for wildlife. Wildlife requires different housing and care than other animals, and only experienced individuals should care for them.

When a good samaritan brings in an injured wildlife, it is important to gather information just like you would a regular client. This is important because if the veterinary clinic thinks the animal may potentially be a carrier of rabies, then the good samaritan may need to follow up with post-exposure prophylaxis at a hospital. The state may also need to be notified of the exposure. It should also be recorded where the animal was found and how long ago it was found.

The good samaritan should not be made to wait in the waiting room. Once all information has been obtained, the good samaritan can leave, and the animal should be brought back and treated. It is important to remember that it is a wild animal, and gloves, masks, and other restraint devices should be used for handling.

Exotic Animals

It is important to learn the normal behavior and physical exam findings for the exotic animals you may see at your practice. Most exotic pets are prey species, and being handled by a stranger could cause them to think you are a predator (Fordham 2007). They may either decide to "fight or freeze" and their behavior could easily worsen their condition. It is important to know that any exotic animal showing any signs of illness, no matter how slight, is likely very sick. There is much thought that prey species do not show signs of illness until they are very sick because in the wild any sign of illness would likely mean being eaten by a predator (Fordham 2007).

The first step to triaging an exotic animal is to simply observe the pet in its own cage (Fordham 2007). It is recommended that clients bring the pet in its normal habitat. Generally, cages are small enough to be transported. If it is too large to be transported, the client should put the animal in something that most closely resembles its normal habitat. This will help to reduce stress and allow you observe the animal in its normal environment. Remember that some exotic animals (e.g., ectotherms) require a constant heat source so you may need to provide one once the pet has arrived at the clinic.

You should observe the animal for breathing difficulties, nasal discharge, level of activity (most exotic animals are very active with the exception of reptiles), and alertness. If there is any fecal matter in the cage, it should be examined whether it is normal. Any change in fecal matter likely indicates there is a problem with the pet. Changes to fecal material include becoming smaller, watery, blood in it, changes in color, or too dry. If the pet appears healthy and happy, it can likely wait with its owner in a quiet exam room with the lights dimmed.

Owners should be asked about the husbandry of the exotic pet: what exactly is in the cage, what bedding is used, where the cage is kept, the lighting the pet receives, what else lives in the cage. They should also be asked what the pet eats and how much water it receives. Lastly, they should be asked about their own observations of the pet's fecal matter, urination, and overall activity.

Mass Casualty Incidents/Disaster Triage

Oftentimes in veterinary medicine we find ourselves triaging one pet at a time. Sometimes it can become busy where we triage four, maybe five pets at a time. Unfortunately, a disaster may occur, and you could find yourself triaging a dozen, maybe even hundreds of animals in a short period of time.

The definition of a disaster is when community resources become overwhelmed, causing inability to function normally. This can be something as large as a hurricane or ice storm or as little as a hazardous material truck turning over on a highway (Fig. 1.6). When local resources are overwhelmed it is a disaster. You may have advance notice of the disaster occurring or you may have no notice. During a disaster, patients must be triaged in a way that will benefit the most animals. Tough choices may need to be made. Picture a truck full of 50 pet-store puppies losing air conditioning on a summer day when it is 95°F outside. As an emergency room technician you do not always get a choice whether you want to be part of the disaster or not (Fig. 1.7).

CHAPTER 1

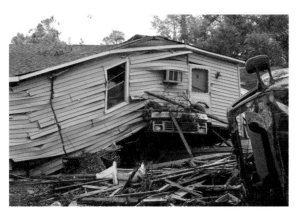

Figure 1.6   A home destroyed from Hurricane Katrina.

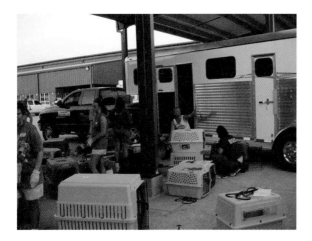

Figure 1.7   Animals being dropped off for medical exam and housing during Hurricane Katrina.

When triaging animals during a disaster, it is important to try and forget about the disaster. If you are thinking about the disaster, you are not completely focused on your patient. Also, if you are overwhelmed by the situation, you may assume all injuries/ diseases are related to the disaster. Preexisting illnesses may be present in several patients or animals may start to acquire new illnesses that are not related to the disaster. For example, the cat that came in for hypothermia also may have pyelonephritis. You should not assume the poor hair coat and emaciation of the cat is solely disaster-related. It is important to always perform a complete physical exam and workup to ensure that each patient is treated separately from the disaster. Stable patients should be transferred to a hospital that is not affected by the disaster so that long-term care can be given to such animals.

Having an organized approach will help ensure that the most patients possible are triaged appropriately. A method must be designed for dealing with numerous patients at once. While there is no designed method to multiple trauma in veterinary medicine, there are two human methods can be used to efficiently triage during a disaster:

Color	Type of Injury
Red	Critical—The patient must receive simple life-saving procedures to ensure survival.
Yellow	The patient should survive as long as simple care is given within a few hours.
Green	Minor injuries—The patient can wait for treatment and still survive.
Black	Dead or dying—The patient's injuries are very severe, and the patient is unlikely to survive regardless of the treatment received.

Figure 1.8   START color code system.

1. Simple Triage and Rapid Treatment (START)
2. Secondary Assessment of Victim Endpoint (SAVE)

Both methods were developed for triaging human casualties during the war. Both START and SAVE are widely accepted in the veterinary community as efficient triage methods for dealing with nonhuman patients (Wingfield and Raffe 2002).

START Method

With the START method, each animal is quickly assessed for respiration, alertness, and perfusion status. This is also known as the RAP status. Using this system, animals are color-coded (red, yellow, green, black) (Fig. 1.8) and moved to their color-coded areas (Wingfield and Raffe 2002). Animals should be marked with the appropriate color. Owners can be given cards for their animals, and unowned animals can be marked with identification bands. The date, time, name of the person who triaged, initial problem, and color should all be listed (Wingfield and Raffe 2002).

As a baseline, animals that are walking are considered green. These are animals that have minimal injuries and are considered stable enough to wait for medical treatment. Having every staff member in the clinic become familiar with the color-coded system will help decrease confusion if and when disaster strikes.

Using the START method, animals can be quickly assessed and brought to appropriate treatment areas to receive the treatment they need. Areas should be set up and staffed to deal with a particularly color-coded animal. Animals may need to be reassessed as time passes. Reassessment times should be agreed upon so that animals will not be forgotten. An animal's status may change, and it may be given a different color code depending on the current condition.

SAVE Method

The SAVE method is much faster than the START method and works well when resources and personnel are limited (Wingfield and Raffe 2002). It will help to conserve resources and personnel by focusing them on patients who have the best chance of survival. Using the SAVE method, patients are divided into three categories:

1. Those who will die regardless of the treatment
2. Those who will survive regardless of treatment or nontreatment
3. Those who will benefit if medical intervention occurs immediately

Only those that fall in groups two and three are given care. As tough as it is, group one can either be humanly euthanized if time allows or left to die on their own. Remember, the goal is to save animals. Time and resources should be given only to those animals that have a chance of survival. Group number two is put on "hold" while group number three is treated. This method is fast and efficient because it allows for all resources to focus on only one group. After group number three has been dealt with, group number two can be reassessed and treated. Placing an animal in one of the groups is a judgment call and can be difficult at times. Decisions must be made quickly to save as many patients as possible.

Conclusion

Triage is one of the most important jobs of an emergency room technician. The ability to triage quickly and appropriately will give your patient the best chance of survival.

References

Archer, E. 2009. *Nursing the Head Trauma Patient. British Small Animal Veterinary Congress Proceedings.*

Davis, H. 2008. *Triage in the Emergency Room. Atlantic Coast Veterinary Conference Proceedings.*

Dodam, J. 2002. *Ventilating the Anesthetized Patient. Western Veterinary Conference.*

Fordham, M. 2007. *Triage of the Exotic Animal Patient. International Veterinary Emergency and Critical Care Symposium Proceedings.*

Fortney, W. 2004. *Triage and Diagnosis for Sick Neonates. Western Veterinary Conference Proceedings.*

Gilger, B. 2006. *Ocular Emergencies: Recognition, Triage and Initial Treatment. Atlantic Coast Veterinary Conference Proceedings.*

Grossman, V. 2003. *Quick Reference to Triage*, 2nd ed. Philadelphia: Lippincott Williams and Wilkins.

Hansen, B. 2005. *Triage and Primary Survey: Where Are Your Priorities? Atlantic Coast Veterinary Conference Proceedings.*

Hughes, D. 2005. *Triage and Major Body Systems. World Small Animal Veterinary Association World Congress Proceedings.*

CHAPTER 1

Mathews, K. 2007. *Veterinary Emergency and Critical Care*, 2nd ed. Guelph, ON: Lifelearn.

Rivera, A. 2003. *Clinical Importance of Triage and Vital Signs. ACVIM Proceedings.*

Sturges, B. 2006. *Neuro 911: Triaging Neurological Emergencies. Veterinary Neurology Symposium Proceedings.*

Wingfield, W, Raffe, M. 2002. *The Veterinary ICU Book.* Jackson Hole, WY: Teton NewMedia.

Shock and Initial Stabilization

2

Jennifer Keefe

Introduction

After being initially assessed and triaged in the emergency room, those patients with shock or immediate life threats need to be stabilized quickly and as completely as possible within the treatment area.

Initial stabilization almost always starts with intravenous catheter placement and preliminary laboratory tests, and may also extend to include fluid therapy, oxygen delivery, ventilation support, sedation, and pain management. All of these topics are introduced in this chapter and then discussed in more detail in later chapters of the book.

Systemic Hypoperfusion (Shock)

Patients in shock are suffering from a state of hemodynamic compromise, which includes reduced systemic tissue perfusion and impaired delivery of oxygen (DO_2) to tissue. More specifically, shock is the inability to meet tissue oxygen consumption demands. *Further discussion of oxygen delivery is provided in the cardiovascular emergencies chapter.* Shock is not a diagnosis in itself but rather is always secondary to an underlying internal or external upset. Many different categorization schemes have been suggested to define shock. For the purpose of this text, four classes of shock are recognized.

Hypovolemic shock is the most common form of shock seen in small animal medicine. It is the result of decreased intravascular volume from blood loss, or from fluid losses due to vomiting, diarrhea, or third spacing. Patient in hypovolemic shock have the predominant problem of decreased cardiac preload.

Obstructive shock results from a physical obstruction in the circulatory system such as heartworm disease, pericardial effusion, and gastric torsion. The result is ultimately decreased cardiac preload returning to the heart.

Distributive shock has initiating causes such as sepsis, anaphylaxis, and systemic inflammatory response syndrome (SIRS). Blood volume is present; however, it is in places it should not be. A hallmark feature of distributive shock is vasodilation.

Cardiogenic shock is shock resulting from heart failure. It is often associated with a decrease in cardiac contractility, increased afterload, and increased cardiac preload. The treatment of cardiogenic shock is discussed in Chapter 6, "Cardiovascular Emergencies."

Pathophysiology of Hypovolemic Shock

Shock is a dynamic and complicated process that involves several compensatory mechanisms. An initial insult (e.g., blood loss) causes a decrease in intravascular volume. This decrease in volume results in a decreased venous return to the heart and a decreased ventricular filling (cardiac preload). The reduction in cardiac preload results in decreased stroke volume, cardiac output, and blood pressure. The decrease in cardiac output along with decreased hemoglobin levels from bleeding results in a decreased delivery of oxygen to tissues and the shock state (Fig. 2.1).

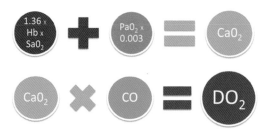

Figure 2.1   Delivery of Oxygen (DO_2) components.

The Neuroendocrine Response and the Renin-Angiotensin-Aldosterone System (RAAS)

Following an initial drop in blood pressure, there is a decreased firing of baroreceptors in the blood vessels in the aortic arch and carotid sinus and mechanoreceptors and volume receptors within the heart and kidneys. The decreased firing of these receptors initiates a dramatic reactive neuroendocrine response that attempts to immediately reestablish normal blood pressure and preserve perfusion and oxygen delivery to vital structures such as the brain, heart, and lungs.

The immediate response following decreased baroreceptor firing is a decrease in autonomic parasympathetic stimulation and an increase in sympathetic stimulation. The sympathetic stimulation results in activation of alpha-1 and beta-1 adrenergic receptors, causing vasoconstriction, increased heart rate, and increased cardiac contractility. These changes aim to improve systemic vascular resistance and cardiac output. Decreased renal blood flow causes activation of the RAAS. The end result of the RAAS is a contribution to systemic vasoconstriction and sodium and water retention, which helps to increase circulating plasma volume and improve stroke volume.

More specifically, the RAAS is initially activated with the release of renin. Renin decreases renal artery perfusion, increases renal tubular sodium concentration, and triggers beta-adrenergic stimulation. Beta-adrenergic stimulation increases cardiac output further by increasing the heart rate and cardiac muscle contractility as previously discussed.

Renin and angiotensin-converting enzyme (ACE) convert angiotensin I to angiotensin II. Angiotensin II is a potent vasoconstrictor. It also stimulates the secretion of adrenocorticotropic hormone (ACTH, also known as corticotropin), aldosterone, and antidiuretic hormone (ADH).

Corticotropin triggers the adrenal cortex to release cortisol. Cortisol works synergistically with epinephrine and glucagon to induce a catabolic state (meaning the body is breaking down reserves for immediate energy needs), stimulates gluconeogenesis (the generation of glucose from non-carbohydrates such as lactate) and insulin resistance, and retains sodium and water by kidney.

Aldosterone contributes to the reabsorption of sodium and water, and exchanges potassium and hydrogen for sodium within the kidney. ADH increases water permeability, decreases water and sodium losses, and preserves intravascular volume. It is also a potent vasoconstrictor.

Stages of Shock and Clinical Signs

The *compensatory phase* of shock starts once a patient suffers the initial insult (i.e., hemorrhage). The body tries to preserve its vital organs such as the heart, brain, and lungs. Therefore, peripheral vessels constrict, and the spleen contracts to move blood into the central arterial circulation. It is because of this that the circulation to extremities is greatly reduced (therefore often cold). Inflammatory cytokines begin to mount in hypoxic tissue. Splenic contraction also may cause the packed cell volume (PCV) to initially remain normal or high in the face of acute hemorrhage.

Clinical signs of the compensatory phase can be difficult to identify but may include tachycardia, injected mucous membranes with a rapid capillary refill time, and bounding pulses, while blood pressure ranges from normal to slight hypertension. Cats do not usually display this response unless they are in tremendous pain (Kirby 2008).

These responses can compensate for mild to moderate decreases in intravascular volume by producing the compensatory stage of shock. If the loss is too great for them to restore normal function or is persistent for prolonged periods of time, the early decompensatory stage of shock begins (Kirby 2008).

The *early decompensatory phase* is the next phase of hypovolemic shock. Reserves are beginning to diminish, and the cytokines from hypoxic tissues are now entering the systemic circulation. This incites SIRS, and SIRS further depletes intravascular volume by causing significant vasodilation and increased capillary permeability.

Clinical signs of this phase include tachycardia, weak pulses, hypotension, pale mucous membranes, prolonged capillary refill time, hypothermia, and normal to decreased mentation. This is where aggressive volume resuscitation is essential to decrease mortality (Kirby 2008).

The *late decompensatory phase* is the final and terminal stage of all forms of shock. It is brought on by prolonged and severe tissue hypoxia that causes adenosine triphosphate (ATP, the energy storage and transfer molecule in the cell) production to resort to anaerobic metabolism. Anaerobic metabolism is nearly 20 times less productive than aerobic metabolism, and, if continued, this phase progresses to circulatory collapse and insufficient blood flow to the brain and heart. Since the heart cannot sustain any kind of compensatory response at this late phase, the animal rapidly declines and dies.

Clinical signs for this phase include bradycardia, severe hypotension, pale to cyanotic mucous membranes, undetectable capillary refill time, weak to absent pulses, hypothermia, and decreased to comatose mentation. Cardiac arrest is at hand without intense intervention (Kirby 2008).

Initial Stabilization

The goal of initial stabilization is of course to rapidly stabilize immediate life threats. The goal of shock therapy specifically is to meet oxygen delivery requirements to tissues and to shut off the neuroendocrine response as quickly as possible. In cases of hypovolemic, obstructive, and distributive shock, therapy is initiated with fluid administration and supplemental oxygen (Davis 2008). Concurrently, laboratory samples are obtained, and pain management is provided for any animal experiencing pain.

Patients presenting with any type of hemorrhage should also have their bleeding slowed or stopped to minimize ongoing hypovolemia. Open lacerations should have pressure bandages applied as soon as possible, and abdominal hemorrhage can be slowed by placing a wrap around the abdomen. Patients suspected of having sepsis should be started on antibiotic therapy ideally within 1 hour of presentation.

Later, following intravenous fluid therapy and oxygen administration, fractures must be addressed as part of initial stabilization. Open fractures should be flushed and bandaged to stabilize the fracture and protect the wound from further contamination.

Intravenous Catheter Placement

The intravenous catheter is the direct line from veterinary paraprofessional to the patient. It allows for rapid fluid administration, and necessary medications can be given with immediate effects. Therefore, intravenous catheterization placement is often the initial priority in any emergent patient even if it is unknown whether or not the patient's owner will pursue treatment. If a patient's owner opts not to pursue further treatment, the intravenous catheter can be used for a humane euthanasia if necessary. One of the few exceptions to placing an intravenous catheter first upon patient arrival is when the patient is in severe cardiac or respiratory distress and any stress may push them into respiratory or cardiac arrest. Therefore, some patients require an initial hands-off minimalistic approach, oxygen therapy, possible sedation or thoracocentesis, and catheterization later (Figs. 2.2 and 2.3).

Severely compromised patients will present more difficulty in catheter placement because not only is the vein difficult, if not impossible, to visualize, but hypotension can prevent blood from appearing in the hub of the catheter when the vein is entered (flash). Performing a venous "cutdown" may be necessary to ensure placement. A cutdown is when the patient's skin is pinched up and away from the vein in order to avoid piercing the vein (Figs. 2.4 and 2.5), while a sterile surgical blade or needle is used to slice across

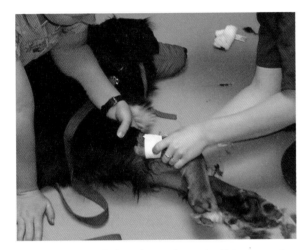

Figure 2.2   Adequate patient restraint, including chemical restraint if necessary, is paramount for successful catheter placement.

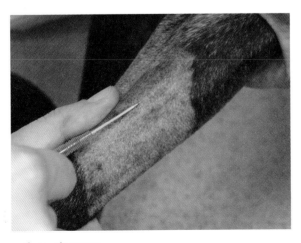

Figure 2.3   Intravenous catheter placement.

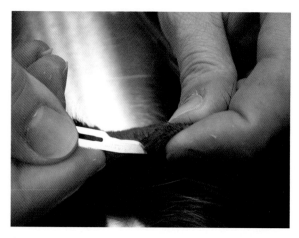

Figure 2.4   Venous cutdown or "facilitation hole": pinch the skin to avoid inadvertently piercing the vein.

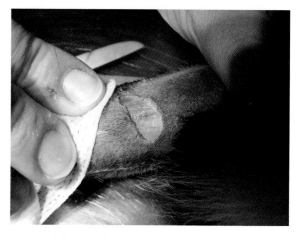

Figure 2.5   Visualize the vein and insert catheter.

the skin, thus making the vein apparent and the catheter more easily visualized entering the vein. Skin glue or suture can be used to close the skin around the catheter.

Further discussion on intravenous catheters and venous access is available in Chapter 3, "Venous Access."

Fluid Therapy

Fluid therapy is imperative in stabilizing patients suffering from most forms of shock, and it aims to bring the mean arterial blood pressure (MAP) to 70–90 mmHg or the systolic blood pressure to 90–110 mmHg. Overshooting these numbers can have deleterious effects.

Physiology

Fluid in the body is either in a cell (intracellular) or outside of a cell (extracellular). The three major fluid compartments are the intracellular, intravascular, and interstitial spaces. The intravascular and interstitial compartments make up the extracellular space. Fluid movement from the intravascular to interstitial and intracellular compartments occurs at the capillary membrane, and this membrane is freely permeable to water and small molecular weight particles. The interstitial compartment is the space between the capillaries and the cells. The intracellular compartment is separated from the interstitial compartment by a cell membrane, which is freely permeable to water but not small or large molecular weight particles.

Fluids to be administered must concentrate within the compartment where the volume deficit lies. Colloids are often used for intravascular volume replacement, while crystalloids help with intravascular and interstitial volume replacement. However, it is important to understand that the majority of crystalloids do not remain in the intravascular space beyond an hour. Crystalloids and colloids can be used together to replace interstitial fluid deficits, but crystalloids should be administered at a reduced dose. Typically a 40%–60% reduction is selected.

Crystalloids

Isotonic crystalloids such as regular saline (0.9% NaCl), Lactated Ringers solution (LRS), and Normosol-R® (Hospira, Lake Forest, IL) are balanced water-based solutions with small molecular weight particles that are freely permeable to the capillary membrane. Approximately 70%–75% of administered isotonic crystalloids move into the interstitial space within 1 hour after administration (Wingfield and Raffe 2002).

The full shock dose of crystalloids is 90 mL/kg for the dog and 55 mL/kg for the cat (Wingfield and Raffe 2002). This is determined by a patient's full blood volume. Administering this entire quantity is known as *large volume resuscitation* and is not commonplace today. Rather, a typical initial fluid bolus for a hypovolemic patient is a fourth to a third of their shock dose over approximately 10–20 minutes (e.g., 20 mL/kg). The patient's condition needs to be reassessed frequently during administration since each patient will respond differently to aggressive fluid therapy. This methodology is referred to as *limited volume* or *end point resuscitation*. After the initial bolus, parameters should be evaluated and additional crystalloid fluid boluses can then be administered as directed by physiological parameters (see "Resuscitation End Point" section later in this chapter). The full shock dose is often not needed in most patients.

Hypertonic crystalloids such as hypertonic saline can also be used in shock therapy when it is difficult to administer large volumes of fluids rapidly enough to resuscitate the patient or when large volumes of fluid are contraindicated. Hypertonic saline causes rapid fluid shifts from the intracellular compartment to the extracellular (DiBartola 2006) because water follows sodium concentration. This results in rapid expansion of the intravascular volume causing improved venous return and cardiac output, vasodilation, and improved tissue perfusion.

A dose of 4 mL/kg IV for both cat and dog given over 5 minutes (Wingfield and Raffe 2002) can be selected. Once intravascular volume is restored, isotonic crystalloids still need to be administered to prevent dehydration because fluid has been taken from the intracellular compartment and shifted to the intravascular compartment.

Hypotonic crystalloids such as half-strength saline (0.45% NaCl) should not be used to treat hypovolemic shock for they contain too much free water and distribute excessively to the intracellular compartment. This can lead to a severe and rapid decrease in serum sodium that is potentially deleterious.

Colloids and blood products

Colloids such as 6% Hetastarch (Voluven, Hespan) are water-based solutions of a larger molecular weight that do not readily pass across the healthy capillary membrane. They are considered better blood volume expanders since 50%–80% of the infused volume remains in the intravascular space after 1 hour. Colloids are indicated when crystalloids are not effectively improving blood pressure, and/or when the total protein or albumin are below 3.5 g/dL or 2.0 g/dL, respectively, and colloidal oncontic pressure (COP) is compromised (Davis 2008; Wingfield and Raffe 2002).

Higher molecular weight hetastarches (e.g., Hespan) can be administered at 5 mL/kg in dogs and 2.5 mL/kg in cats over 5–15 minutes up to four times, or 20 mL/kg rapid infusion once (Gaynor 2007). Lower molecular weight hetastarches (e.g., Voluven) can follow similar dosing regiments but can be administered at doses greater than 20 mL/kg/day when necessary without fear of coagulopathy.

Blood products such as whole blood, packed red blood cells (PRBCs), plasma, and hemoglobin-based oxygen carriers (HBOCs) are considered colloids and will also be useful in initial stabilization. They will be discussed further in Chapter 21, "Transfusion Medicine."

Other Treatments for Hypotension

After restoring volume through the use of intravenous fluid therapy, some patients require the use of drug therapy to improve blood pressure and maximize delivery of oxygen to tissue. Measuring central venous pressure in conjunction with blood pressure is useful to determine when cardiac preload has been adequately restored (e.g., 8–10 cmH$_2$O). A faster route in the emergency room is to perform echocardiography and assess whether or not the heart's volume is adequate. If hypotension remains in the face of adequate cardiac volume, the cause of the hypotension must be due to either decreased cardiac contractility (inotropy) or vasodilation. Therefore, several drug therapies can be used if the patient is still unable to maintain a stable blood pressure after vigorous fluid therapy. *Positive inotropes* are used to adjust cardiac contractility, and *vasopressors* (aka "pressors") are used to adjust vascular tone. It should be noted that such drugs are *never* a substitute for adequate volume restoration in the hypovolemic patient and should be used only after adequate volume resuscitation.

Individual drugs

Dopamine and dobutamine are both inotropic agents, meaning they will strengthen cardiac muscle contractions. Dobutamine is a rapid acting parenteral agent that will cause the heart to have stronger beats. Dopamine, on the other hand, is a catecholamine that has different uses at different doses.

Lower doses (0.5–3 mcg/kg/min) of dopamine may dilate renal mesenteric coronary and vascular beds, which may make it useful in oliguric renal failure. Dopamine at a dose

---

Box 2.1   Shortcut to Calculate a CRI

(Drug dose in mcg/kg/min) × (Body weight in kg) = Drug in mg to put in 250 mL fluid bag. Administer at 15 mL/h.

---

of 5–13 mcg/kg/min can be used to improve blood pressure as it acts as an agonist alpha-1 and beta-1 adrenergic receptors to increase blood pressure (Plumb 2005). Some do not consider it as effective since cats lack the DA1 receptor, and use dobutamine instead (Gaynor 2007). Doses of dopamine over 10 mcg/kg/min have predominantly alpha-1 adrenergic effect and therefore has a mainly vasoconstricting effect.

Dobutamine is a beta-1 adrenergic agonist that is indicated in dogs and cats with hypotension from poor cardiac contractility. The dose range is 4.4–15.4 mcg/kg/min. The dose is reduced or discontinued if tachycardia and arrhythmias occur (Plumb 2005).

Phenylephrine, an alpha-1 adrenergic agonist, is indicated for hypotension when beta adrenergic agonist effects are not desirable. It is contraindicated in hypertension and ventricular tachycardia. It should be used with caution in patients that are geriatric, hyperthyroid, bradycardic, or have cardiac disease. The dose is 1–3 mcg/kg/min (Plumb 2005).

Vasopressin, or ADH, is able to cause vasoconstriction independent of adrenergic stimulation as opposed to most other vasopressors. Vasopressin can be used as a stand-alone drug or in conjunction with other agents for refractory hypotension. This strategy allows for lower doses of other vasopressors to be used concurrently, which can help successfully treat hypotension and poor tissue perfusion while minimizing adverse drug reactions. Vasopressin, when selected is dosed at 1–4 microunits/kg/min.

As time is often of the essence with critically hypotensive patients, a shortcut to calculate a constant rate infusion (CRI) is in Box 2.1 (Battaglia 2001).

Resuscitation End Points

When to stop fluid resuscitation during initial stabilization can be a controversial subject and would ideally be directed by universally established end points based on documented evidence. Unfortunately, such end points do not yet exist in veterinary medicine, and when to stop fluid therapy is often based on clinical judgment. In humans, however, it has been documented that up to 85% of severely injured patients have evidence of ongoing tissue hypoxia despite normalization of vital signs. Unfortunately this suggests that occult oxygen debt and the presence of compensated shock may still exist even after we feel we have finished resuscitating a patient (Abou-Khalil et al. 1994; Marino 1998).

Some traditional end points that are assessed routinely in the veterinary emergency room include improved mentation, decreases in heart rate, improved mucous membrane color and capillary refill time, increased body weight, improved urine output and peripheral pulse quality, and normalization of blood pressure.

Quick evaluation of the heart via ultrasound can also be utilized to assess volume status and the need for additional fluids. Central venous pressure (CVP) also can be used to assess volume status; however, measurements can be labor-intensive and therefore is not often used during initial stabilization. An end point for CVP reflecting adequate volume resuscitation during hypovolemia is suggested at 8–10 cmH$_2$O.

Less frequently used resuscitation end points in veterinary medicine include decreasing plasma lactate levels, pulmonary capillary wedge pressures of 10–12 mmHg, cardiac

Table 2.1   Clinical parameters and resuscitation end points monitored during the treatment of shock (Adapted from Rudloff 2002)

Physiologic Parameter	Normal	Compensatory Stage	Early Decompensatory Stage	Late Decompensatory Stage	Resuscitation End Point
Mentation	Alert	Alert and excited	Normal to decreased	Decreased to comatose	Alert
Heart rate (bpm)	Dog: 60–120 Cat: 170–220	Dog: >140 Cat: variable	Dog: >140 Cat: variable	Dog: <140 Cat: <160	Dog: 80–120 Cat: 170–220
Mucous membrane color	Pink	Brick red	Pale	Grey/blue	Pink
Capillary refill time (seconds)	1–2	<1	>2	>2	1–2
MAP (mmHg)	80–100	>80	Variable	<80	80–100
CVP (cm H$_2$O)	0–2	Variable	<5	Variable	8–10

output > 2 L/min, O$_2$ uptake (VO$_2$) > 100 mL/min/m^2, normalizing base deficit, mixed/central venous oxygen saturation levels, and gastric intramucosal pH [pHi] (Wingfield and Raffe 2002) (Table 2.1).

Plasma lactate

Out of all of the advanced resuscitation end point methodologies previously discussed, monitoring plasma lactate trends have gained the most widespread use in recent years. Monitoring plasma lactate levels has become a cheap, simple bedside test.

Lactate is produced from pyruvate by the enzyme lactate dehydrogenase. This reaction occurs in the cytosol of all cells, predominately during periods of tissue oxygen deficiency and anaerobic metabolism. This reaction is reversible, however, and when aerobic metabolism returns, pyruvate regenerates from lactate. Plasma lactate increases when its production by hypoxic tissue overwhelms its elimination by the liver. Shock states, causing systemic hypoperfusion, therefore, consistency result in hyperlactatemia and plasma lactate levels greater than 2.5 mmol/L. Measurement of plasma lactate levels in the emergency room can therefore be quickly used as an indirect assessment of tissue oxygen balance and as a means of evaluating resuscitation success (Fig. 2.6).

Volume Overload/Fluid Intolerance

The goal of fluid therapy is to successfully resuscitate a patient while minimizing side effects. Administering large amounts of fluids has inherent risks, especially to those with concurrent heart disease and, more specifically, left atrial enlargement and volume overload. All patients must not only be watched closely for the efficacy of fluid therapy, but

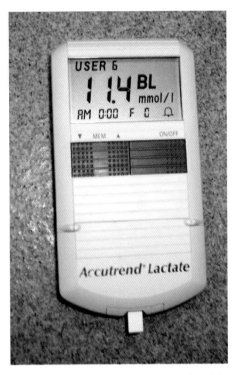

Figure 2.6   Plasma lactate analyzers are inexpensive and can be purchased from many online websites.

also for fluid overload. Signs of fluid overload include clear discharge from the nose, chemosis (swelling of the conjunctiva), pulmonary edema (crackles), a sudden heart murmur or worsening of an existing one, swelling of extremities, increased respiratory effort or distress, and weight gain. Fluids must be discontinued and the patient immediately evaluated if fluid overload and fluid intolerance is suspected.

Dilutional Coagulopathy and Acute Trauma Coagulopathy (ATC)

Patients who have large volumes of fluids administered over a short period of time are also at risk for *dilutional coagulopathy*. This phenomenon occurs due to a dilution of clotting factors and an alteration in clotting factor reserves. Some criticalists have also recently proposed that dogs and cats that experienced severe trauma may actually have an underlining ATC. The exact pathophysiology of this phenomenon has not been elucidated; however, it has been previously recognized in people (Firth and Brohi 2010).

Hypotensive and Small Volume Resuscitation

"Hypotensive resuscitation" and "small volume resuscitation" (Kirby 2008) are two related techniques utilized in situations when aggressive fluid administration can be detrimental to the patient. Examples of this might include pulmonary contusions or patients who are at risk for ongoing hemorrhage. Specifically, cases that were hemorrhaging but

---

Box 2.2   Administration Guidelines for Small Volume Resuscitation (Kirby 2008)

- Isotonic crystalloids:
  - 10–15 mL/kg for dogs rapidly
  - 5–10 mL/kg for cats rapidly
- Colloids (e.g., hetastarch):
  - 5 mL/kg in dogs over 5–15 minutes
  - 2.5 mL/kg in cats over 5–15 minutes
- 7% hypertonic saline
  - 4 mL/kg IV in cats over 5 minutes (Wingfield and Raffe 2002)
  - 4 mL/kg IV in dogs over 5 minutes (Wingfield and Raffe 2002)

---

then formed blood clots (e.g., hemoabdomens) may not benefit from dramatic changes in hydrostatic pressure and clot disruption. The goal of hypotensive and small volume resuscitation, therefore, is to keep the patient away from death but also not make it worse with treatment. In small volume resuscitation, small volumes of fluid are selected to restore physiological parameters in order to minimize interstitial fluid leakage. This is often accomplished by the use of hypertonic saline and or colloids. In hypotensive resuscitation, fluid therapy is directed to not return the patient to normal hemodynamic indices. This strategy aims to fluid resuscitate the patient to a systolic blood pressure of 80–100 mmHg or in some cases tolerate blood pressures that are just subnormal.

Other cases in which small volume resuscitation is indicated include head injury, cardiogenic shock, or oliguric renal failure. The hypothermic patient, especially the cat, also merits special consideration because these animals are prone to pulmonary edema with continued hypotension due to vasoconstriction caused by hypothermia. External warming should be performed once fluid resuscitation has been initiated, and the fluids must be administered with caution (Rudloff 2002).

Oxygen Therapy

Hypoxemia is defined as low arterial partial pressure of oxygen (PaO_2) or, in other words, a low concentration of dissolved oxygen in the blood. Five causes of hypoxemia have been recognized and include:

- Decreased fractional inspired oxygen (FiO_2)
- Hypoventilation
- Ventilation/perfusion (V/Q) mismatch
- Diffusion impairment
- Alveolar shunting

Oxygen supplementation is imperative for any compromised patient suffering from hypoxemia. The fraction of inspired oxygen (FiO_2) in room air is 21%, delivery via flow-by, nasal oxygen cannula, or a filled oxygen chamber is typically 35%–40%, while a patient would require intubation, cuff inflation, and either mechanical or manual ventilation to achieve an FiO_2 of 100% (Willard 2002).

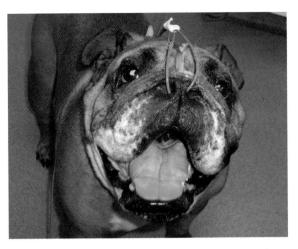

Figure 2.7 Humidification of nasal oxygen is important to avoid irritation of nasal mucosa and improve patient comfort.

The fastest methods of oxygen delivery during initial stabilization are placing the patient in an oxygen cage, or administering flow-by oxygen. Flow-by is delivered by setting the oxygen flowmeter at least at 5 L/minute and either administering the oxygen through a mask with the diaphragm removed, or through the tubing 5–6 in. away from the animal's muzzle. This creates a cone of oxygen that is less irritating to the patient as a strong gust of oxygen can cause the patient to turn away.

Methods for prolonged oxygen supplementation include keeping the patient in an oxygen cage or placing a nasal cannula. Nasal oxygen cannula placement is most commonly performed in the critical care setting. Intratracheal oxygen (placing a nasal cannula that passes the laryngeal folds), or placing a tracheostomy tube (see Chapter 7, "Respiratory Emergencies") can be helpful when the patient needs the oxygen to bypass an upper airway obstruction (i.e., laryngeal paralysis). Very critical cases may require intubation with mechanical or manual ventilation (Fig. 2.7) (Bersenas 2007).

The humidified oxygen flow rate for a patient with a nasal cannula is approximately 100 mL/kg/min, not to exceed 5 L/min as excessive oxygen administration can lead to gastric distention and/or drying of mucous membranes. The flow rate for intratracheal oxygen usually should not exceed 0.5 L/min for a higher rate can cause the tube to oscillate and irritate the trachea.

Sedation for the respiratory distressed

Patients who are too anxious for a thorough evaluation should be placed in an oxygen cage and monitored closely while mild sedation is considered.

A recent study proved the benefit of analgesia and sedation in the respiratory patient. Cats presenting with open mouth breathing had resolution after analgesic therapy (Bersenas 2007). An option for sedation is butorphanol (0.2–0.4 mg/kg) if pain is not the cause of the increased respiratory effort. If analgesia is needed, morphine (0.05–1 mg/kg in dogs and 0.02–0.1 mg/kg in cats) or oxymorphone (0.05–0.1 mg/kg in cats) can be effective. Use lower doses for intravenous administration of these drugs (Plumb 2008). Tranquilizers such as acepromazine (0.025–0.05 mg/kg), diazepam (0.2 mg/kg IV), or

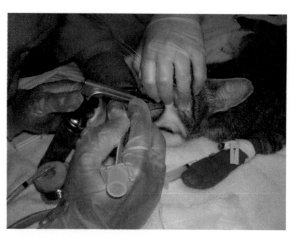

Figure 2.8   A patient is immediately intubated via a propofol rapid sequence intubation (RSI) and an airway is secured. (Courtesy of Thomas Walker DVM, DACVECC.)

midazolam (0.2 mg/kg) have a symbiotic effect with these drugs and can be added if more sedation is desired (Bersenas 2007).

Rapid sequence intubation and ventilation

Patients that have been exerting great effort to breathe for a prolonged time can present in or near respiratory arrest from a combination of exhaustion and suffering from the initial cause of the respiratory compromise. Taking a proactive approach and intervening with anesthetic induction, intubation, and either intermittent positive pressure ventilation (IPPV) or mechanical ventilation before respiratory arrest can aid in decreasing mortality. Most patients do not present in this state, and often, their history and the manner in which they are breathing can help determine how to proceed with stabilization. Once the patient is stable, a complete physical examination and radiographs will help establish a diagnosis.

If the patient is in need of immediate induction and ventilation, rapid sequence induction (RSI) may be the best course of action. RSI is quickly inducing general anesthesia to facilitate intubation. Common agents to use for RSI are propofol or etomidate. If feasible, diazepam can be administered prior to either drug so as to reduce the amount of induction agent used, thus limiting cardiovascular and respiratory side effects. Ketamine and diazepam or alphaxalone are also acceptable RSI techniques (Fig. 2.8).

Thoracocentesis

Thoracocentesis is usually the initial treatment for the patients suffering from pleural effusion or a pneumothorax. It may be beneficial to have preassembled thoracocentesis kits nearby in order to treat severely dyspneic patients quickly.

Analgesia/Sedation

Emergent patients often need analgesia and/or sedation. Administering proper doses of the appropriate drugs in a timely manner will minimize the potential for "wind-up" and chronic pain, thus increasing the likelihood for stabilization and full long-term recovery.

Frequently used analgesic medications include buprenorphine, a partial opioid agonist, hydromorphone, morphine, fentanyl, and oxymorphone which are all pure opioid agonists. Common sedatives in the emergency room include acepromazine, a phenothiazine tranquilizer, for stable, young, and healthy patients (e.g., minor laceration repair on a 5-year-old Lab) and the benzodiazepine tranquilizers diazepam and midazolam for older or less stable patients. Butorphanol is a partial opioid agonist that provides good sedation, but less analgesia than buprenorphine. It can be very useful in the healthy and sick cat alike. All opioids and sedatives can act as cardiovascular and respiratory depressants at varying levels so it is important to dose and monitor carefully (Bersenas 2007).

Stabilization for patients suffering from pleural or pericardial effusion includes procedures such as thoracocentesis or pericardiocentesis. Even though these are compromised animals, they often will benefit from sedation and mild analgesia. Though no sedative or analgesic is without risk, a drug combination such as butorphanol and diazepam IV (do not mix these medications for they will precipitate) can have the desired effect with minimal side effects. Other more stable animals may need mild sedation for radiographs or just to perform a thorough physical exam in order to determine how to proceed with treatment. A combination such as butorphanol and acepromazine may be helpful. For cases requiring more analgesia or more sedation, a drug combination such as hydromorphone IV and midazolam IV is often helpful.

Alpha-2 agonists such as dexmedetomidine are useful sedatives when used in microdoses such as 0.5–1 mcg/kg, and deep sedation can be achieved with higher doses when combined with other medications such as butorphanol, buprenorphine, or bydromorphone. Because of its profound effects, dexmedetomidine is generally avoided in patients that are cardiovascularly compromised, very old, in shock, or debilitated (Plumb 2008). Microdoses of dexmedetomidine (e.g., <1 mcg/kg) are being explored in some populations of critical patients and may be useful in the future.

Preliminary Laboratory Values

Point of care laboratory values can also help guide where treatment should proceed and assess an emergent patient's current status. The "Big 3" is a term used for a PCV, total protein (TP), and blood glucose (BG). These tests yield helpful information with a small amount of blood that can often be obtained from the stylet of an IV catheter, are economical, and most clinics have the capacity to run. *PCV* and *TP* in the acute care setting are predominantly used to monitor hydration status and blood loss. Increases in both PCV and TP are consistent with hemoconcentration and dehydration. Following acute blood loss, splenic contraction may result in a PCV that remains normal or elevated despite significant bleeding. In these cases, evaluation of a decreased TP (<6 mg/dL) in the face of a normal PCV may be a better indication of acute hemorrhage. Both the PCV and TP will be expected to decrease through a dilutional effect after fluid therapy. Increase in *BG* on presentation may be consistent with stress or excitement, especially in cats. Hypoglycemia may indicate a coexisting reason for the shock state, often sepsis. Some practices also run a "Big 4" by also getting a blood urea nitrogen (BUN). *BUN* may be useful to identify azotemia, but further laboratory evaluation is needed to classify the cause of azotemia (e.g., prerenal azotemia from dehydration vs. true renal disease).

Other practices routinely draw blood for larger point of care panels which may include a venous blood gas, electrolytes, and some baseline chemistry values. Nova Biomedical's

CriticalCare Xpress, Idexx's VetStat, and Heska's IStat are examples of such units. Many of these samples, along with a blood smear to obtain an estimated white blood cell and platelet count, can be collected at the time of intravenous catheter placement and sometimes can be collected from the intravenous catheter prior to fluid therapy itself. When time allows later, more extensive laboratory testing such as complete blood counts, full blood chemistries, complete electrolyte panels, complete coagulation panels, urinalyses, and serology panels can be obtained.

Primary and secondary hemostasis

Sometimes in the emergency room, evaluation of primary and secondary hemostasis is necessary. Hemostasis is the interaction between platelets, blood vessels, and the coagulation cascade to form a clot. An interruption in these processes causes coagulopathy, and presenting signs can include epistaxis, petechia, ecchymosis, hematomas, or prolonged bleeding from a venipuncture site. These patients need to be handled gently (Baldwin 2003).

A coagulopathy with *primary hemostasis* is when the problem is suspected with the patient's platelets or vessels. Whole blood or platelet-rich plasma transfusion(s) are indicated to treat related disorders (Grace 2004). Tests include the following:

- A blood smear for a platelet estimate. Estimate 15,000–20,000 platelets per platelet per high power field (hpf), and review 10 fields to average the result. Also scan the feathered edge for platelet clumps to factor in the estimate. A normal patient should have at least 200,000 platelets, or an average of 10 per hpf. Severe bleeding usually does not occur until the platelet count drops to 30,000.
- Buccal mucosal bleeding time (BMBT) can be used to assess platelet function. A template is used to make an incision of standard depth in the buccal mucosa, and a stopwatch tracks the time it takes for the blood to clot. Blood oozing from the incision site can be dabbed away with filter paper or gauze, but the clot forming should not be touched. The normal time for a dog to form a visible clot in the incision is 3–4 minutes.

A coagulopathy with *secondary hemostasis* is when the problem is suspected with the coagulation cascade (clotting factors). Fresh frozen plasma is usually suggested to treat related disorders (Grace 2004). Tests include the following:

- The activated clotting time (ACT) screens for abnormalities in the intrinsic and common pathways by measuring the time for a fibrin clot to form. Available tests include special I-Stat cartridges, or tubes with diatomaceous earth that a normal patient will form a clot within 60–100 seconds.
- The partial thromboplastin time (PTT) measures the intrinsic and common pathways (similar to ACT).
- The prothrombin time (PT) measures the extrinsic and common pathways. These pathways cause the release of thrombin to start the coagulation cascade when there is damage to a blood vessel.

It should be noted that normal times depend on the manufacturer's specifications, shortened times are not indicative of a coagulopathy or hypercoagulation, and proper sampling is imperative for accuracy in these tests. Many clinicians require elevations of 1.5 times the high end of normal before considering a PT or PTT prolonged.

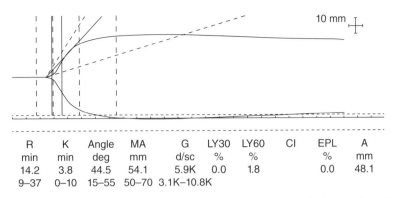

R min	K min	Angle deg	MA mm	G d/sc	LY30 %	LY60 %	CI	EPL %	A mm
14.2	3.8	44.5	54.1	5.9K	0.0	1.8		0.0	48.1
9–37	0–10	15–55	50–70	3.1K–10.8K					

Figure 2.9 A normal equine thromboelastograph (TEG) tracing. (Courtesy of Chris Norkus, BS, CVT, VTS [Emergency & Critical Care/Anesthesia].)

Some larger practices also utilize thromboelastograph (TEG) analysis to better evaluate a patient's clotting as a whole (Fig. 2.9). This global assessment uses citrated whole blood to evaluate all of the steps in hemostasis, including initiation, amplification, propagation, and fibrinolysis, including the interaction of platelets with proteins of the coagulation cascade. It is presently also the only means available in veterinary medicine to evaluate hypercoagulability.

Veterinary technicians should ensure any sample they obtain for hemostatic tests is acquired with a "clean stick," the sample tube provided is properly filled, and, if the sample is being sent out, it is prepared by the laboratory's specifications. The PT/PTT can be run in-house with the proper equipment, or sent out to a lab (Baldwin 2003).

Antibiotic Therapy

In general, antibiotics are not empirically administered in shock states. However, whenever there is disruption of visceral organ perfusion from significant shock states, there is risk of gastrointestinal mucosa damage, barrier breakdown, bacterial translocation, and enteric organism invasion into the circulatory system. Both gram-positive and gram-negative endogenous flora may produce secondary effects that can amplify the shock cycle. Therefore, broad spectrum antibiotic therapy (e.g., cephalosporin) may be selected in such cases.

Additionally, any case that is strongly suspected of having sepsis during the initial stabilization phase of treatment should be started on aggressive antibiotic therapy at once. Septic patients who have delayed time from diagnosis to the start of antibiotic therapy have significantly worse morbidity and mortality. Some initial antibiotics combinations for the treatment of suspected sepsis include clindamycin and amikacin for well-hydrated animals with normal renal function or clindamycin and cefotaxime for geriatric patients or those with questionable renal function.

Anti-Inflammatory Agents

Both corticosteroids and nonsteroidal anti-inflammatory drugs (NSAIDs) have been extensively studied as therapies in shock states. Unfortunately, neither group of drugs

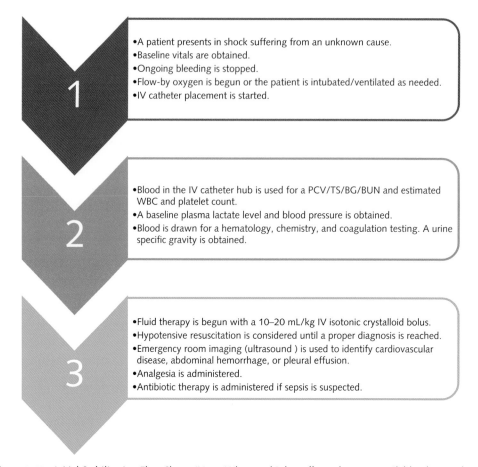

Figure 2.10   Initial Stabilization Flow Sheet. (Note: When multiple staff members are available, these tasks are typically performed concurrently by several people.)
PCV, packed cell volume; TS, total solid; BG, blood glucose; BUN, blood urea nitrogen; WBC, white blood cell.

has shown efficacy in hypovolemic shock to date, and their use has been associated consistently with significant negative side effects such as immunosuppression, gastrointestinal bleeding, and potential nephrotoxicity. As a result, the use of these agents in hypovolemic shock is strongly discouraged. Corticosteroids may have a role, however, in the treatment of some distributive shock states such as anaphylaxis and, at low doses, in sepsis.

Alkalinization

Alkalinization therapy with sodium bicarbonate and other buffering agents has not been shown to be effective for the treatment of shock states. Correcting the underlying perfusion disturbance and restoring normal tissue perfusion is presently considered the best strategy for corrected acid–base imbalances noted during shock states (Fig. 2.10).

Acknowledgment

Special thanks to Leigh Ann Hernandez, DVM, and Ashley Smith, DVM for their help in writing this chapter.

References

Abou-Khalil, B, Scalea, TM, Trooskin, SZ, et al. 1994. Hemodynamic responses to shock in young trauma patients: need for invasive monitoring. *Crit Care Med* 22:633–639.

Baldwin, K. 2003. *Ideal Sample Taking and an Investigation of the Coagulation Panel. American College of Veterinary Internal Medicine Symposium.*

Battaglia, AM. 2001. *Small Animal Emergency and Critical Care: A Manual for the Veterinary Technician*, 1st ed. Philadelphia: W.B. Saunders.

Bersenas, A. 2007. *Managing Emergencies I and II. Western Veterinary Conference.*

Davis, H. 2008. *Nursing Management of the Shock Patient. Atlantic Coast Veterinary Conference.*

DiBartola, S. 2006. *Fluid Electrolyte and Acid-Base Disorders in Small Animal Practice*, 3rd ed. St. Louis, MO: Saunders/Elsevier.

Firth, D, Brohi, K. 2010. The acute coagulopathy of trauma shock: clinical relevance. *Surgeon* 8(3):159–163.

Gaynor, J. 2007. *Blood Pressure Monitoring: What You Don't Know Can Hurt Your Patients—A Practical Approach. Western Veterinary Conference.*

Grace, SF. 2004. *Simplified Approach to Coagulation Disorders. Western Veterinary Conference.*

Kirby, R. 2008. *Shock and Resuscitation: Parts 1 and 2. "Be a Shock Buster!" World Veterinary Congress.*

Marino, PL. 1998. Tissue oxygenation. In *The ICU Book*, 2nd ed., edited by Marino, PL. Baltimore, MD: Williams & Wilkins, pp. 187–203.

Plumb, D. 2005/2008. *Veterinary Drug Handbook*, 5th ed./6th ed. Ames, IA: Wiley-Blackwell.

Rudloff, E. 2002. *Resuscitation from Hypovolemic Shock. World Small Animal Veterinary Association World Congress.*

Willard, S. 2002. *Tips in Obtaining Blood Gases & Interpreting Results. American College Veterinary Internal Medicine (ACVIM) Forum.*

Wingfield, W, Raffe, M. 2002. *The Veterinary ICU Book*, 1st ed. Jackson, WY: Teton NewMedia.

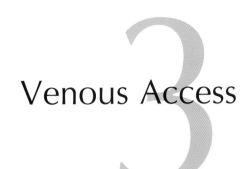

Venous Access

Kara B. Trent

Introduction

Access to the vascular system in the emergent or critical veterinary patient is of paramount importance. It can mean the difference between the success or failure to treat a patient. Access allows the administration of life-saving products such as fluids, medications, blood, and blood products. Knowledge of the advantages and disadvantages to the different types of catheters, sites to be used, techniques to facilitate access, and potential complications associated with them is invaluable to the veterinary team.

CHAPTER 3

Catheter Types

Winged Catheter

Winged catheters are also termed "butterfly catheters." These catheters vary in needle size from 27 to 16 gauge. They have "wings" to hold while placing that can also be used to help secure the catheter. There is also a short length of tubing with a luer adapter at the end to attach to a syringe or fluid line. These catheters are difficult to maintain for long-term use. Typically, butterfly catheters are used temporarily for administration of a medication or small amount of fluids. Another common use is placement for obtaining blood samples. This is helpful with cats and small dogs by placing it in the medial saphenous vein. Advantages include the low degree of technical difficulty to place, and there is no need for clipping of hair and skin preparation. The disadvantages include a high risk of extravasation of medication injected and the difficulty of maintaining for long periods of time. These catheters are typically used in peripheral veins including the cephalic and medial saphenous.

Over-the-Needle Catheters

Over-the-needle catheters are commonly used in veterinary medicine (Fig. 3.1). The technical difficulty of placing theses catheters is minimal. Therefore, over-the-needle catheters are a great option in emergency situations to gain venous access. These catheters come in a variety of lengths and sizes ranging from 10 to 24 gauge (Hansen 2006). A variety of materials are used to manufacture these catheters, including teflon, polypropylene, polyvinyl chloride, and polyurethane (Davis 2009a). These catheters are over-the-needle during placement and the needle is removed once in the vein. These catheters usually can be maintained for approximately 48–72 hours (Hansen 2006). They are used for administration of medications and fluid therapy. Commonly, these catheters are placed in cephalic and saphenous veins but can be placed in almost any superficial vein that is accessible. Advantages of using these catheters include the low technical difficulty to place, low cost, and they give a wider variety of options for placement sites (Hansen 2006). The

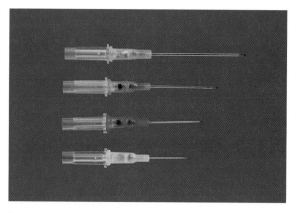

Figure 3.1   Examples of over-the-needle catheters in a variety of sizes. (Courtesy of MILA International, Inc.)

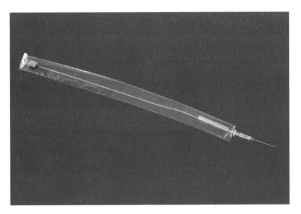

Figure 3.2   Example of through-the-needle catheter; single lumen. (Courtesy MILA International, Inc.)

disadvantages are that the short length limits the use for central venous access and/or aspirating blood for sampling.

Through-the-Needle Catheters

Through-the-needle catheters are long catheters that are used to gain central venous access (Fig. 3.2). These catheters are technically more difficult to place and must be placed with strict sterile technique. This is more time-consuming. Therefore, these catheters are not typically used in emergency situation but rather for critical patients that need long-term venous access. These catheters can be maintained for longer periods of time than shorter over-the-needle catheters. The longer catheters that gain central access can also be used for administration of hyperosmotic solutions and for repeated blood sampling. The external jugular and lateral saphenous veins are used to gain central venous access. Advantages of using through the needle catheters include the ability to gain central access, collect blood samples, administer hyperosmotic solutions, and they have a decreased potential of producing thrombophlebitis over time (Hansen 2006). Disadvantages include the technical difficulty in placement, an increased chance for hemorrhage, and an increased expense when compared with over-the-needle catheters (Hansen 2006).

Other Catheter Types

Other catheters used in veterinary medicine include multilumen catheters and central venous catheters that use a guidewire for placement (Fig. 3.3). Both types are technically more difficult to place, and strict sterile technique is a must. Multilumen catheters are beneficial when simultaneous infusions of incompatible products are necessary. This is inevitable in critical care medicine. Multilumen catheters are commonly used when total parenteral nutrition is necessary because one port can be dedicated to administration and others can be used for other products, blood sampling, and monitoring of central venous pressure (CVP). Multilumen catheters are typically available as having single, double, or triple lumens.

For guidewire placement of catheters, the *Seldinger technique* is commonly used. This technique uses a guidewire to access the vein and avoids the initial puncture into the vein with a large bore needle (Davis 2009b). This technique can be used to initially place catheters or replace an existing catheter. (Davis 2009b)

Catheter and Vein Selection

The decision on which vein should be used for access is dependent on many factors, including the patients needs, technical experience of the person placing the catheter, and availability of specialized catheters (Table 3.1). In true emergency situations, the easiest and quickest way to gain venous access is typically a peripheral vein (cephalic, medial, and lateral saphenous). A short over-the-needle catheter is the least technically demanding and can be placed quickly with little preparation to the insertion site. If one of these commonly used peripheral veins is not accessible, any vein that can be catheterized can be used to administer life-saving medication. Intratracheal and intraosseous (IO) delivery are also options in emergency situations.

If immediate access is not needed, then the patient's other needs should be taken into consideration. When short-term fluid or drug administration is needed, then a short over-the-needle catheter is optimal. An example is a patient undergoing an elective anesthetic procedure. The patient will require venous access for less than 72 hours for administration of fluids and anesthetics. Which peripheral vein is used should also be considered. If a patient has a limb that has an injury such as a laceration, fracture, or infection at the site, it should be avoided. The ability to keep the catheter site clean is considered as well. Limbs that will be affected by vomiting, diarrhea, or other contaminants should be avoided. The size of the catheter should also be considered with fluid administration. When rapid infusions are necessary, to treat shock or hypovolemia for example, then a short, large diameter catheter would be optimal to decrease resistance.

If it is anticipated that the patient's needs include any of the following, then central venous access should be considered:

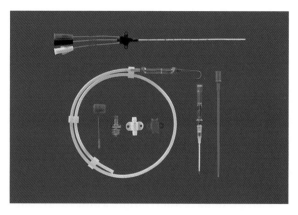

Figure 3.3   Example of guidewire catheter; multilumen. (Courtesy MILA International, Inc.)

Table 3.1 Considerations for selection of catheter placement

Catheter Type	Advantages	Disadvantages
Peripheral access	Technically easy to place	Short-term use (<72 hours)
	Easily accessible	Difficult in compromised patients (poor perfusion, edema, subcutaneous emphysema)
	Requires minimal restraint	
	Decreased risk of complications (hemorrhage, infection, or thrombosis)	Patient can easily access and disrupt placement
		Cannot obtain CVP
	Inexpensive	Cannot obtain blood samples
Central venous access	Long-term use (>72 hours)	Technically more difficult to place
	Can use large bore catheters	Requires restraint during placement
	Can use multilumen catheters	Increased risk of complications (hemorrhage, infection, or thrombosis)
	Can obtain CVP	
	Can obtain blood samples	More expensive
	Can administer hyperosmotic solutions	
	Can administer total parenteral nutrition	

- Long-term (>72 hours) fluid therapy
- Long-term (>72 hours) intravenous medications
- Administration of hyperosmotic solutions
- Administration of potentially irritating drugs (diazepam, mannitol, etc.)
- Administration of parenteral nutrition
- Administration of multiple fluids, medications, or other products that are not compatible (multilumen catheters)
- Multiple blood draws for sampling
- CVP monitoring

To gain central access, a long catheter is placed in the jugular, lateral, or medial saphenous veins. Which technique and catheter type used is also dependent on the patient's needs. Multilumen catheters are optimal for administering multiple fluids, medication, parenteral nutrition, or blood products simultaneously. The ability to administer these products simultaneously in one catheter eliminates the need for multiple catheters when products are incompatible.

IO catheterization is another option in emergency situations. Placement of IO catheters is relatively easy and can be done quickly in emergency situations. This technique is commonly used in neonates or patients with vascular collapse in which intravenous access is not possible. Within the marrow cavity, products administered are absorbed into the sinusoidal network (Hughes and Beal 2000). This route can be used to administer fluids, drugs, blood plasma, and dextrose (Wingfield 2002).

During periods of systemic hypotension intraosseously administered drugs reach peak effect more slowly (Giunti and Otto 2009). This is because of increased vascular resistance and decreased blood flow in the bone marrow (Giunti and Otto 2009). To decrease this effect, a fluid bolus after the administration of drugs or use of a pressurized system to administer fluids is advisable (Giunti and Otto 2009). Once the initial fluid resuscitation or drug administration is completed, typically, peripheral catheterization can be accomplished.

Catheter Placement Techniques

Peripheral Vein (Short; Over-the-Needle)

Peripheral veins are commonly used in emergency situations to gain vascular access. The cephalic, medial, and lateral saphenous veins are all common placement sites. The site is clipped and scrubbed. Aseptic technique is important during catheter placement to decrease the risk of introducing bacteria. Scrub solutions (chlorhexidine, povidine-iodine) require contact time to be most effective. If possible, the area should be continuously in contact with scrub for approximately 2 minutes (Hansen 2006). Alcohol rinsing can then be done. Exam gloves (ideally sterile gloves) are to be worn by the person placing the catheter to avoid any contamination. An assistant is typically necessary to restrain the patient as well as to occlude the vein. Patients that are obtunded may not require restraint and a tourniquet can be used. Whether using an assistant or a tourniquet, the distal leg is held in place with one hand. The catheter in the other hand is held bevel up and angled at approximately 15 degrees (Davis 2009a). The catheter is punctured though the subcutaneous tissue, advanced a short distance, and advanced through the vein. A flash of blood can usually be seen in the hub of the needle, and both the needle and catheter are advanced another 3–5 mm (Hansen 2006). The catheter is slid off the needle and advanced into the vein. The assistant or tourniquet can release the occlusion. A pre-flushed t-port adaptor is secured, and the catheter is flushed with heparin saline. The catheter is secured in place with white tape. A sterile gauze square with or without triple antibiotic ointment is placed over the insertion site, and tape is used to cover the gauze. All tape placed to secure the catheter should be used to anchor the catheter in place. It should be placed

---

Box 3.1   Supplies Needed for Placement of Jugular Catheter

- Appropriate catheter or catheter kit
- Surgical scrub and alcohol gauze
- Sterile gloves
- Sterile drape
- T-port adaptor/cap
- Heparinized saline flushes
- Gauze 3 × 3's
- Triple antibiotic ointment
- Waterproof white tape (1/2 and 1 in.)
- Suture (3-0 Nylon), needleholders
- #11 blade or needle
- Bandaging material—cast padding, gauze, coadhesive

somewhat loosely and pressed in place to avoid swelling distal and/or proximal to the catheter. The ends of the tap should be tabbed to ensure ease of catheter care and removal later. Bandaging material can be used to cover the tape and to prevent direct soiling to the tape.

Jugular Vein (Central Venous Access)

When a long catheter is placed in the jugular vein, there are three commonly used catheter types: through-the-needle, peel away sheath, and guidewire techniques. When placing catheters in the jugular vein, the consequences of introducing foreign material or infectious agents is more serious than with peripheral catheterization (Davis 2009b). Therefore, aseptic technique is extremely important when placing central venous catheters. The area of the neck is clipped and a surgical scrub is performed. The insertion site is infused with a small amount of local anesthetic (e.g., 2% lidocaine). Sterile gloves must be worn, and it is usually necessary to drape the area to avoid dragging the catheter through hair and contaminating it. The patient is placed in lateral recumbency and is restrained by an assistant. The assistant occludes the vein by putting pressure in the thoracic inlet. The jugular vein can be visualized lateral to the trachea and runs between the thoracic inlet and the mandible. The catheter is measured to accomplish appropriate placement. When measuring, the tip of the catheter should end just cranial to the right atrium (Davis 2009b).

Through-the-Needle Catheters

This technique can be used to place single lumen catheters. A small incision or relief hole should be made in the skin with a #11 blade or a needle. This hole will make the insertion of the needle into the subcutaneous space easier. The needle is inserted, beveled up, into the subcutaneous space, and is advanced parallel to the vein for approximately 2 cm (Hansen 2006). Further advancement into the vein is typically confirmed by a "pop" and a flash of blood that can be seen traveling up the catheter. The catheter is then advanced within the sterile plastic through the needle. In some patients, a flash of blood is not seen, especially if the patient is systemically unstable. The catheter can be advanced without a flash, and should advance smoothly. While advancing the catheter, the stylet should be pulled back. If the catheter only advances a short distance, then it is likely in the subcutaneous space and should be retracted and attempted again. Once the catheter is advanced, the needle is pulled back, and slight pressure with gauze is placed over the insertion site to avoid hemorrhage. The needle is covered with the plastic guard, the stylet is removed, and the pre-flushed t-port adaptor is attached. These catheters can often become kinked, so care should be taken when positioning the catheter to avoid this problem. The connections between the needle and catheter, and between the catheter and t-port, can often become loose and disconnect. Care should be taken to secure these connections with tape or glue. The catheter is secured to the skin by suturing either the plastic guard or anchor tape to the skin. Gauze with or without triple antibiotic ointment is placed over the insertion site and multiple (2–3) pieces of tape are wrapped from the catheter around the neck. Cast padding, gauze, and coadhesive material are used to bandage the neck. The t-port is anchored with tape to the outside of the bandage to avoid excessive movement.

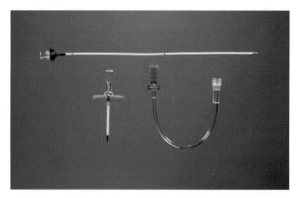

Figure 3.4   Example of peel away sheath catheter; single lumen. (Courtesty MILA International, Inc.)

Peel Away Sheath Catheters

This technique can be used for single or multilumen catheter placement and is available in manufactured kits (Fig. 3.4). An incision made in the skin and the needle, within the peel away sheath, is advanced into the vein as with the through-the-needle technique. Once in the vein, the needle is removed as the sheath is held in place within the vein. The catheter is then fed trough the sheath into the vein and is advanced. A pre-flushed t-port adaptor is attached to the catheter. The sheath is retracted out of the skin, and pressure is placed over the insertion site with gauze. The sheath is peeled away by pulling apart the tabs. The catheter is then secured and bandaged as with the through-the-needle catheters (Fig. 3.5).

Guidewire Catheters (Seldinger Technique)

This technique can be used to place single or multilumen catheters and can be used to reintroduce or replace an existing catheter. These catheters are available in manufactured kits. When using multilumen catheters, the ports should be flushed before starting. Caps are placed on all ports except the distal one. The vein is punctured with the introduction needle, and the guidewire is advanced through the needle into the vein. The wire must not be advanced too far because of the possibility of entering the heart. This can result in atrial injury and cardiac arrhythmias (Beal and Hughes 2000). Once the guidewire is in place, the needle is removed, and the vessel dilator is threaded into the vein. This creates a larger opening into the vein to allow the catheter to pass. The dilator is removed, and the catheter is threaded onto the wire. There is typically some hemorrhage at the insertion site when the dilator is removed. Pressure with gauze can be placed over the site while the catheter is initially being threaded on the guidewire to minimize hemorrhage. Once the wire appears out of the port of the catheter and is held in place, the catheter is advanced into the vein. The wire is then removed. Air is aspirated from the catheter and flushed with heparinized saline. The pre-flushed t-port adaptor is attached, and the catheter is secured and bandaged as described with other jugular catheters (Fig. 3.6).

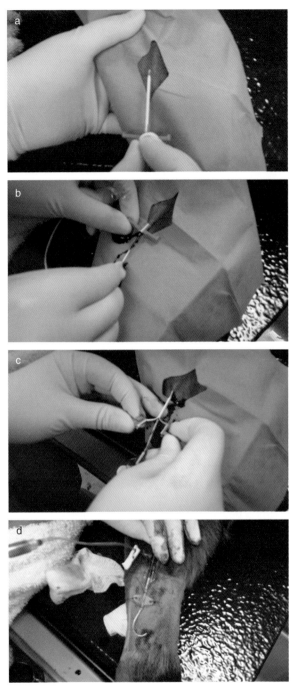

Figure 3.5   Placement of a peel away sheath catheter in the lateral saphenous vein. (a) The area is scrubbed and draped. The vein is visualized. The needle, within the peel away sheath, is advanced into the vein. (b) Once in the vein, confirmed with blood advancing into the hub of the needle, the needle is removed, and the peel away sheath is held in place within the vein. The catheter is fed through the needle into the vein. (c) The sheath is retracted out of the skin and peeled away by pulling apart the tabs. A pre-flushed t-port is attached. (d) The catheter is secured in place by suturing it to the skin. (e) The catheter is bandaged routinely to protect it from movement or contamination.

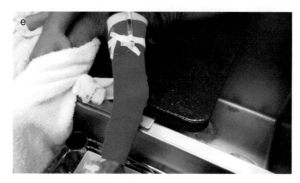

Figure 3.5   *(Continued)*

Venous Cutdown Procedure

Venous cutdown procedures can be used in peripheral or jugular veins. These procedures can be done quickly in emergency situations or in a more controlled situation where venous access has been proven difficult for other reasons such as vascular collapse. In either situation, cutdown procedures are necessary to gain venous access because percutaneous attempts have failed. When possible, aseptic technique must be used. If not possible, the catheter should be removed once the patient is stabilized and another catheter can be placed. If the patient is conscious, a local anesthetic is used along the anticipated incision site. There are two types of cutdown procedures commonly used: a mini cutdown and a full cutdown. Both procedures are similar except that a full cutdown requires a longer incision to accomplish full visualization of the vein. The incision parallel to the vein is made with a #11 blade. Blunt dissection with hemostats is used to expose the vein. Suture is passed around the vein in two locations, one proximal and one distal to the anticipated insertion site. The catheter is then placed directly into the vein. The sutures are then used to secure the catheter directly to the vein. The skin incision is closed by suturing. The catheter and incision is bandaged similar to that of a central catheter.

Interosseus (IO)

IO catheterization is a great option in emergency situations where venous access is challenging because of the small size of the patient or in cases of vascular collapse. This procedure is not technically difficult and can be done quickly. As discussed previously, fluids, drugs, blood, plasma, and dextrose can all be administered effectively (Wingfield 2002). There are multiple sites in which IO catheterizatrion are possible. These sites include the trochanteric fossa of the femur, the greater tubercle of the humerus, wing of the ilium, distal femur proximal to the patella, and the tibial tuberosity (Wingfield 2002). The most common site used is the trochanteric fossa of the femur (Wingfield 2002; Hansen 2006). This site allows easy placement, mobility of the patient, and is usually well tolerated by the patient (Giunti and Otto 2009).

There are commercially available IO needles available, but a bone marrow or spinal needles are also appropriate and commonly used. A nice newer option is a commercially

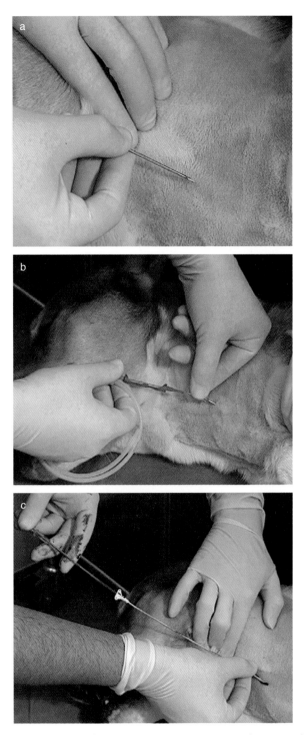

Figure 3.6 Placement of a guidewire catheter. (Courtesy MILA International, Inc.) (a) The area is clipped and scrubbed. The vein is visualized, and the needle is advanced into the vein. (b) The guidewire is advanced through the needle into the vein. The needle is removed, and the vessel dilator is threaded into the vein. The dilator is removed. (c) The catheter is threaded onto the wire. (d) The catheter is threaded into the vein. (e) The catheter is secured in place by suturing it to the skin. The wire is removed, and a pre-flushed t-port is attached. The catheter is bandaged in place routinely.

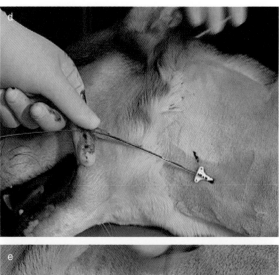

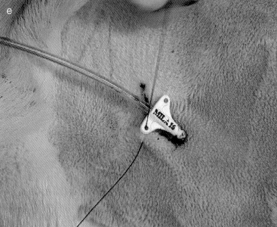

Figure 3.6   *(Continued)*

available interosseous catheter kit, such as the one available through MILA International (www.milainternational.com). This specific kit comes with a power driver that works similarly to an electric drill gun and dramatically quickens the process of smooth IO catheter placement (Fig. 3.7).

In neonates, a simple hypodermic needle can be used (Wingfield 2002; Hansen 2006). The site is clipped and aseptically scrubbed when possible. A local anesthetic (e.g., 2% lidocaine) is infused into the skin, muscle, and periosteum (Wingfield 2002). A small skin incision is made, and the needle is advanced to the periosteum. Initially, gentle pressure with rotation is used to seat the needle into the bone. Pressure is then increased and rotation, clockwise and counter clockwise, is continued. Once in the cortex, a loss of resistance is felt. To assure placement, move the limb and note the needle moving along with it. Aspiration of the needle will often confirm placement by bringing marrow into the syringe. This may not be the case in older animals. Flushing the catheter with saline should yield little resistance. Once the infusion is started, careful monitoring for fluid in the subcutaneous space is necessary. Infusion can be painful when started, but discomfort

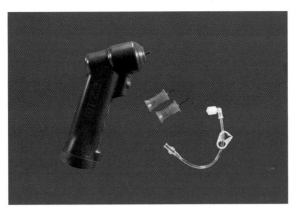

Figure 3.7 A commercially available IO catheter kit and battery-operated needle driver, such as the one here from MILA International, makes rapid and smooth placement of IO catheters easy. (Courtesy MILA International, Inc.)

can be minimized by warming fluids before rapid infusions (Wingfield 2002). The catheter is secured by suturing it to the periosteum. The area is covered with triple antibiotic ointment and bandaged. IO catheters are typically only used in emergency situations for approximately 12–24 hours (Wingfield 2002). The risk of complications is small and with proper maintenance catheters, can remain in place for up to 72 hours (Giunti and Otto 2009). Once the patient is stabilized and it is possible, the catheter is commonly removed and a venous catheter is placed.

Catheter Maintenance

The maintenance of intravenous catheters is extremely important. Improper technique and maintenance can cause a variety of complications. As discussed previously, strict aseptic technique must be used during placement. If in an emergency situation where aseptic technique cannot be used during placement, the catheter should be replaced once the patient has been stabilized. Maintenance of catheters should include monitoring of the area at least every 8 hours. This includes changing of the bandage material and replacement of catheters as necessary. When monitoring the area, observation for swelling, pain, discharge, or soiling of the bandage should be noted. Often, when there is swelling of the toes, the bandage or tape is too tight and is restricting circulation. If swelling is present, the tape/bandage should be loosened. If there is no relief, the tape/bandage should be completely removed and replaced. If pain or discharge is noticed, the catheter should be removed.

There is controversy regarding the length of time an intravenous catheter should be maintained. Commonly short peripheral catheters are replaced every 72 hours. There is little evidence that supports this practice, if appropriate technique and maintenance is followed. There are studies that show there was not an increase in catheter-related infections when catheters were left in place for longer than 72 hours, when compared to those removed before 72 hours (Hughes and Beal 2000). Besides monitoring of the area, every 48 hours, catheter care should be performed (Wingfield 2002; Hansen 2006; Davis 2009a). The bandage and tape should be removed. The insertion area is observed and palpated for any signs of infection, inflammation, or thrombosis. If any signs are observed, the catheter should be removed. Otherwise, the area is cleaned with scrub, dried, and bandaged again. At this time, the catheter should be flushed as well, if there is any leaking of fluid at the insertion site or if there is pain associated with injection, the catheter should be replaced at a different site. If a fever of unknown origin develops during the time a patient has an intravenous catheter in place, the catheter should be considered a source (Hughes and Beal 2000). The catheter should then be removed and submitted for culture and sensitivity testing. After removal of the catheter, the fever will typically resolve. Patency maintained by the use of heparin saline compared to saline alone shows no significant benefit (Hughes and Beal 2000; Hansen 2006). Although patients on continuous infusions of fluids typically do not need the catheter flushed to maintain patency, patients that are receiving intermittent administration of medications do require flushing. This is also the case with small diameter catheters on slow rates of continuous fluids. These catheters should be flushed (with or without heparin) after medication administration or at least every 8 hours. Care should be taken to avoid flushing catheters with higher concentrations of heparin too often in cats and small dogs as it is possible to produce systemic anticoagulation (Hansen 2006). It should also be considered that the occurrence of catheter-related infection is increased with frequent invasion of the injection port (Hughes and Beal 2000).

Complications

There are many complications that can be associated with intravenous catheterization, including extravasation of fluids or medications, infection to tissues and venous system, thrombosis, and air and catheter embolisms. It is important to have knowledge of these potential complications, the signs to look for, and what steps should be taken to prevent complications.

Extravasation

When an intravenous catheter is displaced, extravasation of fluids or medications enter the surrounding tissue. This happens with excessive movement of the area where the catheter is placed, puncture of the catheter tip through the vessel wall, improper placement of the catheter initially, or an occlusion by thrombosis upstream (Hansen 2006; Davis 2009a). The signs to look for when evaluating the patient are swelling, heat, redness, and pain around the catheter site. Signs may be more difficult to evaluate with jugular catheters and may not be obvious until large amounts of fluid have accumulated. When left unnoticed or untreated, there is a potential for more severe complications including necrosis of the surrounding tissue (Hansen 2006).

With jugular catheters, there is the potential for accumulation of mediastinal and pleural fluid resulting in dyspnea (Hansen 2006). There are many precautions that can be taken to decrease the chances of this complication. When placing the catheter, attempt to puncture the vein only once. Having good visualization of the vein and restraint of the patient during placement will help minimize the chances of multiple punctures. To avoid excessive movement of the catheter after placement, it should not be placed near movable joints. If it cannot be avoided, then immobilization with a splint may be necessary

(Hansen 2006). As mentioned previously, the catheter must be monitored frequently. The severity of the complications can be decreased if a problem is detected early on and the catheter is removed.

Infection

An intravenous catheter provides easy access for bacteria to enter the surrounding tissue and venous system. Bacteria can be introduced with improper technique during placement and maintenance of the catheter. Signs of infection at the site include inflammation and cellulitis (Hansen 2006; Davis 2009a). When left unnoticed or untreated, there is a potential for bacteremia and organ infection. Systemic signs include fever and luekocytosis (Hansen 2006).

There are many precautions that can be taken to help prevent infection at the catheter site. As mentioned previously, strict aseptic technique should be practiced while placing the catheter. During placement, the skin should be punctured with the catheter, and the catheter then should be advanced a short distance in the subcutaneous tissue before entering the vein. This "tunneling" can act as a barrier to bacteria that may enter at the insertion site of the skin. Exam gloves, or sterile gloves with central catheters, should be worn when handling the catheter, fluid lines, or injection ports. In studies, catheter colonization has been documented at the exit site of skin, hub connections, and the nursing staff hands (Hansen 2006). Care should be taken to maintain cleanliness within the patient's housing area as well. Precautions for the prevention of the patient chewing or licking at the catheter or fluid line should be taken. If there are any signs of infection, the catheter should be removed and sent for culture and sensitivity testing (Fig. 3.8).

Thrombosis

With intravenous catheterization thrombi can develop on the catheter and/or between the catheter and the vessel wall. This is the result of trauma to the vein (e.g., endothelial

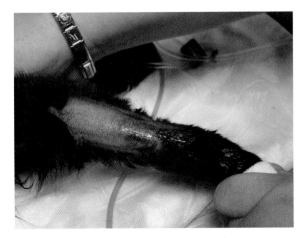

Figure 3.8 Cephalic vein phlebitis following intravenous catheter placement in a cat. (Courtesy of Angela Randals, CVT, VTS [Emergency & Critical Care], VTS [Small Animal Internal Medicine])

damage) or a reaction to the catheter material. When the catheter is removed, the thrombi break free and are sent into circulation. When thrombi are small in size, which is the most common, there is typically not a problem. When thrombi are larger in size, the result can be fatal. The risk of thrombosis is higher in small veins (with low blood flow) or where the catheter passes through a mobile joint (Hansen 2006). There are specific diseases that increase the risk as well. The risk of serious thrombosis and pulmonary thromboembolism is increased in patients with preexisting phlebitis, glomerulonephritis, protein-losing enteropathy, autoimmune hemolytic anemia, and any disorders that cause systemic inflammation (Hansen 2006). The decision to catheterize these patients should be weighed carefully.

Air and Catheter Embolisms

Air embolisms occur when air is introduced into circulation. This can occur when air is injected with a syringe, when air in inappropriately evacuated through fluid lines, or during insertion of a central venous catheter. Small air emboli may go unnoticed, producing no signs or negative effects. Large air emboli may cause respiratory distress, pulmonary edema, or respiratory/cardiac arrest (Hansen 2006). Air emboli can be prevented by taking care to evacuate all air from syringes when administering medications, as well as evacuating all air from fluid lines before connecting to the patient. When placing jugular catheters, the tip of the catheter can be exposed to negative pressure within the chest, and if the hub end is exposed to air, it will create suction. Therefore, the hub should be capped immediately after placement.

Catheter embolisms occur when a portion of the catheter is introduced into circulation. This can potentially occur in multiple situations. When placing over-the-needle catheters, a fragment of the catheter may be introduced into circulation. This can occur after the catheter is partially advanced off of the needle and pulled back over the needle while in the vein. A fragment can be cut off by the needle and then move freely. This can also occur with through-the-needle catheters as well. When pulling the catheter back through the needle, a fragment can be cut.

Other situations that may occur are during catheter removal or bandage change where the catheter is accidentally cut or when the patient chews at the catheter, disconnecting the catheter from the hub. Catheter emboli can be prevented by taking care when placing catheters to not pull the catheter back, over the needle, or through the needle, when in the vein. When removing or replacing bandage material with scissors, the cut should be made well away from the insertion site. When possible, visualization of the catheter insertion site should be confirmed before cutting. Patients that are interested in chewing at the catheter should have an Elizabethan collar placed to prevent damage to the catheter.

References

Beal, MW, Hughes, D. 2000. Vascular access: theory and techniques in the small animal emergency patient. *Clinical Techniques in Small Animal Practice* 15(2):101–109.

Davis, H. 2009a. Peripheral Venous Catheterization. In *Small Animal Critical Care Medicine*, Vol. 1, edited by Silverstein, DC, Hopper, K. St. Louis, MO: Saunders Elsevier, p. 260.

Davis, H. 2009b. Central Venous Catheterization. In *Small Animal Critical Care Medicine*, Vol. 1, edited by Silverstein, DC, Hopper, K. St. Louis, MO: Saunders Elsevier, p. 267.

Giunti, M, Otto, CM. 2009. Intraosseous Catheterization. In *Small Animal Critical Care Medicine*, Vol. 1, edited by Silverstein, DC, Hopper, K. St. Louis, MO: Saunders Elsevier, pp. 263–267.

Hansen, HD. 2006. Technical Aspects of Fluid Therapy. In *Fluid, Electrolyte, and Acid-Base Disorders in Small Animal Practice*, 3rd ed. Vol. 1, edited by DiBartola, S. St. Louis, MO: Saunders Elsevier, pp. 344–375.

Hughes, D, Beal, MW. 2000. Emergency vascular access. *Clinical Techniques in Small Animal Practice* 30(3):491–507.

Wingfield, SG. 2002. Emergency Vascular Access and Intravenous Catheterization. In *The Veterinary ICU Book*, Vol. 1, edited by Wingfield, WE, Raffe, MR Jackson, WY: Teton NewMedia, pp. 59–67.

Monitoring the Critical Patient

Trish Farry

Introduction

Fundamental to the care of the critically ill patient in veterinary practice is consistent, regular, and reliable monitoring by the veterinary technician.

An integral component to monitoring is the accurate and detailed recording of information. These records provide the foundation for case management and are of particular importance in the critical patient whose treatment plans will likely be detailed and complex.

The fragile physiological state and lack of reserve of these patients will result in little tolerance for missed or incorrect treatments.

As technology has provided the veterinary profession with more and more complex and sophisticated monitoring equipment, the role of the veterinary technician has evolved to keep current with these technological advances.

The use of noninvasive and/or invasive monitoring devices can assist the technician in the detection of organ dysfunction, patient compromise, or deterioration. This will enable the technician to alert the veterinarian who can rapidly initiate and/or alter treatment plans.

It is prudent to remember that monitoring devices cannot replace a well-trained, skilled, and observant technician, and are best utilized in conjunction with "hands-on" patient evaluation and observation.

Record Keeping

Accurate and comprehensive record keeping is essential in managing the emergent or critical patient. Records and treatment orders will act as a reminder of physical parameters that need to be assessed as well as prompting the technician to administer scheduled treatments in a timely manner, and help plan patient care when patient numbers are high. Communication and recording of information gained is paramount for management and care of these patients. The technician must be familiar with normal values for the parameters being assessed. Any deviation from normal warrants further communication with the primary care veterinarian. Early recognition of impending physiological decline may facilitate early treatment and prevent further decline in the patients' condition.

The type of patient record and the amount of information recorded will vary depending on the condition and complexity of the patients' illness. Often, there are large staff numbers both veterinary and technical, involved in the ongoing care of a critical patient. The incidence of errors made or things to be missed will increase as staff numbers increase and accurate record keeping becomes paramount in these patients. Critically ill patients have very little physiological tolerance to incorrect treatments or dosages. If at all possible, a system that allows for at least one check should be out in place. The more intensive the treatments, the more detailed the records need to be. The importance of accurate and complete record keeping cannot be overstated in the care of these patients. Patient records can also provide a valuable resource for research and teaching for current and future staff and students.

Some hospitalized patients will only require basic monitoring. Depending on the severity of illness, others may require intensive, more frequent, and advanced monitoring. Figure 4.1 and Boxes 4.1 and 4.2 are examples of monitoring orders and treatment sheets that may be used in a hospitalized patient. These documents are typical of records kept in veterinary practices, and form the foundation of sound record keeping.

Practice of Monitoring

Veterinary practice has evolved with the introduction of monitoring equipment, which can provide valuable information on the physiological status of a patient. All equipment has limitations, and the information provided should only be used in conjunction with a thorough patient examination.

Often, in the critical patient, trends will mean more than individual measurements. Serial observations or trends will often give a more accurate indication of a patient's physiological state. A single measurement can give a baseline against which the effectiveness of any applied treatment can be measured (Keates 2005). It is essential that the technician does not concentrate on one clinical sign or one measured parameter. Several parameters must be monitored to build a more complete picture of physiological function in the individual patient.

Human Senses

The importance of the role played by human senses cannot be overstated in the management of critical patients. By using our senses of sight, touch, hearing, and smell, the technician can quickly and accurately evaluate a patient's physical state. This information

Patient sticker

WEIGHT:
Hosp Day:
Problems List:
To do list:
Date:
UQ VET: STUDENT:
REGULAR VET: UPDATE:
QUOTE: A/C BALANCE:

TREATMENTS		0800	0900	1000	1100	1200	1300	1400	1500	1600	1700	1800	1900	2000	2100	2200	2300	0000	0100	0200	0300	0400	0500	0600	0700
GENERAL	TPR q																								
	Check IV & record fluids in q																								
	Comfort check clean bedding q																								
	Pain score q																								
	Exercise q																								
	Record U/D (calculate UOP) q																								
	Weigh animal and zero fluids q																								
	Catheter care (Ucath/IV) q																								
MEDICATIONS																									
FLUIDS	IV Catheter placement date:																								
LABS																									
OTHER	Water?																								
	Diet?																								
	Eating Y or N																								

Figure 4.1   Basic hospital treatment order sheet.

can form a basis which may be supplemented by additional data provided by modern technology and equipment (Table 4.1).

Monitoring without Monitors

Cardiovascular System

Heart rate and rhythm, MM color, CRT, pulse rate, and pulse quality are utilized as basic evaluation of the cardiovascular system. More advanced monitoring of the cardiovascular system can include arterial blood pressure (ABP), electrocardiography, and CVP.

The use of a stethoscope can provide more than just heart rate. Valuable information on the character of heart sounds, heart rate, and rhythm can be obtained, providing an overview on the cardiovascular status of a patient. If a technician were to rely on a monitor alone, subtleties in the patient's condition may be overlooked. Any variation on normal heart rate and rhythm should warrant further investigation. An elevated heart rate could be a result of something as simple as stress or may signify more serious issues such as sepsis, pain, hyperthermia, or hypotension. A decrease in heart rate may be indicative of hypothermia, hyperkalemia, or shock.

Pulse palpation, usually via the femoral or dorsal pedal arteries can give valuable information about perfusion. The dorsal pedal pulse is found on the cranio-medial aspect

CHAPTER 4

Box 4.1   Nursing Monitoring Orders

- Rectal temperature every 4–12 hours
- Mucous membrane (MM) color, capillary refill time (CRT), pulse quality, and heart rate every 2–12 hours
- Respiratory rate and effort, auscultation of lungs every 2–12 hours
- Note urine output or palpate bladder every 2–6 hours
- Note neurological status and mentation every 2–6 hours
- Note presence of vomiting, regurgitation, or bowel movements every 4–8 hours
- Assess comfort and adequacy of pain control every 2–4 hours
- Turn from side to side if recumbent or stand and walk the patient every 4 hours
- Lubricate eyes with artificial tears if the animal is sedated and unable to blink, every 2–4 hours
- Offer water/and or food (specify food type and amount unless "nil by mouth"), and record volumes ingested
- Check oxygen supplementation percentage every 2–4 hours
- Check that intravenous fluids are the type requested and are running at the correct rate every 2 hours
- Check position, degree of tightness, adequacy of venous drainage, and cleanliness of all bandages every 4–8 hours; replace if necessary
- Flush IV catheters, evaluate patency of all catheters every 4–6 hours
- Packed cell volume, total protein, blood glucose, and blood urea nitrogen every 2–24 hours

Reproduced from the *BSAVA Manual of Canine and Feline Emergency and Critical Care*, edited by Lesley King and Amanda Boag, 2007, Wiley Blackwell, with the permission of BSAVA Publication.

---

of the hindleg just below the hock. If a dorsal pedal pulse is present, a rough estimation of blood pressure can be estimated to be above 80 mmHg systolic. Conversely, if a pulse is absent, the estimate of systolic blood pressure is less than 80 mmHg. Normal pulses should not vary in strength and should be synchronous with the patient's heartbeat. *Pulse deficits* or variation in pulsatile strength may indicate the presence of a cardiac arrhythmia warranting further investigation.

When auscultating a patient, in addition to determining heart rate and rhythm, the technician should identify any abnormal heart sounds. Familiarization with landmarks for auscultating atrioventricular (AV) valves will assist the technician in the detection of murmurs such as mitral regurgitation (Fig. 4.2).

Cardiac arrhythmias are often encountered in the critically ill patient and may represent a significant source of morbidity. Patients with structural heart disease may have an increased risk of developing arrhythmias. Whenever an arrhythmia is detected, an eletrocardiogram (ECG) is indicated.

MM color and CRT can be useful in the assessment of peripheral perfusion. Normal MM color is pink and CRT is less than 2 seconds.

Box 4.2   Advanced Nursing Monitoring Orders (In Addition to Basic Monitoring)

- Continuous or intermittent ECG
- Blood pressure monitoring (direct or indirect), continuous or every 2–12 hours
- Central venous pressure (CVP); continuous or every 2–6 hours
- Pulmonary artery or pulmonary capillary wedge pressure monitoring; continuous or every 2–6 hours
- Pulse oximetry; continuous or every 2–6 hours
- End-tidal capnography; continuous or every 2–6 hours
- Arterial blood gas analysis every 2–12 hours
- Urine output quantitation via closed collection system every 2–4 hours
- Intra-abdominal pressure monitoring very 2–6 hours
- Electrolyte measurement every 4–24 hours
- Colloid osmometry every 4–24 hours
- Nebulize and coupage 10–20 minutes every 4–6 hours
- Check and clean inner cannula of tracheostomy tube every 2–4 hours
- Aspirate chest tubes every 2–4 hours; recording volumes of air/fluid obtained
- Record mechanical ventilator settings; airway pressure and tidal volume every 2 hours
- Peritoneal dialysis; infuse dialysate, dwell and drain every 1–2 hours; record volumes and quantity of fluid obtained

Reproduced from the *BSAVA Manual of Canine and Feline Emergency and Critical Care*, edited by Lesley King and Amanda Boag, 2007, Wiley Blackwell, with the permission of BSAVA Publications.

Respiratory System

The foundation of respiratory system monitoring is auscultation. Auscultation should involve all passages of air movement from the larynx and trachea through to the lung fields. By systematically auscultating each area, the technician should be able to localize any abnormal sounds.

Upper airway obstructions originating from the laryngeal or tracheal area are usually loud, harsh, and high pitched, whereas as lower airway sounds are more quiet and subtle. The most common lower airway sound abnormalities are crackles and wheezes. Crackles are caused by sudden opening and closing of the small airways. Their presence may indicate pulmonary edema resulting from fluid overload, congestive heart failure, or pulmonary fibrosis. Wheezes are the result of airway narrowing and may be due to any condition causing broncho-constriction such as allergic airway disease or feline asthma.

The rate and pattern of respiration are also useful indices in assessment of a patient's respiratory status. The normal resting respiratory rate for a dog or cat is 15–30 breaths per minute. The breathing pattern should be rhythmic, with inspiration of approximately 1 second, with simultaneous expansion of the thorax and the abdomen. Exhalation should be a passive process with no effort or noise. Prolonged inspiration with inspiratory

Table 4.1   Using senses for patient assessment

Sense	Observation	Information
Sight	Mucous membrane color	
	• Pale	Hypoperfusion and vasoconstriction and anemia
	• Pink	Normal
	• Red	Vasodilation, local congestion, sepsis/systemic inflammatory response syndrome (SIRS)
	• Brick red	Hemoconcentration
	• Blue	Cyanosis
	Thoracic movements	
	• Rate	Respiratory rate
	• Amplitude	Tidal volume
	• Type	Respiratory pattern
	Eye	
	• Position	Level of consciousness/responsiveness
	• Lacrimation	
	• Pupil size/response	
	• Position of third eyelid	
	Patient movement	Level of consciousness/responsiveness
	Obvious abnormalities	e.g., Fractures, bleeding
Touch	Pulses	
	• Tone, amplitude	Cardiovascular system, heart rate/rhythm, blood pressure, pulse deficits
	• Rate rhythm	
	• Synchronicity with heart auscultation	
	Capillary refill time	Cardiovascular status: peripheral perfusion
	Palpebral/corneal reflex	Level of consciousness/responsiveness
	Skin temperature	Body temperature
Hearing	Cardiac auscultation	
	• Rate, rhythm, murmurs	Cardiac system: heart rate, rhythm
	Pulmonary auscultation	
	• Rate rhythm, lung sounds	Respiratory system: respiratory rate, integrity
Smell	Presence of abnormal odors	e.g., Ketoacidotic breath, infection, uremia

Adapted and reproduced from the *BSAVA Manual of Canine and Feline Anaesthesia and Analgesia*, 2nd edition, edited by Chris Seymour and Tanya Duke-Novakovski, 2007, Wiley Blackwell, with the permission of BSAVA Publications.

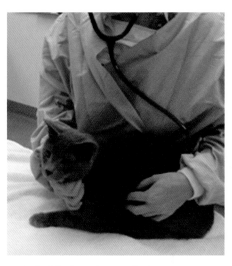

Figure 4.2   Physical examination including thoracic auscultation.

stridor or stertor with a short expiration may indicate upper airway obstruction. Prolonged expiration may be indicative of lower airway disease.

Animals in respiratory distress may display obvious signs such as open mouth breathing, increased abdominal movements, reluctance to sit, or adopt abnormal postures such as an orthopneic stance (Fig. 4.3).

The benefits of examination and treatment of an animal in respiratory distress must be weighed against the deleterious effects of performing such an examination. If the patient's condition is assessed as stable, the provision of supplemental oxygen prior to complete examination and evaluation may be beneficial.

The evaluation of a patient's respiratory status should always include a thorough history, physical examination, and thoracic auscultation. This information can be supplemented by data obtained from monitors utilized in the evaluation of the respiratory system. These include the pulse oximeter and capnograph.

Neurological System

The neurological status of the critical patient must be assessed in conjunction with the other body systems. A patient's mental status and gait should be noted, and any variation from ambulatory, bright, alert, and responsive will necessitate further investigation. Patients may present with many variations in mental status from dullness and depression to hyperexcitability and seizures. Central nervous system (CNS) depression may be a result of primary CNS disease, or may present as a complication from metabolic disorders. Hypoglycemic, or patents with renal or hepatic compromise, may display depressed mentation.

Animals with head trauma may display altered mentation in the form of dullness, stupor, or coma. Pupils may be asymmetrical and nystagmus may be evident. Continually increasing intracranial pressure without treatment may result in brain herniation. In

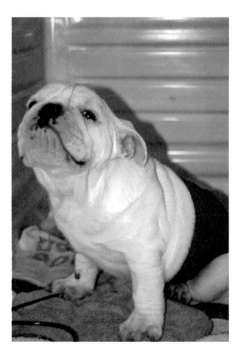

Figure 4.3   A patient demonstrated classic orthopnea posture. A patient with a respiratory obstruction will often adopt a body position that enables them to breathe more comfortably. Usually, it is one in which the patient is sitting up with the elbows abducted.

patients with suspected head trauma, the head should be elevated to ~30° to facilitate venous return and decrease intracranial pressure. Increases in intracranial pressure can be caused by the occlusion of the jugular veins, hence jugular venipuncture is not recommended under these circumstances. Care must be taken to avoid any drugs or situations that may result in coughing or vomiting, as this may also cause increases in intracranial pressure. These patients may also lose their gag reflex, so airway protection via intubation may be warranted (Glass and Kent 2007). Neurological monitoring in the head trauma patient will include:

- Mental status
- Papillary light response
- Pupil sizes
- Palpebral and menace reflex
- Presence of strabismus or nystagmus

Spinal cord injury in the form of intervertebral disc disease is frequently seen in the neurological emergent patient. Spinal trauma, discospondylitis, and fibrocartilagenous emboli are other neurological disorders commonly seen. Patients may present with various stages of neurological deterioration. Ataxia and loss of proprioception may progress to loss of voluntary motor activity and loss of deep pain. These patients require regular, thorough monitoring and serial neurological examinations. The veterinarian should be immediately notified of any deterioration in the ambulation and neurological status of a patient, as further workup, treatment, and/or surgical intervention may be indicated.

Urinary System

One of the most important indicators of renal function is urine output. Urine specific gravity and biochemical analysis of blood urea nitrogen, creatinine, and potassium are also commonly used in the evaluation of renal function.

Urine output is most accurately measured by the placement of an indwelling catheter, although it may also be achieved by weighing bedding that has absorbed urine after bladder voiding. Indications for the placement of an indwelling urinary catheter include patients at risk from acute renal failure and the presence of abdominal trauma that may have potentially damaged the ureters, bladder, or urethra. Catheters are also often utilized in the recumbent patient to prevent urine scalding.

The placement of a urinary catheter is not a benign procedure and should only be placed using a strict aseptic technique. Bacterial infection and urethral trauma are catheter-related complications that can occur if poor technique or maintenance of the indwelling catheter occurs.

Urine output should be assessed and measured every 2–4 hours in the critical patient. Normal urine output should be 1–2 mL/kg/h. Patients on intravenous fluids will have urine output greater than this.

Decreased urine production may result from:

■ Renal failure with anuria or oliguria
■ Dehydration
■ Hypoperfusion/hypotension
■ Urethral trauma
■ Uretal trauma
■ Bladder rupture

In addition to the calculation of urine production, the technician should note the size of the bladder prior to expression and the appearance of the urine, recording color and any presence of abnormal odor (Fig. 4.4).

Integrated Monitoring

Patients do not exist as separate or independent body systems. All body systems are integrated and a change in one system will often influence a change in another. We need to monitor parameters that reflect this integration.

Optimizing tissue perfusion and maintaining adequate oxygen delivery is the main goal in the treatment of the critical patient. The veterinary technician may use various pieces of equipment to monitor the cardiovascular and respiratory systems. This equipment can measure the adequacy of oxygenation, ventilation, and arterial pressure, CVP, and identify cardiac abnormalities.

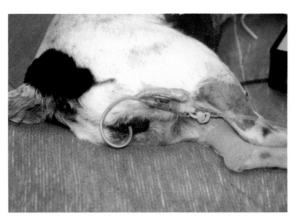

Figure 4.4   A hospitalized case with a closed collection urinary system. A closed collection system is used to accurately monitor urine output. Strict aseptic technique must be used to place and maintain this system as these patients are at risk from nosocomial bacterial infections. The urinary catheter is attached to a sterile collection system.

Monitoring equipment can provide valuable information and act as an extension of the technicians own senses. However, machines can malfunction or fail. The technician should not rely solely on equipment and should physically check the patient at frequent intervals to confirm that the readings are accurate.

Timely detection is crucial in the detection of hemodynamic compromise in the critically ill patient. It is important that the technician understands the principles, practices, and limitations of the more commonly used modalities for monitoring the critically ill.

Blood Pressure

ABP is defined as the product of cardiac output (CO) and total peripheral resistance (Flaherty and Musk 2005).

Arterial pressure is often monitored in the critical patient to provide information on CO. CO is a major determinant of tissue perfusion. ABP is also used to evaluate vital signs and volume status of the patient.

Hypotension is defined as <80 mmHg systolic or <60 mmHg mean arterial pressure (MAP). Blood pressure below these levels should be investigated and treatment instigated. Prolonged hypotension may lead to decreased tissue perfusion and oxygen delivery leading to cellular death. A young, healthy patient may be able to tolerate low blood pressure for a short period of time, but an older, more compromised animal may not have the reserve to recover from a prolonged hypotensive episode.

There are two techniques available for the measurement of blood pressure:

■   Direct
■   Indirect

Direct ABP will give real-time information. Indirect techniques are useful for following trends rather than providing absolute values.

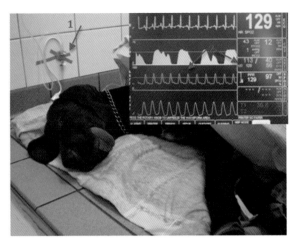

Figure 4.5 Arterial blood pressure (ABP) monitoring is common place in the ICU. Here, a catheter is placed in the dorsal pedal artery and attached to a pressure transducer (1) and multiparameter monitor displaying pulse waveform and ABP (2).

Direct monitoring

Direct blood pressure monitoring is considered the "gold standard," and involves the placement of a catheter in a peripheral artery that is connected to a transducer and monitor. The most frequently used site for arterial catheterization is the dorsal pedal artery. This vessel is usually easily palpable and superficial to the skin's surface. Other commonly used vessels are the coccygeal and carpal arteries. The placement of arterial catheters can be technically challenging, particularly in the emergent patient where peripheral circulation may be compromised (Fig. 4.5).

Indirect monitoring

The two common methods for indirect ABP monitoring are:

- Oscillometry
- Doppler

Oscillometry. In the past, oscillometric blood pressure monitoring in small animal patients has been documented as unreliable. Newer technology and machines have, to some extent, proven to be more reliable in the assessment of blood pressure in small animals.

The oscillometric method involves placing an occlusion cuff over a peripheral artery and attaching the cuff to an electronic monitor. The monitor automatically inflates the cuff to a predetermined pressure before slowly releasing the pressure. As the cuff is deflating, the machine detects oscillations in the artery as pulsatile flow returns. The changes in cuff pressure as the pulsatile flow returns are used to determine systolic (where the oscillations begin), mean (the point of maximum oscillations), and diastolic pressure (where oscillations disappear). The mean pressure is the most accurate of the three values, followed by the systolic measurement, and then diastolic pressure. The advantages of

CHAPTER 4

using oscillometric monitoring are that it is noninvasive, easy to use, and usually the machines can be programmed to take readings at regular intervals. It is important to remember that oscillometry may not be accurate in the presence of arrhythmias, slow pulse rates, or low blood pressure.

Doppler. The Doppler ultrasonic flow monitor method of blood pressure measurement involves placing a piezoelectric probe over a peripheral artery. The probe is attached to a monitor and emits an ultrasonic beam. The monitor amplifies the sound of the blood flow in the vessel under the probe. An occlusion cuff is placed proximally to the probe attached to a sphygmomanometer and inflated until no sound is audible. The reentry of blood into the artery as the cuff is deflated causes a frequency change in sound waves that is known as the Doppler shift. The first audible sound heard as the cuff is being deflated represents systolic pressure. In the canine patient, good correlation has been recorded between Doppler systolic pressure and direct arterial pressure (Weiser 1977). The Doppler has been observed to underestimate systolic pressure in the cat, and a correction factor of 14 mmHg can be added to the recorded reading (Grandy et al. 1992). In cats, the Doppler measurement has been shown to be more closely related to the mean blood pressure (Chaulkett et al. 1998). The advantages of using Doppler are ease of use and affordability. The Doppler is also more reliable than oscillometric monitoring if low pressures and cardiac arrhythmias are present. A disadvantage of the Doppler is that its use is labor-intensive, and it will also only provide information on systolic pressure.

It is important that the occlusion cuff be appropriately sized for each patient. The width of the cuff should be 40% of the circumference of the site where the cuff is placed. An incorrect size cuff will impact greatly on the readings obtained.

Central Venous Pressure (CVP) Monitoring

CVP is the measurement of the hydrostatic pressure in the intrathoracic vena cava. This measurement provides an estimation of blood pressure within the right atrium, which is a reasonable indicator of vascular volume (deSilva 2007). CVP monitoring requires the placement of a central venous catheter, usually via the jugular vein. Catheters placed in the femoral vein in cats and small dogs extending into the abdominal vena cava have been shown to provide fairly accurate measurement of CVP (Berg et al. 1992). In a clinical setting, CVP is utilized to provide information about intravascular blood volume and cardiac function. It is most routinely used as a monitoring tool for the efficacy of fluid

---

Box 4.3   Rules for Cuff Selection for Indirect Blood Pressure Monitoring

- Occlusion cuff should be ~40% of the circumference of the appendage
  - Too large cuff = false low readings
  - Too small cuff = false high readings
  - Too tight cuff = false low readings
  - Too loose cuff = false high readings

therapy, and as indicator for patients at risk from volume overload. As with many modalities of monitoring in the critical patient, isolated CVP readings are of limited value. A trend in readings is much more significant and should be viewed in conjunction with other parameters (blood pressure and urine output.) By monitoring trends in CVP, early detection of intravascular volume abnormalities will aid in effective, timely management and treatment.

Limitations

CVP measures the pressure in the right side of the heart. Measurement of the left side will provide more accurate pressures, as the left side supplies systemic circulation. This measurement, pulmonary arterial pressure (PAP) is achieved by placing a pulmonary artery catheter. This can be technically challenging, time consuming, and costly, thus making CVP is an acceptable alternative.

Patients with head trauma, intracranial disease, coagulopathies, or are at a high risk of thromboembolic disease (e.g., immune-mediated hemolytic anemia [IMHA]) are contraindicated for the placement of a central venous catheter (Waddell and Brown 2009).

Normal ranges for CVP are:

- Low < 0 cm H_2O
- Normal 0–10 cm H_2O
- High > 10 cm H_2O

Indications for CVP monitoring

CVP monitoring is beneficial in any patient that presents with hypovolemia or is at risk from volume overload. Trauma, shock, hemoabdomen, gastric dilation, and volvulus are common presenting causes of hypovolemia. Patients that are at risk of volume overload may include those who require high volume diuresis, patients with preexisting cardiac disease requiring intravenous fluid therapy, or those with right ventricular congestive heart failure.

There are two methods of CVP monitoring, the water manometer and the electronic transducer system. A water manometer can be used to provide intermittent readings and can be constructed by using lengths of sterile drip tubing, a ruler, bag of intravenous fluids, and a three-way tap. The transducer system requires specialized equipment and displays continuous readings on a monitor.

A low CVP (less than 0 cm H_2O) may indicate inadequate intravascular filling, which may be due to fluid loss or vasodilation.

A high CVP (greater than 10 cm H_2O) may be indicative of intravascular volume overload, right-sided cardiac dysfunction, or increases in intrathoracic pressure, which may be resultant from pleural effusions, pneumothorax, or positive pressure ventilation (Hansen 2000).

Pulse Oximetry

Pulse oximeters are one of the most frequently utilized monitors in the critical and emergent patient. Pulse oximetry provides a noninvasive means of measuring oxygenation. These bedside monitors are easy to use, require minimal training, and work well in most species of veterinary patients. The pulse oximeter probe is usually well tolerated by the patient and is most commonly attached to a nonpigmented area, such as the tongue, lip, vulva, prepuce, axilla, inguinal area, pinna, or between the digits. The pulse oximeter provides clinically useful measurements of hemoglobin saturation. The oximeter can also provide continuous monitoring for the hypoxemic patient. Pulse oximetry has a definite place within practice when the "gold standard" of arterial blood gas analysis is not indicated or available. This piece of equipment will provide a useful indication of arterial oxygen saturation, particularly through serial measurements.

The Beers–Lambert law, which associates the concentration of a solution to the intensity of light transmitted through the solution, forms the foundations of pulse oximetry (Severinghaus and Kehheher 1992).

The pulse oximeter probe emits red (940-nm) and infrared (660-nm) light several hundred times per second by two light emitting diodes. Oxyhemoglobin (hemoglobin bound to oxygen) and deoxyhemoglobin (hemoglobin not bound to oxygen) absorb red and infrared light at different wavelengths. The amount of light absorbed at each wavelength is measured, and the absorbance is expressed as a percentage of oxygenated to total hemoglobin. The saturation value obtained is abbreviated to SpO_2. Most pulse oximeters will display heart rate as well as information about the strength of the signal that the oximeter is receiving. This may be shown as a display of bars, rising and falling, or though pulse waveforms.

SpO_2 measurements give an indication of the adequacy of ventilation and circulation. Circulation must be adequate to perfuse the lungs so that hemoglobin can be exposed to oxygen, and circulation to peripheral tissues must be adequate for the pulse oximeter sensor to detect a pulsatile blood flow. Ventilation must also be adequate to provide oxygen exchange.

Normal oxygen saturation should be above 95%. Less than 90% may equate with a large decrease in partial pressure of oxygen in arterial blood (PaO_2). This is displayed by the oxygenation–hemoglobin dissociation curve. The graph illustrates the nonlinear relationship between SpO_2 and PaO_2. The flat, upper part of the curve (PaO_2 between 60–100) demonstrates that large changes in PaO_2 result in minimal changes of SpO_2. When SpO_2 levels drop below 90%, the curve rapidly becomes steep. This demonstrates that below 90% small decreases in SpO_2 are equivalent to large drops in PaO_2. It is also important to realize that the pulse oximeter is therefore a late indicator of hypoxemia. This is especially evident with patients on oxygen supplementation (Fig. 4.6).

A decrease in oxygen saturation requires immediate response. Ventilation should be assessed by evaluating patency of airway, presence of adequate respiration, respiratory rate, and tidal volume.

For pulse oximeters to provide useful information, patients must have reasonable cardiovascular function and hemoglobin concentrations. The information from a pulse oximeter should be interpreted in conjunction with other information that may be relevant. A major limiting factor for the use of pulse oximetry is adequate tissue perfusion. Patients with poor perfusion due to shock, hypotension, or the administration of drugs that affect peripheral circulation (e.g., alpha-2 agonists) may display a falsely low SpO_2. An anemic patient may also display a low SpO_2 reading, but have a normal PaO_2. Likewise, an anemic patient may have significantly decreased ability of the blood to carry oxygen (CaO_2) and therefore a decreased delivery of oxygen to tissue (DO_2) but a normal SpO_2.

Measurement errors may occur from any other substance that also absorbs light at these wavelengths. These include intrinsic substances such as methemoglobin,

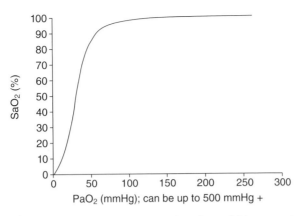

Figure 4.6 The oxyhemoglobin dissociation curve displays hemoglobin saturation at varying oxygen tensions.

carboxyhemoglobin, and some intravascular dyes. Some more common extrinsic factors that may affect pulse oximetry accuracy are patient movement, presence of ambient light, use of heat lamps, and electrocautery.

Capnography

Obtaining an arterial blood sample and performing blood gas analysis most accurately assesses the adequacy of patient ventilation. The limitations of this technique are that it can be technically challenging, it is invasive, and requires expensive equipment for analysis. While it is considered the gold standard method and has a definite place in veterinary practice, capnography provides a noninvasive, and technically less challenging method of obtaining valuable information on the ventilatory status of a critical patient. Capnography will provide a graphic display of carbon dioxide concentration versus time or expired volume during a respiratory cycle (Pypendop 2009). Alveolar gas equilibrates with arterial blood, and thus, end tidal carbon dioxide ($EtCO_2$) measurements are a relatively accurate reflection of $PaCO_2$, under most circumstances. $EtCO_2$ measurements usually reflect a difference of ~5 mmHg less than $PaCO_2$. It is useful to utilize arterial blood gas analysis intermittently to determine the accuracy of the $EtCO_2$ value.

The use of capnography in the critical patient is most frequently used in intubated and ventilated patients. Samples of gas are obtained from removing a sample from the circuit (sidestream sampling) or by passing the total volume of gas through a sensor (direct sampling). The most commonly used monitors utilize sidestream sampling. An adapter is usually placed between the endotracheal tube and breathing circuit and gases are sampled from the circuit. The sample gas is analyzed by one of three methods: infrared absorption, mass spectrometry, or colometric detection. Infrared absorption is the most common method of respiratory CO_2 analysis in veterinary practice. This technology is based on the principle that gases that have two or more dissimilar atoms in the molecule have unique and specific absorption of infrared light (Pypendop 2009). Normal $EtCO_2$ values are 35–45 mmHg.

Hyperventilation is the most common cause of low $EtCO_2$. A low $EtCO_2$ value (<20 mmHg) is called *hypocapnia*. A sudden decrease in $EtCO_2$ may indicate a change in lung perfusion, and may be due to a pulmonary embolism or an impending cardiac arrest as cellular metabolism may be compromised. The delivery of CO_2 to the lungs requires blood flow, thus one of the earliest signs of cardiovascular collapse is an abrupt decrease in $EtCO_2$. Hyperventilation will also result in vasoconstriction of cerebral blood vessels resulting in decreasing intracranial pressure, but may also compromise cerebral oxygen delivery.

A high $EtCO_2 > 60\,mmHg$ (*hypercapnia*), resulting in respiratory acidosis, may be indicating hypoventilation, increased metabolism, or a physical or functional airway obstruction.

Serious organ dysfunction can result from extended periods of hypercapnia. As CO_2 is a potent cerebral vasodilator, prolonged high CO_2 values may result in increased intracranial pressure (ICP) and may result in brain damage (Levine et al. 1997).

Most current monitors display a waveform (capnogram) that will give valuable information and aids in the detection of various abnormalities related to the patient or equipment.

To identify abnormalities, the technician must first be able to identify the components of a normal waveform (Fig. 4.7).

As previously mentioned, $EtCO_2$ measurements are most usually closely correlated with PCO_2 values. Increased dead space ventilation may increase the gradient between $EtCO_2$ and PCO_2.

Box 4.4   Increased CO_2: Possible Causes

- Hypoventilation
- Rebreathing
- Increased CO
- Increased CO_2 production, increased metabolism
  - Shivering, hyperthermia, seizuring, pheochromocytoma
- Endobronchial intubation
- Malignant hyperthermia

Box 4.5   Decreased CO_2: Possible Causes

- Hyperventilation
- Decreased metabolism
  - Hypothermia, hypothyroidism
- Decreased CO
  - Sequelae to cardiac arrest
  - Pulmonary embolism
- Disconnection of breathing circuit, sampling line
- Esophageal intubation

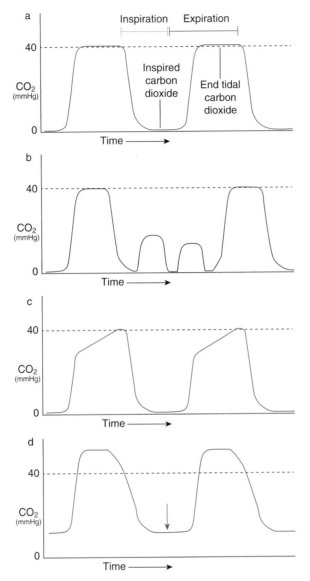

Figure 4.7   Commonly encountered capnograms. (a) Normal capnogram. (b) Capnogram displaying spontaneous breaths during mechanical ventilation. (c) Capnogram displaying airway obstruction (bronchospasm or obstructive pulmonary disease. (d) Capnogram displaying rebreathing with elevated baseline. Reprinted with permission of John Wiley & Sons, Inc. From *Anesthesia for Veterinary* Technicians, edited by S. Bryant, 2010. Images by Mele Tong, CVT, VTS (Anesthesia).

Electrocardiogram (ECG) Monitoring

ECG monitoring is used to assess cardiac rhythm and detect conduction disorders in the veterinary patient.

The heart generates an electrical field during depolarization and repolarization of the myocardium. These electrical signals can be detected on the surface of the body. The signal can be amplified and displayed on a screen with the use of leads and electrodes.

The ECG only monitors the electrical activity of the heart. It does not provide any information on the mechanical function of the heart (i.e., contractility) or the state of circulation (Macintire et al. 2005a,b).

Three bipolar leads (I, II, and III) and the augmented leads (aVR, aVL, and aVF) are the standard leads utilized in the critical patient. Each lead will produce a record of the electrical activity of the heart from a different angle. By using a combination of leads, the information gained can assist in the diagnosis of conduction and rhythm disturbances.

When attaching the ECG leads, good contact is required between the leads and the patient. The leads can be attached directly to the skin of the patient, or alternatively, commercially made self-adhesive electrodes are available. If the leads are attached directly to the patient, some type of gel or alcohol must be used to aid in conduction. For long-term ECG monitoring, it is beneficial to use self-adhesive electrodes, as these cause less discomfort to the patient. To ensure good contact, hair should be clipped before placing the electrodes or they can be applied directly to the pads on the distal limbs. Generally, the leads are placed on the right and left forelegs and the left hindleg.

Lead II is most frequently used in rhythm evaluation in veterinary patients. In the critical patient, it may be necessary to evaluate several leads as the signal strength may vary greatly between leads. Extension discussion on arrhythmias and ECG interpretation is found in Chapter 6, "Cardiovascular Emergencies."

Conclusion

Monitoring devices *can never* and *should never* replace a well-trained, intuitive technician. The most important monitoring technique is clinical assessment by the technician's own senses. All too often, mistakes are made with catastrophic consequences when too much emphasis is placed on information provided from monitoring equipment and not enough attention is focused on patient physical examination. Monitors are only as good as the people using and interpreting the information from them. The technician will need to be familiar with equipment and have some expertise in the recognition of abnormalities that require urgent attention. A proficient technician will have the intuition and ability to detect subtle changes in a patient's clinical condition. Using both the information gathered from physical examination and monitoring devices will enable the technician and veterinarian to analyze a situation and intervene if necessary.

References

Berg, RA, Lloud, TR, Donnerstein, RL. 1992. Accuracy of central venous pressure monitoring in the intraabdominal vena cava: a canine study. *J Pediatr* 120:67.

Chaulkett, NA, Cantwell, SL, Houston, DM. 1998. A comparison of indirect blood pressure monitoring techniques in the anaesthetized cat. *Vet Surg* 27:370–377.

deSilva, A. 2007. Anesthetic monitoring. In *Basics of Anesthesia*, 5th ed., edited by Stoelting, R, Miller, R. Philadelphia: Churchill Livingstone Elsevier, pp. 309–310.

Flaherty, D, Musk, G. 2005. Anaesthetic monitoring equipment for small animals. *In Prac*, 27(10):512–521.

Glass, EN, Kent, M. 2007. Neurologic System Emergencies. In *Small Animal Emergency and Critical Care for Veterinary Technicians*, edited by Battaglia, AM. St. Louis, MO: Saunders Elsevier, pp. 339–355.

Grandy, JL, Dunlop, CI, Hodgson, DS, Curtis, CR, Chapman, PL. 1992. Evaluation of the Doppler ultrasonic method of measuring systolic arterial blood pressure in cats. *Am J Vet Res* 53:1166–1169.

Hansen, B. 2000. Technical aspects of fluid therapy. In *Fluid Therapy in Small Animal Practice*, 2nd ed., edited by DiBartola, SP. Philadelphia: WB Saunders, pp. 281–306.

Keates, HL. 2005. *Anaesthesia teaching notes provided for undergraduate veterinary students*. The University of Queensland.

Levine, RL, Wayne, MA, Miller, CC. 1997. End-tidal carbon dioxide and outcome of out-of-hospital arrest. *N Engl J Med* 337:301–306.

Macintire, DK, Drobatz, KJ, Haskins, SC, Saxon, WD. 2005a. Monitoring critical patients. In *Manual of Small Animal Emergency and Critical Care Medicine*. Philadelphia: Lippincott Williams and Wilkins, pp. 72–73.

Macintire, DK, Drobatz, KJ, Haskins, SC, Saxon, WD. 2005b. Cardiac emergencies. In *Manual of Small Animal Emergency and Critical Care Medicine*. Philadelphia: Lippincott Williams and Wilkins, pp. 160–188.

Pypendop, BH. 2009. Capnography. In *Small Animal Critical Care Medicine*, edited by Silverstein, DC, Hopper, K. St. Louis, MO: Saunders Elsevier, pp. 875–877.

Severinghaus, JW, Kehheher, JF. 1992. Recent developments in pulse oximetry. *Anesthesiology* 76:1018–1038.

Waddell, LS, Brown, AJ. 2009. Hemodynamic monitoring. In *Small Animal Critical Care Medicine*, edited by Silverstein, DC, Hopper, K. St. Louis, MO: Saunders Elsevier, pp. 861–863.

Cardiopulmonary Cerebral Resuscitation

5

Christopher L. Norkus

Introduction

Cardiopulmonary arrest (CPA) is an abrupt complete failure of both the respiratory and circulatory systems. The lack of successful cardiac output and delivery of oxygen to tissue (DO_2) can quickly produce unconsciousness and systemic cellular death from anoxia. If left untreated, cerebral hypoxia results in complete biological brain death within 4–6 minutes of CPA (Safar 1986, 1988). Therefore, prompt cardiopulmonary cerebral resuscitation (CPCR) and advanced cardiac life support (ACLS) interventions are imperative. Veterinary technicians play a key role in ensuring that patients receive this treatment within that period.

Etiology and Recognition

In dogs and cats, common causes of CPA include anesthetic overdose, vagal stimulation, severe trauma (e.g., hypovolemia, pneumothorax), unstable cardiac arrhythmias (e.g., unstable ventricular tachycardia), severe electrolyte disturbances (e.g., hyperkalemia), cardiorespiratory disorders (e.g., congestive heart failure, hypoxemia, pericardial tamponade), and debilitating or end-stage diseases (e.g., sepsis, cancer, etc). Rapid pursuit and treatment of the underlining CPA cause, if possible, is paramount to long-term survival.

Potential signs of impending CPA include dramatic changes in the effort, rate, or rhythm of breathing (e.g., agonal breathing, decreased rate, and sudden increased rate), absence of pulse, significant hypotension with a systolic blood pressure < 50 mmHG, irregular to inaudible heart sounds, dramatic changes in heart rate or rhythm, absence of surgical bleeding, changes in mucous membrane color (e.g., white or cyanotic), fixed and dilated pupils, distressed vocalizations, and patient collapse.

All animals admitted to the hospital should have a designated resuscitation code assigned. Such a resuscitation code is assigned to a patient only after practical discussion with a pet's owners explaining prognosis, cost, and ethical considerations of performing CPCR. Often "do not resuscitate" (DNR) is assigned the color code of *red*, full resuscitation efforts, including open chest efforts, the color code of *green*, and limited resuscitation efforts excluding open chest efforts the color *yellow*. If ever a patient has not been assigned a resuscitation code and experiences a CPA while in hospital, the patient is treated with full resuscitation efforts until directed otherwise.

Initial Interventions

Rapid assessment of the patient is crucial if CPA is suspected. Initially, the rescuer should page for help and quickly note the time. The response by all of the veterinary team to a potential arrest must be immediate. Before CPCR is initiated, it is essential to quickly evaluate the patient's responsiveness, breathing, and pulse. Those patients in CPA will be nonresponsive and apneic, with nondetectable pulses. Taken from human emergency medicine, veterinary CPCR is initiated in three tiers: basic life support (BLS), advanced life support (ALS), and ongoing postresuscitative care (Pablo 2003). The BLS phase involves establishing an open and clear airway, providing assisted ventilation, and performing effective chest compressions. These steps are often called the ABCs—airway, breathing, and circulation. The ALS stage includes such advanced care as endotracheal intubation, venous access, interpretation of an electrocardiogram (ECG), drug administration, and defibrillation. Postresuscitative care includes ongoing intensive monitoring as well as cardiovascular and ventilatory support.

Patients experiencing CPA will need to be placed in an accessible location that is adjacent to an oxygen source. In some instances this may require moving a patient to a central hospital location or treatment room. A designated resuscitation area, or "crash cart" (Table 5.1) should have treatment and diagnostic supplies at the ready. Typically patients are placed in right lateral recumbancy, but some research has suggested dorsal recumbancy is better for larger patients. While this positioning may be more effective, practically, it can be very difficult positioning to maintain in a large dog and is therefore not often used (see Figs. 5.1–5.3).

Table 5.1 Author's recommended contents for crash carts

General	ECG or Multiparameter Monitor
	Defibrillator
	Suction unit
	ECG or ultrasound jelly
	Stethoscope
	Timer

Airway and breathing	Laryngoscope and blades
	Clear endotracheal tubes (various sizes)
	Endotracheal tube ties (e.g., Cut IV line)
	A tool for grasping objects obstructing the airway (e.g., doyen intestinal clamp)
	Tracheostomy tubes
	Thoracocenties setup (60 cc syringe, butterfly catheters, extension sets, 3-way stop cock)
	Ambu bags

Circulation	3 or 5 French red rubber feeding tube for IT drug administration
	IV catheters of various sizes (including central venous catheters)
	Tape
	IV catheter caps
	Crystalloid fluid bag(s) with IV line attached
	Colloid fluid bag(s)
	7% Hypertonic saline
	Slam bags

Drugs	Syringe (variety of sizes) with large bore hypodermic needs attached (e.g., 20 g)
	Atropine
	Epinephrine 1:1000 (depending on manufacture, may need to be refrigerated)
	Vasopressin
	Lidocaine (without epinephrine!)
	Propofol
	Calcium gluconate
	Sodium bicarbonate
	Magnesium chloride
	50% Dextrose
	Naloxone
	Non-heparinized flushes (so can be used to flush drugs IT)

Miscellaneous	Gauze
	Surgical gloves
	Scalpel blades
	Minor surgical pack

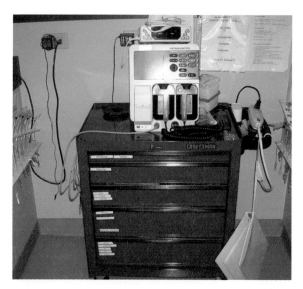

Figure 5.1 A well-stocked crash cart should be located in a central area of the hospital with access to an oxygen source. (Courtesy of Thomas Walker, DVM, DACVECC.)

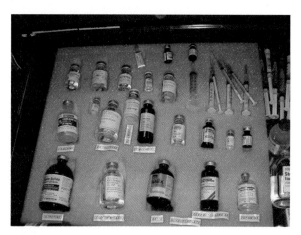

Figure 5.2 Injectable drugs stored in the crash cart should be kept to an absolute minimum to avoid confusion at times of crisis. (Courtesy of Thomas Walker, DVM, DACVECC.)

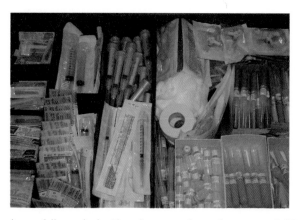

Figure 5.3 Crash cart drawer fully stocked with catheter supplies make everyone's life easier when seconds count. (Courtesy of Thomas Walker, DVM, DACVECC.)

Basic Life Support (BLS)

Airway Management

Initial airway management involves extending the patient's neck to straighten the airway and pulling the patient's tongue forward. The veterinary staff quickly examines the upper airway and initiates suctioning, if necessary. All foreign material or vomit observed in the patient's oropharynx should be cleared immediately.

If the patient's airway is fully obstructed, sharp abdominal thrusts and digital finger sweeps of the pharynx can help dislodge the obstruction. An emergency tracheotomy may be necessary if the airway obstruction is not promptly resolved. Percutaneous insertion of a needle or intravenous (IV) catheter directly into the trachea distal to the obstruction, along with oxygen administration, can be lifesaving while a tracheotomy is being performed. In some cases, material fully obstructing the airway (such as a tennis ball) can be successfully manually removed with long hemostats or Doyen intestinal clamps.

Breathing

After the patient's airway has been cleared, an endotracheal tube should be placed. Tube placement must be confirmed and the tube secured and cuffed. The patient is then ventilated with 100% oxygen. Proper ventilation is a critical component of BLS. Published recommendations for veterinary patients have cited patients receive 100% oxygen at a rate of 10–24 breaths/min (Henik 1992; Kruse-Elliott 2001). Hyperventilation has been shown to be significantly detrimental in humans because it can result in decreased myocardial and cerebral perfusion (Aufderheide et al. 2004; Plunkett and McMichael 2008). Therefore, choosing a rate on the lower end of the 10–24 breaths/min scale or slightly below are likely advised. In humans, the most current recommendations (American Heart Association 2010 CPCR Guidelines) recommend a ventilation rate of 1 breath per every 6–8 seconds or 8–10 breaths per minute.

Veterinary patients can be easily and safely ventilated with a bag-valve mask (AMBU bag). Using an anesthesia machine can be slow and ineffective because the pop-off valve must be opened and closed repeatedly. Peak airway pressure should be less than $20\,cmH_2O$ (Kruse-Elliott 2001). Lack of chest wall motion, poor ventilation, or absence of lung sounds should prompt an immediate search for a poorly positioned tube or a severe pleural space disorder (e.g., pneumothorax, hemothroax). In these cases, immediate thoracotomy is typically necessary.

Acupuncture also has been used to treat CPA (Schoen 2003). Needling the acupuncture point Governing Vessel 26 (GV26) can help stimulate respiration and increase cerebral oxygen (Janssens et al. 1979; Looney 2001). This point can be stimulated by inserting a regular 25-gauge needle or acupuncture needle into the nasal philtrum to a depth of about 10–20 mm and performing jabs in a henpecking motion while monitoring for improvement in respiration (Looney 2001) (Fig. 5.4).

The usage of impedance threshold devices (ITDs) also has shown promise in both humans and animal models (Yannopoulos and Aufderheide 2007). The ITD is a small, inexpensive device that is placed on the proximal end of an endotracheal tube during resuscitation to create an increase in negative pressure during the chest-recoil phase of chest compression. This increase in negative pressure creates a vacuum that results in more blood being pulled into the heart and, therefore, more blood output during the next

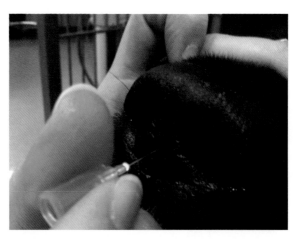

Figure 5.4   A needle is used to show the correct location (nasal philtrum) to perform GV26. (Courtesy of David Liss, RVT, VTS [Emergency & Critical Care].)

compression. ITDs include a timing light that helps the rescuer ventilate the patient at the proper rate to avoid hyperventilation.

Circulation

The goal of circulatory support during CPCR is to maximize myocardial and cerebral perfusion. Chest compressions should be performed immediately in patients without a pulse. External cardiac massage (ECM) at a rate of 80–120 compressions/min is recommended (Plunkett and McMichael 2008), but higher rates within that range seem to work better (Kern et al. 1987). Based on the American Heart Association's 2010 guidelines for CPCR, the rescuer performing chest compressions should push hard, push fast (a minimum of 100 compressions/minute), allow full chest recoil after each compression, and minimize interruptions in chest compressions. It is also critical that chest compressions be continuous and not stopped once they are started (Fig. 5.5).

Small patients weighing less than 15 lb (7 kg) should receive compressions directly over the heart (*cardiac pump theory*), whereas larger patients should receive more caudal compressions that are directed over the widest part of the chest (*thoracic pump theory*). The cardiac pump theory asserts that arterial blood flow is a result of direct compression of the ventricles and, therefore, makes sense in small patients with thin compliable chest walls. Closed-chest compressions in large patients, however, generally are inadequate in actually compressing the ventricles. Therefore, the thoracic pump theory is used and theorizes that forward blood flow in larger patients is actually the result of a generalized increase in intrathoracic pressure.

Interposed abdominal compressions, or abdominal compressions over the cranial abdomen, at a rate of 70–90 compressions/min can be alternated with chest compressions and have been shown to increase cardiac output (Ralston et al. 1982; Voorhees et al. 1984). Guidelines for open-chest internal cardiac massage (ICM) typically recommend its immediate use in all patients weighing more than 40 lb (18 kg), in other patients after 10 minutes of CPCR regardless of their size, and in all cases of trauma and/or hemorrhage, such as patients with pneumothorax, hemothorax, or cardiac tamponade (Henik 1992; Barton and Crowe 2000). ICM allows direct visualization of the heart, aortic compression

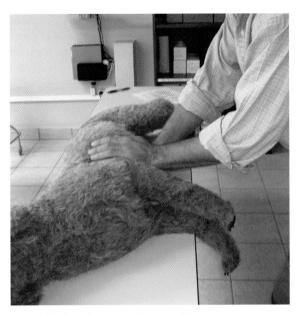

Figure 5.5 Remember to "push hard, push fast, and don't stop" for chest compressions to be effective. (Courtesy of Thomas Walker, DVM, DACVECC.)

or cross-clamping, and internal defibrillation. ICM also can increase cardiac output, blood pressure, coronary perfusion pressure, and cerebral perfusion pressure compared with closed-chest CPCR and has been associated with the increased return of spontaneous circulation (ROSC) and improved neurologic outcomes in animal models (Kern et al. 1987; Feneley et al. 1988).

The veterinary staff should regularly assess the effectiveness of CPCR by palpating for the presence of pulses during compressions and by using a Doppler ultrasound transducer. However, if this comes at the expense of stopping chest compressions then this step should be avoided. With sufficient water-based lubricant, a Doppler transducer can be placed directly over one of the patient's open eyeballs. The presence of a "swooshing" wave sound from the Doppler unit during concurrent chest compressions can provide a crude estimate of whether forward blood flow is reaching the brain. If chest compressions are not generating adequate forward blood flow, the patient should be repositioned or the resuscitation technique changed to increase intrathoracic pressure, or ICM should be considered.

Advanced Life Support

Establishing venous access is important, but it should never interfere with chest compressions or the delivery of defibrillation. Venous access can be established by using such methods as intraosseus catheter placement and venous cutdown. The jugular vein typically yields well to catheterization during CPA and provides the shortest transit time for drugs to reach the heart (Emmerman et al. 1988). If a resuscitation drug is administered by a peripheral venous route, administer the drug by bolus injection and follow it with a 20-mL bolus of IV fluid. Then, elevate the extremity for 10–20 seconds to facilitate drug delivery to the central circulation (Emmerman et al. 1988).

After venous access has been established, aggressive fluid administration should be considered if hypovolemia existed before the CPA event or if the patient is experiencing blood loss. The can quickly be evaluated by ultrasound examination of the heart. However, overzealous fluid administration in patients with normal body fluid volume may be detrimental (Ditchey and Lindenfeld 1984). Fluid resuscitation can include hypertonic saline, crystalloids, colloids, blood products, and hemoglobin-based oxygen-carrying solutions (Emmerman et al. 1988).

If an IV catheter cannot be placed initially, emergency drugs, such as lidocaine, epinephrine, atropine, naloxone, and vasopressin can be administered through the endotracheal tube (Emmerman et al. 1988; Wenzel et al. 1997). Typically, a long red rubber catheter is inserted down the endotracheal tube, and drugs are administered through the catheter. Drug doses are typically increased two- to threefold and are followed by a small saline chaser to ensure successful drug passage into the lungs (Cole et al. 2003). Intracardiac injection of medication is contraindicated, especially during closed-chest CPCR. Inaccurate injection and complications, such as vessel or cardiac laceration and hemorrhage, are common (Sabin et al. 1983; Jespersen et al. 1990).

Drugs and Defibrillation

Specific treatment of cardiopulmonary arrest (CPA) depends on the type of arrhythmia, which can be effectively differentiated on an ECG only. The two most common arrhythmias in veterinary patients appear to be ventricular asystole and pulseless electrical activity (PEA), also known as electromechanical dissociation. Ventricular fibrillation (VF), the most common arrhythmia in humans, appears to not be as commonly observed in cats and dogs (Rush and Wingfield 1992). This may in part be due to the fact that humans commonly experience cardiac arrest for different reasons (i.e., myocardial infractions) than veterinary patients.

CPA Rhythms

Ventricular Asystole

Asystole, also known as "flatline," is a result of the complete absence of electrical or mechanical activity from the ventricles. A rare P wave may be observed, reflecting atrial activity, but no QRS complexes are seen (Fig. 5.6).

Transcutaneous electrical pacing is immediately initiated in human medicine, although it has not gained widespread use in veterinary patients. Routine veterinary treatment

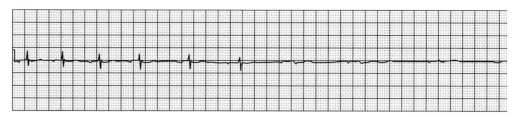

Figure 5.6   An EKG tracing showing a patient deteriorating to ventricular asystole. CPCR must be started immediately. (Courtesy of Diane Hudson, RVT, VTS [Anesthesia].)

includes IV epinephrine administered at 0.01–0.02 mg/kg every 3–5 minutes and IV atropine administered at 0.02–0.05 mg/kg every 3–5 minutes (Cole et al. 2003). A single dose of IV vasopressin at 0.2–0.8 U/kg should also be considered (Schmittinger et al. 2005; (Scroggin and Quandt 2009). Atropine is not routinely administered in the rabbit because this species uniquely produce atropine esterase which limits the drug's clinical effectiveness. Glycopyrrolate is preferred in the rabbit and works quickly. Of additional interest, atropine has been removed from the 2010 AHA CPCR recommendations for the treatment of asystole stating that is not believed to be of therapeutic benefit.

Pulseless Electrical Activity (PEA)/Electromechanical Dissociation

The ECG of patients with PEA is relatively normal, reflecting the presence of electrical activity in the heart. Consequently, P waves, QRS complexes, and T waves may be observed. However, lack of mechanical activity in the heart prevents effective cardiac output and forward perfusion to the body (Fig. 5.7).

Routine veterinary treatment includes administration of IV epinephrine at 0.01–0.02 mg/kg every 3–5 minutes and IV atropine at 0.04–0.05 mg/kg every 3–5 minutes (Cole et al. 2003). A single dose of IV vasopressin at 0.2–0.8 U/kg should also be considered (Schmittinger et al. 2005; (Scroggin and Quandt 2009). Interestingly, atropine has been removed from the 2010 AHA CPCR guidelines for PEA treatment because it is not believed to offer additional benefit. The use of different therapies, such as naloxone, dexamethasone, and calcium, to aid in PEA treatment has been advocated. However, little published information supports regular use of these agents. The key to treatment of PEA is rapid identification and correction of the underlining offending problem.

Ventricular Fibrillation (VF)

In patients with VF, the ECG waveform is erratic and chaotic. No clear P waves, QRS complexes, or T waves are observed (Fig. 5.8).

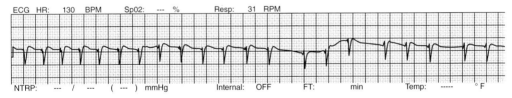

Figure 5.7 An EKG tracing showing an example of pulseless electrical activity (PEA). This rhythm sometimes (and with fatal consequences) is mistaken for a normal sinus rhythm. (Courtesy of Diane Hudson, RVT, VTS [Anesthesia].)

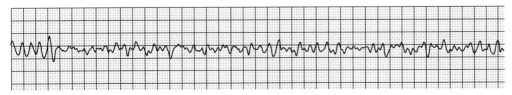

Figure 5.8 An example of ventricular fibrillation. Immediate electrical defibrillation is required. (Courtesy of Diane Hudson, RVT, VTS [Anesthesia].)

Treatment of VF involves immediate electrical defibrillation. An initial shock of 3–5 J/kg is recommended. Human 2010 CPCR guidelines from the American Heart Association (AHA) recommend that CPCR should then be continued for 2 minutes following initial defibrillation before a second defibrillation attempt or drug therapy. This allows some oxygen delivery to the myocardium and promotes more effective defibrillation. These recommendations are based upon the understanding that biphasic defibrillators are readily used in human medicine. As biphasic defibrillators are not yet frequently utilized in veterinary medicine, literature based on older AHA guidelines may be more appropriate. Older guidelines would recommend that an initial shock should be repeated in immediate succession at a 50% higher setting two additional times if the heart rhythm does not respond. Then, following the three progressively higher-voltage shocks and unsuccessful conversion to a stable rhythm, chest compressions and ventilation are continued for 1–2 minutes (Cole et al. 2003). Biphasic defibrillation has been documented in the small animal patient and will likely become the preferred method of small animal defibrillation in the future (Bright and Wright 2009). Which initial defibrillation strategy to currently employ in our veterinary patients is up for debate.

Following unsuccessful defibrillation low-dose epinephrine at 0.01 mg/kg and vasopressin at 0.8 U/kg then can be administered. Such drugs may make successful defibrillation more likely. Defibrillation may then be resumed at 5–10 J/kg, followed by administration of an additional drug, such as amiodarone, magnesium chloride, or lidocaine. After each new drug has been administered, defibrillation is again attempted at the 5- to 10-J/kg setting to restore a normal perfusing rhythm (Cole et al. 2003).

It is difficult to successfully treat VF without a defibrillator. A sharp precordial thump administered to the chest wall may convert VF to a sinus rhythm in small patients but is unlikely to be effective in larger patients. In the author's hands, this technique has proved lifesaving in the cat. Although pharmacologic defibrillation using such agents as potassium chloride, insulin/dextrose, and acetylcholine has been suggested in other texts, clinically their use is almost never, if ever, effective (Fig. 5.9).

Additional Considerations

Many additional drugs have been explored in the treatment of CPA. Currently, the use of doxapram for respiratory arrest is not recommended. The drug has been shown to increase cerebral and myocardial oxygen demand and reduce cerebral blood flow, and therefore, potentially worsen outcomes in animals and humans (Soma and Kenny 1967; Miletich et al. 1976; Bruckner et al. 1977; Dani et al. 2006). Sodium bicarbonate should only be administered during cardiopulmonary cerebral resuscitation (CPCR) to manage severe metabolic acidosis diagnosed before the arrest, preexisting hyperkalemia, or the lactic acidosis generated by prolonged anaerobic metabolism in hypoxic tissues during CPCR efforts (>10 minutes). The routine use of calcium during CPCR is no longer advised. Its use may be justified in patients with hyperkalemia, hypocalcemia, or affected by a calcium channel blocker overdose. Routine use may potentiate cellular damage secondary to ischemia (van Pelt and Wingfield 1992).

Unfortunately, most patients in CPA cannot be resuscitated even if CPCR is performed perfectly. End-tidal carbon dioxide measurements (ETC02) higher than 15 mm Hg are reportedly associated with higher survival rates (Callaham and Barton 1990). In humans,

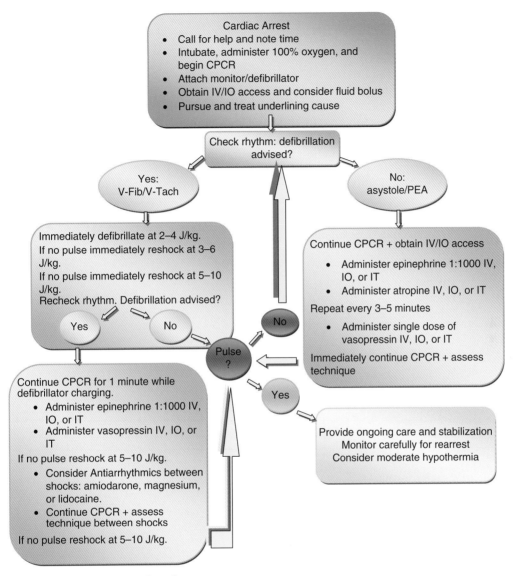

Cardiac Arrest
- Call for help and note time
- Intubate, administer 100% oxygen, and begin CPCR
- Attach monitor/defibrillator
- Obtain IV/IO access and consider fluid bolus
- Pursue and treat underlining cause

Check rhythm: defibrillation advised?

Yes: V-Fib/V-Tach

No: asystole/PEA

Immediately defibrillate at 2–4 J/kg.
If no pulse immediately reshock at 3–6 J/kg.
If no pulse immediately reshock at 5–10 J/kg.
Recheck rhythm. Defibrillation advised?

Yes   No

Pulse?

No

Yes

Continue CPCR + obtain IV/IO access
- Administer epinephrine 1:1000 IV, IO, or IT
- Administer atropine IV, IO, or IT

Repeat every 3–5 minutes
- Administer single dose of vasopressin IV, IO, or IT

Immediately continue CPCR + assess technique

Continue CPCR for 1 minute while defibrillator charging.
- Administer epinephrine 1:1000 IV, IO, or IT
- Administer vasopressin IV, IO, or IT

If no pulse reshock at 5–10 J/kg.
- Consider Antiarrhythmics between shocks: amiodarone, magnesium, or lidocaine.
- Continue CPCR + assess technique between shocks

If no pulse reshock at 5–10 J/kg.

Provide ongoing care and stabilization
Monitor carefully for rearrest
Consider moderate hypothermia

Figure 5.9 Veterinary CPCR flow chart.

post ROSC hypotension is predictive of in-hospital death and is associated with diminished functional status among survivors (Trzeciak et al. 2009). Some have suggested that asystole should not be treated for more than 5 minutes or with more than two rounds of epinephrine, although there are no published studies confirming that premise. Other types of arrhythmia usually can be treated until they progress to asystole, unless the patient's owner declines further resuscitation efforts. Patients who present to the hospital suffering from severe hypothermia should be fully rewarmed before resuscitation efforts are deemed unsuccessful. In humans, the remarkable ability to resuscitate patients with hypothermia even hours after their cardiac arrest has promoted the saying that "you aren't dead until you're warm and dead."

Box 5.1   CPCR Considerations

Always During CPCR
- Push hard and fast (ideally 100 compressions/minute).
- Ensure full chest recoil.
- Minimize interruptions in chest compressions.
- Avoid hyperventilation (ideally 8–12 breaths/minute).
- Secure airway and confirm placement.
- Rotate rescuer performing chest compressions every 2 minutes to prevent fatigue.
- Search for and treat contributing factors
    - Hypovolemia
    - Hypoxia
    - Hydrogen ion (acidosis)
    - Hyperkalemia/hypokalemia
    - Hypoglycemia
    - Hypothermia
    - Toxins
    - Trauma
    - Tamponade, cardiac

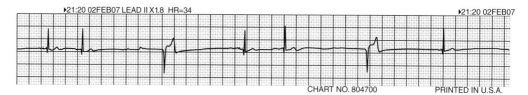

Figure 5.10   An EKG tracing showing ventricular escape beats. These beats should never be suppressed with lidocaine.

Postresuscitative Care

Patients that are restored to a perfusing cardiac rhythm commonly experience rearrest often within minutes to several hours, especially if the original cause of the CPA event has not been identified and resolved. Therefore, resuscitated patients usually require significant cardiovascular and ventilator support during the period following CPA. Stable and perfusing ventricular escape rhythms should never be suppressed with drug therapy (e.g., lidocaine) (Fig. 5.10).

Mild to moderate (28°C–32°C) hypothermia after resuscitation from CPA decreases cerebral oxygen demand and has been shown to improve outcomes in dogs and humans (Nozari et al. 2004, 2006). Inducing mild to moderate hypothermia in the patient should be considered a therapeutic option and has recently started to be explored (Hayes 2009). Hyperglycemia has been shown to be associated with worse neurologic outcomes in human patients and should be avoided after a CPA event (Steingrub and Mundt 1996). Neurological recovery is maximized by achieving normotension as well as by treatment with Mannitol for CPA-related cerebral edema. Corticosteroids are not presently recommended.

The poor perfusion state present during CPA also may precipitate brain injury, disseminated intravascular coagulation, gut reperfusion syndrome, and renal or other organ failure. Therefore, intensive monitoring and aggressive supportive care are required to optimize blood pressure, cardiac output, oxygenation, ventilation, and vital organ perfusion (Steingrub and Mundt 1996; Nozari et al. 2004).

Prognosis

After CPA, the success rate for recovery of veterinary patients is generally poor (Kass and Haskins 1992; Wingfield and Van Pelt 1992; de Vos et al. 1999). A 1-week survival rate of less than 4% for both cats and dogs that received CPCR following full arrest has been reported (Kass and Haskins 1992). However, functional recovery has been reported in most animals that survive CPA (Waldrop et al. 2004). Based on current research, resuscitation appears to be most successful in patients that are treated quickly, are treated by multiple rescuers, have a reversible underlying disease process, such as anesthetic overdose, upper airway obstruction, hemorrhage, or electrolyte abnormalities; and, ideally, are not in full CPA (Kass and Haskins 1992; de Vos et al. 1999; Waldrop et al. 2004; Hofmeister et al. 2009).

References

American Heart Association. 2010. CPR & ECC Guidelines. www.heart.org/cpr.

Aufderheide, TP, Sigurdsson, G, Pirrallo, RG, et al. 2004. Hyperventilation-induced hypotension during cardiopulmonary resuscitation. *Circulation* 109:1960–1965.

Barton, L, Crowe, DT. 2000. Open chest cardiopulmonary resuscitation. In *Kirk's Current Veterinary Therapy XIII*, edited by Bonagura, JD. Philadelphia: WB Saunders, pp. 147–149.

Bright, JM, Wright, BD. 2009. Successful biphasic transthoracic defibrillation of a dog with prolonged refractory ventricular fibrillation. *J Vet Emerg Crit Care (San Antonio)* 19(3):275–279.

Bruckner, JB, Hess, W, Schneider, E, et al. 1977. Doxapram-induced changes in circulation and myocardial efficiency. *Anaesthesist* 26(4):156–164.

Callaham, M, Barton, C. 1990. Prediction of outcome of cardiopulmonary resuscitation from end-tidal carbon dioxide concentration. *Crit Care Med* 18(4):358–362.

Cole, S, Otto, C, Hughes, D. 2003. Cardiopulmonary cerebral resuscitation in small animals—a clinical practice review. *J Vet Emerg Crit Care* 13(1):13–23.

Dani, C, Bertini, G, Pezzati, M, et al. 2006. Brain hemodynamic effects of doxapram in preterm infants. *Biol Neonate* 89(2):69–74.

de Vos, R, Koster, RW, de Haan, RJ, et al. 1999. In-hospital cardiopulmonary resuscitation: prearrest morbidity and outcome. *Arch Intern Med* 159(8):845–850.

Ditchey, RV, Lindenfeld, J. 1984. Potential adverse effects of volume loading on perfusion of vital organs during closed-chest resuscitation. *Circulation* 69(1):181–189.

Emmerman, CL, Pinchak, AC, Hancock, D, et al. 1988. Effect of injection site on circulation times during cardiac arrest. *Crit Care Med* 16(11):1138–1141.

Feneley, MP, Maier, GW, Kern, KB, et al. 1988. Influence of compression rate on initial success of resuscitation and 24 hour survival after prolonged manual cardiopulmonary resuscitation in dogs. *Circulation* 77(1):240–250.

Hayes, G. 2009. Severe seizures associated with traumatic brain injury managed by controlled hypothermia, pharmacological coma, and mechanical ventilation in a dog. *J Vet Emerg Crit Care* 19(6):629–634.

Henik, RA. 1992. Basic life support and external cardiac compressions in dogs and cats. *J Am Vet Med Assoc* 200(12):1925–1931.

Hofmeister, EH, Brainard, BM, Egger, CM, et al. 2009. Prognostic indicators for dogs and cats with cardiopulmonary arrest treated by cardiopulmonary cerebral resuscitation at a university teaching hospital. *J Am Vet Med Assoc* 235(1):50–57.

Janssens, L, Altman, S, Rogers, PA. 1979. Respiratory and cardiac arrest under general anaesthesia: treatment by acupuncture of the nasal philtrum. *Vet Rec* 105(12): 273–276.

Jespersen, HF, Granborg, J, Hansen, U, et al. 1990. Feasibility of intracardiac injection of drugs during cardiac arrest. *Eur Heart J* 11(3):269–274.

Kass, PH, Haskins, SC. 1992. Survival following cardiopulmonary resuscitation in dogs and cats. *J Vet Emerg Crit Care* 2(2):57–65.

Kern, KB, Sanders, AB, Badylak, SF, et al. 1987. Long-term survival with open-chest cardiac massage after ineffective closed-chest compression in a canine preparation. *Circulation* 75(2):498–503.

Kruse-Elliott, KT. 2001. Cardiopulmonary resuscitation. Strategies for maximizing success. *Vet Med* 16(1):51–58.

Looney, AL. 2001. Current thoughts on cardiopulmonary arrest and resuscitation. *Atlantic Coast Veterinary Conference Proceeding*.

Miletich, DJ, Ivankovich, AD, Albrecht, RF, et al. 1976. The effects of doxapram on cerebral blood flow and peripheral hemodynamics in the anesthetized and unanesthetized goat. *Anesth Analg* 55(2):279–285.

Nozari, A, Safar, P, Stezoski, SW, et al. 2004. Mild hypothermia during prolonged cardiopulmonary cerebral resuscitation increases conscious survival in dogs. *Crit Care Med* 32(10):2110–2116.

Nozari, A, Safar, P, Stezoski, SW, et al. 2006. Critical time window for intra-arrest cooling with cold saline flush in a dog model of cardiopulmonary resuscitation. *Circulation* 113:2690–2696.

Pablo, LS. 2003. Current concepts in cardiopulmonary resuscitation. *World Small Animal Veterinary Association World Congress Proceeding*.

Plunkett, SJ, McMichael, M. 2008. Cardiopulmonary resuscitation in small animal medicine: an update. *J Vet Intern Med* 22(1):9–25.

Ralston, SH, Babbs, CF, Niebauer, MJ. 1982. Cardiopulmonary resuscitation with interposed abdominal compression in dogs. *Anesth Analg* 61(8):645–651.

Rush, JE, Wingfield, WE. 1992. Recognition and frequency of dysrhythmias during cardiopulmonary arrest. *J Am Vet Med Assoc* 200(12):1932–1937.

Sabin, HI, Coghill, SB, Khunti, K, McNeill, CO. 1983. Accuracy of intracardiac injections determined by a post-mortem study. *Lancet* 2(8358):1054–1055.

Safar, P. 1986. Cerebral resuscitation after cardiac arrest: a review. *Circulation* 74(6 Pt 2):IV138–IV153.

Safar, P. 1988. Resuscitation from clinical death: pathophysiologic limits and therapeutic potentials. *Crit Care Med* 16(10):923–941.

Schmittinger, CA, Astner, S, Astner, L, et al. 2005. Cardiopulmonary resuscitation with vasopressin in a dog. *Vet Anaesth Analg* 32(2):112–114.

Schoen, AM. 2003. Veterinary medical acupuncture in critical care medicine. *World Small Animal Veterinary Association World Congress Proceeding*.

Scroggin, RD Jr., Quandt, J. 2009. The use of vasopressin for treating vasodilatory shock and cardiopulmonary arrest. *J Vet Emerg Crit Care* 19(2):145–157.

Soma, LR, Kenny, R. 1967. Respiratory, cardiovascular, metabolic, and electroencephalographic effects of of doxapram hydrochloride in the dog. *Am J Vet Res* 28(12): 191–198.

Steingrub, JS, Mundt, DJ. 1996. Blood glucose and neurological outcome with global brain ischemia. *Crit Care Med* 24(5):802–806.

Trzeciak, S, Jones, AE, Kilgannon, JH, et al. 2009. Significance of arterial hypotension after resuscitation from cardiac arrest. *Crit Care Med* 37(11):2895–2903.

van Pelt, DR, Wingfield, WE. 1992. Controversial issues in drug treatment during cardiopulmonary resuscitation. *J Am Vet Med Assoc* 200:1938–1944.

Voorhees, WD 3rd, Ralston, SH, Babbs, CF. 1984. Regional blood flow during cardiopulmonary resuscitation with abdominal counterpulsation in dogs. *Am J Emerg Med* 2(2):123–128.

Waldrop, JE, Rozanski, EA, Swanke, ED, et al. 2004. Causes of cardiopulmonary arrest, resuscitation management, and functional outcome in dogs and cats surviving cardiopulmonary arrest. *J Vet Emerg Crit Care* 14(1):22–29.

Wenzel, V, Lindner, KH, Prengel, AW, Lurie, KG, Strohmenger, HU. 1997. Endobronchial vasopressin improves survival during cardiopulmonary resuscitation in pigs. *Anesthesiology* 86:1375–1381.

Wingfield, WE, Van Pelt, DR. 1992. Respiratory and cardiopulmonary arrest in dogs and cats: 265 cases (1986–1991). *J Am Vet Med Assoc* 200(12):1993–1996.

Yannopoulos, D, Aufderheide, TP. 2007. Use of the impedance threshold device (ITD). *Resuscitation* 75(1):192–193.

CHAPTER 5

Section 2

Specific Organ System Disorders

Cardiovascular Emergencies

Christopher L. Norkus

Introduction

Heart disease is one of the leading causes of morbidity in both human and veterinary medicine and is a common problem for which animals are presented to the emergency department. Recent research would suggest that the prognosis for acute congestive heart failure (CHF) in dogs and cats may be better than previously documented. When treated appropriately, up to 80% of cases presenting to the emergency room with acute CHF may survive to discharge (Goutal et al. 2010) With this encouraging figure, it is paramount, therefore, that technicians be knowledgeable in cardiovascular disorders and well versed in their management to continue to maximize patient survival.

Anatomy of the Pericardium and Heart

The heart is the muscular pump of the cardiovascular system. Collectively, the musculature and conducting system of the heart are known as the myocardium. The heart is a cone-shaped organ and is obliquely placed in the thorax so that its base faces dorsocranially and its apex is directed ventrocaudally (Evans 1993).

The heart is divided internally by a longitudinal septum into a cranioventral (right) and a caudaldorsal (left) part. The left heart consists of the left atrium and left ventricle, which together receive blood from the lungs and pump it to all parts of the body. The right side of the heart is made up of the right atrium and right ventricle, and together they receive blood from all parts of the body, including the heart itself, and pump it onward to the lungs for oxygen uptake.

The heart forms a part of the mediastinum, which acts as a partition to separate the two pleural cavities. The heart extends from the third rib to the caudal boarder of the sixth rib (Evans 1993). However, it is important to recognize that variations in position can exist among breeds, individuals, and in the presence of pathology.

The pericardium is the fibroserous sac that surrounds the heart. The pericardial cavity is located between the pericardium and the heart and normally contains between 0.3 and 1 mL of a clear, light yellow fluid (Evans 1993).

Within the heart itself, the atrioventricular (AV) valves are intake valves to the ventricles. They prevent blood from returning to the atria during the systolic phase of cardiac contraction. These valves are structurally anchored by chordae tendineae. The right AV valve, also known as the tricuspid valve, separates the right atria from the right ventricle. Tricuspid valve lesions cause heart murmurs that are usually heard most distinctly at the fourth right intercostal space at the level of the costochondral junction (Evans 1993). The left AV valve, also known as the mitral or bicuspid valve, separates the left atria from the left ventricle. Heart murmurs associated with lesions in this part of the heart generally are most intense at the fifth left intercostal space above the middle of the lower third of the thorax (Evans 1993).

Blood leaving the right ventricle must pass through the pulmonic valve before entering the lungs. Heart murmurs resulting from lesions of the pulmonic valve are best heard at the third intercostal space more ventrally than the point of the shoulder. Blood leaving the left ventricle must pass through the aortic valve before being pumped into the ascending aorta. Lesions of the aortic valve typically produce heart murmurs that are located loudest at the fourth left intercostal space slightly below the point of the shoulder. Both the aortic and pulmonic valves are semilunar valves and do not have chordate tendineae. Blood being pumped from the left ventricle proceeds onward into the aorta where the left and right coronary arteries take blood to the heart, where the brachiocephalic trunk and left subclavian artery bring blood to the limbs and cranial sections of the body, and where the descending aorta transports blood to the caudal half of the body (Evans 1993).

Electrical Conductance and Generation of the Electrocardiogram (ECG) Wave

No part of the canine or feline conduction system can be adequately identified via routine gross dissection. Each component of an ECG wave reflects an electrical event occurring

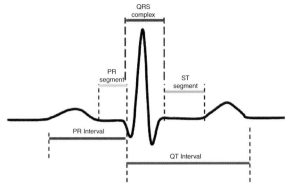

Figure 6.1   An ECG wave form showing intervals, segments, and the QRS complex. (Courtesy of Kristen Cooley, BA, CVT, VTS [Anesthesia].)

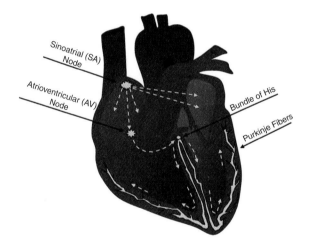

Figure 6.2   Normal electrical conductance in the heart begins at the SA node, moves on to the AV node, travels on to the AV bundle, and finally down to the Purkinje fibers. (Courtesy of Kristen Cooley, BA, CVT, VTS [Anesthesia].)

in a specific part of the heart. In the healthy heart, the sinoatrial (SA) node, located in the right atrium, initiates the heart's electrical activity. This impulse then spreads through both atria and down the heart, causing both atria to contract and resulting in the formation of the *P wave* on an ECG tracing. Electrical activity proceeds down the heart reaching the AV bundle, a mass of Purkinje fibers that begin as the AV node at the floor of the right atrium.

At the AV node, the electrical impulse depolarizing the heart is intentionally delayed, allowing the atria to finish their contracting. This period of rest is reflected on the ECG as a flat segment between the P wave and QRS complex. The AV node also acts as an effective gatekeeper, preventing unwanted atrial impulses (e.g., atrial premature complexes [APCs], atrial fibrillation) from crossing to and activating the ventricles. Once having crossed the AV node, an electrical impulse travels through the ventricles by way of the His-Purkinje system and allows the ventricles to contract. The His bundle then divides into right and left bundle branches at the apex of the heart, which diverts electrical activity to their respective ventricle. Overall, the depolarization of the ventricles is apparent on the ECG as the *QRS complex*. Atrial repolarization is not visible on an ECG as it occurs masked by the QRS complex. Ventricular repolarization is seen as the *T wave* on the ECG (Figs. 6.1 and 6.2).

Blood Pressure (BP) and Delivery of Oxygen to Tissue

Arterial BP is most simply defined as the pressure exerted by circulating blood on the walls of blood vessels. BP is made up of a systolic and a diastolic component. The systolic component is created at the end of the cardiac cycle when the ventricles are contracting and represents a peak pressure in the arteries. Conversely, diastolic pressure is the minimum pressure in the arteries, occurring at the beginning of each cardiac cycle when the ventricles are fully filled with blood.

Upon closer examination, arterial BP is the approximate product of two different components: systemic vascular resistance (SVR) and cardiac output (CO) (Ettinger and Feldman 2005, p. 472). The formula $BP = SVR \times CO$ can be derived. SVR refers to the degree of peripheral resistance, predominantly dilation (vasodilation) or constriction (vasoconstriction) of systemic blood vessels. CO is the volume of blood being pumped by the heart in a given minute.

CO itself is the product of another two separate components: stroke volume (SV) and heart rate (HR) (Ettinger and Feldman 2005, p. 472). As SV increases, CO increases as well. SV is the volume of blood being pumped from the heart at each pump. HR is simply the number of times the heart pumps a minute. As a result, a new formula is created: $CO = HR \times SV$. Increases in HR increase CO linearly until a plateau is reached. Further increases in HR result in a decrease in CO (Ettinger and Feldman 2005, p. 472) (Fig. 6.3).

Looking further, we learn that SV itself is also made up of three contributors: *cardiac preload*, *cardiac contractility*, and *cardiac afterload* (Ettinger and Feldman 2005, p. 472). Cardiac preload is the force acting to stretch the ventricular fibers at the end of diastole and is estimated as being the end-diastolic volume. Because it reflects the degree of ventricular filling just before contraction, it can be thought of as the blood volume returning to the heart. Afterload is the resistance created by the vasculature that the heart must overcome for blood to leave the heart. Cardiac contractility is the intrinsic property of the myocardial cell, or simply put, the strength or ability of the heart to contract.

SV increases with increases in preload and contractility and decreases in afterload. Increases in SVR cause a decrease in cardiac compliance and increases in afterload. With decreased compliance, there is an increase in energy cost to maintain blood flow and an increase in myocardial oxygen consumption (MVO_2).

CO is of critical importance because it is also a specific component of how oxygen is delivered to tissue. The delivery of oxygen to tissue (DO_2) is the product of CO and arterial oxygen content (CaO_2). Thereby, $DO_2 = CO \times CaO_2$. CaO_2 is a component of hemoglobin's saturation with oxygen (SaO_2), the amount of hemoglobin available (Hgb), a constant that dictates the amount of hemoglobin that can be bound by hemoglobin (1.36), the amount of oxygen dissolved in the blood (PaO_2), and a solubility constant (0.003). Thus, $CaO_2 = (SaO_2 \times Hgb \times 1.36) + (PaO_2 \times 0.003)$. Defects to any of these components lead to decreased systemic oxygen delivery to tissue (*hypoxia*) and systemic hypoperfusion.

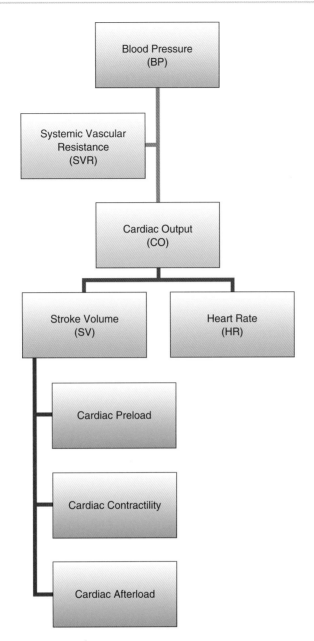

Figure 6.3 Blood pressure components.

Pathophysiology of Heart Failure

Heart failure is a clinical syndrome in which impaired cardiac pumping results in decreased ventricular output, venous return, and CO. During such a state, the heart cannot effectively pump to deliver oxygen requirements to the body. The hemodynamic consequences of heart failure are complicated by the fact that many cases of heart failure have concurrent biochemical and pathological changes to the myocardial cells. These changes accelerate deterioration of the myocardium and in turn alter myocardial contractility and relaxation and therefore transform heart failure into a progressive disease.

Essentially, the heart has limited means of failure. The heart may fail to pump enough blood out into the aorta or pulmonary artery to maintain SV, CO, and arterial BP. This has previously been referred to as *systolic failure, forward heart failure,* or *low output heart failure.* These cases manifest themselves with signs of decreased CO and BP such as hypotension, weakness, and lethargy. Additionally, there may be inadequate ventricular filling, often referred to as *diastolic heart failure* or, previously, *backward heart failure.* Or the heart may not be able to adequately empty itself and its venous reservoirs. This is referred to as *congestive heart failure* (CHF). These cases manifest themselves with signs of congestion: pulmonary edema, pleural effusion, or ascites.

Heart failure can additionally be separated into left, right, or bilateral based upon which side of the heart is working ineffectively. Left-sided heart failure is associated clinically with signs of congestion such as pulmonary edema and dyspnea. Right-sided heart failure is associated with backup of systemic circulation and may manifest itself in ascites and peripheral edema. Bilateral heart failure, therefore, shares clinical signs of both left- and right-sided disease.

Systolic Heart Failure

Systolic heart failure is characterized by a normal filling of the ventricles but a decrease in the forward SV. A decrease in stroke volume may be the result of either decreased cardiac contractility (inotropy) or an increased ventricular pressure (pressure overload) or volume (volume overload).

Common etiologies of decreased myocardial function and contractility include primary and secondary causes. Primary causes include conditions like dilated cardiomyopathy (DCM), myocardial infarction, and doxorubicin toxicity. Secondary causes stem from chronic volume or pressure overload within the heart and the adaptive changes that result. Decreased cardiac contractility results in a decrease in SV and decrease in CO and BP.

Volume overload causes of systolic heart failure include valvular diseases (e.g., chronic mitral valve insufficiency [CMVI], infectious endocarditis [IE], ruptured chordae tendineae, congenital heart diseases such aspatent ductus arteriosus [PDA], atrial or ventricular septal defect), hyperthyroidism, and chronic anemia. Cardiac volume overload leads to an increase in wall stress. This insult causes a stretching of the heart wall and results in eccentric ventricular hypertrophy and fibrosis. These changes lead to further decrease in cardiac function.

Frequent pressure overload causes of systolic heart failure include congenital heart diseases (e.g., pulmonic stenosis, subaortic stenosis), systemic hypertension, heartworm disease, pulmonary thromboembolism, and primary pulmonary hypertension. Pressure overload results in concentric hypertrophy of the ventricular muscle. The hypertrophied muscle is prone to ischemia, fibrosis, and increased collagen formation. These changes lead to further decreases in cardiac function.

Diastolic Heart Failure

Diastolic dysfunction results from impairment in ventricular filling. Diastolic heart failure occurs when pulmonary venous congestion and clinical signs occur in the presence of normal systolic function. Diastolic failure may result from several offending factors, including abnormal cardiac relaxation, external constraint by the pericardium, or abnormal cardiac compliance.

Conditions that lead to abnormal ventricular chamber or muscle properties include ventricular hypertrophy (e.g., hypertrophic cardiomyopathy [HCM], subaortic stenosis, pulmonic stenosis, systemic hypertension, heartworm disease), DCM, myocardial infarction, obstruction of ventricular filling (e.g., intracardiac neoplasia), and pericardial diseases (e.g., cardiac tamponade).

Adaptive Physiological Changes to Heart Failure

Most clinical signs observed in heart failure are due to the chronic activation and adaptive physiological response to restore and maintain homeostasis. Regardless of the cause, the progression of heart failure results in a decrease in CO and a fall in arterial BP. Changes in arterial BP are sensed by baroreceptors in the aortic arch and carotid sinus and mechanoreceptors and volume receptors within the heart and kidneys. The decreased firing of these receptors initiates a reactive neuroendocrine response that attempts to reestablish normal BP.

The immediate response is a decrease in autonomic parasympathetic stimulation and an increase in sympathetic stimulation. The sympathetic stimulation results in activation of alpha-1 and beta-1 adrenergic receptors, causing vasoconstriction, increased HR, and increased cardiac contractility. These changes aim to improve SVR and CO. Decreased renal blood flow causes activation of the renin-angiotensin-aldosterone system (RAAS) (Fig. 6.4). The result is a contribution to systemic vasoconstriction and sodium and water retention, which helps to increase circulating plasma volume and improve SV.

CHAPTER 6

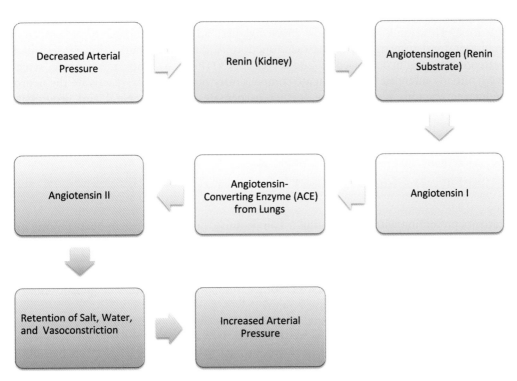

Figure 6.4   The renin-angiotensin-aldosterone system (RAAS).

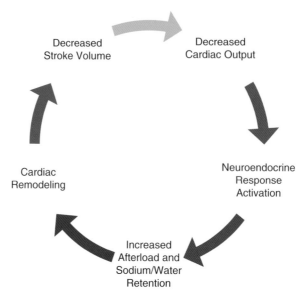

Figure 6.5 Vicious cycle of heart failure.

These mechanisms are very effective compensatory means for acute insults to the body. During heart failure, however, these compensatory mechanisms are chronically activated and result in adverse long-term effects. Chronic adrenergic stimulation, for example, leads to prolonged increases in afterload and MVO_2, ventricular arrhythmia, and promotes cardiac remodeling (Ettinger and Feldman 2005, p. 923). Continued RAAS activation leads to prolonged increases in afterload, too, as well as prolonged sodium and water retention. This results in an increase in cardiac preload and a volume and pressure over-load that are detrimental to the cardiac function. Additionally, afterload increases, inadvertently resulting in decreased SV and decreased CO (Fig. 6.5). These mechanisms, which were initially intended to be for acute compensatory purposes only, reactivate the neuro-endocrine response and therefore further perpetuates the detrimental and progressive cycle. Heart failure is therefore a progressive and vicious cycle. Treating patients for heart failure aims to counterbalance the body's adverse response.

Emergency Treatment of Heart Failure

Patients presenting with cardiovascular compromise, including those in heart failure, are extremely fragile and should be handled with a gentle hand. Struggling, anxiety, and stress can contribute to increases in sympathetic nervous system activation, worsening of arrhythmias, decreased myocardial perfusion, and can quickly result in patient death. Therefore, stressful procedures such as thoracic radiographs and other diagnostic endeavors may have to wait until the case is stable.

As the pulmonary interstitial space and alveoli become flooded with fluid, inadequate ventilation and functional shunting occur. This leads to dyspnea. Clinically cardiac disease cases, therefore, may be easily confused with primary respiratory disease. The NT-proBNP test may be helpful to differentiate between the two (Oyama et al. 2009).

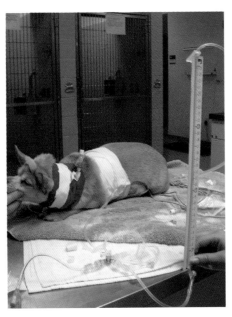

Figure 6.6   Central venous pressure (CVP) monitoring in the ICU. (Courtesy of Thomas Walker, DVM, DACVECC.)

Oxygen administration should be provided to combat the resulting hypoxemia in patients with heart failure. An oxygen cage lends itself nicely to minimize restraint. Oxygen via face mask, nasal cannula, or hood can be considered, but only if they do not stress the patient.

Placement of an intravenous catheter should be considered, but never at the expense of stress to the patient. Intravenous fluid therapy is not typically warranted in patients with heart failure because these patients typically have high cardiac preload and are volume and pressure overloaded from the start. Patients who are dehydrated or are in hypovolemic shock should be treated with conservative low-dose crystalloid fluids until physiological parameters improve. Ultrasound to assess left atrial enlargement or central venous pressure (CVP) monitoring will be essential to monitor for volume overload in these cases (Fig. 6.6). Upon hydration and normovolemia, solutions such as 0.45% NaCl or 5% dextrose in water (D5W) can be considered for maintenance if fluids are absolutely necessary.

Most dogs and cats presenting in heart failure are stressed and anxious. Many will benefit from low-dose sedation. Butorphanol 0.1–0.4 mg/kg IM, SQ, IV yields itself nicely in the cat (Ettinger and Feldman 2005, p. 1077). Morphine 0.25 mg/kg IM, SQ yields itself well in the dog (Plunkett 2001). Morphine may also have the added advantage of being a pulmonary vasodilator.

The loop diuretic furosemide is typically a mainstay of treatment for the heart failure patient as it acts to reduce cardiac preload, decrease pulmonary hydrostatic pressure, and remove pulmonary edema. When given intravenously, furosemide may also result in pulmonary vasodilation. Depending on what the patient permits, IV or IM furosemide at 2–8 mg/kg IV q2-8h is administered in the dog (Ettinger and Feldman 2005, p. 1033). Furosemide via constant rate infusion (CRI) may be an adventitious alternative at 0.1–1 mg/kg/h (Rozanski and Rush 2007). In the cat, 2–4 mg/kg q1h IV or IM q1-2h is selected (Ettinger and Feldman 2005, p. 1094; Rozanski and Rush 2007). Furosemide administration may cause dehydration, hypovolemia, azotemia, and electrolyte disturbances such as hypokalemia, especially in the cat (Ettinger and Feldman 2005, p. 472).

Nitroglycerine paste can also be considered as a venodilator, thereby reducing cardiac preload; however, its benefit in the dog and cat has recently come into question (Ettinger and Feldman 2005, p. 472). In the dog, 1/4–3/4 in. applied cutaneously every 8–12 hours may be selected. In the cat, 1/8–1/4 in. may be administered every 4–6 hours (Ettinger and Feldman 2005, p. 1077). Due to poor peripheral perfusion at the time of administration, locations such as the ear should be avoided and be replaced by core locations such as the thorax or inguinal region. Nitroglycerin should be avoided or administered with great care in cases with systolic BPs < 100 mgHg. Technicians administering nitroglycerin must wear gloves and carefully label the site of administration to prevent accidental human exposure.

Afterload reduction can be achieved by the administration of a CRI of nitroprusside, an ultrarapid short-acting balanced arterial and venous dilator. Administered at 2–10 mg/kg/min in dogs, the drug requires careful monitoring of BP to achieve accurate titration and safe use (Ettinger and Feldman 2005, p. 1033). In the cat, 0.5–3 mcg/kg/min is used (Rozanski and Rush 2007). BPs below 90 mmHg should be avoided (Rozanski and Rush 2007). Hydralazine is an arterial dilator that can be administered orally at 1–2 mg/kg in the dog rather than utilizing injectable agents Ettinger and Feldman 2005, p. 1033). Nitroprusside and hydralazine should be administered with great care, if at all, in cases with systolic BPs < 100 mgHg.

After the aforementioned therapy, positive inotropes can be considered to increase cardiac contractility and improve systolic function. Dobutamine via CRI at 1–10 mcg/kg/min is often considered in the dog (Rozanski and Rush 2007). In the cat, 1–3 mcg/kg/min may be selected (Rozanski and Rush 2007). BP and ECG monitoring should be continued during dobutamine administration. Oral pimobendan, a newer inodilator, has the advantage of providing the patient with positive inoptropy as well as reducing afterload. In the dog, 0.25 mg/kg q12h PO is initially selected. Some are beginning to use this drug orally in the emergency setting. Other potential agents to augment systolic performance include dopamine and the bipyridines amrinone and milrinone. Amrinone and milrinone have not been widely explored within veterinary medicine to date. Dopamine, acting as a precursor to norepinephrine, raises concern about high risk for cardiac arrhythmias and can potentially worsen afterload via alpha-1 agonism. It is therefore generally not a first-line agent.

Mechanical ventilation should be considered in select cases at imminent risk of cardio-pulmonary arrest. Mechanical ventilation allows for full control over the airway, avoidance of respiratory failure, and positive end expiratory pressure (PEEP), which is helpful in clearing pulmonary edema (Rozanski and Rush 2007). Unfortunately, mechanical ventilation requires special equipment, operator skill, significant time, and financial resources, and usually requires some degree of chemical restraint in an already compromised patient. Drug combinations such as an opioid (e.g., fentanyl) and/or a benzodiazepine (e.g., midazolam) can be utilized to facilitate intubation in such critical cases. Etomidate can also be utilized with minimized alterations to cardiac or respiratory function.

Specific cardiac arrhythmias should be addressed concurrently if they are affecting CO. Thoracocentesis should be performed in dogs and cats with pleural effusion. Overall, the treatment goal for cats with HCM and heart failure tends to focus predominantly on relieving venous and pulmonary congestion through preload reduction and on removing pleural effusion via thoracocentesis to improve oxygenation and ventilation. Although response in the individual patient should always be the end goal, augmentation of systolic function or significant afterload reduction is often not a key strategy employed in the feline patient.

Cardiovascular Nursing

Monitoring by the dedicated paraprofessional is vital for successful patient outcome with cardiovascular cases. Nursing orders typically include frequent assessment of temperature, mucus membrane color, capillary refill time, HR, pulse rate and character, respirator rate and character, skin turgor, mentation, body weight, CVP, pulse oximetry, ECG and telemetry, and BP monitoring.

Respiratory rate and effort and increasing body weight can be excellent early indications of volume overload in the dog and cat. Additional signs of volume overload include serous nasal discharge, labored breathing, moist cough, chemosis, exophthalmos, nausea, vomiting, ascites, tachycardia, subcutaneous edema, pulmonary crackles, pleural effusion, depression, and polyuria. CVPs > 13 cmH$_2$O or an increase of >3 cm in 1 hour are also suspicious of volume overload.

Extra care needs to be taken to keep cardiac patients calm and in minimal stress environments to prevent sympathetic nervous system stimulation and worsen their disease. Patients with cardiac disease are often distressed and anxious to begin with. When therapy has been effective in treating pleural effusion or pulmonary edema, patients typically have their respiratory rate decrease, mucous membrane color improve, and are able to lie down and sleep. Improvement on radiographs usually follows long after clinical signs improve.

Specific Cardiac Emergencies

Chronic Valvular Heart Disease (CVHD)

CVHD, also known as endocardiosis, is a progressive degenerative disease of the AV valves, most commonly the left AV valve (mitral valve). CVHD is quite common in the dog and has been estimated to account for as much as 80% of all canine cardiac disease (Ettinger and Feldman 2005, p. 1022). The prevalence in cats appears low. Although potentially found in all breeds, CVHD has the greatest prevalence in dogs of small to medium size such as the King Charles Spaniel and Papillon (Fig. 6.7).

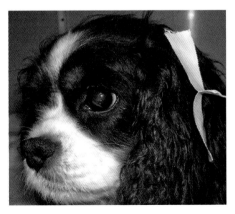

Figure 6.7   A Cavalier King Charles Spaniel being treated for endocardiosis. (Courtesy of Thomas Walker, DVM, DACVECC.)

CHAPTER 6

CVHD is a slow progressive disease that often takes many years to evolve to severe disease with CHF. Many dogs with CVHD are not clinically affected by the disease within their lifetime. Still, CVHD has been reported to account for 75% of the cases of CHF in dogs (Ettinger and Feldman 2005, p. 1022).

Mild to moderate CVHD is usually not associated with any signs of disease. Exercise intolerance and cough may have been subtle changes noticed by the owner. As the condition progresses, pulmonary edema, tachypnea, and dyspnea occur. Upon presentation to the emergency room, these dogs are often anxious and restless. Lethargy, anorexia, and cardiac cachexia may also be reported in the history. Syncope and tachyarrhythmias may also be noted on the exam or within the patient's history. Jugular vein distention (JVD) may be present.

Upon auscultation, pulmonary wheezes and crackles may be heard best at the end of inspiration. Mucous membranes are normal, cyanotic, or grayish. The most prominent feature of CVHD will be a holosystolic heart murmur on the left apex over the fourth intercostal space. With intensity, the murmur may radiate over to the right side of the thorax. In cases of severe heart failure, the heart sounds and murmurs may be muffled by pleural effusion or pericardial effusion. Frequent findings on ECG include sinus arrhythmia, atrial premature depolarizations (APDs), atrial tachycardia, atrial fibrillation, and ventricular arrhythmias.

Radiography is of value to assess the sequelae of CVHD. Additionally, it helps to rule out other possible causes of the clinical signs such as bronchial disease. Left atrial enlargement is an early and consistent radiographic feature of CVHD. With progression of the disease, the left atrium and left ventricle continue to enlarge, and signs of pulmonary congestion and edema typically develop. Echocardiography is necessary to confirm the diagnosis but is not helpful in evaluating for the presence of CHF. There are no specific therapeutic recommendations for the emergency treatment of CVHD other than standard heart failure therapy.

Dilated Cardiomyopathy (DCM)

Today, DCM is a primary myocardial disease of the dog characterized by cardiac enlargement and impaired systolic function. Taurine deficiency was previously discovered as the predominant cause of dilated cardiomyopathy in cats, essentially eliminating the disease in that species. It appears that a wide variety of myocardial insults can result in DCM: genetic, toxic (e.g., doxorubicin), nutrition, and viral. Generally, DCM is a disease of adult large and medium-sized dog breeds. The owners may have noticed a gradual development of exercise intolerance and weight loss (Ettinger and Feldman 2005, p. 1077); however, for many, a diagnosis is not made until CHF develops and the patient is presented to the emergency room for coughing, tachypnea, dyspnea, and potentially ascites.

Upon physical exam, a soft systolic heart murmur that is consistent with mitral valve regurgitation and/or a gallop rhythm may be auscultated at the left cardiac apex (Ettinger and Feldman 2005, p. 1077). Tachyarrhythmias may also be noted. ECG findings may reveal left atrial and ventricular enlargement and sinus tachycardia, atrial fibrillation, or frequently, ventricular dysrhythmias. Radiographic findings confirm left atrial and ventricular enlargement and often pulmonary edema. Echocardiography is the diagnostic test of choice for definitive diagnosis. There are no specific emergency therapeutic recommendations for the treatment of DCM other than standard heart failure therapy.

Caval Syndrome of Heartworm Disease

Heartworm caval syndrome is a rare but serious complication of a heavy worm burden (often >60) from canine heartworm disease. A strong male predilection for the condition appears to be present (Ettinger and Feldman 2005, p. 1132). Following heavy infection with adult heartworms, the parasites obstruct the inflow to the right heart and interfere with tricuspid valve function. These events significantly reduce cardiac preload and therefore CO. Cardiac arrhythmias may also occur. Because of trauma to red blood cells (RBCs) from the worms, intravascular hemolysis occurs, followed by hemoglobinemia, hemoglobinuria, hepatic and renal dysfunction, and disseminated intravascular coagulation (DIC) in many dogs. Without treatment, death frequently ensues within 24–72 hours.

Patient history may include a sudden onset of anorexia, lethargy, mild cough, dyspnea, hemoptysis, and hemoglobinuria. On physical exam, patients may demonstrate pale mucous membranes, JVD, ascites, weak pulses, hepatosplenomegaly, abnormal lung sounds, gallop rhythm, and systolic heart murmur over the right thorax at the fourth intercostal space.

Laboratory findings will often include hemoglobinemia and microfilaria, a mild regenerative anemia, an inflammatory leukogram, and elevations to hepatic enzymes, bilirubin, and renal function indices. CVPs are elevated in 80% of cases with a mean of $11.4\,cmH_2O$ (Ettinger and Feldman 2005).

Prognosis is poor unless the right heart and caval (vena cava) heartworms are removed. Even with direct venotomy and worm retrieval, mortality can be approximately 40% (Ettinger and Feldman 2005).

Fluid therapy should be administered to combat hypovolemia but must be carefully titrated as to not precipitate signs of CHF. Monitoring CVPs is essential to allow the most aggressive fluid therapy possible. Rarely, whole blood or transfused coagulation factors (e.g., plasma) may be indicated. Ultimately, venotomy, often not requiring more than local anesthesia, is performed in left lateral recumbency. An effort should be made to remove as many worms as possible, often totaling 35–50. Fluoroscopic guidance, when available, is useful for this procedure. Worm embolectomy is frequently successful in stabilizing the dog, allowing adulticide therapy to be instituted to destroy the remaining heartworms at a later date.

Hypertrophic Cardiomyopathy (HCM)

HCM is a common disease of the cat characterized by thickening of the left ventricular wall and papillary muscles. As a result, concentric hypertrophy (thickening of the heart wall creating a small chamber size) occurs. A male predisposition for HCM has been reported (Ettinger and Feldman 2005, p. 1077). The exact cause of feline HCM has not been elucidated, but a possible genetic link has been identified.

Cats with HCM often initially have no signs until they are presented to the emergency room in moderate to severe heart failure or have developed systemic thromboembolism. Cats with HCM may die suddenly with often no prior clinical signs suggestive of heart disease and no obvious trigger. Early signs are subtle and can include a systolic murmur heard best over the midsternum or left apex beat (Ettinger and Feldman 2005, p. 1077). A gallop rhythm can sometimes be auscultated with HCM cases. Radiographic findings may be unremarkable or may include left atrial enlargement, pulmonary edema, and pleural effusion. The diagnosis of HCM is almost always made via echocardiography.

There are no specific therapeutic recommendations for the emergency treatment of HCM other than standard heart failure therapy. In the cat, less emphasis is placed on improving systolic function and reducing afterload, and more priority is paid to relieving pleural effusion via thoracocentesis.

Systemic Thromboembolism (STE)

A systemic thrombus, or blood clot within the vasculature, becomes a thromboembolism when it breaks free from a primary site of origination and migrates to a distant site in the vasculature where is becomes lodged or embolized. Now partially or completely occluding the blood vessel, blood flow distal to the thromboembolism is blocked, and oxygen and nutrient delivery to distal tissue is compromised.

Although systemic thromboembolism can occur in any patient, more than 70% of cases seen in veterinary medicine are in cats with cardiomyopathy (Ettinger and Feldman 2005, p. 1098). Usually, these cats have left atrial enlargement, and their thrombus forms in the left atrium as well. Most cats with STE (approximately 90%) have the thromboembolism lodged at the terminal abdominal aorta (Ettinger and Feldman 2005). The thrombus commonly extends down the external iliac arteries, giving the appearance of a saddle. The term "saddle thromboembolism" therefore is sometimes used.

STE of the terminal aorta rapidly causes acute caudal limb weakness (paraparesis), paralysis (paraplegia), and severe pain. Femoral pulses are lost, cold extremities, and pale or cyanotic pads result from the lack of perfusion. Upon physical exam, a heart murmur or gallop rhythm are frequently present. Many cats are concurrently in heart failure and therefore simultaneously have dyspnea. Cats with STE are typically hypothermic. The cranial tibialis and gastrocnemius muscles are most severely affected and are commonly intensely painful, swollen, and tight. Urine retention may occur. Many cats, however, retain their ability to move their tails. Depending on time of presentation, regions of tissue necrosis and muscle contracture may be present.

In the acute stages, Doppler blood flow measurement will reveal the absence of successful blood flow. A toenail on an affected limb will also fail to bleed when freshly cut. The diagnosis of STE in cats is predominantly made based on history and clinical signs. Diagnostic imaging of the affected vessels by angiography or nuclear medicine is needed for definitive diagnosis. Echocardiogram may be useful to identify the underlying cardiac disease and document severely compromised circulation via color flow imaging.

Most cats with STE have blood work changes consistent with muscle necrosis and stress hyperglycemia. Significant increases in blood urea nitrogen (BUN) and creatinine may suggest that the thrombus had embolized in the region of the renal arteries and has affected renal perfusion.

The short-term prognosis for cats with STE but without heart failure is guarded. Heart failure and cats with rectal temperatures lower than 98.9°F may likely have a worse prognosis (Ettinger and Feldman 2005, p. 1102). Long-term prognosis appears highly variable and depends on the individual patient's response to treatment and the ability to control the underlying cause. In general, however, prognosis for STE is not favorable. Even after successful treatment, a large percentage of cats unfortunately will still develop repeated STE.

Treatment should initially include addressing the underlying cause whenever possible. Euthanasia should be considered in cases of STE that have a poor prognosis due to severe cardiomyopathy or other debilitating disease. As STE results in extreme pain, aggressive pain management is of critical importance. Multimodal analgesia, including mu agonist opioids (e.g., fentanyl, hydromorphone, morphine), is preferred. Agents such as butorphanol and buprenorphine likely do not provide adequate analgesia. Beyond analgesia, specific treatment options for STE are often palliative, including supportive care and the administration of drugs with unfounded benefit (Ettinger and Feldman 2005).

Palliative therapy may only include pain control and cage rest or may involve administering drugs such as aspirin, heparin, or low molecular weight heparin (LMWH), antiplatelet drugs (e.g., clopidogrel), and arteriolar dilators such as acepromazine and hydralazine. Heparin when used does not aid in thrombolysis but rather may prevent new thrombus formation on top of existing ones. As these cases are often in heart failure, fluid administration is generally not indicated.

Unfortunately, definitive therapy for clot removal has typically proved unrewarding in the cat. Surgical removal of STE is generally thought to be associated with high mortality and is not frequently performed. Balloon embolectomy, a procedure of choice in humans, has been utilized but tends to be associated with significant reperfusion syndrome that may not ultimately improve outcome. Thrombolytic therapy, which is also widely used in human medicine, includes drugs such as tissue plasminogen activator (t-PA), streptokinase, and urokinase. Both t-PA and streptokinase have been investigated in cats with STE with discouraging results. Severe reperfusion injury is common, and sudden arrhythmic death has occurred (Moore et al. 2007). The use of urokinase appears to have shown some promise in cats. Although further investigation of different dosages and possible different agents continues at this time, thrombolytic drugs are typically considered unsuccessful and are associated with increased risk of morbidity and mortality for the vast majority of patients. Rheolytic thrombectomy is a new interventional radiology therapy that may show promise in treating STE cases in the future.

Myocardial Infarction

Unlike in humans, acute myocardial infarction ("heart attack") is an uncommon occurrence in dogs and cats. A main reason for this appears to be because humans have a high incidence of atherosclerosis while dogs and cats do not. When the condition has occurred in dogs and cats, it appears to most commonly have been associated with a concurrent systemic disease that has lead to a hypercoagulative and thromboembolic state. Such conditions might include neoplasia, renal disease, sepsis, immune-mediated disease, pancreatic disease, and endocarditis.

Pericardial Effusion

Pericardial effusion is an abnormal accumulation of fluid in the pericardial cavity. When fluid accumulation is significant and compresses the heart, the condition is referred to as *cardiac tamponade*. As intrapericardial pressure is increased, ventricular filling in diastole is impaired. Decreased ventricular filling results in decreased preload, decreased SV, and decreased CO.

There are many potential causes of pericardial effusion. Common causes of acquired pericardial effusion include mesothelioma, cardiac hemangiosarcoma, chemodectomas, bacterial, fungal, or viral infections, foreign body penetration, feline infectious peritonitis (FIP), left atrial rupture and hemorrhage, lymphosarcoma, rhabdomyosarcoma, coagulopathy, and idiopathic pericardial effusion.

Pericardial effusion occurs primarily in older, large breed dogs, but can occur with any signalment (Ettinger and Feldman 2005, p. 1109). Cases may present to the emergency room with a wide variety of presenting chief complaints and signs. Lethargy, dyspnea, anorexia, collapse, abdominal distention, and vomiting may be observed. Common physical exam findings include muffled heart sounds, weak pulses, pale mucous membranes, and ascites. Additional findings may include JVD and pulsus paradoxus.

Thoracic radiographs in these cases are often diagnostic. Pericardial effusions are frequently described as having a round, enlarged, globoid cardiac silhouette. Tracheal elevation and widening of the caudal vena cava may also be observed. Echocardiography is excellent at evaluating suspected cases. Pericardial effusion appears as an anechoic space surrounding the heart. Most dogs with pericardial effusion have ECG findings of either sinus tachycardia or a normal sinus rhythm. Ventricular arrhythmias may also be observed. Unique to pericardial effusion cases is the pathognomonic ECG finding of *electrical alternans* (Fig. 6.8). Electrical alternans is a beat-to-beat variation in the amplitude of the QRS and ST-T complexes (Ettinger and Feldman 2005, p. 1110). This unique phenomena occurs because of a swinging of the heart once every other heartbeat in large pericardial effusions (Fig. 6.9).

Emergency therapy for pericardial effusion includes fluid therapy to combat hypovolemia and careful pericardiocentesis with concurrent ECG monitoring (Fig. 6.10). Treatment for cardiac arrhythmias before and during this procedure may be necessary, and may be indicative of an increased mortality (Humm et al. 2009). Aspirated pericardial fluid should be collected and analyzed, but may not always help yield a clear specific inciting cause (Ettinger and Feldman 2005). Ultimately though, pursuit and treatment of the underlying cause must be addressed.

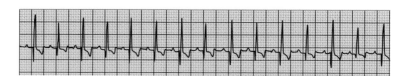

Figure 6.8   An ECG tracing showing electrical "alternans" consistent with pericardial effusion. (Courtesy of Jennifer Keefe, CVT, VTS [Emergency & Critical Care], VTS [Anesthesia].)

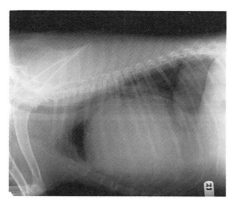

Figure 6.9   A lateral chest radiograph showing a large globoid cardiac silhouette consistent with pericardial disease. (Courtesy of Jennifer Keefe, CVT, VTS [Emergency & Critical Care], VTS [Anesthesia].)

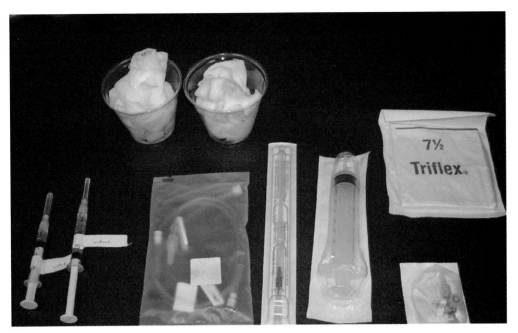

Figure 6.10   Materials commonly used to set up for pericardiocentesis. (Courtesy of Thomas Walker, DVM, DACVECC.)

Infectious Endocarditis (IE)

IE is a fairly uncommon disorder resulting from colonization of the cardiac endocardium by microorganisms. Bacteremia is the most frequent etiology. The result of the endocarditis is eventual destruction of the valve and internal structures of the heart. Vegetative growth may cause thromboembolism if it migrates from the heart and additionally may result in metastatic infection of many body organs.

Medium to large breed male dogs, often purebred, are reported to be predisposed. Because the condition can easily spread to multiple body organs, a wide production of clinical signs may occur. This can make clinical signs variable and diagnosis difficult. Commonly reported signs include fever, newly developed heart murmurs, lameness, lethargy, anorexia, weight loss, and gastrointestinal (GI) disturbances (Ettinger and Feldman 2005). Predisposing factors in combination with clinical signs should raise high suspicion of IE. Such factors include immunosuppression (e.g., corticosteroid administration, diabetes mellitus, hyperadrenocorticism), indwelling catheters, aortic stenosis, recent surgery, trauma to oral mucosa or genital tract, and current infection such as prostatis, abscesses, infected wounds, and pyoderma.

On ECG, arrhythmias may be noted in a large portion of dogs with IE (Ettinger and Feldman 2005). Radiography often will not add additional specific information to help diagnose IE. Valvular vegetative growth may be evident on echocardiogram. Laboratory findings may include a mild non-regenerative anemia, an inflammatory leukogram, and evidence of metastatic spread to any potential organ system.

Ultimately, blood cultures are the gold standard for diagnosis of IE. A consistent positive finding through repeated sampling is valuable to exclude accidental sample contamination. In dogs, frequent microorganisms known to cause IE include *Staphylococcus aureus, Escherichia coli, Pseudomonas aeruginosa, Corynebacterium* spp., *Bartonella vinsonii*, and *Erysipelothrix rhusiopathiae*. Culture and antibiotic sensitivity testing is paramount for correct diagnosis of the offending microorganism and treatment of IE (Ettinger and Feldman 2005). Criteria for definitive diagnosis includes a positive culture from two separate samples plus clinical signs evident of cardiac involvement.

Management of IE is directed at eradicating the offending infective microorganisms and treating all of their secondary systemic consequences. While awaiting culture and antibiotic sensitivity results, high dosages of bactericidal antibiotics should be started intravenously and then later followed by a minimum of 6 weeks on the effective antibiotic. Factors that influence a worse prognosis include gram-negative infection, late diagnosis and late start of antibiotic therapy, septic embolization, aortic valve vegetation, and heart or renal failure that does not respond to therapy (Ettinger and Feldman 2005, p. 1039).

Trauma-Associated Myocardial Injury

Trauma-associated myocardial injury, commonly referred to as traumatic myocarditis or myocardial contusion, is a common occurrence 12–36 hours following thoracic trauma that manifests in cardiac arrhythmias, most frequently of ventricular origin. The pathophysiology of the trauma-induced arrhythmias is unclear but may result from decreased myocardial perfusion after shock and subsequent reperfusion injury. Pharmacological intervention is often not necessary and prior to any antiarrhythmic drug therapy, patients should have their BP normalized, oxygenation deficits corrected, pain management addressed, and electrolyte–acid–base disorders restored.

Indications for treatment with a stabilizing bolus of lidocaine at 2–4 mg/kg IV followed by 50–80 mcg/kg/min CRI in the dog include HRs at or greater than 180 bpm, R on T phenomena, or any arrhythmia that is causing a decrease in CO. Other agents such as procainamide, amiodarone, or esmolol may be selected in refractory cases but most cases respond well to lidocaine when needed. Cases with trauma-associated myocardial injury typically resolve on their own within 2–4 days. Patients are sometimes sent home on oral mexiletine, atenolol, sotalol, or some combination thereof.

Cardiac Arrhythmias

The diagnostic modality of choice for clinical evaluation of cardiac arrhythmias is the ECG (Fig. 6.11). As previously discussed within this chapter, each component of the ECG tracing reflects a specific electrical event within the working heart. The clinical impact of cardiac arrhythmias may range from harmless to potentially life-threatening.

Alterations of sinus excitability

Sinus bradycardia. Sinus bradycardia is a sinus rhythm in which the HR is abnormally low (Fig. 6.12). A 1:1 ratio of normal-appearing QRS complexes and P waves exist. Sinus bradycardia is generally a result of predominance of the parasympathetic system on the heart. The arrhythmia may result from physiological causes or pathological causes. Within the emergency room, frequent causes include athletic individuals, rest or sleep, drugs (opioids, alpha-2 agonists), hyperkalemia, severe hypertension, structural cardiac disease, and feline shock.

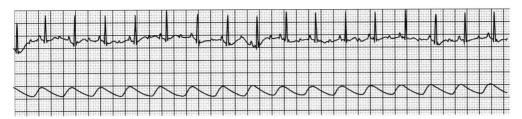

Figure 6.11 An ECG tracing showing a normal sinus rhythm (NSR). (Courtesy of Darci Palmer, RVT, VTS [Anesthesia].)

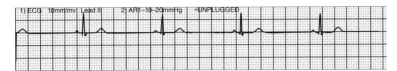

Figure 6.12 An ECG tracing showing sinus bradycardia. (Courtesy of Kristen Cooley, BA, CVT, VTS [Anesthesia].)

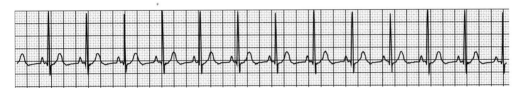

Figure 6.13 An ECG tracing showing a sinus tachycardia. (Courtesy of Kristen Cooley, BA, CVT, VTS [Anesthesia].)

In general, this is a benign arrhythmia that does not require treatment other than identification and, if indicated, treatment of the underlying cause. Only severe bradycardias that diminish BP or results in overt clinical signs (e.g., syncope, weakness) warrant specific therapy with drugs or pacemaker implantation. Antiarrhythmic drugs to consider include parasympatholytics such as atropine or glycopyrrolate and sympathomimetics such epinephrine, dopamine, or isoproterenol. Pacemaker implantation is rarely needed.

Sinus tachycardia. Sinus tachycardia is a sinus rhythm that occurs at an above normal HR (Fig. 6.13). Diagnosis of this arrhythmia on an ECG can be difficult if the rate is very high. A vagal maneuver such as carotid sinus massage or ocular pressure may temporarily slow the rate enough to determine if the rhythm is sinus in origin.

The causes of sinus tachycardia are diverse but ultimately result from activation of the sympathetic nervous system. Frequent reasons from sinus tachycardia seen in the emergency room include pain, anxiety, and excitement, need to urinate, shock states, hyperthyroidism, drug therapy (e.g., ketamine), and other systemic disturbances.

Treatment for sinus tachycardia involves identifying and addressing the underlying cause. This typically includes providing oxygen, fluid therapy, and analgesia.

Atrial disturbances

Atrial standstill. Atrial standstill is characterized by the total absence of atrial depolarization. Therefore, the ECG appearance is of a regular rhythm that lacks a detectable P wave. Causes of atrial standstill include severe hyperkalemia, disease of the atrium, and ECG artifact. Treatment is directed at the underlying cause. Immediate assessment of electrolyte status is warranted and, if indicated, treatment of hyperkalemia.

APDs. APDs, also known as atrial extrasystoles, premature atrial contractions, and APCs or atrial premature contractions, are premature depolarizations that originate in an ectopic part of the atrium. Identification of APDs is made by identifying prematurity of the P-QRS-T sequence, QRS complexes that are narrow and similar in appearance to the sinus QRS complexes (having "supraventricular appearance"), and P waves that are of a different amplitude than the sinus P wave.

The pathogenesis of APDs is not only most commonly related to a structural cardiac (atrial) lesion, but also includes hyperthyroidism, atrial tumors, digitalis toxicity, and other systemic disturbances (Ettinger and Feldman 2005). The clinical repercussions of APDs are generally insignificant unless they occur in repeated bursts (i.e., atrial tachycardia). Treatment is directed at addressing the underlying cause rather than specific drug therapy.

Atrial tachycardia. Atrial tachycardia (supraventricular tachycardia) is a series of three or more APDs in rapid sequence at a rate greater than the sinus rhythm. The arrhythmia may be intermittent or continuous. Causes of atrial tachycardia are the same as for APDs. The clinical impact of atrial tachycardia depends on its duration, rate, and underlying cause. Atrial tachycardia often can precede atrial fibrillation (Ettinger and Feldman 2005). Specific treatment for atrial tachycardia is directed at the identifying cause. Antiarrhythmic drugs to consider include digoxin, class II antiarrhythmics (e.g., propanolol, esmolol), or class IV antiarrhythmics (e.g., diltiazem). Electrocardioversion can also be used for sustained atrial tachycardia (Fig. 6.14).

Atrial fibrillation. Atrial fibrillation is a common arrhythmia that can have potentially serious hemodynamic consequences. Atrial fibrillation is characterized by a complete electrical disorganization at the atrial level. The result is a rapid and uncoordinated series of atrial depolarizations ranging from 400–1200 bpm. The AV node successfully acts as a "gatekeeper" and prevents this erratic atrial activity from spreading to and affecting the ventricles. The AV node, therefore, takes over some control of the ventricular rate.

The ECG characteristics of atrial fibrillation include an absence of P waves, the presence of f (fibrillation) waves, an irregular R-R interval, and a supraventricular-appearing QRS complex (Fig. 6.15). Atrial fibrillation is one of the few cardiac arrhythmias that may be strongly suspected based upon cardiac auscultation. During auscultation, the

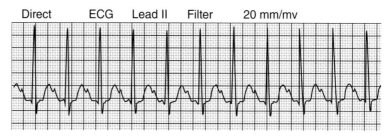

Figure 6.14 An ECG tracing showing atrial tachycardia. (Courtesy of Kristen Cooley, BA, CVT, VTS [Anesthesia].)

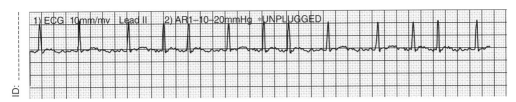

Figure 6.15 An ECG tracing showing atrial fibrillation. (Courtesy of Kristen Cooley, BA, CVT, VTS [Anesthesia].)

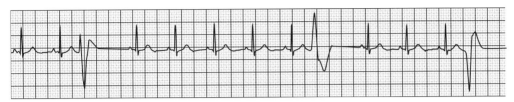

Figure 6.16 An ECG tracing showing a ventricular premature depolarization (VPD). (Courtesy of Kristen Cooley, BA, CVT, VTS [Anesthesia].)

cardiac rhythm is irregular and chaotic, potentially mimicking the sound of shoes in a washing machine or "jungle drums."

Atrial fibrillation in dogs is most often due to an underlying cardiac disease but may also occur in structurally normal heart under anesthesia, with hypothyroidism, pericardiocentesis, GI disease, and volume overload (Ettinger and Feldman 2005). In cats, atrial fibrillation is most commonly due to atrial enlargement secondary to cardiac disease (Ettinger and Feldman 2005).

Two predominant goals exist in the treatment of atrial fibrillation. The first goal is treatment of the underlying cause. The second is aimed at maximizing CO by slowing the rate of conduction through the AV node and therefore slowing the HR. Emergency therapy for atrial fibrillation effecting CO includes digoxin, class II antiarrhythmics (e.g., propanolol, esmolol), or class IV antiarrhythmics (e.g., diltiazem). Lidocaine and electrocardioversion may also be considered.

Ventricular disturbances

Ventricular Premature Depolarizations (VPDs). VPDs (previously known as premature ventricular contractions [PVCs] VPC) are ventricular extrasystoles or depolarizations that occur from an ectopic ventricular location. These arrhythmias are one of the most common rhythm disturbances observed in emergency and critical care settings.

VPDs can be identified on an ECG by the premature wide (>0.07 seconds in the dog) and bizarre looking QRS complex that they generate (Ettinger and Feldman 2005, p. 1060) (Fig. 6.16). Additionally there is P wave dissociation and often a compensatory pause after a single VPD.

The causes for VPDs are extensive. Virtually all cardiac and systemic disorders can result in VPDs. They are most commonly observed in cases with valvular heart disease, cardiomyopathies, congenital heart disease, anemia, hypoxia, gastric dilatation-volvulus syndrome, abdominal masses (e.g., splenic neoplasia), acidosis, hypokalemia, sepsis, myocarditis, trauma, toxicities, anesthetic agents (e.g., thiopental), excessive sympathetic stimulation, and pain.

CHAPTER 6

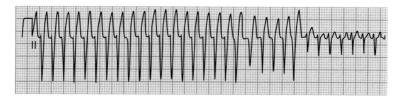

Figure 6.17   An ECG tracing showing ventricular tachycardia. (Courtesy of Trish Farry, CVN, VTS [Emergency & Critical Care], VTS [Anesthesia], Cert IV [TAA].)

Clinical signs of VPDs may be absent or include those of decreased CO: weakness, syncope, and potentially sudden death. VPDs are one of the few arrhythmias that can be tentatively diagnosed via cardiac auscultation. VPDs typically sound as irregular "dropped" beats that occur earlier than expected.

Treatment of isolated or occasional VPDs is likely not necessary. In general, the primary treatment goal for VPDs is to address or eliminate the inciting cause and then control the rhythm and rate so that CO is maximized. Initial treatment for VPDs should include evaluation of oxygenation and oxygen therapy as necessary, fluid therapy to ensure normotension, appropriate analgesia, and evaluation and correction of acid/base/electrolyte disturbances. Specific antiarrhythmic therapy, if required, include class I (lidocaine, procainamide), class II (propanolol, esmolol), and class III (amiodarone) antiarrhythmic agents, or potentially electrical defibrillation.

Ventricular Tachycardia (VT)/Flutter and Accelerated Idioventricular Rhythm (AIVR). VT is defined as three or more VPDs in rapid sequence that occur at an HR at or above 160 bpm (Fig. 6.17). A specific subset of VT, known as AIVR or slow VT, occurs at HRs between 70 and 160 bpm. Ventricular flutter, on the other hand, is a rapid prefibrillatory stage of VT. The causes of VT, AIVR, and ventricular flutter are the same as for VPDs.

The decision as to when to treat arrhythmias of ventricular excitability, such as VT, is a controversial subject. Much of the veterinary recommendations are based upon human literature which may not necessarily extrapolate well to cats and dogs. As VT occurs at higher HRs, the increased ventricular firing rate eventually results in decreased CO, decreased ventricular filling time, and decreased myocardial perfusion. Because of this, VT should likely be treated with drug therapy if the HR is high: >160 bpm in large dogs, >180 bpm in small dogs, and >240 bpm in cats (Ettinger and Feldman 2005). Other proposed indications for drug treatment of ventricular excitability include when "R on T phenomena" is observed, when VPDs are highly polymorphic, or whenever CO appears compromised.

Because ventricular flutter is a severe form of VT and rapidly deteriorates into ventricular fibrillation, it warrants immediate treatment. Although the causes and appearance of AIVR are the same as with VT, AIVR does not require treatment because the slower ventricular rate does not compromise ventricular filling time and therefore is generally well tolerated by the patient.

Treatment for unstable VT and ventricular flutter are identical to that of VPDs. Lidocaine is often selected as an initial drug of choice in the dog, being initially administered at 2 mg/kg IV and repeated as necessary up to a total dose of 8 mg/kg. When the VT or ventricular flutter has converted to a more stable rhythm, a CRI of lidocaine at 40–75 mcg/kg/min is selected (Rozanski and Rush 2007). If the lidocaine is initially ineffective, another drug should be selected. Because of concern of lidocaine toxicity in cats, many either do not use lidocaine as their first choice of antiarrhythmic drug for VT and ventricular flutter in cats, often selecting propanolol instead, or just use lidocaine at a reduced dose. Patients who do not respond to drug therapy should also have their electrolyte levels checked with specific attention paid to potassium and magnesium. Deficiencies in these electrolytes may need to be corrected before drug therapy will be successful.

Torsades de Pointes. Torsades de Pointes is an uncommon form of VT that arises from a prolongation of the QT interval (Ettinger and Feldman 2005). The appearance of Torsades de Pointes on the ECG is that of a ribbon. Causes of the disturbance include hypokalemia, hypocalcemia, and antiarrhythmia drug toxicity (Ettinger and Feldman 2005). Treatment for the rhythm is highly specific and includes discontinuation of all antiarrhythmic drugs and administration of intravenous magnesium sulfate at 20–30 mg/kg IV slowly (Ettinger and Feldman 2005).

AV blocks

AV blocks are disturbances of conduction between the atria and ventricle. Such conduction disturbances can be as simple as a delay or as profound as a complete stoppage. As a result, clinical signs can vary from nonexistent to potentially life-threatening.

First degree AV block. First degree AV block is a simple delay of conduction from the atria to the ventricles. Although conductance is slowed, each impulse does successfully cross to the AV node. A prolonged PR interval with a normal sinus appearing QRS complex is necessary for the diagnosis. There are no clinical manifestations of first degree AV block, and the arrhythmia requires no treatment.

Second degree AV block. Second degree AV block is the result of a complete but transient interruption of conductance from the atria to the ventricles. As a result, P waves are present for every QRS complex but a QRS complex does not exist for every P wave. Second degree AV block is further divided into two subclasses: *Mobitz Type 1*, which is characterized by a progressive lengthening of the PR interval which ultimately results in a P wave that occurs without a QRS complex (Fig. 6.18), and *Mobitz Type 2*, which demonstrates perfectly regular PR intervals for all QRS complexes, but one or more P wave lacks a corresponding QRS complex (Fig. 6.19).

Depending on the ventricular rate and its impact on CO, clinical signs may be absent and require no treatment whatsoever or may produce exercise intolerance, lethargy, syncope, or hypoxic seizures (Stokes–Adams seizures) and require drug intervention.

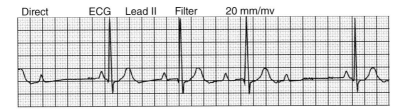

Figure 6.18   An ECG tracing showing a Mobitz Type 1 second degree AV block. (Courtesy of Kristen Cooley, BA, CVT, VTS [Anesthesia].)

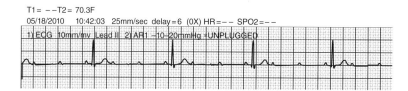

T1= – –T2= 70.3F
05/18/2010   10:42:03   25mm/sec delay=6 (0X) HR=– – SPO2=– –
1) ECG 10mm/mv Lead II 2) AR1 –10–20mmHg UNPLUGGED

Figure 6.19   An ECG tracing showing a Mobitz Type 2 second degree AV block. (Courtesy of Kristen Cooley, BA, CVT, VTS [Anesthesia].)

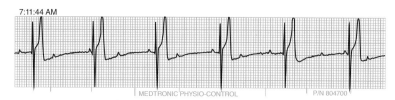

7:11:44 AM

MEDTRONIC PHYSIO-CONTROL   P/N 804700

Figure 6.20   An ECG tracing showing a complete third degree AV block.

The common causes of second degree AV block may include high resting vagal tone, antiarrhythmic agents, opioids, alpha-2 adrenergic agonists, cardiac disease with atrial dilation, and AV nodal lesions (Ettinger and Feldman 2005).

Treatment, if necessitated by diminished CO or clinical signs, is first directed at the underlying cause whenever possible. Acute drug therapy includes parasympatholytic agents (e.g., atropine, glycopyrrolate) and sympathomimetic agents (e.g., dopamine, dobutamine, isoproterenol, epinephrine). Cases that do not respond to drug therapy require pacemaker implantation.

Third degree AV block. Third degree AV block is a complete failure of conductance and total dissociation of the atria and the ventricles (Fig. 6.20). On ECG, there is no consistent PR interval. P waves occur variably with or without QRS complexes. In some cases, P waves may even occur during a QRS complex. The ventricular rate during third degree AV block is generally slow. As a result, marked lethargy, exercise intolerance, weakness, and syncope may result. Some patients may not always exhibit clinical signs (e.g., cats) and may not require treatment.

The causes of third degree AV block include alpha-2 agonist administration, hyperkalemia, cardiac glycoside toxicity, Lyme disease, endocarditis, traumatic myocarditis, cardiomyopathies, endocardiosis, or myocardial fibrosis (Ettinger and Feldman 2005).

Treatment for third degree AV block is aimed at the underlying cause. Drug therapy includes parasympatholytic agents (e.g., atropine, glycopyrrolate) and sympathomimetic agents (e.g., dopamine, dobutamine, isoproterenol, epinephrine) but is generally unrewarding. Symptomatic cases that fail to respond to drug therapy require pacemaker implantation.

References

Ettinger, SJ, Feldman, EC. 2005. *Textbook of Veterinary Internal Medicine*, 6th ed. St. Louis, MO: Elsevier Saunders.

Evans, H. 1993. *Miller's Anatomy of the Dog*, 3rd ed. Philadelphia: Saunders.

Goutal, C, Keri, I, Kenney, S. 2010. Evaluation of acute congestive heart failure in dogs and cats: 145 cases (2007–2008). *J Vet Emerg Crit Care* 20(3):330–337.

Humm, K, Keenaghan-Clarke, E, Boag, A. 2009. Adverse events associated with pericardiocentesis in dogs: 85 cases (1999–2006). *J Vet Emerg Crit Care* 19(4):352–356.

Moore, K, Morris, N, Dhupa, N, et al. 2007. Retrospective study of streptokinase administration in 46 cats with arterial thromboembolism. *J Vet Emerg Crit Care* 10(2):103–106.

Oyama, MA, Rush, JE, Rozanksi, EA, et al. 2009. Assessment of serum N-terminal pro-B-type natriuretic peptide concentration for differentiation of congestive heart failure from primary respiratory tract disease as the cause of respiratory signs in dogs. *J Am Vet Med Assoc* 235:1319–1325.

Plunkett, SJ. 2001. *Emergency Procedure for the Small Animal Veterinarian*, 2nd ed. Philadelphia: W.B. Saunders.

Rozanski, EA, Rush, JE. 2007. *Small Animal Emergency and Critical Care Medicine*, 1st ed. London: Manson.

CHAPTER 6

Respiratory Emergencies

Dana Heath and *Lori Baden Atkins*

Introduction

Respiratory disorders are common in small animals and account for a significant number of emergency visits and hospitalizations. Respiratory distress or dyspnea may be a direct result of toxin exposure, trauma, an acute exacerbation of chronic conditions, secondary to infectious processes, or fluid shifts.

Patients in respiratory distress are often anxious and are easily stressed. Physical examination, diagnostics, and treatments may need to be staged and the patient allowed to rest in an oxygen-rich environment between procedures. Overzealous handling of respiratory distress patients, particularly felines, may significantly worsen dyspnea and can have fatal consequences.

Anatomy of the Respiratory System

The main function of the respiratory system is to provide the body with a continuous source of gas exchange between the inspirited air and the circulatory system. This gas exchange system includes supplying the body with oxygen during inspiration and removing carbon dioxide (CO_2) during expiration. Room air at sea level contains 21% oxygen. Upon inspiration, oxygen enters the body through the nose or mouth, travels through the pharynx and on to the trachea. The trachea enters the chest thoracic cavity and then divides at the carina into two bronchi and enters the lungs. Each *bronchi* serves to provide oxygen to one lung; the left bronchi supporting the left lung and the right bronchi supporting the right lung. The left lung is made up of a cranial, middle, caudal, and accessory lung lobe. The left lung, however, is composed only of a cranial and caudal lobe, with the cranial lobe having a cranial and caudal portion. With each lung lobe, their respective bronchi then divide further into smaller *bronchioles*. Finally at the end of each smaller bronchiole are clusters of alveoli. It is here at the alveoli where gas exchange with the circulatory system occurs via the *alveolar–capillary membrane*.

The pleura is a thin membrane that encases the lungs and covers the inner walls of the thoracic cavity. This membrane is covered with a thin film of serous fluid, which provides lubrication as the lungs expand and contract within the thoracic cavity. The area within the pleura is called the pleural cavity and is normally in a state of negative pressure. This negative pressure or vacuum causes the lungs to expand and contract in conjunction with the expansion and contraction of the thoracic cavity. Loss of the normal negative pressure within the thoracic cavity typically results in respiratory distress and may lead to collapse of one or more lung lobes.

Mechanics of Normal Respiration

Normal respiration is dependent upon the contraction and relaxation of the diaphragm, the contraction and relaxation of the chest and abdominal muscles, and the negative pressure that exists within the pleural cavity. Inspiration occurs as contraction of the diaphragm, and forward, outward movement of the ribs and chest muscles enlarge the thoracic cavity. The abdominal muscles relax, allowing the abdominal organs to move caudally as the diaphragm contracts. The expansion of the thoracic cavity causes expansion of the lungs, and air is drawn in through the bronchial tree and into the alveoli. Following inspiration, the muscles of the abdomen contract and push the abdominal organs forward into the caudal aspect of the diaphragm. The diaphragm is pushed forward into the thoracic cavity as it returns to its normal, resting position. The muscles of the chest draw the ribs inward toward the chest. These actions decrease the size of the thoracic cavity and expel air out of the lungs in expiration.

Respiratory Physiology

Delivery of Oxygen

Adequate tissue oxygenation is governed by a combination of processes including external respiration, oxygen transport, and internal respiration. Any impairment of these processes may lead to inadequate oxygenation of the tissues and subsequent cellular damage or death.

External respiration involves the inhalation of oxygen into the lungs, diffusion of oxygen molecules onto the red blood cells, and exhalation of CO_2. During normal respiration, air is drawn into the nasal passages where is it warmed and humidified as it passes over the nasal turbinates en route to the lungs. Once air reaches the alveoli, oxygen diffuses through the alveolar–capillary membrane, where it binds with the hemoglobin (Hb) in the red blood cells (RBCs) to form oxyhemoglobin (HbO_2).

Oxygen transport involves the ability to move oxygen from the alveoli to the tissues. Hb is the primary carrier of oxygen; each molecule has the capacity to carry four oxygen molecules. Under normal physiological conditions, it is assumed that Hb will bind oxygen to all four sites and will have an oxygen saturation (SaO_2) of >97%. Once oxygen is bound by Hb, it is transported to the tissues as blood is circulated throughout the body by the cardiovascular system.

At the cellular level, oxygen molecules disassociate from the Hb and diffuse into the cells. Approximately 80%–90% of the oxygen diffused into the cell is consumed by the mitochondria during production of adenosine triphosphate (ATP), which is then utilized by cell for energy.

CO_2

CO_2 is the major by-product of cellular oxygen metabolism. Although often thought of as a waste product, CO_2 actually plays a significant role in maintaining acid–base balance. CO_2 combines with water (H_2O) to form carbonic acid, which quickly dissolves into hydrogen ions (H^+) and bicarbonate ions (HCO_3^-). The pH is directly affected by the ratio of CO_2 to HCO_3^-.

The primary route for excretion of CO_2 is through exhalation following transport to the alveoli. After conversion of CO_2 into HCO_3^-, a chloride shift occurs as HCO_3^- are released into the plasma by the RBCs in exchange for chloride ions. Bicarbonate is transported to the alveoli in the plasma, where it combines with hydrogen ions to form carbonic acid, and is then separated into CO_2 and water. The CO_2 diffuses across the alveolar–capillary membrane and is exhaled as a waste gas. A small amount (~20%) of CO_2 binds to Hb as carbaminohemoglobin and is exchanged for oxygen at the alveoli without further chemical conversion.

Hypoxemia versus Hypoxia

There are a number of terms used to describe oxygenation and ventilation; an understanding of these terms is essential.

Oxygenation—Saturation with oxygen.
Ventilation—The exchange of oxygen and CO_2 through inhalation and exhalation.
Hypoxemia—Deficiency of oxygen within the blood. Patients breathing room air at sea level are considered hypoxemic when the partial pressure of oxygen in arterial blood (PaO_2) is less than 80 mmHg.
Hypoxia—Decreased oxygenation of the tissues.
Anemic hypoxia—Decreased oxygenation of the tissues secondary to decreased level of Hb. Anemic hypoxia may also be observed in conditions where the Hb

is unable to bind and transport oxygen such as methemoglobinemia and carboxyhemoglobinemia.

Ischemic hypoxia—Decreased oxygenation of the tissues secondary to decreased perfusion. Ischemic hypoxia may be global as demonstrated by hypovolemic or cardiogenic shock or local as demonstrated by thromboembolic disease.

Causes of Hypoxemia

Hypoxemia may be caused by any number of conditions that interfere with the body's ability to access oxygen during respiration and transport the oxygen molecules to the RBCs. A *decreased fractional inspired oxygen concentration* (FiO_2) may result in hypoxemia. A healthy patient breathing room air ($FiO_2 = 21\%$) is expected to have a PaO_2 of 80–100 mmHg ($PaO_2 = 4$–$5 \times FiO_2$). This is sometimes referred to as the *5 times inspired rule*. When the concentration of inspired oxygen is decreased, the patient's PaO_2 should decrease in a corresponding manner. Increasing the percentage of inspired oxygen easily treats this form of hypoxemia.

Hypoventilation may result in hypoxemia as CO_2 replaces oxygen within the alveoli, with a subsequent decrease in the PaO_2. Hypoventilation is manifested by an increase in the partial pressure of CO_2 in arterial blood ($PaCO_2$); patients with a $PaCO_2 > 40$ mmHg are considered to be hypoventilating. Oxygen therapy may be temporarily beneficial in the hypoventilatory patient, but definitive treatment requires assisted or mechanical ventilation to allow the removal of CO_2. The arterial CO_2 concentration provides the primary impetus for alveolar ventilation. In the normal patient, ventilation increases as the $PaCO_2$ rises and conversely decreases as the $PaCO_2$ falls. This homeostatic mechanism may not be functional in certain conditions and disease states including depression of the respiratory center by certain drugs or anesthetics, diseases affecting the central nervous system (CNS), and diseases of the respiratory muscles or chest wall. Patients with these conditions are not able to compensate by increasing ventilation as the $PaCO_2$ rises. Oxygen therapy, without assisted ventilation, should be used cautiously in these patients. In the presence of severe hypercapnia ($PaCO_2 > 80$ mmHg), regulation of ventilatory drive in response to CO_2 fails and hypoxia becomes the trigger for ventilation.

Hypoxemia is often secondary to conditions that interfere with oxygen diffusion through the alveoli and into the capillaries. Diffusion is typically discussed as the relationship between alveolar ventilation (V) and pulmonary blood flow or perfusion (Q); inequality in this relationship denotes impaired diffusion and is termed *V/Q mismatch*. Pulmonary thromboembolism results in a very high V/Q mismatch as the lung is adequately oxygenated while perfusion is decreased. Asthma, pneumonia, pulmonary edema, and any other pulmonary disease that results in poor ventilation or partial alveolar collapse may result in a low V/Q mismatch due to decreased oxygen availability with adequate perfusion. Other causes of V/Q mismatch include pulmonary dead space and pulmonary shunting. Oxygen therapy may be efficacious for low V/Q mismatch but frequently needs to be augmented by positive end expiratory pressure (PEEP) in order to maximize the oxygen delivery to the alveoli.

Causes of Hypoxia

Hypoxia frequently develops following hypoxemia, unless effective intervention is employed. Anemia is a common initiator of hypoxia. Any functional decrease in the number of RBCs or the Hb concentration of the RBCs results in a net decrease in the oxygen-carrying capacity of the blood. The normal Hb concentration for dogs and cats is ~12–15 g Hb/dL. Additionally, any chemical change that impairs the Hb from binding with oxygen molecules may cause a significant decrease in the oxygen-carrying capacity of the blood. Patients exposed to carbon monoxide will form carboxyhemoglobin. Due to its high affinity for Hb (~218× greater than oxygen), carbon monoxide will bind to the Hb molecules, rendering them nonfunctional in an oxygen-carrying capacity. Methemoglobinemia may be observed secondary to acetaminophen toxicity in cats and other toxins such as nitrites, phenol, sulfites, and naphthalene in both cats and dogs. Every 1.5 g/dL of methemoglobin is equivalent to a 5 g/dL decrease in functional Hb. Treatment of anemic hypoxia should involve replacement of functional RBCs or Hb through blood transfusion or Oxyglobin® (OPK Biotech LLC, Cambridge, MA) and concurrent oxygen supplementation. Treatment of the underlying cause of anemia is typically required to achieve a long-term positive outcome.

Ischemic hypoxia results from inadequate perfusion, resulting in decreased tissue oxygenation. Conditions such as hypovolemic shock, circulatory failure, and severe hemorrhage classically result in decreased tissue perfusion throughout the body and a corresponding decrease in the delivery of oxygen to the tissues. Localized hypoxia may result from loss of perfusion to specific organs or regions as seen in thromboembolic disease. Treatment of ischemic hypoxia involves increasing perfusion. In addition to volume replacement, effective treatment of hypovolemic shock must also address the underlying cause. Bleeding due to laceration may be controlled by the use of a pressure bandage, while hemorrhage caused by hepatic or splenic rupture will typically require immediate surgical intervention. Treatment of circulatory failure must focus on improving cardiac output, thereby restoring tissue perfusion and oxygenation. Oxygen therapy should be instituted concurrently with restoration of perfusion.

Assessment of Oxygenation and Ventilation

Observation of either increased or depressed respiratory effort is a common indicator of hypoventilation and possible hypoxemia. Conditions that lead to decreased lung compliance such as pneumonia, pleural effusion, and pulmonary edema are typified by a pattern of rapid, shallow breathing; obstructive conditions such as asthma and laryngeal paralysis are characterized by slow, deep breaths. Observations should be made regarding the phase of ventilation requiring increased effort: is the patient working harder during the inspiratory phase or the expiratory phase? Increased inspiratory effort is consistent with diseases of the upper airway such as laryngeal paralysis while increased expiratory effort is associated with obstructive conditions of the lower airway such as asthma. Observation of a significant abdominal effort with minimal thoracic excursions during ventilation may be indicative of hypoventilation. Dyspneic patients frequently modify their posture to reduce airway resistance; elevation of the head and extension of the neck straightens the trachea while abduction of the elbows minimizes compression of the chest wall.

Physical evaluation of the clinically dyspneic patient must be approached with caution, especially in the cat. These patients are often very unstable; diagnostics and treatments are usually performed in stages to avoid further stress to the patient. Mucous membrane (MM) color and capillary refill time (CRT) may be easily assessed and may yield significant information regarding the patient's oxygenation and perfusion status. Cyanotic mucous membranes indicate severe hypoxemia; the SaO_2 of arterial blood is typically <80% in patients with clinical cyanosis. Cyanosis may not be evident in anemic patients; the blue color associated with cyanosis is not detectable in desaturated Hb concentrations of <5 g/dL. Patients with poor perfusion secondary to shock or anemia will typically demonstrate pale mucous membranes and cyanosis may not be readily apparent. Carbon monoxide poisoning is typified by cherry red mucous membranes, while chocolate brown mucous membranes are indicative of methemoglobin; both indicate a change in the ability of the Hb to bind and transport oxygen. Prolonged CRT is indicative of poor perfusion.

Auscultation of the thorax may reveal crackles indicative of fluid within the alveoli secondary to pulmonary edema or pneumonia. Wheezes are indicative of narrowed respiratory passages secondary to inflammation, mucous accumulation, or other obstructive processes. Pneumothorax, pleural effusion, diaphragmatic hernia, and other pleural spaces diseases often result in diminished or absent lung or heart sounds upon auscultation. Cardiac auscultation may reveal murmurs or arrhythmias, which may be indicative of decreased perfusion.

Measurement of packed cell volume (PCV) will give an estimation of the number of RBCs and the patient's ability to transport oxygen via the Hb in the RBCs. Pulse oximetry, capnography, and arterial blood gases (ABGs) are additional methods of measuring oxygenation and ventilation. They will be discussed in further detail in later chapters within this book.

Tracheostomy Tubes

A temporary tracheotomy tube may be placed in severe respiratory conditions that compromise the upper airway or when surgical procedures within the upper airway do not allow for orotracheal intubation.

Care of the tracheostomy is as important as the placement procedure itself (Figs. 7.1 and 7.2). Tracheostomy tubes require intensive care and continuous monitoring to prevent life-threatening complications such as inadvertent tube removal or occlusion from blood or mucus.

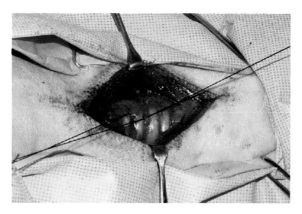

Figure 7.1   When time allows, a tracheostomy tube should be placed surgically under sterile conditions. In some cases, with a patient dying before your eyes, time does not allow for this.

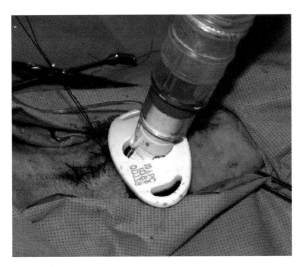

Figure 7.2   There is an old adage that the best time for clinicians to place a tracheostomy tube is when the thought first crosses their mind. Waiting longer may compromise patient survival.

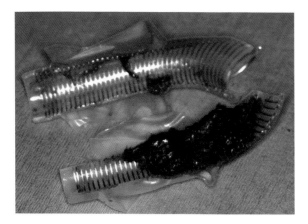

Figure 7.3   Regular tracheostomy tube care is important to prevent complications. Here, a large obstruction was identified obstructing air passage upon tube removal.

Maintenance of a temporary tracheostomy requires intermittently removing and cleaning the tube or inner cannula (every 4–6 hours), suctioning the trachea carefully as needed, cleaning the stoma, and providing humidification. Normally, the upper airway system humidifies air as it is inhaled. Breathing air directly into the trachea bypasses the normal humidification system, causing mucosal irritation and increased mucus secretion.

Suctioning is performed aseptically with a small sterile suction catheter or red rubber tube and should only last for approximately 10 seconds. Oxygen should be supplied to the patient during the suctioning procedure to minimize hypoxia and stress. Initially, the bandage should be changed and the stoma cleaned twice daily or when visibly soiled. Humidification should be provided hourly by instilling 0.2 mL/kg of sterile saline into the tube or by nebulization. Humidification is very important and will help to prevent secretions from becoming too thick to be cleared by normal means (Fig. 7.3).

Specific Respiratory Disorders

Upper Airway

Laryngeal paralysis

Laryngeal paralysis occurs when innervation of the intrinsic laryngeal muscles is disrupted, resulting in complete or partial failure of the arytenoid cartilages and vocal folds to abduct during inspiration and adduct during expiration. Acquired idiopathic laryngeal paralysis is the most common form, with congenital forms reported to affect certain breeds including Bouvier des Flandres, Siberian huskies, Labrador retrievers, Dalmatians, Rottweilers, English setters, and English bull terriers.

Clinical signs. Signs of laryngeal paralysis are progressive inspiratory stridor, noisy respirations, voice changes, exercise intolerance, heat intolerance, and various levels of dyspnea, cyanosis, and panting. Severe cases may exhibit hyperthermia, coughing, or gagging associated with ingestion of food or water, vomiting, restlessness, and anxiety. Exercise, excitement, obesity, and high temperatures may exacerbate the condition. The severity of the disease usually correlates with the degree of abduction, unilateral versus bilateral paralysis, and the level of exertion. Severely affected animals present with marked respiratory distress, cyanosis, and collapse. A common complication of laryngeal paralysis is aspiration pneumonia; this may be the first indication of the condition in previously undiagnosed patients.

Diagnosis. Lateral cervical and thoracic radiographic images are essential to rule out other abnormalities and evaluate for aspiration pneumonia. A definitive diagnosis requires the evaluation of laryngeal function under a light plane of general anesthesia (e.g., thiopental or propofol). Oxygen supplementation via flow-by is crucial during evaluation of the arytenoids and larynx; the patient is intubated once the evaluation is complete. Patients affected by unilateral paralysis will only move one side of their arytenoids while bilateral paralysis affects both sides.

Treatment. Asymptomatic laryngeal paralysis often requires no treatment, but owners should be counseled regarding the need to maintain their pets at a healthy weight and avoid excessive exercise and overheating as these may exacerbate the condition. Patients with moderate to severe respiratory distress presenting to the emergency room require oxygen supplementation, sedation (e.g., acepromazine and butorphanol), corticosteroids to reduce inflammation, and cooling measures if the patient is hyperthermic; severely dyspneic animals may require immediate rapid sequence induction (RSI) and intubation until upper airway inflammation resolves. When not in crisis, these animals should be maintained in a quiet, non-stressful environment and handled with minimal restraint to prevent struggling which may increase oxygen consumption. The only definite therapy for laryngeal paralysis is corrective surgery. A unilateral cricoarytenoid lateralization, or "tieback," can be performed and involves changing the anatomy of the larynx by permanently fixing it in a semi-open position by suture prosthesis. This allows for more normal flow of oxygen to the patient's lungs.

Collapsing trachea

The trachea is a flexible tubular structure made up of smooth muscle, soft tissue, and C-shaped, circular cartilaginous rings connecting the upper (oral, nasal, pharyngeal, and laryngeal sections) airways and the lower (bronchial and bronchiolar) airways. The trachea spans both the extrathoracic and intrathoracic portions of the respiratory tract. In the dog, "tracheal collapse" refers to a condition of excessive collapsibility of the trachea, usually resulting in a flattening of the tracheal lumen (O'Brien et al. 1966; Amis 1974; Done and Drew 1976; Nelson 1993; Hedlund 1991). Tracheal collapse is associated with tracheal trauma, compressive extraluminal masses, tracheal hypoplasia, and intraluminal masses. The tracheal cartilages lose the ability to maintain their rigidity, leading to the upper portion of the trachea collapsing during inspiration and the thoracic trachea collapsing during expiration. The resulting collapse reduces the tracheal lumen size, thereby interfering with or obstructing airflow from reaching the lungs.

Tracheal collapse is a common cause of airway obstruction and is typically diagnosed in middle-aged toy and miniature breeds such as Yorkshire terriers, toy Poodles, Pugs, Pomeranians, Chihuahuas and Maltese. Collapsing trachea in large breed dogs is typically associated with tracheal trauma, intraluminal or extraluminal masses, or deformity.

Clinical signs and diagnosis. Patients may present showing clinical signs ranging from mild to severe respiratory distress. Symptoms may include exercise intolerance, abnormal respiratory noises (wheezing, hacking, coughing), and stridorous breathing; severe cases often exhibit a characteristic "goose honk" cough, respiratory distress, cyanosis, syncope, open mouth breathing, and abduction of forelimbs with labored breathing. Clinical signs may be more severe in obese patients. Exercise, excitement, drinking, eating, tracheal infections, tracheal compression (neck collars), or hot, humid weather frequently elicits or exacerbates clinical symptoms.

Diagnosis. Diagnostic imaging techniques including lateral radiographs (both inspiratory and expiratory) of neck and thorax, tracheal ultrasound, and fluoroscopy usually demonstrate excessive narrowing of the trachea and are considered diagnostic for tracheal collapse. Tracheobronchoscopy may reveal the presence of a mass or anatomical defect. Submission of tracheal secretions for cytology and culture and sensitivity can also provide valuable diagnostic information (Fig. 7.4).

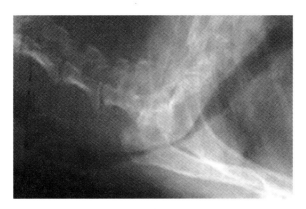

Figure 7.4   Because collapsing trachea is a dynamic disease, both inspiratory and expiratory thoracic radiographs are needed to evaluate the condition's presence. Even then, some cases can be overlooked.

Treatment. Methods for therapy are conservative medical management and surgical correction. Affected dogs should be maintained in an environment free of respiratory irritants, smoke, or allergens and be encouraged to lose weight. Medical therapy often provides transient relief and rarely impedes the disease progression.

Surgical intervention with the placement of tracheal stents and prosthesis are two options potentially available for correction. The feasibility and success of these procedures are dependent on the degree and location of the tracheal collapse.

Lower Airway

Pulmonary contusions

Pulmonary contusions are a frequent finding following thoracic trauma; damaged capillaries within the lung tissue hemorrhage into the alveoli and bronchioli. Blood and fluid accumulate in the alveoli creating a barrier preventing normal gas exchange across the alveolar–capillary membrane and resulting in venous admixture and hypoxemia. Additional factors which may increase the severity of respiratory compromise include decreased cardiac output from shock or cardiovascular injury and hypoventilation secondary to pain.

Clinical signs and diagnosis. Clinical signs of pulmonary contusions vary in severity and include thoracic pain and mild to severe dyspnea. Coughing, cyanosis, and hemoptysis (coughing up blood) are typically indicative of severe pulmonary contusions. While radiographs are helpful to confirm a diagnosis of pulmonary contusion, it is important to note that radiographic changes are not usually apparent for the first 6–12 hours following the traumatic incident. Diagnosis is based on clinical signs and physical exam findings, radiographs, and a history of thoracic trauma; auscultation often reveals increased bronchovesicular sounds or crackles. ABG monitoring is beneficial to determine the severity of hypoxemia and to monitor therapy.

Treatment. Hypoxemia is treated with supplementation of oxygen via nasal cannula or oxygen cage; severe cases may require mechanical ventilation. Analgesics are imperative to reduce pain and improve ventilation. Intravenous fluids may be required to improve cardiac output and improve perfusion; fluid therapy should be carefully monitored to avoid overload and leakage into the pulmonary interstitial. While diuretics are not generally indicated for treatment of pulmonary contusions, they may be required to treat fluid overload or pulmonary edema. Corticosteroids and antibiotics do not provide benefit to patients with pulmonary contusions.

Feline asthma

The term feline asthma is typically used to describe a hypersensitivity reaction in cats characterized by pulmonary bronchoconstriction, eosinophilic airway inflammation, and airway edema.

Symptoms and diagnosis. Symptoms of feline asthma vary in severity from chronic, mild inflammation to acute, severe disease. Mild cases may be characterized by occasional cough, which may be exacerbated by environmental changes. Patients with severe disease may present with significant dyspnea, crackles, or harsh lung sounds; the classic respiratory pattern is a prolonged expiratory phase, and wheezes are frequently auscultated during this phase.

Diagnosis is based on symptoms and physical exam. Radiographs may demonstrate alveolar or interstitial infiltrates, air trapping, peribronchial cuffing, and flattening of the diaphragm; normal radiographs do not preclude a diagnosis of feline asthma. Samples collected via bronchoalveolar wash are typically inflammatory. Eosinophilia may be noted on the leukogram.

Treatment. Cats presenting in respiratory distress are extremely fragile and require very gentle handling. The patient should be placed in an oxygen cage or treated with supplemental oxygen via mask or flow-by. Administration of an inhaled bronchodilator (e.g., albuterol) often demonstrates rapid, dramatic improvement of respiratory symptoms; best results are achieved by utilization of a metered dose inhaler attached to a spacer and a mask designed for cats. An injectable bronchodilator such as terbutaline or aminophylline may also be selected.

Corticosteroids are considered the primary treatment for feline asthma. Inhaled steroids generally have fewer systemic side effects and may be preferred over systemic drugs. Moderate to severe cases may be treated with a course of oral prednisone or intravenous dexamethasone in acute exacerbations.

Near drowning

In human medicine, the term drowning is used to describe a fatality within 24 hours of a submersion incident. Near drowning is used to describe an incident in which the victim survives for more than 24 hours following submersion. The salinity of the water involved in the incident is a primary determinant of the ensuing pathophysiology.

Salt water aspiration

Aspiration of salt water typically results in alveolar flooding as fluid moves from the capillary beds into the alveoli due to increased osmolarity. Hypoxemia ensues as the fluid in the alveoli forms a barrier that interferes with normal gas exchange across the alveolar–capillary membrane.

Another prominent feature of salt water aspiration is hypovolemia and hypotension secondary to redistribution of intravascular fluid. In cases involving aspiration of large quantities of salt water, hypernatremia and other electrolyte abnormalities may be significant.

Fresh water aspiration

The primary concern in fresh water aspiration is dilution of alveolar surfactant with subsequent collapse of the alveoli and pulmonary atelectasis. Severe hypoxemia is attributable to several factors including the presence of fluid in the alveoli and ventilation-perfusion (V/Q) mismatch with intrapulmonary shunting secondary to alveolar collapse and atelectasis.

Dry drowning

In a small number of victims, severe laryngospasm occurs during submersion and prevents aspiration of any significant quantity of water. Hypoxemia develops rapidly, and the victim loses consciousness; if the laryngospasm persists, severe hypoxia leads to cardiac arrest. Patients that survive the initial submersion often develop noncardiogenic pulmonary edema secondary to intrathoracic pressure changes associated with continued respiratory efforts in the presence of persistent laryngospasm.

Cold water immersion

Hypothermia develops rapidly following submersion in frigid water. Blood is preferentially shunted to cerebral and coronary circulation through peripheral vasoconstriction. Severe bradycardia ensues, and the metabolic rate drops significantly, decreasing the oxygen requirement and protecting the vital organs from some of the effects of hypoxemia. Prolonged hypothermia may result in fatal cardiac conduction disturbances and arrhythmias.

Clinical signs and diagnosis. Symptoms of drowning vary slightly depending upon the salinity and temperature of the water, but there are several prominent features. All drowning victims have had some degree of contact with water or fluid in a volume sufficient to immerse the nares and oral cavity. Typical symptoms include dyspnea, tachypnea, tachycardia or bradycardia, hypothermia, anxiety, altered level of consciousness, metabolic acidosis, coughing, pink-tinged or frothy fluid in oropharynx, apnea, and cardiac arrest.

Near drowning should be suspected in patients presenting with any of these symptoms and a history of exposure or access to water. These animals should be closely examined and monitored for hypoxemia and other complications.

Treatment. The initial treatment in drowning or suspected drowning is administration of 100% oxygen. Patients that are unable to maintain a $PaO_2 > 80\,mmHg$ on a FiO_2 of 100% may require assisted or mechanical ventilation.

Submersion in water typically results in hypothermia as body temperature drops approximately 25 times faster in cold water as compared to air at the same temperature. Warming measures including dry blankets, circulating warm water or air blankets, and warm IV fluids should be instituted. In severe hypothermia, more aggressive core-warming strategies including warm peritoneal lavage and pleural irrigation may be required. In the event of cardiac arrest in the severely hypothermic patient, resuscitation efforts must be continued until the patient is normothermic.

ABGs, acid–base status, and electrolytes should be closely monitored. During submersion, patients often ingest significant quantities of water. Fresh water aspiration and ingestion may lead to significant hemodilution as water moves into the intravascular spaces; salt water aspiration and ingestion frequently leads to hypovolemia as fluid shifts into the alveoli and stomach due to the higher osmolarity of the salt water. IV fluid therapy should be tailored to meet the needs of the individual patient.

Bronchospasm or bronchial irritation is common following fluid aspiration. Patients should be monitored closely and may benefit from administration of an IV or inhaled bronchodilator.

A significant number of patients will vomit or regurgitate stomach contents and are at substantial risk of aspiration pneumonia following the initial incident. Other complicating factors in near drowning may include aspiration of contaminants, chemicals, infectious organisms, or foreign materials from the water. Early and aggressive antibiotic therapy is warranted if signs of infection develop. Bronchoaveolar lavage (BAL) is indicated in patients demonstrating signs of respiratory infection; samples should be submitted to identify organisms and susceptibilities.

Smoke inhalation

In addition to extreme heat, fire produces numerous toxic by-products of combustion including carbon monoxide, hydrogen cyanide, nitrogen dioxide, hydrogen chloride, benzene, aldehydes, and ammonia (Demling and Desanti 2005). Victims of smoke inhalation frequently exhibit airway injury secondary to thermal or chemical burns as well as systemic manifestations of chemical poisoning from substances such as carbon monoxide and hydrogen cyanide.

Primary hypoxia may also result from a significant decrease in FiO_2. Fire within an enclosed area rapidly consumes oxygen and produces CO_2; the total percentage of oxygen may drop to 15%.

Thermal injury. Inhalation of superheated gases causes direct thermal injury to the oral cavity and upper airways. Swelling and edema formation typically develop within 1–12 hours but may be delayed up to 72 hours following the initial injury and may be moderate to life-threatening dependent upon the severity of the damage. Deep burns of the neck and face frequently exacerbate the degree of swelling and airway obstruction.

Chemical injury. Significant irritation and chemical burns are induced by inhalation of noxious by-products of combustion. Hydrogen chloride reacts with the moisture in the mucous membranes to form hydrochloric acid. Both acrolein, an aldehyde by-product of wood, and hydrochloric acid cause protein denaturation and cell death upon contact with pulmonary tissues. Initial symptoms include bronchospasm and bronchorrhea (excessive mucous production in the bronchi) and are evidenced by wheezing, dyspnea, and chest pain. Chemical irritation of the airway leads to inflammation and pulmonary edema formation 2–48 hours following exposure. V/Q mismatch and hypoxia develop secondary to airway constriction.

Systemic toxicities. Carbon monoxide and hydrogen cyanide are highly toxic; a high rate of fatalities associated with inhalation of these gases is well documented in human medicine. Carbon monoxide competitively binds with Hb in the red blood cells to create carboxyhemoglobin, which dramatically decreases the ability to transport oxygen. Hb has a much higher affinity for carbon monoxide (200–250×) than for oxygen; therefore, even a small percentage can have profound effects. Hypoxia is further exacerbated as carboxyhemoglobin shifts the HbO_2 dissociation curve to the left, decreasing the ability of Hb to release bound oxygen to the tissues (Dobratz 2002). Carbon monoxide can also bind to myoglobin and may lead to cardiac toxicity and renal failure. Cyanide poisoning inhibits aerobic metabolism in the tissue cells, resulting in lactic acidosis and cellular hypoxia.

Clinical signs. Signs of smoke inhalation vary depending upon the chemicals and gases inhaled, length of exposure to smoke and high temperatures, and underlying conditions. Initial symptoms include ocular irritation and tearing, coughing, wheezing, laryngospasm, and bronchospasm. Prolonged exposure results in significant hypoxia, and patients may present with altered mental status, seizures, or loss of consciousness. Dermal burns, especially on the face or neck, are indicative of significant exposure to extremely high temperatures and corresponding thermal trauma to the airway should be presumed.

Diagnosis. Any patient presenting with a history of exposure to smoke or fire should be closely monitored at least 24 hours for signs of smoke inhalation injury. Diagnosis is based on history and clinical symptoms. Since carboxyhemoglobin does not significantly affect PaO_2 or SaO_2 measurements, blood gas analysis is not a dependable method for diagnosis of carbon monoxide toxicity. The use of pulse oximetry is also unreliable as it cannot differentiate between HbO_2, methemoglobin, and carboxyhemoglobin. Carbon monoxide toxicity can be diagnosed through evaluation of arterial blood samples in a co-oximeter or by measurement of serum carboxyhemoglobin levels.

Persistent metabolic acidosis in patients following fluid volume resuscitation and restoration of sufficient cardiac output is suggestive of impaired oxygen transport and may be attributable to carbon monoxide or cyanide toxicity.

Thoracic radiographs may show various changes including alveolar, interstitial, and peribronchial.

Treatment. Early and aggressive oxygen therapy is essential for treatment of smoke inhalation injuries and associated hypoxia. FiO_2 levels of 100% accelerate the rate at which carbon monoxide disassociates from Hb, decreasing the elimination half-life from 4–6 hours at room air to 40–60 minutes (Serebrisky et al. 2010). Pharyngeal and laryngeal swelling and edema can occur rapidly; severe cases may result in asphyxiation due to airway occlusion. Emergency intubation or tracheostomy is indicated if the airway is significantly compromised.

Bronchoconstriction is common due to thermal and chemical irritation of the airways. Administration of IV or inhaled bronchodilators may ease constriction and assist in clearance of mucous and particulate matter from the airways. Administration of humidified oxygen, along with nebulization and coupage, will also help to clear secretions.

Judicious intravenous fluid therapy with a balanced electrolyte solution is indicated to restore and maintain tissue perfusion. Hydration status should be closely monitored to avoid fluid overload and minimize the risk of pulmonary edema. Administration of corticosteroids is controversial; there is no strong evidence that their use is beneficial at this time.

Many victims of smoke inhalation will develop significant ocular irritation which may progress to corneal ulcerations. Treatment consists of topical, broad-spectrum antibiotics and prevention of self-trauma. Systemic antibiotics are indicated if pulmonary infections develop; patients requiring mechanical ventilation are especially susceptible and should be monitored closely.

Pneumonia

Pneumonia is an inflammation of the pulmonary parenchyma which typically results in exudate infiltration of the alveoli. Bacterial pathogens are the most common cause of pneumonia in small animals; other less common etiologies include viral, fungal, protozoal, and parasitic organisms, aspiration of gastric contents, chemical irritants, and smoke inhalation (Reiss and McKiernan 2002).

Certain patient populations are considered to be at higher risk for development of pneumonia. Animals with impaired immunity secondary to diabetes mellitus, Cushing's disease, renal disease, and leukopenia are more susceptible to infectious organisms, as are patients receiving immune-suppressive therapeutics. Viral infections including feline leukemia virus, feline immunodeficiency virus, and parvovirus weaken the immune system and predispose patients to infectious agents.

Functional factors that may increase the risk of developing pneumonia include brachycephalic anatomy, laryngeal paralysis, and megaesophagus. The gag reflex may be impaired following sedation or in the presence of neuromuscular paralysis (i.e., botulism, coonhound paralysis), increasing the risk of aspiration pneumonia (Reiss and McKiernan 2002).

Other at-risk groups include pediatric and geriatric patients, animals with preexisting respiratory disease or trauma, patients requiring mechanical ventilation, severely debilitated or malnourished animals, and postoperative patients following laryngeal or tracheal surgery.

Clinical signs. Typical signs include lethargy, anorexia, moist cough, and exercise intolerance. Severe cases may exhibit dyspnea with a rapid and shallow respiratory pattern, audible wheezing, postural adaptations, and cyanosis. Although not a consistent finding, patients with bacterial pneumonias are often febrile; absence of fever does not rule out pneumonia.

Diagnosis. Diagnosis of pneumonia is based on clinical symptoms, physical exam findings, radiographic images, and laboratory findings. Fine to coarse crackles are typically noted on auscultation; wheezing or respiratory clicks may be noted dependent upon the extent of bronchial inflammation. Consolidation of any portion of the lungs will result in significantly decreased or absent sounds over that area. Concurrent tracheal irritation may be present; tracheal palpation may elicit coughing. Pulse oximetry may demonstrate normal to decreased Hb saturation. Patients are frequently dehydrated secondary to decreased appetite and fluid intake along with increased respiratory effort and associated fluid loss.

Radiographic images are the primary diagnostic tool for determination and evaluation of pneumonia. Radiographic findings are variable depending upon the etiological agent and may not be apparent for 24–48 hours following the onset of pneumonia. Typical findings include alveolar, bronchial, or interstitial patterns, evidence of alveolar infiltrates, consolidation, and air bronchograms. Infiltrative patterns in the right cranial or middle and the left cranial lung lobes are characteristically indicative of aspiration pneumonia.

Laboratory findings vary depending upon the etiological agent and the severity of disease. Assessment of PaO_2 and SO_2 through ABG analysis can be a good indicator of disease severity and response to treatment. Respiratory cultures should be collected by transtracheal wash (TTW) or bronchoalveolar lavage (BAL) and submitted for identification and sensitivity testing (Fig. 7.5).

Treatment. Patients exhibiting tachypnea, respiratory distress, low PaO_2 (<60 mmHg), or low SaO_2 (<90%) require supplemental oxygen (Reiss and McKiernan 2002).

Fluid therapy should be aimed toward restoration and maintenance of tissue perfusion. Adequate hydration is essential to maintain moisture in the airways and facilitate clearance of respiratory secretions.

Antimicrobial therapy is based on culture and sensitivity results; broad spectrum antibiotics may be initiated while results are pending.

Nebulization with 0.9% sodium chloride solution thins the respiratory secretions and facilitates clearance. Coupage further assists clearance by inducing coughing and loosening mucous and debris. Patients stable enough for exercise benefit from moderate walks to facilitate removal of secretions, improve psychological status, and maintain muscle tone (Fig. 7.6).

CHAPTER 7

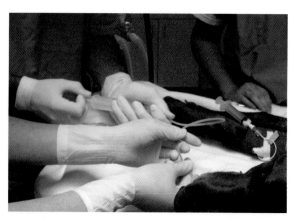

Figure 7.5   Here an airway wash is being performed on a dog with suspected aspiration pneumonia. (Courtesy of Thomas Walker, DVM, DACVECC.)

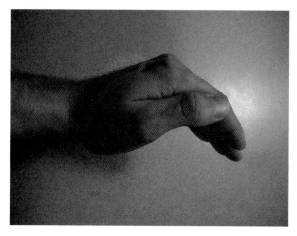

Figure 7.6   Correct hand technique for coupage is important to maximize its benefit. (Courtesy of Christopher Norkus, BS, CVT, VTS [Emergency & Critical Care], VTS [Anesthesia].)

Acute respiratory distress syndrome (ARDS)

ARDS and acute lung injury (ALI) describe a generalized inflammatory process characterized by pulmonary edema and infiltration of inflammatory cells. ALI varies in severity from mild to moderate with a PaO_2 FiO_2 ratio of 300 or less; ARDS comprises the most severe form and yields a PaO_2 FiO_2 ratio of 200 or less. Accumulation of neutrophils and macrophages within the lungs, along with interstitial and alveolar edema, are characteristic of ALI. Progression of the inflammatory response leads to ARDS which is characterized by formation of hyaline membranes within the alveoli, excessive production of type II pneumocytes, and interstitial fibrosis.

The lungs are highly susceptible to inflammatory insult and ALI/ARDS may be triggered by direct injury to the lungs or by systemic conditions. Aspiration pneumonia, smoke inhalation, pulmonary contusions, and chemical pneumonitis all result in direct pulmonary injury and inflammation. Systemic inflammatory response syndrome (SIRS) is commonly implicated in ALI/ARDS; other causative agents include pancreatitis, sepsis, and necrosis secondary to torsion or obstruction.

Clinical signs. ALI patients typically present with mild to moderate respiratory distress and hypoxia; ARDS patients exhibit severe dyspnea, profound hypoxia, and cyanosis. A moist cough may be present; foamy, pink-tinged fluid may be expectorated. Harsh lung sounds are a frequent finding in ALI; crackles are prevalent in ARDS.

Diagnosis. Diagnosis is based on clinical symptoms, laboratory findings, and radiographs. ABG samples typically demonstrate decreased PaO_2; in ARDS, the PaO_2 may be profoundly decreased and is often accompanied by decreased $PaCO_2$ secondary to hyperventilation. Other significant findings may include leukopenia secondary to sequestration, metabolic acidosis from hypoxemia and anaerobic metabolism, coagulopathies, and hypoproteinemia.

Radiographs are a key tool in the diagnosis of ALI/ARDS. Patients with ALI typically exhibit interstitial and peribronchial patterns; in ARDS patients, all lung fields are affected and exhibit diffuse, bilateral alveolar infiltrates. Differential diagnoses include fluid volume overload, cardiogenic pulmonary edema, pneumonia, intrapulmonary hemorrhage, and neoplasia. The primary diagnostic indicator of ARDS is severe dyspnea and pulmonary edema with normal cardiac function.

Treatment. Oxygen supplementation may be administered by mask, nasal cannula, or oxygen cage for patient with mild to moderate ALI symptoms. ARDS patients usually require positive-pressure ventilation. ABG monitoring is helpful to assess therapeutic efficacy.

IV fluid therapy should be geared toward maintenance of perfusion; excessive fluid volume may worsen pulmonary edema. Colloids and or plasma are often required to maintain intravascular fluid volume in the presence of hypoalbuminemia and increased vascular permeability secondary to inflammatory mediators. Fresh frozen plasma provides active coagulation factors and albumin as well as colloid support. Diuretic use should be reserved for cases of volume overload.

Treatment of the underlying cause is necessary to minimize the progression which initiated ALI/ARDS. The use of corticosteroids remains controversial in human literature. Several studies have demonstrated that early administration of corticosteroids may reduce ventilator time and improve oxygenation and lung compliance as compared with patients not receiving corticosteroids. However, the study also noted that patients receiving corticosteroids were more likely to have to be placed back on the ventilator, and there was no difference in mortality between the two groups (Hudson and Meduri 2005).

Further care is supportive; while many patients respond to treatment for ALI, ARDS carries a grave prognosis.

Pneumothorax

Pneumothorax occurs when there is an accumulation of air or gas in the pleural space in sufficient quantity to cause collapse of the lung and marked reduction in ventilation. *Open pneumothorax* occurs when there is open communication between the external environment and the pleural space; *closed pneumothorax* occurs when air accumulates due to leakage from the pulmonary parenchyma, bronchial tree, or esophagus. *Traumatic pneumothorax* can be classified as open or closed and is a result of a traumatic event in which air accumulates in the pleural space; *spontaneous pneumothorax* occurs in previously healthy animals as a result of air leakage from the lung into the pleural space due to an unknown cause without trauma. *Tension pneumothorax* is a collection of air or gas in

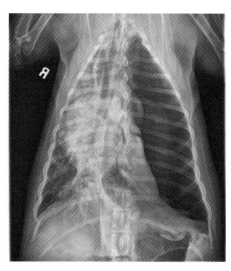

Figure 7.7   Radiograph demonstrating a severe left-sided pneumothorax. Rapid thoracocentesis is imperative for this patient.

the pleural cavity of the chest between the lung and the chest wall. Usually as a result of trauma, a flap of tissue acts as a one-way valve so that there is a continuous influx of air into the pleural cavity on inspiration that does not return to the lung on expiration. Tension pneumothorax is an immediate life-threatening condition and requires urgent treatment and resolution.

Clinical signs and diagnosis. Symptoms of pneumothorax are an acute onset of dyspnea and various degrees of respiratory distress ranging from a mild form to more severe and life-threatening. Thoracic auscultation may reveal decreased heart and lung sounds. Traumatic injuries such as rib and limb fractures, pulmonary contusions, and sucking chest wounds often support a diagnosis of traumatic pneumothorax.

Identification of free air in the pleural space through imaging techniques such as thoracic radiographs or ultrasound is diagnostic for pneumothorax. Alternatively, diagnostic thoracocentesis is often significantly less stressful for a dyspneic patient and may be therapeutic as removal of air decreases the pressure on the lungs and heart. Once the animal's condition is stabilized, a more through diagnostic evaluation may be performed to identify the cause of the pneumothorax (Fig. 7.7).

Treatment. A significant percentage of pneumothorax patients may be managed medically; surgical intervention is typically required for spontaneous cases and those with extensive wounds to the thoracic wall or internal pulmonary structures. Medical management involves oxygen supplementation, removal of air from the pleural space, and administration of appropriate analgesics.

The method chosen to evacuate air from the thoracic cavity is dependent upon the volume of air present, the speed of air accumulation, the severity of traumatic defects, and the likelihood of persistent or recurrent pneumothorax. Small amounts of air can frequently be managed with periodic needle thoracocentesis until the pneumothorax is resolved; large or persistent accumulations typically warrant chest tube placement. Intermittent suctioning of the chest tube is appropriate for patients with slow or minimal air

---

Box 7.1   Supplies Required for Thoracocentesis

- Clippers
- Povidine or chlorhexidine scrub solution
- Alcohol
- 3-way stopcock
- Butterfly catheter (19 g or 21 g)
- Extension set (optional)
- IV catheter or needle (optional)
- 3 mL syringe
- Collection syringe (20, 35, or 60 mL) dependent upon the size of the patient
- Bowl or graduated cylinder
- Ethylenediaminetetraacetic acid (EDTA) tubes
- Aerobic and anaerobic culturettes or media

---

buildup; continuous drainage should be considered when dealing with large traumatic defects or persistent pneumothorax as this method allows for quicker resolution of dyspnea.

Oxygen supplementation is often beneficial, especially in animals with pulmonary trauma. Analgesics should always be considered for animals with soft tissue trauma or fractured ribs. Patients receiving analgesic therapy are more likely to breath comfortably and typically demonstrate improved ventilatory effort.

Surgical intervention is indicated when extensive wounds are present and require closure or repair to facilitate healing. Patients presenting with an open chest wound benefit from a sterile adhesive dressing being placed over the wound(s) initially followed by immediate evacuation of air from the chest via thoracocentesis; surgical closure may be performed once the patient is stable. Surgical correction is also indicated in spontaneous pneumothorax due to the high incidence of recurrence with medical management.

Hemothorax

Hemothorax is the accumulation of blood in the pleural space usually as a result of blunt force or penetrating thoracic trauma or coagulopathy.

Clinical signs and diagnosis. Clinical signs at presentation range from mild dyspnea to tachycardia, pale mucous membranes, and decreased capillary refill time associated with hypovolemic shock. Auscultation typically reveals muffled heart and lung sounds.

A tentative diagnosis of hemothorax may be made based on history and physical exam. Thoracic radiographs and ultrasound will typically reveal the presence of fluid within the pleural space; aspiration of blood from the thoracic cavity is confirmatory.

Treatment. Treatment of hemothorax requires identification and resolution of the underlying cause while minimizing dyspnea. Traumatic hemothorax may resolve with medical management; persistent hemorrhage or arterial bleeds typically require surgical correction. Coagulopathies require immediate replacement of active clotting factors; this is best achieved through transfusion with fresh frozen plasma, frozen plasma, or fresh whole

---

Box 7.2   Thoracocentesis Procedure

1. Gently restrain patient; lateral recumbency is recommended for pneumothorax, while sitting, standing, or sternal positions are often best for collection of fluid.
2. Clip and aseptically prep the area from the sixth through the tenth intercostal spaces. If pneumothorax is suspected, the highest portion of the chest wall should be prepped. The collection site for pleural effusion is lower on the chest wall, approximately the level of the costochondral junction.
3. Attach the 3-way stopcock to the syringe; attach the butterfly catheter or extension set and needle to the stopcock. Verify that the stopcock is "turned off" toward the needle.
   - Remember that when using a 3-way stopcock, wherever the arrow points, is "off." The stopcock should always be "turned off" to the patient unless you are actively aspirating the pleural space.
4. The needle is inserted into the thoracic cavity at the cranial edge of the eighth or ninth rib in order to avoid the intercostal vessels.
5. Once the needle has been introduced, position it laterally so that the needle rests against the chest wall with the bevel open to the thoracic cavity in order to minimize the risk of laceration during lung expansion.
6. Turn the stopcock so that the arrow points away from the needle and the syringe.
7. Apply light traction to the syringe to aspirate the fluid or air. When the syringe is filled, turn the stopcock back toward the needle and expel the fluid or air collected out through the side port of the stopcock.
8. Fluid may be expelled into a bowl or graduated cylinder to facilitate quantitation of volume aspirated. Fluid samples should be saved in EDTA tubes for cytological evaluation; aerobic and anaerobic culture samples should also be obtained and may be saved in sterile red top tubes.
9. It may be necessary to redirect the needle or reposition the patient to effectively aspirate pockets of fluid or air.

---

blood followed by vitamin K_1 therapy. It is not advisable to remove large quantities of blood via thoracocentesis unless the patient is experiencing respiratory compromise; blood remaining in the thoracic cavity will be reabsorbed. In many cases, blood that is aspirated from the pleural space can be autotransfused back into the patient.

Pleural effusion

The term pleural effusion is used to define an accumulation of excessive fluid within the pleura, the fluid-filled space that surrounds the lungs. It occurs when the rate of fluid accumulation exceeds the rate of absorption. Effusion may result from right heart failure, infection (pyothorax), lymph (chylothorax), neoplasia, or hemorrhage (hemothorax); it is commonly attributed to chronic chylothorax or pyothorax.

Clinical signs and diagnosis. The most common signs of pleural effusion are dyspnea and exercise intolerance; classically, respiration is marked by forceful inspiration with delayed expiration. This respiratory pattern makes the animal appear as though it is holding its breath and is particularly noticeable in cats.

Box 7.3   Supplies Required for Chest Tube Placement

- Clippers
- Prep materials: povidine or chlorhexidine scrub solution, alcohol
- Sterile chest tube or red rubber catheter, size is dependent upon the patient
  - Cats or very small dogs: 14–16 Fr
  - Small dogs: 18–22 Fr
  - Medium dogs: 22–28 Fr
  - Large dogs: 28–36 Fr
- Lidocaine 2% solution for local anesthetic block
- Sterile surgical pack or chest tube pack
  - Scalpel handle
  - Olsen-Hagar or Mayo-Hagar needle holders
  - Curved and straight hemostats
  - Gauze sponges
  - Towel clamps
- Scalpel blade
- Surgical attire including cap, mask, gown, and sterile gloves
- C-clamp
- Christmas tree adapter
- 3-way stopcock
- Sterile, nonabsorbable suture
- Bandage materials

Recognition of the characteristic respiratory pattern and auscultation of muffled heart and lung sounds in the presence of dyspnea point to pleural effusion. The presence of fluid within the pleural space may be confirmed with various diagnostic imaging techniques including thoracic radiographs, ultrasound, magnetic resonance imaging (MRI), or computed tomographic (CT) scan. Therapeutic thoracocentesis may be indicated before a more through diagnostic imaging can be performed. The removal of air or fluid prior to taking radiographs will help to stabilize the patient and allow for improved visualization of the heart and lungs. Fluid obtained via thoracocentesis may be submitted for cell count, cytology, chemical analysis (e.g., triglyceride level), and culture and sensitivity; laboratory analysis often provides valuable diagnostic information to classify the type of effusion (Fig. 7.8).

Treatment. Initial treatment of pleural effusion focuses on minimizing patient stress, providing supplemental oxygen, and resolution or reduction of dyspnea as fluid is evacuated by thoracocentesis. Definitive therapy is aimed as identification and treatment of the underlying cause.

Flail chest

Flail chest occurs secondary to blunt trauma when multiple adjacent ribs are each fractured in more than one place; the resulting flail segment is not attached to either the sternum or spine and moves independently of the nonfractured ribs. In the absence of a pneumothorax, negative pressure in the thoracic cavity pulls the flail segment inward while the rest of the chest wall moves outward during inspiration.

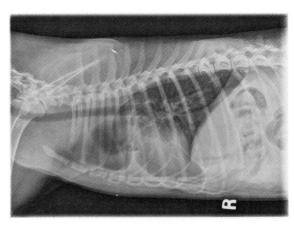

Figure 7.8   Radiograph demonstrating a significant pleural effusion. Thoracocentesis is performed, and the effusion is submitted for fluid analysis, cytology, and potentially bacterial culture.

Clinical signs and diagnosis. Patients with flail chest injuries typically present with a rapid, shallow respiratory pattern, tachypnea, tachycardia, and anxiety.

Diagnosis of flail chest is based on patient history, symptoms, observation of paradoxical chest movement, and radiographic evidence of fractures. The respiratory compromise seen in flail chest is associated with pain and concurrent pathology such as pulmonary contusions, pneumothorax, hemothorax, and/or cardiovascular trauma.

Treatment. Initial treatment is supportive, typically consisting of oxygen supplementation and analgesic therapy (e.g., intercostals nerve blocks). Positioning the patient in lateral recumbency with the flail segment down may decrease pain and improve respiratory function; chest wraps should be avoided as they tend to compress the chest wall and decrease compliance while providing minimal support of the flail segment. Patients with significant pulmonary contusions or lung pathology may require ventilatory support. Once the patient's hemodynamic and respiratory status is stable, the flail segment may be surgically stabilized.

Diaphragmatic hernia

Thoracic trauma frequently results in tearing of the diaphragm and possible displacement or entrapment of abdominal contents into the thoracic cavity. Respiratory distress secondary to traumatic diaphragmatic hernias varies from subclinical to severe depending upon the extent of abdominal organ displacement.

Clinical signs and diagnosis. Typical symptoms include tachypnea, a rapid shallow respiratory pattern, and cyanosis; auscultation may reveal decreased heart and lung sounds or bowel sounds within the thoracic cavity. Myocardial irritation secondary to displaced abdominal contents often results in cardiac arrhythmias (e.g., ventricular premature depolarizations).

Diagnosis of diaphragmatic hernia is based on patient history, clinical symptoms, and diagnostic imaging. Radiographic evidence of intestinal loops, stomach, or other abdominal organs within the chest is definitive. Changes in the cardiac silhouette, displacement of lung fields, loss of diaphragmatic outline, and pleural effusion should be considered suspicious, and further imaging may be indicated. Contrast media may be utilized to enhance radiographic images. Barium sulfate or iodine contrast media administered orally will define the location of the stomach and intestines; barium is contraindicated if gastrointestinal perforation is suspected. Nonionized iodinated contrast material (e.g., iohexol) should be selected if gastrointestinal perforation is suspected.

Ultrasound may definitively demonstrate the presence of abdominal organs within the thorax or, more subtly, changes in the demarcation between the lungs and the liver often suggest diaphragmatic hernia.

Diaphragmatic hernia may be a late finding (months to years) after trauma. Hernias that have been asymptomatic for an extended period of time may manifest acutely. Obtaining a detailed history frequently assists in the identification of the underlying etiology of the hernia. Chronic hernia may involve greater risk of morbidity and mortality (Nelson, personal communication).

Treatment. Treatment involves stabilization of life-threatening conditions and supportive care including fluid therapy for correction of shock and cardiovascular support, oxygen therapy, and pain management. Surgical repair of the diaphragm is performed once the patient is stable. Herniation of the stomach into the thorax requires close monitoring; these animals are at significant risk of severe respiratory compromise secondary to gastric distension, and emergency surgery may be required.

Postoperative complications include pneumothorax, organ necrosis secondary to loss of perfusion, and peritonitis or sepsis due to leakage from gastrointestinal perforations. Re-expansion pulmonary edema can be a serious complication following rapid re-inflation of lung tissue during atelectasis.

CHAPTER 7

References

Amis, TC. 1974. Tracheal collapse in the dog. *Aust Vet J* 50:285–289.

Demling, RH, Desanti, L. 2005. Burns: resuscitation phase (0–36 hours). In *Principles of Critical Care*, edited by Hall, J, Schmidt, G, Wood, L. New York: McGraw Hill, p. 3e.

Dobratz, KJ. 2002. Smoke inhalation. In *The Veterinary ICU Book*, edited by Wingfield, WE, Raffe, MR. Jackson Hole, WY: Teton NewMedia, pp. 983–988.

Done, SH, Drew, RA. 1976. Observations of the pathology of tracheal collapse in dogs. *J Small Anim Pract* 17:783–791.

Hedlund, CS. 1991. Tracheal collapse. *Probl Vet Med* 3(2):229–238.

Hudson, LD, Meduri, GU. 2005. *Corticosteroids in ARDS—The Debate Goes On*. July 9, 2010, from Pulmonary Reviews.com, Vol. 10, No. 6.

Nelson, AW. 1993. Diseases of trachea and bronchi, and lungs. In *Textbook of Veterinary Surgery*, 2nd ed., edited by Slatter, DH. Philadelphia: WB Saunders, pp. 858–888.

O'Brien, JA, Buchanan, KW, Kelly, DF. 1966. Tracheal collapse in the dog. *J Am Vet Radiol Soc* 7:12–19.

Reiss, AJ, McKiernan, BC. 2002. Pneumonia. In *The Veterinary ICU Book*, edited by Wingfield, WE, Raffe, MR. Jackson Hole, WY: Teton NewMedia, pp. 643–654.

Serebrisky, D, Nazarian, EB, Connolly, H. 2010. *Inhalation Injury: Treatment & Medication*. July 8, 2010, from eMedicine Specialties. emedicine.medscape.com/article/1002413-treatment#Medication.

Gastrointestinal Emergencies

8

Amy Campbell

Introduction

Gastrointestinal emergencies affect the esophagus, stomach, small and large intestine. Patients present with a wide range of clinical signs ranging from mild to life-threatening. Dysphagia, regurgitation, gagging, vomiting, nonproductive retching, diarrhea, flatulence, borborygmus, dyschezia, hematemesis, hematochezia, constipation, and abdominal pain are all indicative of a disease of the gastrointestinal (GI) tract. A careful patient history and thorough physical examination are both instrumental in identifying the specific issue at hand and will aid in the diagnosis, treatment, and recovery of the patient.

Assessment of the Gastrointestinal Emergency

It is the responsibility of the veterinary technician to determine if a patient requires immediate medical intervention based on the symptoms and owner complaint at the time of triage. When assessing animals, the veterinary technician needs to consider the major body systems: respiratory, cardiovascular, neurological, and renal. Following initial stabilization, a diagnostic plan, developed by the veterinary team, is put into motion to identify the disease and whether to pursue surgical versus medical intervention. Quick assessment and stabilization are crucial in the prevention of serious complications including septic peritonitis or systemic inflammatory response syndrome (SIRS) and multiple organ dysfunction syndrome (MODS).

Perhaps the most important tool when evaluating the animal that presents with acute abdominal pain is the accurate medical history taken from the owner. Information that should be extracted from the owner should include any dietary indiscretions including any possibility that the animal has ingested a foreign body. Has the animal been exposed to any toxins? Are there other animals in the home, and if so, are they affected as well? Does the animal have any significant medical history? Is the patient intact? Has the animal experienced any trauma? Is he/she currently taking any medications? When was the animal last normal? When was the onset of symptoms? The client often holds the answer to many of the veterinary team's questions.

The physical examination is a process that is ongoing throughout the treatment of the patient. A primary evaluation is performed at presentation. Should the patient present in an unstable condition, treatment is initiated immediately. After the onset of emergency stabilization, a secondary evaluation may be required before client communication begins. Many times, the physical examination, onset of treatment, diagnostic tests, imaging, and consultation with client are done simultaneously to expedite patient care.

As with any critically ill patient, full attention must be given to assess the cardiovascular, central nervous, and respiratory systems (heart, brain, and lungs). When dealing with the acute abdomen, a careful abdominal palpation is crucial and may reveal a specific area of pain which in turn will aid in the diagnostic approach. The area under the tongue should be evaluated for the presence of a linear foreign body (Fig. 8.1).

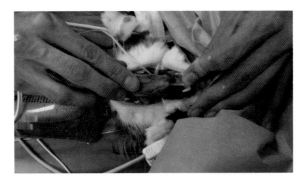

Figure 8.1 This image demonstrates the importance of the oral examination. This patient had a linear (string) foreign body that was caught under the tongue. Most of the time, the patient requires surgery to repair the damage done by the linear foreign body. Occasionally, however, the linear foreign body need only be cut and allowed to pass through the body.

If the patient is too fractious for a thorough oral exam, sedation may be required. The oral examination should not be skipped because the patient is not compliant. Examination of the reproductive systems is important. Discharge from the vulva may be indicative of a pyometra. A rectal examination will reveal the presence of melena, masses, or uroliths in the urethra, as well as prostatic enlargement or pain.

A minimum emergency database should be collected for any animal presenting with an acute abdomen. A packed cell volume (PCV) and total solids (TS) will alert the veterinary team to a potential hemorrhage or anemia versus dehydration. An elevation in both the PCV and TS is indicative of dehydration and is perhaps the most common finding in dogs and cats that present with an acute abdomen. Protein loss from the vasculature is suspected when a patient has a normal to increased PCV with decreased TS.

An animal that has experienced a hemorrhage may have decreased PCV and TS though this may not be recognized until the patient has received some fluid resuscitation. A patient that presents with acute abdominal pain with hypoglycemia is indicative of a septic abdomen. Evaluation of blood lactate helps to determine tissue perfusion and will be reflective of resuscitation efforts as well. Elevations in blood urea nitrogen (BUN) may reflect renal disease, and the technician should obtain a urine sample to evaluate urine specific gravity (USG). The patient's electrocardiogram (ECG) should be evaluated starting at presentation for the presence of arrhythmias. As with every portion of the database, the continual monitoring of the ECG will aid in evaluating the response to treatment initiated. Blood pressure measurement serves to assess the degree of hypotension in the shock patient. Though not specific to the acute abdomen, a pulse oximetry measurement and assessment of blood gas is helpful in detecting underlying lung disease and whether or not the patient requires oxygen therapy. A thorough understanding of the GI tract, its function, and effects on the body's systems are crucial in the treatment, monitoring, and nursing care of the patient with GI disease.

CHAPTER 8

Esophagus

The esophagus connects the oropharynx to the stomach. Its primary function is to carry ingesta from the oral cavity to the stomach by swallowing.

Esophagitis

Esophagitis is an acute or chronic inflammatory disorder of the esophageal mucosa. In severe cases, the inflammation can extend into the deeper layers of the esophagus. Esophagitis is usually a result from the ingestion of a corrosive agent, ingestion of a foreign body, thermal burns, persistent vomiting, or gastroesophageal reflux (GER).

Often the patient will present with owner complaints of gagging, inappetence or anorexia, ptyalism, regurgitation, exaggerated swallowing motion, odynophagia, lethargy, and sometimes weight loss. Physical examination as well as blood work will prove to be unremarkable. Occasionally, there will be evidence of aspiration pneumonia. Mild esophagitis is generally treated by withholding food for 24–48 hours, and dispensing an oral sucralfate suspension. While there have been no definitive studies proving sucralfate to be effective in patients with esophagitis, it does have cytoprotective properties when it binds to an eroded or ulcerated site. Further, it is recommended that the patient be given an H2 receptor antagonist (such as famotidine, ranitidine, or cimetidine) or a proton pump inhibitor (such as omeprazole) to aid in the repression of gastric acid production. Patients with more severe cases of esophagitis may require advanced diagnostics and thus may be referred to an internal medicine specialist for an esophagram under fluoroscopy, endoscopy, and biopsies of the esophagus.

Esophageal Obstructions

Esophageal foreign bodies are a far more common occurrence in the dog than the cat. Dogs typically present with foreign bodies such as bones, fish hooks, and improperly chewed food boluses while cats generally have fish hook or sewing needle esophageal foreign bodies. The foreign body will typically come to rest in an area of the esophagus that is the least distensible, specifically the thoracic inlet, heart base, and the lower esophagus. Patients present with a history of regurgitation, dysphagia, retching, gagging, ptyalism, or odynophagia. Sometimes, the owner will have been witness to the ingestion of the foreign object, which aids the diagnostic process. Thoracic radiographs may reveal the foreign body, though a contrast study may be required to detect radiolucent foreign bodies. An esophageal perforation may cause a pneumothorax or pneumomediastinum which would be evident on radiographs. Endoscopy is the preferred method of retrieving the foreign body if there is no perforation of the esophagus. Ideally, the foreign object can be removed through the mouth, but in many cases, endoscopy will only serve to push the foreign body into the stomach where it may be retrieved via surgical gastrotomy. Once the foreign body has been removed, many animals require no further medical therapy. Those with moderate esophageal damage may be treated as they would if they had esophagitis: administration of H_2 blockers or proton pump inhibitors, sucralfate solution to aid in mucosal healing, and an antibiotic such as metronidazole. Additionally, the patient may be given pain management so as to prevent discomfort when eating for several days following the retrieval of the foreign body.

Megaesophagus

Megaesophagus is a regional or diffuse dilation of the esophagus with minimal or non-existent peristalsis. This disorder is either congenital or acquired. Congenital megaesophagus occurs rarely in young dogs potentially secondary to developmental abnormalities. Breeds of dog predisposed to this disorder include wire-haired Terriers, Schnauzers, Great Danes, Golden Retrievers, German Shepherds and the Shar-pei. The prognosis is not known for these dogs, but there have been reports of spontaneous improvement.

Adult onset idiopathic megaesophagus occurs in dogs between the ages of 7 and 15, and while it has been reported more frequently in larger breeds of dog, there is no specific breed predisposition. The cause of this disorder is yet unknown. Aspiration pneumonia is a common side effect of this disorder and is known to be a poor prognostic indicator.

Secondary megaesophagus can result from a number of other disorders that affect neuromuscular function, such as myasthenia gravis, hypothyroidism, lead toxicity, immune-mediated polyneuritis, polymyositis, adrenocorticol insufficiency, and dysautonomia. Regardless of the etiology, the most common clinical sign of megaesophagus is regurgitation. The appetite is usually always unaffected by this disease unless there is concurrent aspiration pneumonia present. Radiographs generally reveal a diffusely dilated esophagus that may be filled with air, food, and sometimes fluid. In a study of 49 dogs, about 25% seemed to tolerate this disorder well with few complications.

Treatment is generally aimed at treating the symptoms if the underlying cause has not been determined. Therapy generally involves feeding the patient medium-sized meatballs of canned food while they are sitting and facing upward. Dogs that develop secondary esophagitis can be treated with sucralfate suspension and antacids. Because the canine esophagus is composed of skeletal muscle, drugs such as metoclopramide or cisapride will be of no help to dogs. However, since the feline distal esophagus consists of smooth muscle, these drugs may prove to be helpful, though there are no current clinical studies to prove it at this time. Surgical treatment of megaesophagus, gastroesophageal myotomy, has proven to have poor results and is not a recommended treatment of the disorder. Owners of dogs with this disease must be educated of possible complications such as aspiration pneumonia as well as the use of a harness rather than a neck lead. These clients need to understand that they must be vigilant in the care of their dog throughout the remainder of his/her lifetime.

Stomach

The primary functions of the stomach are storage, mechanical and enzymatic processing, and transportation of partially digested food into the small intestine. The stomach is both muscular and glandular. The muscular action of the stomach functions to break down food boluses that arrive via the esophagus in order to promote duodenal digestion and absorption. The glandular portion of the stomach acts by producing gastric acid to aid in the liquefying of food so that it may be gradually released into the small intestine. The gastric mucosal barrier within the stomach is continually damaged by decreases in pH, mechanical irritation, and digestive enzymes. This barrier protects itself by secreting bicarbonate and mucus. The epithelial cells within the gastric mucosal barrier contain a significant amount of hydrophobic phospholipids that repel gastric acid. This protects the stomach from autodigestion by the gastric acid. Additionally, these epithelial cells are high in intracellular bicarbonate that neutralizes acid. The gastric mucosa has the ability to repair itself because the turnover rate of epithelial cells is very high, leading to quick regeneration of injured cells (Steiner 2008). Nonsteroidal anti-inflammatory drugs (NSAIDs) block the production of prostaglandins, which are the first in the chain of events described above that serve to protect the lining of the gastrointestinal (GI) tract from the harsh stomach environment. The effect of this blockade is a decreased ability of the body to withstand acidic stomach contents resulting in gastritis and GI ulcers (Bill 2008).

Acute Gastritis

Acute gastritis is defined as inflammation of the lining of the stomach. This disorder is the most common cause of vomiting in both canine and feline patients, primarily due to the inability of the stomach's mucosal barrier to protect itself. Ingestion of spoiled foods, foreign objects, or gut-irritating drugs such as NSAIDs are common causes of gastritis. Gastritis can also be a result of a viral infection, such as parvovirus, distemper or infectious hepatitis, or resulting from a parasitic infection. Because of their affinity for eating things other than food that is presented to them, dogs are affected more often than cats. Clinical signs associated with acute gastritis include vomiting and anorexia. Abdominal discomfort and fever are often absent in these patients.

Diagnosis of gastritis is one of exclusion unless the animal was seen ingesting a gastric irritant. Depending on the severity and duration of the vomiting, the patient may have decreases in potassium, sodium, and chloride. Poor perfusion may lead to an increase in lactate resulting in a metabolic acidosis. The majority of patients will have limited changes in blood work. Overall, these patients will respond favorably to treatment.

Therapy for the patient with acute gastritis consists of fluid therapy, restricting food and water intake for 12–24 hours, limiting afferent input from the inflamed stomach by decreasing gastric acid secretion by administering an H_2 antagonist, and providing mucosal protection with the administration of sucralfate. Centrally acting antiemetics such as metoclopramide may be included in the treatment plan if vomiting persists. If vomiting continues, the patient will require IV fluid administration with potassium supplementation. The oral intake of water is first introduced when oral restriction has been discontinued. If the patient is able to drink without vomiting, then small amounts of a bland diet (boiled chicken and rice, cottage cheese) is offered. The bland diet should continue for several days until the animal has fully recovered. Once improved, then the animal's normal diet may be slowly reintroduced over the course of several days to prevent recurrence of the gastritis.

The prognosis for acute gastritis is excellent, assuming that electrolyte balance has been maintained.

Gastric Dilatation-Volvulus (GDV)

GDV, commonly referred to as bloat, is characterized by the malposition (usually clockwise) of the stomach when it fills with gas and rotates within the abdominal cavity. The effects of this syndrome are systemic and life-threatening, requiring medical and surgical intervention. Blood vessels connect the spleen to the stomach, so when the stomach rotates, the spleen is taken with it. Rotation of the stomach compresses the vena cava, thus decreasing venous return to the heart as well as portal blood flow. Ultimately, the decrease in venous return results in a profound decrease in cardiac output, blood pressure, and tissue perfusion affecting all organs including the heart. Decreased perfusion to the twisted stomach results in gastric necrosis and ischemic injury.

The cause of GDV is yet unknown. The disorder has been known to occur in as much as 60,000 dogs annually in the United States alone. Thoracoabdominal dimension has been shown to play a part in the disorder. Large breed, deep-chested dogs are typically affected (Great Dane, Akita, Saint Bernard, Irish setter). Dogs are usually 7 years of age or older. Environmental risk factors that have been reported include diet (including eating from an elevated food bowl), gastric gas accumulation, anesthesia, and stress. There have also been studies that have shown that gastric ligament laxity may play a role in GDV. Nevertheless, there have been no definitive studies that have proved a singular cause for the disorder.

Clinical signs include nonproductive retching, abdominal distention, and restlessness. If allowed to progress, this condition will cause the dog to collapse due to hypovolemic shock. The treatment of shock is of the utmost importance upon presentation.

Intervention begins with IV catheter placement, crystalloid boluses, colloid boluses, antibiotic administration, and pain management. The gas-filled stomach may put increased

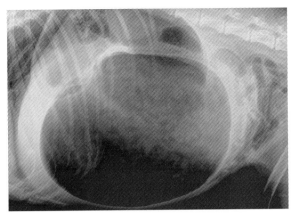

Figure 8.2 Right lateral abdominal radiograph of a dog with gastric dilatation-volvulus (GDV). GDV is characterized by the classic "double bubble" radiographic image seen here.

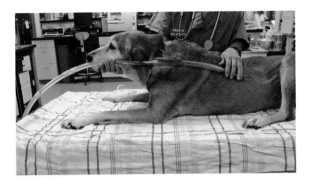

Figure 8.3 Prior to oral insertion, the orogastric tube is measured from the tip of the nose to the last rib.

pressure on the diaphragm causing inadequate lung expansion resulting in respiratory distress and as such, oxygen therapy should be initiated immediately. Preliminary electrocardiogram (ECG) and blood work is obtained. Blood lactate levels greater than 9 mmol/L is indicative of the severity of ischemic disease due to GDV and carries a significantly worse prognosis (Zacher et al. 2010). The standard diagnostic tool for GDV is a right lateral abdominal radiograph. Normally, the pylorus is seen on the down side of the abdomen on radiographs. In dogs with GDV, the pylorus has moved from the right side of the abdomen, and when viewed in right lateral recumbency, the pylorus is seen on the up side of the abdomen as a separate gas-filled structure dorsal to the stomach. A characteristic gas pattern described as a double bubble (Fig. 8.2), boxing glove, or curling rock is indicative of GDV. Once the diagnosis of GDV is confirmed, steps are taken for surgical repair of the twisted stomach.

Gastric decompression is initiated first to alleviate the pressure put on the vena cava and portal vein, thereby improving cardiac output and blood pressure. The patient is intubated and the orogastric tube is measured from the nose to the last rib and marked as such (Fig. 8.3).

Firm pressure and twisting motion is required when advancing the tube into the stomach. Esophageal and gastric tears are complications of this procedure so care must be taken to not force the tube down the throat of the patient. If attempts to pass the orogastric tube are unsuccessful, a gastrocentesis may be necessary to release some of the gas from the stomach. Generally after this release, a tube can be successfully placed into the stomach, allowing its contents to flow out of the tube into a nearby bucket. Lavaging the stomach will aid in the expulsion of all the stomach contents prior to surgery.

The purpose of surgery in these patients is to decompress and return the stomach to its normal position within the abdominal cavity. The stomach and spleen are assessed for viability. In some cases, a splenectomy is indicated. If the surgeon finds that there is significant, irreversible tissue damage, then a partial gastrectomy is performed. A gastropexy is indicated to prevent the event from recurring by creating a permanent adhesion between the stomach and the body wall. Recurrence rates as high as 80% have been reported when no gastropexy is performed.

The technician must be mindful of the risk factors associated with the postoperative GDV patient. The primary goal when caring for these patients is to maintain adequate tissue perfusion. Generally, these animals will receive higher fluid rates for the first 48 hours because of the significant fluid losses into the peritoneal cavity and GI tract. Usually, the patient is placed on a continuous ECG monitor as they are susceptible to ventricular arrhythmias. These are primarily a result of ischemic injury to the myocardium during the GDV event and the subsequent release of reperfusion products into the bloodstream. Electrolyte abnormalities may also play a role in these arrhythmias, as will pain, acidosis, and disseminated intravascular coagulation (DIC). Ventricular arrhythmias are not often treated unless they are determined to be multifocal and the patient is cardiovascularly compromised. If the patient is found to have impaired cardiac function, a heart rate in excess of 160 bpm, weak pulses, prolonged capillary refill time (CRT), obtunded mentation with poor mucous membrane color, then the arrhythmia is usually treated with an intravascular bolus of lidocaine. If the patient responds to the bolus, then it is started on a lidocaine constant rate infusion (CRI). Complete elimination of the arrhythmia may not occur, but it is are often decreased in severity. Ventricular arrhythmias in these patients are usually self-limiting and will decrease over the course of hospitalization.

Anemia and hypoproteinemia may also occur in postoperative GDV patients. Ischemic injury to the stomach may result in hemorrhagic gastritis. Intraoperative blood loss or aggressive fluid therapy results in anemia. Hypoproteinemia is often secondary to gastric inflammation resulting in the loss of proteins. The decrease in plasma proteins may result in decreased colloidal oncotic pressure and can delay wound healing. If either anemia or hypoproteinemia persists, then blood products need to be considered as part of the postoperative treatment plan.

During the GDV event, many inflammatory mediators are released and or activated as a result of the introduction of bacteria, endotoxins, or tissue hypoxia. As a result, the veterinary team must always be on the lookout for the development of sepsis or systemic inflammatory response syndrome (SIRS). The patient that is hypotensive, tachycardic, hypovolemic, hypothermic, or febrile with either elevated or decreased white cell count is a prime candidate for septic shock, especially if there is evidence of multiple organ involvement. In these cases, the goal is to treat and correct the underlying problem, support the patient's needs, whether it be with oxygen, nutritional support, pain management, wound care, and patient comfort requirements. Further, any patient that is suspected to have SIRS or sepsis should be monitored for signs of DIC. The patient is watched closely for petechia, ecchymosis, hypercoagulability, and bleeding from venipuncture sites. Platelet estimates can be performed in-house while complete coagulation profiles are sent to an outside laboratory. Treatment for DIC includes heparin therapy, administration of blood products, and supportive care.

Postoperative GDV patients with or without minimal complications can begin the oral intake of fluids within 12 hours of surgery. If water is well tolerated, then small amounts of a bland diet may be introduced around the 24-hour period. Dogs are weaned from their fluid therapy over a 24- to 48-hour time period. NSAIDs are contraindicated in these patients because they inhibit prostaglandins and may worsen an already high incidence of gastric mucosal compromise. Furthermore, H_2 receptor antagonists such as famotidine and coating drugs such as sucralfate are often prescribed postoperatively.

Hemorrhagic Gastroenteritis (HGE)

HGE is an acute disease that occurs in dogs. The etiology of the disease is unknown, though anaphylactic reactions to enteric toxins have been suspected as being involved in the pathogenesis (Steiner 2008). Small breed, middle-aged dogs are typically affected. HGE is characterized by an acute onset of explosive, bloody diarrhea. A classic "raspberry jam" appearance is noted with the feces. Animals with this disease tend to decline rapidly in health and typically present with moderate to severe dehydration. Without appropriate therapy, these patients will continue to deteriorate and die.

Clinical signs of HGE include the aforementioned diarrhea along with vomiting, anorexia, generalized depression, and rarely fever. These patients lose a significant amount of fluid from their GI in a short amount of time and therefore may present in hypovolemic shock. Some patients present in septic shock with a normal or subnormal body temperature. Abdominal discomfort is often apparent in these animals, causing them to moan or cry out. They may not be able to find a comfortable position in which to lie down. Abdominal palpation may reveal fluid- or gas-filled loops of bowel which will elicit pain when touched.

Ruling out other causes such as parvovirus, pancreatitis, GI foreign body obstruction, Addison's disease, GI parasites, or bacterial infections is key before arriving at a diagnosis of HGE. Packed cell volume (PCV) in these patients is typically elevated to higher than 60% with little to no increase in total proteins. This hemoconcentration is due to hypovolemia or splenic contraction. Total protein levels remain unchanged because of GI loss of serum proteins or redistribution of body water into the vascular space.

Aggressive fluid therapy should be initiated immediately with these patients as rapid decompensation may occur. The goal is to replace quickly the fluid losses from vomiting and diarrhea and then maintain ongoing hydration. The GI tract is the shock organ of the dog, and lack of proper perfusion causes worsening of GI inflammation, bacterial translocation, sepsis, and DIC. These patients often require both crystalloid and colloid fluid therapy. One very important aspect of treatment for HGE is the management of pain that accompanies the disease. Antiemetics as well as antibiotics are also included in the treatment plan. Often, food and water are withheld for 24–48 hours, followed by the slow reintroduction of water first, then a bland diet free of fats and sugars.

Keeping these patients clean and dry while hospitalized is not often an easy task. They may require frequent bathing, and care must be taken when taking a rectal body temperature as this may cause the patient to experience pain. The application of topicals such as A&D ointment is helpful in treating the sore rectal area. Once food is reintroduced, it may prove difficult to get these dogs to eat anything. The patient may need to be coaxed to eat. It is important that these animals be eating before they are discharged from the hospital. Often these patients are discharged from the hospital with an H_2 blocker such as famotidine, a broad spectrum antibiotic such as metronidazole and owner instructions to feed small, frequent meals of a bland diet for several days. Once the patient is symptom-free, their normal diet may be reintroduced over the course of 3–5 days.

Intestinal Tract

The intestinal tract is the entry point for all metabolic energy into the animal. It has a number of functions, all of which are essential for normal digestion. Five of the primary functions of the intestines are as follows (Steiner 2008):

1. Motility—The intestines aid in the movement of ingesta from the stomach through the intestines, and lastly expel the remains as feces.
2. Secretion—The intestines secrete electrolytes, enzymes, and fluid into the intestinal lumen.
3. Digestion—Pancreatic digestive enzymes mediate the breakdown of ingesta in the cranial small intestine.
4. Absorption—The nutrients left over after the breakdown of ingesta are organized and introduced into the body's circulation.
5. Barrier function—This serves to prevent the translocation of bacteria and digestive enzymes into circulation. Further, it serves to prevent the loss of plasma proteins.

The GI tract is under direct control of its own complex enteric nervous system (ENS), which is an autonomic system. It communicates continually with the central nervous system (CNS) by receiving efferent and sending afferent signals. Studies have demonstrated that when the vagus nerve is severed, the ENS does not cease functioning (Breton 2008).

The role of the GI tract in the body's immune system is significant. The small intestine is essentially an enormous area of mucosal tissue that is constantly exposed to the external environment, which translates into it being a major potential entry point for allergens, bacteria, and viruses. Immune system cells and mast cells are located throughout the GI tract, acting as natural killers. Because the system is continually exposed to innumerable antigens, it is said to be in a constant state of inflammation; it is only when the inflammation becomes excessive that a disease becomes evident, as is the case with inflammatory bowel disease (IBD).

There are numerous types of bacteria that exist normally within the intestinal lumen. They function to assist in the normal digestive and absorption processes. They also serve to prevent pathogenic bacteria from colonizing within the GI tract and to positively affect the enteric immune system. Each individual animal seems to have a different set of flora within their GI tract, and it has been found that cats have a greater number and diversity of bacteria within their intestinal tract. While all of the bacteria that normally exist within the GI tract are essential for normal GI function, they are also pathogens and are hugely detrimental should they cross the GI mucosal barrier into the bloodstream. Any number of disorders can leave the body vulnerable to GI mucosal disturbances, and the intestinal tract continually plays a balancing act to maintain optimal function.

Canine Parvovirus (CPV)

CPV is a highly contagious virus that is the primary cause of enteric disease in puppies. There are two strains of the virus, CPV-1 and CPV-2. The latter has proven to be the more pathogenic virus that continues to infect dogs to this day. It is primarily transmitted via contaminated feces and is very hardy in the environment with an incubation period in the field of 7–14 days. Breeds that have been reported to have an increased risk of being infected by this virus include the Doberman, Rottweiler, Staffordshire terrier, German shepherd, Labrador retrievers, and Alaskan sled dogs. It is generally seen in dogs less than 6 months of age and commonly occurs in puppies between 6 and 20 weeks of age.

The virus itself is a small, nonenveloped single stranded DNA virus. It infects rapidly dividing cells, such as those that exist in the bone marrow and GI tract. It enters the body through the oronasal lymphoid tissue and spreads through plasma circulating through the body. Clinical signs usually begin to appear 4–10 days post infection.

These patients generally present with reported history of sudden onset of vomiting, diarrhea, depression, anorexia, and abdominal pain. It is the destruction of the intestinal cells that cause intestinal bleeding and associated hematochezia. It is this and the neutropenia caused by bone marrow suppression that makes puppies extremely susceptible to bacterial translocation. In severe cases, sepsis, septic shock, multiple organ dysfunction syndrome (MODS), and SIRS can result from the endotoxins and bacteria released into the bloodstream. Clinical signs in these patients are tachycardia, hypoperfusion, poor pulse quality, prolonged CRT, cool extremities, and profound depression. Often, mucous membranes are pale but may be injected if the patient presents with SIRS.

In-house snap tests are available and are enormously useful in the diagnosis of the virus (Fig. 8.4).

However, false negatives can occur if the test is performed too early in the disease process, and as such, the test should be repeated 36–48 hours later if clinical signs are indicative of CPV.

Alternatively, a false positive on the in-house snap test can occur if the animal has received a live parvoviral vaccine within the preceding 2 weeks. If an animal is suspected of having CPV but has a negative result on the in-house snap, then a polymerase chain reaction (PCR) should be submitted to a lab for confirmation.

A complete blood count will reveal a neutropenia resulting from peripheral consumption and also from destruction of white blood cell (WBC) precursors in the bone marrow.

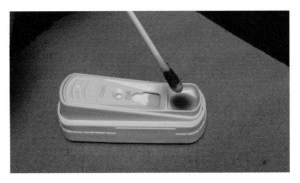

Figure 8.4   In-house snap test that is available for in-house testing for canine parvovirus (CPV). A fecal sample is needed for this test.

CHAPTER 8

Additional blood work may reveal hypoproteinemia, hyperbilirubinemia, increased liver enzymes, hypokalemia, hypoglycemia, and a prerenal azotemia. Patients that are severely affected will have prolonged clotting times and thrombocytopenia that is highly indicative of DIC. However, a hypercoagulability has been noted in dogs with CPV without DIC. This is presumably due to a reduction in antithrombin activity and hyperfibrinogenemia. Diagnostic imaging is useful in ruling out other conditions such as an intestinal obstruction and intussusception as well as detecting aspiration pneumonia if present.

Treatment of canine parvovirus is aimed at supportive care with fluid therapy, antibiotics, and antiemetics along with nutritional therapy and pain management. Current recommendations in the treatment of parvovirus indicate that the patient should be treated as a patient with gram-negative sepsis. Initial IV fluid therapy is directed at treating hypoperfusion and then at treating dehydration. Ongoing losses from vomiting, diarrhea, and insensible losses need to be taken into consideration as well. Dextrose and potassium (KCl) supplementation in IV fluids is almost always a requirement, with KCl supplementation not to exceed 0.5 mEq/kg/h. Colloidal fluid therapy is indicated when the patient is hypoproteinemic, is septic, or if it has vasculitis that can result in extravasation of albumin. Should the patient develop anemia or severe hypoproteinemia, then blood products are indicated such as whole blood or plasma.

Antibiotics are warranted in all dogs with parvovirus. This is because of the bacterial translocation that usually occurs. Ampicillin and enrofloxacin together are commonly used, though the use of enrofloxacin in puppies is debatable as it may cause cartilage abnormalities in growing animals. Many feel that short courses of the drug may be acceptable. Third-generation cephalosporins are beneficial. If renal function is good and the patient is adequately hydrated, an aminoglycoside such as gentamicin or amikacin may also be included in the treatment plan. If an aminoglycoside is used, it is important to perform a urinalysis daily to look for granular casts, an early sign of renal toxicity.

Metoclopramide is a common antiemetic used in treating dogs with CPV, as vomiting is a major issue with these patients. One of the risks associated with metoclopramide is intussuseption as it increases gastric emptying. Additionally, metoclopramide increases the production of prolactin which may cause increased cytokine production and may promote the imflammatory response. Prochlorperazine and chlorpromazine are also antiemetics used in the treatment of CPV, and they can produce adverse side effects similar to metoclopramide. Further, they have sedative properties which are undesirable in a vomiting animal as well as vasodilation properties which, in an inadequately fluid-resuscitated patient, could prove to be detrimental. Maropitant is an antiemetic given once daily as a subcutaneous injection. Care should be taken by the technician when administering this drug as it may cause pain during or just after injection. Ondansetron and dolasetron are two other highly effective and commonly used antiemetic agents.

The use of antiviral drugs has not been thoroughly investigated for the specific treatment of CPV. However, in recent years, oseltamivir (Tamiflu), a neuraminidase inhibitor, has received a lot of attention in the treatment of CPV. The drug is used for the treatment of influenza in humans. Because the influenza virus is dependent on neuramidase to invade cells and reproduce, it has been theorized that oseltamivir is an effective drug in the treatment of CPV. However, CPV does not rely on neuramidase for its pathogenesis. In fact, neuramidase may be beneficial in combating bacterial adhesion. Additional studies need to be completed to find out if oseltamivir is indeed effective in the treatment of CPV (Petrollini-Rogers and Otto 2009).

There have been attempts to develop strategies to enhance the immune function of patients with CPV by way of immune modulation. One method is to collect serum from dogs that have recovered from the virus and administer it to those with the disease. This may improve the outcome by way of passive immunity, though there have not yet been any clinical trials to prove this to be true. Another attempt at improving immune function of infected dogs is the use of human recombinant granulocyte stimulating factor. However, in a 1998 clinical trial to investigate this drug, no positive result was demonstrated (Rewerts et al. 1998). Feline interferon (type omega) has been approved for use in Japan, Australia, New Zealand, and Europe (Humm 2009). One study has shown the drug to decrease clinical signs and also decrease mortality rates (Ishiwata et al. 1998). However, this therapy may need to be initiated very early in the disease for it to have any significant benefit.

It was thought for some time that puppies with CPV should have food and water withheld until vomiting ceased. However, recent studies have shown that feeding these patients throughout the course of the disease has beneficial effects. Dogs that receive nutritional support early in the onset of treatment have shown to demonstrate clinical improvement sooner than those that have not been provided with nutritional support (Mohr et al. 2003). Furthermore, nutritional support has shown to decrease the intestinal permeability, thus decreasing the chance of bacterial translocation.

Dogs infected with CPV are to be kept isolated from all other patients in the hospital. One technician per shift should be designated to care for the patient. Recommendations are to burn any bedding used by these patients and all organic material should be removed from the hospital immediately. When cleaning and disinfecting an area where a CPV-positive dog has been, contact time is critical as the virus can live for several months in the environment in the absence of sunlight. A 5% bleach solution is recommended with a contact time of 10 minutes (Stavisky 2009).

Puppies that survive a CPV-2 infection are reportedly protected from reinfection for a minimum of 20 months, if not for the remainder of their lives. The disease can continue to be shed for up to 14 days after recovery; therefore, it is crucial to educate the owner and instruct them to not socialize their puppy with other dogs for a minimum of 2 weeks following discharge from the hospital.

Gastric and Intestinal Obstruction

Gastric and intestinal obstruction results in the inability of food to progress normally through the GI tract. Commonly, this is caused by neoplasia, intussusception, or by the ingestion of a foreign object. Presenting clinical signs include anorexia, vomiting, straining to defecate or diarrhea, and abdominal pain. Measures that should be taken at the time of presentation include IV catheter placement, preliminary blood work (PCV/TS, electrolytes, blood glucose, lactate, and blood urea nitrogen [BUN]), blood pressure, and initiation of IV fluid therapy, pain management, and diagnostic imaging. A diagnosis is typically made via abdominal radiographs and/or abdominal ultrasound, though some foreign bodies may be palpated. A contrast study may or may not be necessary depending on initial imaging results.

Patients that present with an intestinal obstruction may be in shock, requiring aggressive fluid resuscitation and correction of electrolyte imbalances. The animal may arrive at the hospital in stable condition, in hyper- or hypodynamic shock. While the goal is to stabilize the patient before proceeding to surgery, in some instances, the patient may not be fully stabilized until the obstruction is repaired. The major concern with any animal with this condition is perforation. If perforated, then additional patient concerns include septic peritonitis. If the foreign object is a toxin, such as lead or zinc, this leads to concerns of toxicity as well.

Surgery for a gastric obstruction should consist of a gastrotomy alone. When the foreign object is obstructing the small or large intestines, then an enterotomy is performed, sometimes several. If a portion of the intestinal tract has suffered a significant amount of damage due to poor perfusion or trauma, then the surgeon may need to perform a resection and anastomosis of the intestine.

Nursing care for the postoperative enterotomy patient include continued IV fluid therapy, appropriate pain management, antiemetic therapy if indicated, and nutritional therapy. Care should be taken to protect the abdominal incision from urine or feces. Enteral nutrition should be initiated as soon as possible based on the patient's clinical status. The prognosis is generally dependent on the severity of the obstruction. Most patients can tolerate removal of up to 70% of their small intestines.

Intussusception

Intussusception is described as the invagination of one portion of the bowel into another. The proximal segment always invaginates into the distal bowel. The invagination typically occurs in the jejunum, ileum, or ileocolic junction. This disorder is common in puppies and kittens but can occur in animals of any age. Common causes are GI parasite infections, small bowel hypermotility, and those with severe bacterial or viral enteritis.

Clinical signs are similar to symptoms of intestinal obstruction, vomiting, anorexia, and diarrhea. The clinical signs are generally milder than those associated with a complete obstruction. Treatment is very similar to that of an intestinal foreign body obstruction.

Rectal Prolapse

This disorder is seen most frequently in puppies and kittens secondary to intestinal parasite infections and viral enteritis. However, it can occur in animals of any age due to neoplasia, perineal hernia, constipation, dystocia, urolithiasis, prostatitis, or foreign body. The diagnosis is made on physical examination. An everted tubular portion of the rectum is visualized protruding through the anus with tenesmus. It is important to differentiate a rectal prolapse from an intussuseption. A lubricated thermometer cannot be advanced between the rectal wall and prolapsed tissue in cases of rectal prolapse. Should the thermometer (or blunt probe) advance easily, then an intussuseption should be suspected.

If the rectal mucosa is not very irritated or edematous then treatment is fairly easy. The area should be lavaged with warm isotonic fluid, lubricated, and gently massaged until it is reduced. If edema makes this difficult, then a 50% dextrose solution can be applied to reduce the edema. A loose purse string is applied to the anus to allow for the passage of stool without a relapse of the rectal prolapse. The patient should be fed a low residue diet and prescribed a stool softener such as lactulose or docusate sodium. Once the underlying cause of the prolapse is identified and corrected, the purse string may be removed in 2 week's time.

In severe cases, surgical repair is necessary. A resection and anastomosis is performed if there is necrotic or devitalized tissue. If the prolapse continues to recur, then a colopexy may be indicated (Macintire et al. 2006). The use of rectal thermometers in the postoperative period is contraindicated in these patients (Macintire et al. 2006).

Pancreatitis

In dogs and cats, the pancreas is a long, narrow structure that is not easily discernible. The right limb of the pancreas lies next to the duodenum, and the left limb is next to the spleen. The pancreas has both endocrine and exocrine functions. The primary function of the exocrine pancreas is to synthesize and secrete a number of regulatory polypeptides, the most important of these being insulin and glucagon. It also produces digestive enzymes that are released into the duodenum through a duct system.

Pancreatitis is the most common exocrine pancreatic disease in dogs and cats. It is described as inflammation of the pancreas and is classified as either acute or chronic. Both classifications can be associated with systemic complications. Commonly, the acute form of pancreatitis is seen in patients that present in veterinary emergency rooms. Often the cause is unknown; however, it is generally thought that pancreatitis occurs when digestive enzymes are activated that cause autodigestion of the pancreas. Pancreatic inflammation can extend to the stomach, duodenum, liver, and colon. It is one of the most common causes of bile duct obstruction. Vasoactive mediators are released into the systemic circulation of the animal and can lead to a number of effects commonly associated with severe pancreatitis including liver and kidney damage, pulmonary edema, DIC, and hypotension (Gaynor 2009).

There is no specific cause of pancreatitis, though low-protein, high-fat diets have been shown to induce the disease. Hyperlipidemia typically precedes pancreatitis in both humans and dogs. Some drugs are suspected to aid in the development of pancreatitis, though there have been no studies to prove this as of yet. These drugs include corticosteroids, furosemide, thiazide diuretics, tetracycline, sulfonamides, and azathioprine. Accidental trauma such as blunt force from a car impact or high-rise syndrome can lead to pancreatitis. Pancreatitis may occur simply from the handling of the pancreas during surgery or obtaining a sample for biopsy. Hypotension during anesthesia may cause sufficient ischemia to the pancreas to cause the disorder. An in-house snap test aids in diagnosing pancreatitis (Fig. 8.5).

Etiology

Abnormal fusion of normally segregated lysosomes with zymogen granules occurs within acinar cells. The result is the premature activation of trypsinogen to trypsin and changes in intracellular ionized calcium (iCa). Other proenzymes are activated by trypsin and a cascade of local and systemic effects are set into motion resulting in the clinical signs of acute pancreatitis. Localized ischemia and oxygen free radicals contribute to the disruption of cell membranes resulting in pancreatic necrosis and hemorrhage and increased capillary permeability. Increases in pancreatic vascular permeability can lead to fluid losses, comprising perfusion and stimulating the recruitment of additional inflammatory cells and mediators, resulting in a vicious cycle that leads to SIRS and MODS.

Dogs with acute pancreatitis may present with anorexia, weakness, and occasionally, diarrhea. Often, they will show signs of abdominal discomfort. Alternatively, cats often no not always exhibit clinical signs of abdominal discomfort. Physical examination may reveal the patient to be febrile, icteric, dehydrated, and painful on abdominal palpation. Bowel sounds may be undetectable on auscultation as a result of concurrent peritonitis

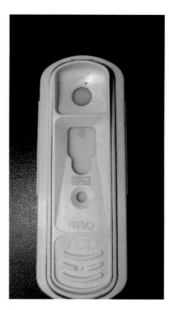

Figure 8.5   In-house snap test available for aiding in the diagnosis of pancreatitis (SNAP® cPL™ Test [canine pancreas-specific lipase], IDEXX Laboratories, Westbrook, ME]).

or intestinal ileus. There may be evidence of systemic involvement at the time of presentation, including bleeding disorders, cardiac arrhythmias, dyspnea, oliguria, shock, and collapse. Baseline information taken from samples at the time of presentation should include urinalysis, urine culture and sensitivity, thoracic and abdominal radiographs, blood gas, lactate, iCa, and coagulation times. A multi-lumen catheter should be placed to allow for serial monitoring of the above values to spare the patient the discomfort of multiple venipunctures. Further, depending on the severity of the disease, parenteral nutrition may need to be included as a part of the patient's treatment plan.

The diagnosis of pancreatitis can be challenging. In-house lab work can be helpful, but it alone will not provide a definitive diagnosis. Lab work may reveal a neutrophilic leukocytosis with a left shift, thrombocytopenia, anemia (more commonly seen in cats than in dogs), an increased PCV reflective of dehydration, increased liver enzymes indicative of concurrent hepatic disease, prerenal azotemia, hyperglycemia or hypoglycemia as a result of hepatic disease, SIRS or sepsis, hypocalcemia, and hypomagnesemia, potentially reflective of peripancreatic fat saponification. Decreased iCa in cats has been shown to be a poor prognostic indicator. There may be hypoalbuminemia resulting from GI losses. Additionally, lab work results may include hypokalemia, hypercholesterolemia, hypertriglyceridemia, and hyperlipidemia which may be grossly obvious and can interfere with other blood serum chemistry values.

Elevations in lipase and amylase have historically been diagnostic markers for acute pancreatitis; however, these values may stem from extrapancreatic sources as with azotemia or GI disease. Further, these values may be within normal limits, particularly in cats. Trypsin-like immunoreactivity (TLI) is suggestive of acute pancreatitis but may result from azotemia or GI disease in cats and again can be within normal limits in confirmed cases of pancreatitis. Currently, pancreatic lipase immunoreactivity (PLI) assays are the diagnostic test of choice. This test is species-specific, and the results are not affected by extrapancreatic lipase activity. The recent introduction of an in-house snap test to detect canine-specific pancreatic lipase has proved useful in quickly confirming a diagnosis of acute pancreatitis in the dog.

Radiographs are useful in ruling out conditions such as intestinal obstruction. Increased density and diminished contrast of the right cranial abdomen may be noted with displacement of the stomach to the left. The area between the stomach and duodenum may appear to be widened as well. Abdominal ultrasound may reveal an enlarged, hyperechoic pancreas as well as hyperechoic peripancreatic tissue. A study of the accuracy of diagnosing pancreatitis based on abdominal ultrasound found it to be 68% effective. This seems to be largely dependent on operator skill level, however, and is most definitely a better diagnostic tool than the measurement of amylase and lipase alone. Ultrasound can detect subtle changes and is useful in the sampling of fluid or tissue for pathologist review. Computed tomography (CT), while the gold standard in human medicine for diagnosing pancreatitis, has not been studied sufficiently to prove its accuracy in detecting acute pancreatitis in the veterinary patient (Gaynor 2009).

Patients with pancreatitis can decompensate quickly at any time and as such, continual monitoring is required. Initial treatment is aimed at resuscitation of the hemodynamically unstable patient. Shock rate replacement fluids and increased maintenance rates may be required to replace ongoing losses due to vomiting, insensible losses, or third spacing into the GI tract.

Aggressive pain management is required for patients suffering from pancreatitis. It not only decreases stress hormone levels and improves ventilation, but it also may improve GI motility if ileus is present as a result of severe pain. Thus, the administration of pain medication is indicated even if the patient is not displaying overt clinical signs of pain. A CRI of an opioid such as fentanyl may be initiated at a dose of 3–5 mcg/kg/h for moderate pain. In the case of severe pain, the fentanyl can be increased to 5–10 mcg/kg/h, and ketamine is supplemented at a dose of 0.2–0.4 mg/kg/h. As with any animal receiving an opioid, the patient's respiratory function needs to be continually evaluated. Low-dose lidocaine may also be added to the pain management regime for multimodal pain management. Lidocaine has the added benefit of having promotility effects and as such is helpful in patients with severe ileus. On the other hand, lidocaine CRIs may also make patients nauseated and less interested in eating. Additionally, the use of ketamine and lidocaine in the treatment of pancreatitis may prove beneficial when considering the oxidative damage that is associated with this disease (Gaynor 2009).

Historically, patients with acute pancreatitis have been non per os (NPO) for up to several days, the idea being to rest the pancreas for a period of time. In fact, there has been no evidence to support not feeding patients that are not vomiting. Furthermore, there is no evidence to show that feeding a patient with pancreatitis stimulates pancreatic secretions. Animals with severe acute pancreatitis are typically in a hypercatabolic state and require enteral nutrition early in treatment. There are a number of benefits of enteral feeding, including improved gut mucosal function, decrease chances of bacterial translocation, less cost to the client, decreases in hospitalization time, and far fewer complications than with parenteral feeding.

"If the Gut Works, Use It"

Ideally, the patient will take food willingly. If the patient is not taking enough nutrition orally on their own, then syringe feeding is an option. However, a number of patients

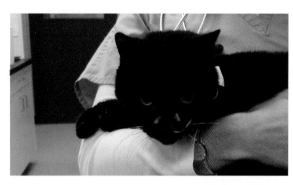

Figure 8.6   This cat has had a nasoesophageal (NE) tube placed for the administration of nutrition in the absence of oral intake.

may not be compliant with this method. If this is the case, then a feeding tube may be placed to provide enteral feeding that meets the patient's nutritional requirements. Nasoesophageal (NE) tubes are the most desirable option as often the patient does not require anything other than light sedation for placement (Fig. 8.6).

Another option is an esophagostomy tube as some patients will require long-term nutritional support, and these tubes are easily tolerated by the patient. Placement is relatively simple and requires only a short time under anesthesia. Another benefit is that the patient can be released to the client with this tube in place for at-home management. If the patient is unable to tolerate either of the above feeding tubes, then a gastrostomy or jejunostomy tube is yet another option for enteral feeding. A gastrostomy tube may be placed by either the percutaneous endoscopic gastrostomy (PEG) technique or via laparotomy. Both of these techniques require general anesthesia, with the laparotomy technique requiring lengthy anesthesia and surgical incision into the abdomen. The advantage of the laparotomy technique is that an abdominal exploration is performed and biopsies can be obtained. Similarly, a jejunostomy tube requires a laparotomy and extended anesthesia times. This type of feeding tube bypasses the stomach and pancreas altogether, and feeding is introduced directly into the jejunum. This tube requires a CRI of nutrition. The more invasive the feeding tube, the more complications there are, such as infection of the insertion site and peritonitis upon tube removal.

Total parenteral nutrition (TPN) or partial parenteral nutrition (PPN) is indicated when the nutritional needs of the patient cannot be met by enteral feeding or if continued vomiting prevents the use of the feeding tubes mentioned above. In these cases, the diet is based on the individual patient's nutritional requirement and administered intravenously through a specially designated catheter lumen. Unfortunately, the cost to the client is considerable, and the risk of sepsis is significantly increased.

Antibiotic therapy is recommended only when a documented infection is present. The prophylactic use of antibiotic therapy has not been shown to improve the outcome of acute pancreatitis. However, an experimental study in dogs has demonstrated some improved survivability. A number of clinicians opt to administer a second generation cephalosporin or a combination of enrofloxacin and ampicillin with these animals.

A number of antiemetics are available for use with patients with acute pancreatitis and should be administered to stop ongoing fluid losses from vomiting. Metoclopramide has shown to improve GI tone and is generally administered as a CRI (0.01–0.02 mg/kg/h). One of the benefits of this drug is that it can be administered orally and as such can be prescribed to the client so therapy may continue at home after the patient is discharged. Dolasetron can be administered once daily as an IV injection (0.6–1 mg/kg). Maropitant is another antiemetic that is given as a subcutaneous injection once daily (1 mg/kg). This drug has both central and peripheral effects and has been reported to have the added benefit of blocking visceral pain. It is important to note that maropitant may cause pain during or just after injection in some animals and as such care should be taken when administering this drug.

Animals that recover from acute pancreatitis may continue to have flare-ups throughout their lives. They are at risk of developing diseases such as diabetes mellitus, chronic pancreatitis, and exocrine pancreatic insufficiency. According to studies, dogs that have had acute pancreatitis may have continued subclinical pancreatic inflammation.

Liver Disease

The liver is one of the largest organs in the body. In adult dogs and cats, it accounts for approximately 3% of the total body weight. It has deeply incised lobes that are easily discernable. The visceral surface of the liver is in contact with the stomach. Changes in size or shape of the liver can cause displacement of the stomach, which may explain why vomiting is often a clinical sign for many liver diseases.

Hepatic Lipidosis

Hepatic lipidosis is not a primary GI disease nor does it affect the GI system. However, disturbances within the GI system can lead to hepatic lipidosis, particularly in cats. Fat accumulation in the liver can result in all species, specifically as a result of diabetes mellitus. In cats, however, idiopathic hepatic lipidosis is the most common form of the disease. Overweight cats seem to be most predisposed to this disease, though any cat that consumes insufficient calories or becomes completely anorexic is at risk. Certain amino acids such as arginine and methionine may play a role in lipid accumulation. When the amount of carbohydrates consumed is less than what is required for body maintenance, fatty acids are mobilized from the body fat. These fatty acids are released into the blood and end up in the liver where they are first converted into triglycerides and then further converted into lipoproteins. The fat content in a normal feline liver is about 5%, whereas the liver of a cat with lipidosis may double or triple in size due to retained fat.

Cats with hepatic lipidosis usually present with a history of anorexia, weight loss, lethargy, vomiting, and weakness. Often, the physical examination will reveal icterus, hepatomegaly, cachexia, and dehydration. The degree of jaundice should not be used as a prognostic indicator as the liver has the ability to make a full recovery despite severe elevations in liver enzymes.

Blood work will usually reveal an increase of liver enzymes. Total bilirubin concentrations can range up to 20 mg/dL, and there may be a mild to moderate nonregenerative anemia present, as well as increases in alanine aminotransferase and alkaline phosphatase. Hyperglycemia may be mild to moderate, and in severe cases, hyperammonemia may be present. The synthesis of alpha and beta globulins occurs in the liver. Prothrombin is perhaps the most important alpha globulin produced by the liver. Because prothrombin along with thrombin is necessary for coagulation, any injury to the liver hinders the body's ability to form clots. It is therefore crucial that clotting times be within normal range before liver biopsies and multiple venipunctures be performed, specifically those involving larger vessels such as the jugular veins.

Radiographs may only reveal an enlarged liver. Abdominal ultrasound provides clearer information about the liver and will allow for liver aspirates. A diagnosis of hepatic lipidosis may only be made by evaluating the hepatic cells. One retrospective study found that in over 90% of cases of feline hepatic lipidosis, there were concurrent diseases such as IBD, septic peritonitis, inflammatory liver disease, and pancreatitis, among others.

Because lack of nutrition promotes lipolysis and glycogenolysis, it is important to institute nutritional therapy as soon as possible. Nutritional therapy will likely be necessary for several weeks to months. If the patient is stable enough to endure general anesthesia, then an esophagostomy tube or PEG tube may be placed to provide nutrition. In the unstable patient, an NE tube is an acceptable route of nutrition administration. Non-lactate- and non-glucose-containing IV fluid therapy will treat dehydration, as it decreases hepatic circulation and impairs detoxification. Attention should be paid to improve and/or maintain serum potassium, phosphate, and magnesium levels, as decreases in these can be a result of refeeding syndrome. Antiemetic therapy along with the administration of vitamin K may be required. Half of cats suffering from hepatic lipidosis have prolonged clotting times and will need supplemental vitamin K.

Hepatic Encephalopathy (HE)

HE is defined as a dysfunction of the brain secondary to hepatic dysfunction. This disorder occurs in both dogs and cats and represents a number of complex neurological symptoms. HE is classified as either acute, severe total hepatic failure, or chronic, which may be subclinical or severe, and is the more common form of HE. Cats can have a form of HE related to a deficiency of essential amino acids and the subsequent development of hepatic lipidosis. This form can be successfully managed with amino acid supplementation.

Mild cases of HE can be managed by feeding the patient a low protein diet high in carbohydrates, thus leading to a reduction of the associated ammonia and amino acid load. It is important to be mindful of the animal's nutritional requirements. More severe cases of HE are treated with lactulose, antibiotics, and potentially colonic retention enemas (e.g., povidone-iodine).

Lactulose is not absorbed in the small intestine and is fermented to volatile free fatty acids by colonic bacteria. This results in shifting the equilibrium to a nonabsorbable ionized ammonia, and increased colonic motility (Steiner 2008). Metronidazole and neomycin are antibiotics that are often selected as they reduce the flora in the intestine, reducing toxic by-products produced by bacteria in the gut. Colonic enemas with povidone-iodine work in a similar fashion by reducing large bowel bacteria.

Septic Peritonitis

Peritonitis is defined as the inflammation of the peritoneal cavity and has many etiologies. In the presence of bacteria, it is referred to as septic peritonitis. Causes of septic peritonitis include penetrating injury (as from a stick or bullet), ruptured GI, necrotic tumor, ruptured uterus or urinary bladder, prostatic, splenic, and hepatic abscesses, and sepsis. The most common cause of this disease is from some form of disruption from the GI tract, frequently due to the presence of a foreign body that has perforated the intestines. GI leakage may also occur from ulceration of the stomach wall, neoplasia, ischemic damage, and dehiscence of a previous surgical incision. NSAID administration has been associated with gastroduodenal perforation. Bacteria that are absorbed by the peritoneum have systemic effects including SIRS, shock, DIC, hypotension, acid–base disturbances and electrolyte derangements that can affect cardiac function resulting in decreased cardiac output. Azotemia results from renal hypoperfusion and insufficiency, and acute renal failure can result from direct renal damage from bacteremia.

Animals with septic peritonitis typically present with a nonspecific history. Owners may report anorexia, depression, vomiting, diarrhea, or collapse. Septic peritonitis should be high on the list of differentials for any patient that has recently undergone abdominal surgery. Animals may be recumbent or ambulatory at presentation, reflecting the severity of systemic involvement. Those that are standing may be in what is known as the "praying position" in which the back is arched while the front posture is lowered. Physical examination findings include fever, tachycardia, weak peripheral pulses, and abdominal pain on palpation. It is noteworthy to mention that one study found that only 62% of cats with septic peritonitis exhibited pain when their abdomen was palpated. Patients may present in varying stages of hypovolemic and cardiovascular shock, with either pale or injected mucous membranes, prolonged CRT, weak pulses with tachycardia and, depending on the state of perfusion, hypothermia or hyperthermia. A small percentage of cats may present both bradycardia and hypothermia, which according to a recent study is consistent with a markedly decreased survival rate. Additionally, hyperlactemia in cats with septic peritonitis has been shown to be a poor prognostic indicator.

Because many of these patients present collapsed, treatment and diagnosis start simultaneously. Emergency diagnostics and stabilization measures should be instituted within 5 minutes of presentation. Preliminary blood work should include PCV and TS, coagulation times, blood gas that includes BUN, blood glucose, lactate, pH, and electrolytes. An abdominocentesis should be performed (regardless of ultrasound availability), and the fluid should be microscopically evaluated for septic suppurative inflammation (increased neutrophil count and bacteria). Measurement of glucose and lactate levels from abdominal fluid may also be useful when compared in conjunction with those from peripheral blood to support the diagnosis.

Intravenous catheters are placed and fluid therapy is initiated. Because hypoproteinemia is common in patients with septic peritonitis, large volumes of crystalloids may result in edema. Therefore, a combination of crystalloid and colloid fluid therapy, which may include blood products such as fresh frozen plasma, is preferred. The end goal is to have the patient resuscitated to the point that they are able to go to surgery within 6 hours of presentation, as is the goal in human medicine.

Abdominocentesis is indicated when there is free fluid within the abdomen. The patient is positioned in left lateral recumbency and an area of approximately 6 in. is clipped and aseptically prepared around the umbilicus (Fig. 8.7).

Using the following technique and wearing sterile gloves, a 22 or 20 gauge needle is inserted into four quadrants: cranial and to the right, cranial and to the left, caudal to the right, and caudal to the left (Fig. 8.8).

The needle is twisted gently as it is inserted so as to push abdominal organs away from the tip. An over-the-needle catheter the same as the gauge mentioned above may also be utilized in this technique. Usually, fluid will flow freely from one or more of the needle hubs. If not, then a 3- or 6-mL syringe is attached to one of the needles, and the fluid is

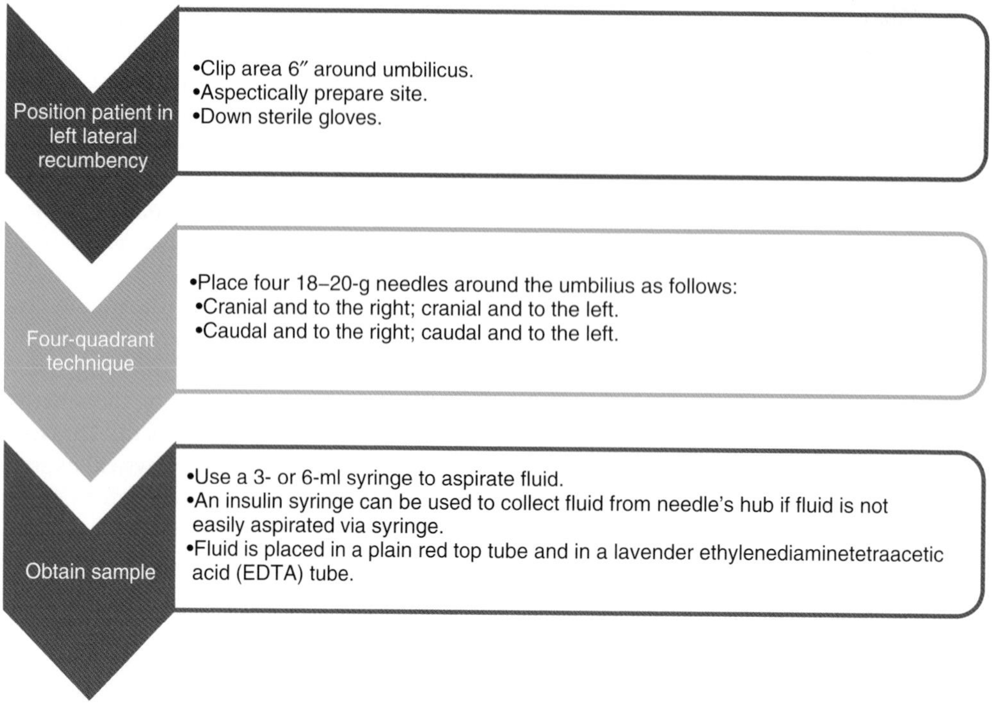

Position patient in left lateral recumbency
- Clip area 6″ around umbilicus.
- Aspectically prepare site.
- Down sterile gloves.

Four-quadrant technique
- Place four 18–20-g needles around the umbilius as follows:
- Cranial and to the right; cranial and to the left.
- Caudal and to the right; caudal and to the left.

Obtain sample
- Use a 3- or 6-ml syringe to aspirate fluid.
- An insulin syringe can be used to collect fluid from needle's hub if fluid is not easily aspirated via syringe.
- Fluid is placed in a plain red top tube and in a lavender ethylenediaminetetraacetic acid (EDTA) tube.

Figure 8.7   Abdominocentesis technique.

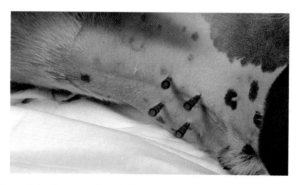

Figure 8.8   Four quadrant abdominocentesis technique.

aspirated from the abdominal cavity. If there is appreciable peritoneal effusion, either visible on radiographs or on ultrasound, then a blind abdominocentesis should yield a sufficient sample for analysis. However, if a patient arrives early in the disease process, there may be very little fluid in the peritoneum. In cases such as this, an ultrasound-guided abdominocentesis is indicated. If minimal volumes of fluid make a definitive diagnosis impossible, then a diagnostic peritoneal lavage (DPL) is indicated.

While there are commercial kits available for DPL, they are expensive and are often unnecessary as most veterinary hospitals have the required tools to perform the technique. The ventral abdomen is clipped and aseptically prepared as described above. Multiple side ports are cut into an 18- or 16-gauge over-the-needle catheter while wearing sterile gloves. It is of importance to note to not cut more than half the circumference of the catheter as it may weaken and could potentially break off inside the patient's abdominal cavity. The catheter is inserted into the peritoneal cavity just caudal and to the right of the umbilicus and is directed dorsally and caudally. Warmed sterile saline (0.9% NaCl, 22 mL/kg) is then infused into the peritoneal cavity. The catheter is then removed. The patient is monitored for respiratory distress as the increase in intraabdominal pressure may put pressure on the diaphragm and impair respiratory function. Ambulatory patients should be walked while their abdomen is concurrently massaged so that the fluid is distributed throughout the peritoneal cavity. If the patient is nonambulatory, then it should be gently rolled from side to side. The abdomen is then again aseptically prepared, and abdominocentesis is performed to obtain a fluid sample. In cases that require DPL, biochemical analyses can be artificially decreased as a result of dilution.

Fluid samples should be submitted for pathologist review, aerobic and anaerobic culture, and sensitivity. An in-house cytology is useful in diagnosing the cause of the peritonitis. Increases in WBCs (greater than 2000 cells per microliter) along with intracellular bacteria are indicative of septic peritonitis. Fluid from patients that have recently undergone abdominal surgery may show signs of significant inflammation. In these animals, 7000–9000 WBCs per microliter is suggestive of a moderate peritonitis. Furthermore, animals that have been receiving antibiotics may have no observable bacteria in their peritoneal fluid samples despite having contamination.

In addition to in-house analysis of peritoneal fluid using a microscope, measuring glucose and lactate concentrations has proved to be useful in the diagnosis of septic peritonitis in dogs. Studies have shown that a glucose concentration difference of greater than 20 mg/dL between a peripheral blood sample and peritoneal fluid is 100% specific for a diagnosis of septic peritonitis. A blood-to-fluid lactate difference less than 2 mmol/L is assumptive of a diagnosis of septic peritonitis in dogs; however, the same does not apply to cats.

A complete blood count may reflect a leukocytosis with or without a left shift, anemia, and thrombocytopenia. A serum chemistry including lipase and amylase should be run in-house using both peripheral blood samples and peritoneal fluid. A coagulation profile should be run and monitored throughout the course of treatment. All results are taken into account and are useful in determining specific organ involvement.

Once the patient is hemodynamically stable, survey abdominal radiographs are obtained. Usually, these will reveal a loss of detail (as with abdominal effusion) or pneumoperitoneum. Evidence of intestinal obstruction or bowel placation can be ruled out. If films are not conclusive and ultrasound is unavailable, then an upper GI contrast study can be performed to confirm a GI rupture. Barium sulfate should not be utilized in cases where GI rupture is strongly suspected as it will cause lesions in the peritoneum. Rather, a nonionic iodinated contrast medium such as iohexol should be used. Abdominal ultrasound is the preferred diagnostic choice when imaging and is often useful in determining the underlying cause of the peritonitis.

The goals in treatment of septic peritonitis include stabilizing the patient, identifying and addressing the source of contamination, correcting the infection, initiating appropriate antibiotic therapy, and establishing peritoneal drainage. After pre-therapy blood and urine samples are obtained, fluid resuscitation is initiated. Shock doses of crystalloids and colloids are administered to correct hypovolemia and electrolyte imbalances. Broadspectrum antibiotics are administered empirically as studies have demonstrated that patients that receive empirical antibiotic therapy have an increased chance of survival as compared to those that do not. If renal function in the patient has been determined to be normal, then an aminoglycoside such as gentamycin or amikacin coupled with a first-generation cephalosporin such as ampicillin may be administered. Cefoxitin, a second-generation cephalosporin, may be administered as a single agent or combined with ampicillin or cefazolin concurrently with enrofloxacin or an aminoglycoside. Metronidazole may also be added to the treatment plan in the event that extended anaerobic therapy is required. Bactericidal drugs are preferred over bacteriostatic drugs as patients with septic peritonitis are immunocompromised. Once the patient is stable enough for general anesthesia, a celiotomy is indicated.

The purpose of surgery in the patient is to resolve the source of infection, decrease the contaminated load via peritoneal lavage, and, if indicated, provide the patient with a method for enteral feeding. Once the source of infection has been surgically corrected, large volumes of warm sterile isotonic fluid are used to lavage the abdominal cavity.

Care of postoperative septic abdomen patients is complex, as these animals are critically ill and at risk of a number of complications. As with any critically ill patient, a multi-lumen catheter should be placed at the time of presentation if possible; if not, then postoperative placement is acceptable. The multi-lumen catheter allows for serial blood draws with no patient discomfort, central venous pressure (CVP) measurement, multiple fluid type administration, as well as parenteral nutrition administration if necessary. Additionally, a urinary catheter, if not placed prior to surgery, should be placed immediately following when the patient is returned to the critical care unit. The urinary catheter will serve multiple purposes: prevent contamination of incision sites or open abdomen, maximize patient comfort as well as measurement of urinary output. Monitoring urine output (UOP) is crucial in helping to maintain an adequate fluid balance in the postoperative septic abdomen. The amount and types of fluids administered to the postoperative septic abdomen are dependent on several factors, including CVP, blood pressure, body weight, maintenance requirements, and continued fluid losses, concurrent infusions such as blood products, parenteral or enteral nutrition, and UOP.

Maintaining adequate blood pressure and subsequently adequate tissue perfusion in the postoperative septic abdomen patient can be difficult, as some of the inflammatory mediators released during sepsis have hypotensive effects. If the patient has had adequate fluid resuscitation and is still unable to maintain a normal blood pressure, then it is determined to be in septic shock and will require the administration of vasopressors. Dopamine improves renal and mesenteric perfusion at lower doses. As doses increase, vasoconstriction increases as does myocardial contractility. Further increases in dosages result in constriction of renal arteries, decreasing renal perfusion and causing irreversible kidney damage. Dobutamine enhances myocardial function and increases cardiac output. Norepinephrine and vasopressin are both potent vasoconstrictors and are generally only reserved for cases that do not respond to the above vasopressors.

When caring for the postoperative septic abdomen patient (or any critically ill animal), Kirby's Rule of 20 should be considered at all times.

While it may appear daunting, it helps to guide the veterinary team as they tailor their treatment plans according to each patient. With the septic peritonitis patient, just about every rule applies with postoperative nursing care. The veterinary technician is responsible for maintaining patient comfort, administering a number of medication and fluids, as well as advocating for the patient, such as when pain control is inadequate. Monitoring the patient's heart rate, rhythm, UOP, blood pressure, CVP, and laboratory values are only a part of the technician's role.

CHAPTER 8

Box 8.1   Kirby's Rule of 20

- Fluid balance
- Oncotic pull
- Glucose
- Electrolyte and acid–base balance
- Oxygenation and ventilation
- Mentation
- Perfusion and blood pressure
- Heart rate, rhythm, and contractility
- Albumin level
- Coagulation
- Red blood cell and hemoglobin concentration
- Renal function
- Immune status, antibiotic dosage and selection, WBC count
- GI motility and mucosal integrity
- Drug dosages and metabolism
- Nutrition
- Pain control
- Nursing care and patient mobilization
- Wound care and bandage change
- Tender loving care

References

Bill, R. 2008. *NSAIDS-Keeping Up with All the Changes. Atlantic Coast Veterinary Conference Proceedings.*

Breton, A. 2008. *Gastrointestinal Technician Multidisciplinary Systems Review. International Veterinary Emergency and Critical Care Symposium Proceedings.*

Gaynor, A. 2009. Acute pancreatitis. In *Small Animal Critical Care Medicine*, edited by Editor, DS, Editor, KH. St. Louis, MO: Saunders, pp. 537–541.

Humm, K. 2009. Canine parvovirus infection. In *Small Animal Critical Care Medicine*, edited by Editor, DS, Editor, KH. St. Louis, MO: Saunders, pp. 482–485.

Ishiwata, K, Minagawa, T, Kajimoto, T. 1998. Clinical effects of the recombinant feline interferon-omega on experimental parvovirus infection in beagle dogs. *J Vet Medical Science* 60(8):911–917.

Macintire, D. 2006. *Treatment of Parvoviral Enteritis. Western Veterinary Conference Proceedings.*

Macintire, D, Drobatz, K, Haskins, S, et al. 2006. *Manual of Small Animal Emergency and Critical Care Medicine.* Hoboken, NJ: Wiley-Blackwell.

Mohr, A, Leisewitz, A, Jacobson, L et al. 2003. Effect of early enteral nutrition on intestinal permeability, intestinal protein loss, and outcome in dogs with severe parvoviral enteritis. *J Vet Intern Medicine* 17(6):791–798.

Petrollini-Rogers, E, Otto, C. 2009. *Canine Parvovirus.* International Veterinary Emergency and Critical Care Symposium Proceedings.

Rewerts, J, McCaw, D, Cohn, L, et al. 1998. Recombinant human granulocyte colony-stimulating factor for treatment of puppies with neutropenia secondary to canine parvovirus infection. *J Am Vet Medical Assoc* 213(7):991–992.

Stavisky, J. 2009. *Parvovirus Disease*. British Small Animal Veterinary Congress Proceedings.

Steiner, J. 2008. *Small Animal Gastroenterology*. Hannover, Germany: Schlutersche Verlagsgesellschaft mbH & Co.

Zacher, LA, Berg, K, Shaw, SP, Kudeg, RK. 2010. Association between outcome and changes in plasma lactate concentration during presurgical treatment in dogs with gastric dilatation-volvulus: 64 cases (2002–2008). *J Am Vet Med Assoc* 236(8): 892–897.

Urogenital Emergencies

9

Andrea M. Steele

Introduction

Numerous conditions of the urogenital tract can cause a patient to present as an emergency. These conditions can be of primary or secondary causes. It is important for veterinary technicians to have a firm grasp of disorders of the urogenital system, and an understanding of how to differentiate between primary and secondary conditions. This chapter will concentrate on the anatomy and physiology of the kidneys, reasons why they are susceptible to damage, and give examples of common emergencies seen in veterinary medicine. Nursing strategies for renal patients will also be discussed.

Renal Anatomy

Location

The kidneys lie in the retroperitoneal space in dogs and cats. They lie in a sheltered area under the strong dorsal muscles along the back, and are surrounded by protective adipose tissue. Renal fascia holds the kidneys in place, and the right kidney lies slightly more cranial than the left in all species. The kidneys of the cat are quite mobile, and easily moved on palpation, whereas in dogs they are more firmly affixed (Christie 2003). The length of the kidney in both species is proportional to the size of the animal and when assessed radiographically, is compared to the length of the second lumbar vertebrae (L2). In both species, normal kidneys are considered to be 2.5–3 times the length of L2, and both kidneys should be the same size (Dennis et al. 2001; Christie 2003).

Gross Anatomy

In the gross anatomy of the dog and cat kidney, there are two layers: the cortex (outer layer) and the medulla (inner layer). The kidney of the dog and cat is termed "unilobar" or one lobe (Moffat 1975).

Other important structures within the dog kidney include the renal pelvis, a large collecting channel for urine that terminates in the ureter, and a fibrous capsule that surrounds the entire kidney. In the cat, the anatomy is quite similar; however, cats have a serosal capsule, not the strong fibrous sheath of the dog (Christie 2003).

Renal Blood Supply

The blood supply of the kidney arises from the aorta via the renal artery and terminates at the caudal vena cava via the renal vein. The two renal arteries branch from the caudal aorta, with one going to each kidney. In some dogs, two renal arteries going to the same kidney have been identified (Marques-Sampaio et al. 2007). The kidney is a very vascular organ, and the artery branches into several interlobar arteries, then smaller arterioles and capillaries within the kidney tissue. The capillary beds terminate in the beginning of the venous circulation as small venules and finally end in the renal vein, which flows into the caudal vena cava.

Microscopic Anatomy

Microscopically, the anatomy of the kidney is highly specialized. The structural and functional unit of the kidney is the nephron. The nephron is a multicellular structure composed of several distinct areas, each with its own function (Fig. 9.1).

The nephron is composed of Bowman's space (also referred to as Bowman's capsule), glomerulus, proximal tubule, the loop of Henle (ascending and descending limbs), and the distal tubule. Dogs and cats differ in the number of nephrons per kidney; dogs have approximately 415,000 nephrons per kidney, and cats have approximately 190,000 nephrons per kidney (Christie 2003). Numerous nephrons connect to collecting tubules,

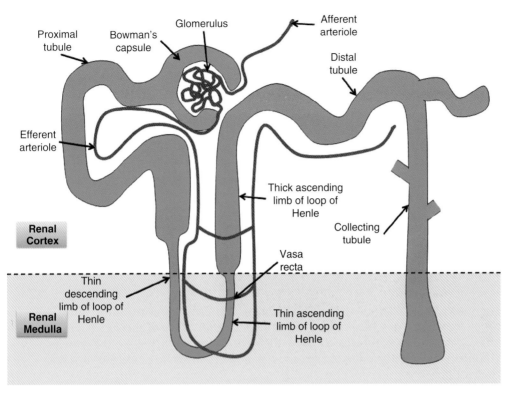

Figure 9.1   Schematic view of the renal nephron. The nephron is a hollow structure where filtrate enters at the glomerulus and moves through the proximal tubule, loop of Henle, distal tubule, and finally into the collecting tubules. The filtrate is adjusted throughout its journey through the nephron and collecting tubules to ultimately form urine. Modified from Rennke and Denker (2007).

eventually depositing urine into the renal pelvis for delivery to the bladder via the ureters.

Two of the principal features of the nephron are the glomerulus and Bowman's space. The glomerulus is a capillary bed that is fed by the afferent arteriole, which arises from the renal artery. The blood enters the glomerulus, circulates through very quickly, then exits through the efferent arteriole. The efferent arteriole then continues to supply blood to the remainder of the nephron and carry away reabsorbed solutes and water from the tubules.

Bowman's capsule is a hollow structure that surrounds the glomerulus. The epithelial structure of Bowman's capsule is intimately associated with the glomerular capillary membrane, allowing rapid movement of ultrafiltrate into the space (DiBartola 2006). Bowman's space is contiguous with the lumen of the proximal tubules, the next structure of the nephron.

The proximal tubule is a long, convoluted tube with an inner lumen covered in microvilli to increase surface area. The proximal tubule terminates in the loop of Henle, a "hairpin" curve shaped structure which is divided into the thin descending, thin ascending, and thick ascending sections. The loop of Henle extends from the kidney cortex to deep in the medulla, before curving back and into the kidney cortex. Finally, the thick ascending loop of Henle becomes the distal convoluted tubule, which terminates at the collecting duct.

Renal Physiology

The kidneys play a vital role in maintaining the volume and composition of body fluids. In the normal animal, while at rest, and in a thermoneutral environment, water balance is maintained: water intake is equal to water lost. Kidneys clean the body fluids of end products such as urea, uric acid, and creatinine, while also conserving solutes such as proteins, amino acids, and glucose in the body. They produce hormones such as erythropoietin, renin-angiotensin, and calcitriol, and have metabolic functions such as participating in the *degradation of peptides*. Thus, any disruption in their ability to perform these functions can have a far-reaching impact upon the body.

Urine Production

The most important function of the kidney is the production of urine, the process by which the kidneys rid the body of end products of metabolism and toxins and reabsorb water. The kidney reabsorbs 99% of the plasma water filtered by the tubules. Urine production relies on two factors: proper function of the nephron and blood supply to the glomerulus.

The nephron is where urine production takes place and the glomerulus, surrounded by Bowman's capsule, initiates the filtration process. The glomerulus delivers approximately 20 times the patient's extracellular fluid volume to the nephrons each day, resulting in a glomerular filtration rate (GFR) of 3–5 mL/min/kg for dogs and 2.5–3.5 mL/min/kg for cats (Brown 2003; DiBartola 2006). Both the glomerulus and Bowman's capsule are single cell in thickness, and their close proximity allows the rapid movement of small and mid-weight molecules and water from the glomerulus to the capsule (DiBartola 2006). The mean renal arterial pressure is 100 mmHg, for both dogs and cats, while the pressure within the glomerular capillary is 55 mmHg in dogs and 59 mmHg in cats. The pressure within the glomerular capillary is substantially higher than the pressure within Bowman's space, thus leading to a difference in hydrostatic pressure of 35 mmHg, facilitating rapid filtration through the glomerular capillary wall (DiBartola 2006). The glomerular capillary wall has both size and charge selectivity. Size selectivity excludes all molecules greater than 4 nm. Charge selectivity allows positively charged molecules to pass easily through the membrane, electrically neutral molecules meet with mild resistance, and negatively charged molecules experience the greatest resistance to filtration (DiBartola 2006).

Filtration is the initial step in urine production via the passive movement of protein and cell free plasma from the glomerular capillaries into Bowman's space to form a plasma ultrafiltrate. The ultrafiltrate moves into the tubules and is modified as it moves through the nephron:

1. The *proximal tubule's* large surface area allows for reabsorption of 50%–55% of filtered water and sodium, and virtually all of the glucose, phosphate, and amino acids found in the ultrafiltrate (DiBartola 2006; Rennke and Denker 2007). Reabsorption of solutes uses mechanisms of active transport, while water moves passively

along the concentration gradient as solutes move out of the tubule lumen and into the tubular cells (DiBartola 2006).

2. The *Loop of Henle* continues to reabsorb sodium and chloride as well as calcium and magnesium. Reabsorption within the loop requires an active transport mechanism. A concentration gradient is no longer established following the removal of solutes (glucose, phosphate, and amino acids) in the proximal tubules. Very little water is reabsorbed in the loop of Henle as the cells are relatively impermeable to water. The reabsorption of sodium, without reabsorption of water, causes a dilution of the filtrate and a hyposmotic fluid (DiBartola 2006; Rennke and Denker 2007).

3. The *distal tubule* is similar to the ascending limb of the loop of Henle as it is relatively impermeable to water but continues to reabsorb sodium and chloride. Parathyroid hormone acts on the distal tubules to regulate calcium reabsorption (DiBartola 2006; Rennke and Denker 2007).

4. The fluid reaching the *collecting duct* is hyposmotic to plasma with an osmolality of approximately 100 mOsm/kg. Under the influence of antidiuretic hormone (ADH), released from the posterior pituitary, the collecting ducts begin to reabsorb water. Without ADH, the collecting ducts are relatively impermeable to water. The osmolality of the urine can increase from 100 mOsm/kg to greater than 300 mOsm/kg, with approximately two-thirds of water being resorbed (DiBartola 2006; Rennke and Denker 2007).

Fluid in the collecting ducts is deposited in the renal pelvis as urine, where it enters the ureter and finally the bladder, where it awaits micturition.

The kidney's blood supply arises from the renal artery, to become the intrarenal arteries, which further bifurcate into smaller and smaller vessels. Approximately 90% of the renal blood flow (RBF) is directed to the renal cortex, the zone in which the glomeruli are found. This blood flow is actively involved in filtration (Dibartola 2006). On a microscopic level, each nephron is intimately associated with an afferent arteriole (which supplies the glomerulus), the efferent arteriole, and the vasa recta. The vessels of the kidneys are uniquely suited to protecting RBF, and thus supporting a maximal GFR. If an animal can maintain mean arterial blood pressures (MAPs) of 80–100 mmHg, the kidney can maintain a constant RBF and GFR that varies less than 10% (DiBartola 2006; Rennke and Denker 2007). This protective ability is referred to as *autoregulation* and is intrinsic to the kidney tissue, resulting in constriction or dilation of the afferent or efferent arterioles in response to varying mean arterial pressures.

If an animal becomes hypotensive with mean arterial pressures of 70 mmHg or less, RBF and GFR decline linearly, and autoregulation becomes ineffective (DiBartola 2006).

The kidneys are highly sensitive organs and can easily be damaged. They receive 20% of the cardiac output, and 90% of that blood goes to the kidney cortex, where key structures of the nephron are exposed to toxins concentrated in the blood. While autoregulation is used to keep RBF, and therefore GFR at a constant level, periods of hypotension (MAP < 70 mmHg) can cause an interruption of oxygen delivery to the kidney. Cells of the proximal tubule and thick ascending loop of Henle are particularly sensitive to ischemia as they have a very high metabolic rate (Grauer 2009).

Fortunately, the normal kidney has far more capacity than is required to perform its many functions, providing a substantial reserve. If the kidneys are damaged, they must lose 66% of their function before clinical signs of renal insufficiency will appear, and 75% before developing renal failure and blood work changes. After a hypoxic or toxic insult, the kidneys have the ability to regenerate tubular cells, and many patients will regain full or partial function. In veterinary patients, the goal is to support the patient through the crisis period, until sufficient function is restored (Rennke and Denker 2007).

The Renin-Angiotensin System (RAS)

The kidney has endocrine functions which are vital to the maintenance of extracellular fluid volume, red blood cell production, and maintenance of calcium homeostasis through the excretion of renin, erythropoietin, and calcitriol (DiBartola 2006). The RAS is of particular importance in emergency and critical care; it is very important to have a thorough understanding of the RAS and the response to hypovolemia and/or hypotension. Figure 9.2 summarizes the cause and effect of the RAS.

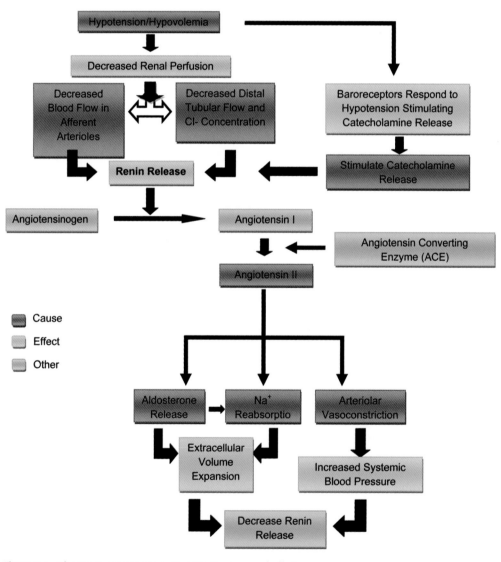

Figure 9.2   The Renin-angiotensin system (RAS), cause and effects.

Azotemia

Azotemia is recognized by an abnormal concentration of urea and creatinine in the blood. Azotemia can be related to a diminished capacity of the kidney to remove these substances, but equally as common, it can be related to conditions that affect the volume of blood reaching the kidneys, or impaired outflow of urine. As such, azotemia, and consequently, acute renal failure, are categorized as prerenal, intrinsic renal, or postrenal in origin.

Prerenal Azotemia

Prerenal azotemia literally translates to "before the kidney" azotemia, and implies a failure of blood supply to reach the glomerulus and subsequent reduction of solutes that move through the nephron. Classic prerenal causes of azotemia include conditions affecting intravascular volume such as hypovolemic shock or third space losses, decreased cardiac output, high protein diet, or gastrointestinal bleeding (Mathews 2007; Langston 2009).

Prerenal azotemia can quickly resolve if treatment is instituted and the inciting cause is removed. Typical treatments will include aggressive fluid therapy with the use of crystalloids, as well as synthetic colloids and/or blood products as indicated.

A common sequel to a severe hypotensive insult is damage to the kidney itself. This can result in acute intrinsic renal insufficiency or failure, which will be discussed next.

Acute Intrinsic Renal Failure (ARF)/Acute Kidney Injury (AKI)

ARF, also referred to as AKI, can be caused by different etiologies, and it is often difficult to determine the exact cause. The most common causes are ischemia, nephrotoxins, or infectious agents. ARF also occurs secondary to other disease processes (Ross et al. 2002).

Presentation

There are three phases involved in ARF, namely, (1) initiation, (2) maintenance, and (3) recovery. The stage that the patient is in will affect the presentation and diagnostics. In many or even most cases, however, the specific insult to the kidney is not known, and the patient may present with less specific symptoms. Symptoms may include change in urination patterns (increased or decreased), anorexia, restlessness, vomiting, diarrhea, ataxia, and seizures. Be aware that the owner may not know of a recent toxin exposure. Findings on physical examination may also be nonspecific and may include dehydration or overhydration, depression, hypothermia or hyperthermia, injected sclera, small bladder, and firm, large kidneys which are often painful. Blood work may show only mild changes in the initiation phase (Ross et al. 2002).

Unfortunately, because of the nonspecific signs of renal failure, many patients present at the end of the initiation phase or in the maintenance phase. Since the damage has already occurred, careful management is required to allow the kidneys to repair while avoiding complications. In most cases of moderate to severe ARF, patients would not survive to the recovery stage without veterinary intervention.

Box 9.1   Common Insults Resulting in Renal Insufficiency/ARF (Mathews 2007)

Toxins
- *Lillium* spp.
- Grapes and raisins
- Ethylene glycol
- Nonsteroidal anti-inflammatory drugs (NSAIDs)
- Antibiotics
  - Aminoglycosides
  - Polymyxin B
  - Sulfonamides
  - Tetracyclines
- Amphotericin B
- Heavy metals
- Radiocontrast media
- Hemoglobin
- Myoglobin

Ischemia
- Anesthesia
- Dehydration
- Hypotension
- Hypovolemia
- Renal vascular thrombosis
- Renal parenchymal injury

Infectious Agents
- Leptospirosis
- Bacterial or fungal pyelonephritis
- Babesiosis
- Borreliosis

Other Systemic Disease
- Disseminated intravascular coagulation
- Diabetes mellitus
- Hyperadrenocorticism

Initial diagnostics

Initial diagnostics may show several critical findings such as hypokalemia/hyperkalemia, severe dehydration or overhydration, severe metabolic acidosis, and severe hypocalcemia, all which must be addressed promptly. Obtaining necessary blood work prior to initiating intravenous therapy is very important to provide a baseline from which to reference future blood work. Initial packed cell volume/total solid (PCV/TS), blood gases, electrolytes, glucose, blood urea nitrogen (BUN), activated clotting time (ACT), complete blood count (CBC), biochemical profile, electrocardiogram (ECG), blood pressure (BP), urinalysis, and an accurate body weight would be considered the minimum database for any patient suspected of ARF (Ross et al. 2002; Mathews 2006a,b; Mathews 2007).

Initial interventions

Placement of a peripheral intravenous catheter will allow fluid resuscitation and administration of drugs. Placement of a central venous catheter may be indicated, as it will allow the measurement of central venous pressures (CVPs). CVP is used in many institutions as a means to direct fluid therapy (see Chapter 4, "Monitoring the Critical Paient"). Several types of catheters can be used as central venous catheters; the use of multi-lumen catheters (placed with the Seldinger technique) allow the measurement of CVP, blood sampling, as well as administration of fluids, parenteral nutrition, and drugs. Since these patients are often admitted for 2 weeks or more, the expense of these types of catheters is outweighed by their longevity (may be in place 30 days or more) and versatility (Ross et al. 2002; Mathews 2007).

Many ARF patients will present with oliguria, which generally appears in the maintenance phase of ARF. This oliguria is considered pathologic in nature and is characterized by a small urine volume with a low urine specific gravity (USG), indicating the kidney has lost the ability to concentrate urine. Patients may also present as polyuric. This is more common with nephrotoxic insults than with ischemic events, and carries a slightly better prognosis. Some patients may also present or develop anuria, which is often a brief stage until the patient becomes appropriately hydrated. However, if anuria persists, the patient is assigned the gravest prognosis (Ross et al. 2002; Mathews 2007).

Postrenal Azotemia

Postrenal azotemia occurs when there is an impediment to the flow of urine out of the body. The most common veterinary example is the urethral obstruction of the male cat; however, other examples include ruptured or herniated bladder, ruptured urethra, urinary blockage from neoplasia of the urethra, bladder, or surrounding tissues, prostatic disease, and uroliths (Mathews 2007).

Trauma patients should be thoroughly evaluated for urinary tract trauma to ensure that the system is intact with no leakage. Leakage commonly occurs into the abdomen, but urethral trauma can result in urine leakage into the hind limbs and inguinal areas. Trauma resulting in urine leakage will likely require surgery (Mathews 2007).

As the most common cause of postrenal azotemia, obstructive feline lower urinary tract disease (FLUTD) is an emergency commonly seen in every veterinary practice. Reported incidence is between 1% and 10% of cats presenting for veterinary care (Lee and Drobatz 2003).

Owners frequently delay treatment because they think that the cat straining in the litter box is simply constipated. Thus, cats often present in crisis. Prior to complete obstruction, the owner may have noticed the cat urinating outside of the litter box, excessively grooming the genitalia, vocalizing, having hematuria or dysuria (Drobatz 2009). Subsequent to the onset of an obstruction, systemic signs may take 24 hours to manifest, and postrenal azotemia may develop within 48 hours (Mathews 2007).

Upon presentation and suspicion of urethral obstruction, it is important to assess the cat thoroughly. A moderate to large sized, hard bladder is typically palpated; however, in the case of bladder rupture, the bladder may no longer be palpated. Many of these cats present cardiovascularly unstable secondary to fluid deficits and metabolic derangements. Oxygen should be administered, intravenous access, and minimum database (PCV,

TS, blood glucose, BUN stick, venous blood gas, and electrolytes) obtained. An ECG strip should be evaluated for classical signs of hyperkalemia including bradycardia or inappropriately low heart rate, tall T waves, absent P waves, prolonged P-R intervals and widened QRS complexes. It is important to note that not all cats will exhibit these classical signs, despite having life-threatening hyperkalemia, and therefore, blood K$^+$ levels should be evaluated quickly (Drobatz 2009). Other metabolic concerns are a typical metabolic acidosis and hypocalcemia, both of which can increase cardiotoxicity of hyperkalemia and thus need to be addressed (Lee and Drobatz 2003). Fluid resuscitation with a balanced electrolyte solution should *not* be withheld until the obstruction is relieved, and should be bolused as necessary with reassessments every 5–10 minutes to stabilize the patient. Choice of fluid is often the preference of the clinician; many will choose 0.9% NaCl, while others will choose an alkalinizing isotonic replacement solution. Emergency treatment of hyperkalemia should also be instituted prior to relieving the obstruction (Mathews 2007; Drobatz 2009). Hyperkalemia resulting in bradycardia is considered life-threatening and must be treated immediately. Treatment of hyperkalemia has two specific goals: (1) protect the heart and (2) reduce the serum potassium. These two goals are achieved by (1) the administration of calcium gluconate. Calcium gluconate acts to reduce the impact of high serum potassium on myocardial conduction; (2) administration of intravenous regular (Toronto) insulin and dextrose. Insulin acts to encourage cellular potassium uptake, thus reducing serum potassium. Glucose also moves into cells in the presence of insulin; therefore, an exogenous source of glucose is required to prevent hypoglycemia. Therefore, dextrose is generally given as an intravenous bolus, followed by a constant rate infusion (CRI) for 12–24 hours. In general, insulin and dextrose are administered along with intravenous fluids at a rate determined by the calculated fluid deficit of the patient. Finally, in some cases, insulin and dextrose are insufficient to reduce serum potassium, and intravenous sodium bicarbonate may be given. Sodium bicarbonate acts to increase serum pH, subsequently causing potassium to be driven intracellularly. Sodium bicarbonate administration is not without risks and will only be given when other options have failed or are inadequate and the clinician has fully assessed the patient's acid–base status.

Once the patient has been assessed, intravenous catheter placed, minimum database obtained, and fluid therapy instituted as necessary, relieving the obstruction should take place immediately. While catheterization of the obstructed cat can be difficult, the general procedure is the same as that presented in Box 9.2, Placement of Urinary Catheters in Dogs and Cats.

While many very ill cats may not require sedation, many will, and it will be necessary to provide some chemical restraint. Chemical restraint has the added benefit of relaxing the urethral sphincters, allowing the catheter to pass more easily.

If a mucous plug is causing the obstruction, the catheter will usually pass easily into the bladder. If uroliths or crystals are present, catheterization will be more difficult, and will likely require retropulsing with sterile saline in syringes. The catheter is advanced to the point of resistance (an open-end tomcat catheter works best), and a 12 mL syringe of 0.9% saline is attached. While advancing the catheter, an assistant can maintain a constant flow of flush into the catheter, hopefully causing the urolith or crystals to retreat into the bladder. This flushing and advancing may need to be repeated several times. Once the catheter is successfully placed in the bladder, urine should be drained using a syringe, and the bladder should be flushed numerous times with sterile saline until the bladder is free of debris. The tomcat catheter should be replaced with a 3.5 or 5 Fr feeding tube for longer term use (Mathews 2007; Drobatz 2009).

Box 9.2   Placement of Urinary Catheters in Dogs and Cats

General Supplies Needed for Urinary Catheter Placement:

- Chlorhexidine soap and/or 0.05% aqueous chlorhexidine solution
- Sterile gloves
- Sterile catheter:
  - Male dogs: flexible 5 or 8 Fr PVC feeding tube, 6 or 8 Fr × 55 cm silicone Foley catheter
  - Female dogs: Foley catheter, 8–12 Fr, 10–12 in. in length
  - Male or female cats: flexible 3.5 or 5 Fr PVC feeding tube, or tomcat catheter
- Sterile saline for Foley balloon inflation, usually 1–5 mL
- Sterile lubricant
- Sterile 2% lidocaine jelly in syringe
- Suture material
- 20 G needle
- Closed collection system
  - a "just-emptied" IV fluid bag and *new* 10 drop/s IV line with *all* clamps removed
  - a commercial urine collection system with one way valve

Sources: (Battaglia 2007; Mathews 2007; Smarick 2009a,b).

CHAPTER 9

If catheterization attempts are unsuccessful, cystocentesis may be considered using a 22 G needle. Cystocentesis should be considered a last resort to stablilize the cat prior to a surgical cystotomy, as it has been associated with increased risk of bladder rupture (Mathews 2007; Drobatz 2009).

Following catheterization, many cats develop a postobstructive dieresis, becoming extremely polyuric. Fluid assessment must be done continually, until the kidneys begin to regain their concentrating ability and kidney parameters return to normal. Many cats will become hypokalemic and may have other electrolyte derangements during this period, and it is important to supplement as necessary (Drobatz 2009). Nursing strategies will be discussed further in the following section.

Nursing Care of the Renal Patient

Any patient that is acutely azotemic is in need of further care. Interpretation of physical examination findings and diagnostics (blood work, ultrasound, radiographs, etc.) will determine the cause of the azotemia and indication for further treatment. In most cases, a patient such as this will be hospitalized and on fluid therapy, and will be watched closely with respect to vital signs, hydration status, body weight, urine output, and renal parameters. There are several strategies that can be used to manage the renal patient, keeping in mind that these patients are often very intensive, requiring extended care for periods of time.

Monitoring

Patients with renal compromise require frequent vital sign monitoring, the frequency of which needs to be tailored to the individual patient. For example, the stable, postobstructed cat may benefit from frequent (q 1–2 hour) check of mentation and respiration but have a full temperature, pulse, and respiration (TPR) and BP performed twice daily. A highly unstable peritoneal dialysis (PD) ARF patient (PD will be discussed later in the chapter) may require hourly mentation, TPR, blood gas and electrolytes, and continuous ECG and invasive blood pressure (IBP).

Of course, these *scheduled* events will be ordered by a veterinarian; however, it is important for every technician to realize that when it comes to critical care, the patient is *always* assessed. Expect the unexpected and never become complacent, or just do what is asked. Walking into the room, the eyes of a technician should observe every patient and keenly ascertain the condition of each patient. A patient that appears to be in worsening condition should always benefit from a full set of vital signs, and the veterinarian should be notified of any concerns. Technicians should always be on the watch for changes in patient condition: something as simple as an elevation in respiratory rate should warrant further investigation.

Monitoring Fluid Balance

Fluid therapy and subsequent urine volume are very important parameters to measure in the renal patient. Ensuring that the patient remains hydrated, has adequate intravascular volume, and thus maintains effective RBF and GFR are paramount to the success of treating a renal patient.

One of the most important factors in monitoring fluid balance of the renal patient is to quantify urine output. Urine output for a normally hydrated patient should be 1–2 mL/kg/h. While the actual definition of oliguria is <0.27–0.5 mL/kg/h, any patient producing < 1–2 mL/kg/h while on intravenous fluids may be oliguric (Mathews 2007; Langston 2009).

Urinary Catheterization

One of the first requirements for nursing an ARF patient may be the placement of an indwelling urinary catheter with a closed collection system (see Box 9.2 for placement of various catheters).

Perhaps the most reliable method of quantifying urine output, it is also the most invasive. Urinary catheterization of both male and female cats and dogs is relatively easy, with a little practice (Fig. 9.3).

Indwelling urinary catheters are invasive and are not without risks, the most important of which is the development of urinary catheter-associated urinary tract infection (CAUTI). CAUTI can arise via either intraluminal (through the inside of the catheter) or extraluminal (along the outside of the catheter) means. Most often in veterinary patients, contamination comes from feces on the urinary line or through self-grooming behavior.

The use of indwelling urinary catheters in ARF patients can be relatively long-term; therefore, asepsis upon placement and routine maintenance to avoid contamination is of the utmost importance. Standard urinary catheter maintenance includes cleaning the catheter beginning at the prepuce or vulva, then the entire line to the collection bag, every 8 hours or as needed with 0.05% chlorhexidine tincture; avoid elevating the urinary drainage bag above the level of the patient to avoid retrograde flow of urine into the bladder; avoid contaminating the outflow port of the urine bag (Mathews 2006a,b; Smarick 2009a); avoid placing the urine bag in direct contact with the floor, and never reinsert a catheter that is migrating out of the urethra—it should be removed and replaced instead. At our institution, the collection bags and lines are changed every 72 hours, and a sample of urine for culture and sensitivity is obtained at that time (Fig. 9.4) (Mathews 2007).

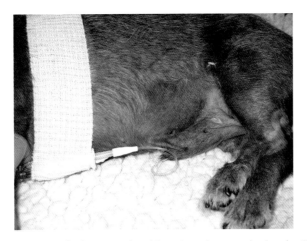

Figure 9.3 Urinary catheter in male dog. Note that this catheter is secured using the "finger trap" suture tie and is stabilized to the body with an elastic bandage belly wrap.

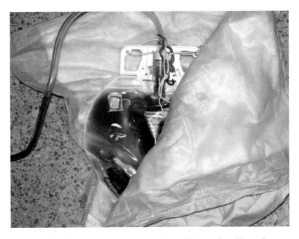

Figure 9.4 Example of a closed collection system urine bag. This style of bag features an anti-reflux valve to prevent retrograde flow of urine. Note the bag is wrapped and is not directly on the floor. The use of a diaper pad (blue outer wrap) acts as a barrier, keeps the bag clean, and absorbs any leaks. It also provides a visual cue, helping to avoid bags being stepped on. Many institutions may use containers for this purpose. A day of week sticker placed on the bag is an easy reminder to change the bag every 72 hours.

CHAPTER 9

In anuric or oliguric patients with little to no urine, an injection port used to cap the urinary catheter will allow periodic removal with a needle and syringe for more accurate assessment of urine volume. If the patient becomes polyuric, it is important to remember to aspirate the catheter more frequently, connect to a closed collection system, or remove the catheter and use another method of quantification.

When emptying the closed collection system, the volume of urine should be measured with a syringe or a measuring cup, rather than the volume on the collection bag. These bags are approximate volumes only, and with relatively small volumes, are highly inaccurate (Smarick 2009b).

Most important when quantifying urine output with a urinary catheter is *that urine output should never* = 0! Zero should never be written in a patient's records without a secondary note stating that the technician assessed the catheter for patency and assessed bladder size. If the urine output is zero, or less than the parameters given, the veterinarian must be immediately notified. Methods of assessing the patency of a urinary catheter are (1) flushing the catheter with 5–10 mL of 0.9% sterile NaCl. The volume should not only easily flow in, it should easily be aspirated out. If the volume will not flow in, the catheter is kinked or obstructed, and must be removed and replaced. If urine easily flows in, but cannot be aspirated out, the catheter placement is suspect (likely not in far enough). A bladder ultrasound or radiograph will verify catheter placement. If the catheter is not in the bladder, the catheter should be removed and replaced (if still necessary); (2) palpating the bladder for size. This is easily done in most small dogs and cats but may be more difficult to assess in larger dogs.

As urinary catheters are invasive and have inherent risks, they should be removed as soon as the patient is able to tolerate other means of assessing urine output.

Other collection methods

Dogs can be walked outdoors and the urine collected and measured. This is particularly useful for polyuric animals, although it can become quite labor-intensive when they have to urinate every half an hour. For most male dogs, urine can be collected directly into a measuring cup, and female dogs with a kidney bowl or pie plate.

For cats, the use of a nonabsorbent litter often works well, or for those that resist different types of litter, the clean litter pan and litter can be weighed at the time of placement into the cage and weighted again after urination to get an approximate volume (*assumption that 1 g = 1 mL*).

A method particularly useful for young puppies that are notoriously difficult to quantify urine is a metabolic cage. Urine is directed to a central drain for collection. Providing that the patient can be kept clean and dry with a small bed area, these types of cages work very well.

For recumbent patients, diaper pads are a good option, as long as they can be changed frequently to avoid the patient becoming wet. The pads are weighed prior to and after use to assess urine volume. Targeted placement of the pads under the prepuce or vulva allows the patient to remain clean and dry without the risk of lying in urine.

Regardless of the method chosen to collect and quantify urine, it is good practice to also acquire a USG at every opportunity (Mathews 2007). A USG can be useful for trending in conjunction with urine output, and provides information on the concentration ability of the kidney. It takes minimal time and effort to perform and is a valuable piece of information.

Measuring Ins and Outs

Accurate calculations of the fluid volume in (fluids, parenteral nutrition, and enteral water) and volume out (urine, vomitus, diarrhea), also known as "Ins and Outs," is very important in patients with renal concerns. This may be assessed every 1–4 hours. In the anuric or oliguric renal failure patient, iatrogenic overhydration is very common. By monitoring the volume in and volume out, overhydration can be prevented by only replacing the patient's insensible losses and measured volume out. In the polyuric renal failure patient, dehydration can become a problem, as the kidney is not able to concentrate urine, and thus, conserve water. Some patients may urinate 25–40 mL/kg/h, causing them to dehydrate very quickly (Mathews 2007). Often "matching ins and outs" is practiced, where the volume of urine out in one time period is the fluid volume given in the next time period. Patients can be receiving several times their daily maintenance fluid rate and must be monitored closely.

Body Weight

Assessing body weight on a frequent basis (ideally 2–4 times per day) will also assist in quantifying hydration and will verify the accuracy of "in and out" calculations (Langston 2009). Having an accurate scale is very important. If there is more than one scale available, the scale used should be noted on the patient's flow sheet to maintain consistency.

Peripheral Edema

Monitoring the patient for peripheral edema, often first noticed in the hocks, is another indicator of overhydration (Fig. 9.5).

This could also indicate that albumin levels are low and should be assessed. Skin turgor often changes when a patient becomes edematous, and their skin takes on a jiggly consistency.

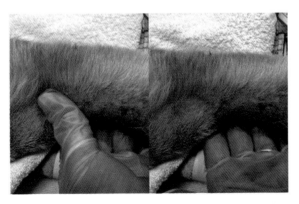

Figure 9.5   Assessment for peripheral edema. Most commonly develops in the initial stages over the metatarsals. Digital pressure results in an area of compression as noted in the picture.

CHAPTER 9

Auscultation

Frequent auscultation of patients with renal compromise is an important way to assess for overhydration. Crackles from pulmonary edema may be one of the first signs of overhydration. For acute renal failure patients that become overloaded, this can be a serious concern, as the kidney may not have the ability to remove the excess fluid. It is important for the technicians to assess the lung sounds frequently in any ARF patient to familiarize themselves with the "normal" sounds of the patient, allowing them to rapidly identify a change. A gradual or sudden increase in respiratory rate may also be an indication of overhydration.

Auscultation of the heart is also very important to consider, as ARF patients can develop arrhythmias. Any concerns in rate or rhythm should be assessed via an ECG strip, and the veterinarian notified.

Central Venous Pressure (CVP)

As previously mentioned, the placement of a central venous line may assist in determining appropriate fluid volumes for the patient. CVP is the measurement of the hydrostatic pressure in the intrathoracic vena cava, and estimates right atrial pressure (RAP). A central venous catheter can be placed in the jugular vein, or a longer catheter through the medial or lateral saphenous vein (femoral vein) can be used. Ideal placement is in the cranial or caudal vena cava, just outside the right atrium of the heart (Waddell and Brown 2009). Upon placement of a central venous line, the CVP waveform must be assessed. Radiographic confirmation of catheter placement will provide more confidence in the CVP reading. CVP in normovolemic patients is considered to be 0–5 cmH$_2$O. It is important to note, however, that many monitors measure CVP in mmHg, and a conversion factor of 1.36 (x mmHg/1.36 = y cmH$_2$O) is used. CVP is most used in a trending fashion, rather than using the individual readings as we would arterial BP. Patient position and position of the catheter will affect the CVP reading; therefore, in an ideal world, the patient will be measured in the same position each time.

Laboratory

Renal patients can have rapid changes in electrolytes and blood gases, and must be closely monitored. Life-threatening hyperkalemia, hypocalcemia, and severe metabolic acidosis can develop. Frequent assessment of renal parameters is necessary for assessing the patient's condition, and daily trending of urea and creatinine will give an indication of the patient's response to therapy.

Nutrition

Providing nutrition to renal patients is an extremely important nursing consideration. While some patients may continue to eat, most often, enteral or parenteral supplementation is required. In human ARF patients, early nutrition support has been shown to decrease morbidity (Langston 2009). The placement of a nasoesophageal or nasogastric tube is recommended for short-term supplementation in patients that are not vomiting. In cases in which long-term supplementation of water and food might be required, placement of an esophagostomy or percutaneous endoscopic gastrostomy (PEG) tube may be indicated, as owners can continue to supplement as necessary once the patient is discharged. Providing partial or total parenteral nutrition (PPN) should be considered if the enteral route is not available (see Chapter 22, "Nutrition for the Critically Ill"). Interestingly, some strongly feel that patients with renal failure have a preference for sweet foods. In some cases, muffins, fruit (melon, banana, etc.), yogurt, cupcakes, and doughnuts have been greatly desirable to patients who were previously thought to be anorexic.

Peritoneal Dialysis (PD)

Many patients in ARF would only survive if treated with dialysis. PD is the method most commonly used in veterinary medicine; however, several hemodialysis units at major referral centers have opened in recent years. Hemodialysis is considered the "gold standard"; however, the location of various clinics, and cost, may make it prohibitive for many owners. PD is the most widely used and is available in any clinic with an advanced level of care; therefore, the focus of this chapter will be the special nursing considerations associated with PD.

PD has been used in human medicine since 1923 (Labato 2000). It continues to be used in humans for both acute and chronic renal failure, toxin exposure, and a multitude of other conditions. In veterinary medicine, PD is primarily used for the treatment of acute renal failure, although it is also less commonly used for acute toxin exposure (of dialyzable toxins) and for extreme volume overload (Labato 2000; Fischer 2009).

PD is based on fluid and solute exchange across a semipermeable membrane. In using an appropriate solution, or dialysate, of varying osmolality, molecules in high concentration in the body such as urea and creatinine, as well as ions such as sodium and potassium, can be drawn across the semipermeable membrane until they reach equilibrium (equal concentrations on both sides of the membrane) (Fischer 2009).

The peritoneal membrane is an ideal semipermeable membrane for dialysis as it is permeable to uremic toxins, has a tremendously vascular surface, and has limited permeability to molecules over 30,000 MW (Labato 2000).

As the name implies, PD is the process in which a dialysate is infused into the peritoneal cavity, initiating osmosis across the peritoneal membrane. The technique itself is relatively simple; however, placement and maintenance of the PD catheter, maintaining sterility, and patient monitoring require advanced skill.

The placement of a PD catheter is performed as a surgical procedure by the veterinarian. Occasionally for very short term use, a temporary catheter may be placed which is often a single lumen, long term style catheter placed percutaneously with the Seldinger technique and local anesthetic. Unfortunately, while simple to place, these catheters do not last for long-term PD. The omentum often clogs the holes of the catheter or they become kinked. They may be chosen as a "middle of the night" solution to get PD underway rapidly, rather than surgically place a catheter while the patient may be too unstable. Other short-term options for catheters include tube catheters with stylets such as "pigtail" catheters.

A long-term PD catheter is often chosen by clinician preference and may also be driven by cost. PD catheters are widely available from human medical supply companies. These catheters are specific to the task, and include Dacron cuffs that are placed in the rectus muscle and subcutaneous layers to promote adhesion to the body wall and prevent leakage (Labato 2000; Fischer 2009). These catheters stay in place many months to years in human PD patients, although their purpose is generally in the management of chronic renal failure. In veterinary patients, the main thrust of use for PD is for acute renal failure.

While commercial dialysate solutions are widely available, they can be expensive, and large quantities are used with each patient. Many find it less expensive and more convenient to make their own. Lactated Ringers solution (LRS) is a balanced isotonic crystalloid solution, which is an ideal dialysate with the additions of dextrose and heparin. Dextrose is added in varying concentrations of 1.5%–4.25% depending on the volemic state of the patient. Heparin may be added to avoid fibrin clogging the tube fenestrations. However, if heparin is used, it is usually only used for the first 1–2 days (Fischer 2009).

Peritonitis is the most common complication of PD and is most often associated with contamination through handling. Several considerations for prevention of infection are associated with PD, and must be strictly adhered to by nursing staff. The following section discusses how infection may be prevented.

Preparation of dialysate. Bags of dialysate should be prepared as needed, not several in advance. Single-dose vials of dextrose and heparin should be used, and aseptic technique must be adhered to when preparing the dialysate, including the use of sterile gloves. Fluid should be warmed to body temperature (38°C) in a warming cabinet prior to infusion. Warm fluid is more comfortable for the patient and also promotes vasodilation of the peritoneal capillaries (Labato 2000; Fischer 2009).

The veterinarian will determine the appropriate prescription for dialysate. Typically, dextrose is used as the osmotic agent in PD, enhancing ultrafiltration and removal of water across the membrane due to its hypertonicity. Varying the concentration of dextrose will allow for tailoring of the osmotic draw relative to the condition of the patient. Dextrose concentrations of 1.5% is used in dehydrated or normovolemic patients, 2.5% is used for mildly overhydrated patients, and 4.25% is generally reserved for those that are severely overhydrated (Labato 2000).

Strict asepsis. The PD catheter is placed under strict asepsis, often in the surgical suite. Maintenance of the tubes and insertion site are very important means of preventing infection. Often the PD site will leak fluid, and a sterile absorbent dressing must be applied over the site and changed frequently. The site and tubes must be handled with sterile gloves, and the tube and lines wiped with a chlorhexidine solution several times daily (usually q 8 hours) to minimize bacteria.

Collection system. A closed Y-type system where a stopcock is used to divide into infusion and recovery lines has been shown to be efficacious in avoiding contamination. The stopcocks and lines must be handled with sterile gloves, and chlorhexidine or povidone-iodine-soaked gauze is wrapped around any connections or ports and changed twice daily. Prior to infusion into the abdomen, a flush of fresh dialysate is allowed to exit via the recovery line. The closed collection system in veterinary medicine is often created by piecing together various tubes and lines, including IV dripsets (10 drops/s), extension sets, and a stopcock. A stopcock is imperative to separate infusate and exfusate. The exfusate collection bag can be a purchased sterile IV infusion bag or an IV fluid bag that has been emptied aseptically for the purpose (Fig. 9.6) (Dzyban and Labato 2000; Labato 2000).

Infusion procedure

A cycle of infusion into the abdomen, and subsequent drainage from the abdomen, is called a "dwell." The fluid must remain in the abdomen for approximately 40 minutes to reach equilibrium and maximize removal of water and solutes. Typical dialysate volumes are 30–40 mL/kg, and this may be reduced by half in the first 24 hours to minimize abdominal distension and leakage (Dyzban and Labato 2000; Labato 2000; Fischer 2009).

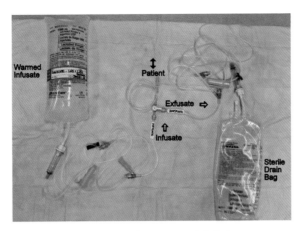

Figure 9.6   Example of Y-closed collection system for peritoneal dialysis.

Technicians are generally entrusted with the dwell procedure, and it is important to ensure that the dwell is appropriately timed to maximize effectiveness. The use of a cageside timer is ideal in keeping track of time. For consistency, only one technician should perform the PD throughout the shift whenever possible. In our institution, our goal in the initial 24 hours is to try to stay on a 1-hour schedule: 5 minutes for infusion, 40 minute to dwell, 15 minutes to drain. If the infusion does not flow well by gravity, an infusion pump can be used to deliver the volume. Some animals will react to rapid infusion of the dialysate, and the rate must be slowed. The drain volume should be assessed each time, with the expectation of draining 90%–100% of the infusate (Labato 2000). In cases that 4.25% dextrose containing dialysate is being used, the drain volume may be more than the infusate volume.

Maintaining accurate records by recording the volume in, volume out, dwell time, and calculating the net difference in fluid volumes should be standard practice with each "dwell." The veterinarian should be alerted if the patient is retaining dialysate. Changes in the color, turbidity, or odor of peritoneal fluid may be very significant and affect patient outcome. Technicians should assess the fluid with every flush, and the veterinarian should be notified of any changes.

Once clinical signs and laboratory values begin to show improvement, the frequency of dwells is reduced, and the dwell time is increased, as prescribed by the veterinarian. PD is discontinued once the patient can maintain a normal fluid balance, urine output improves, and is non-uremic.

References

Battaglia, AM. 2007. Urologic emergencies. In *Small Animal Emergency and Critical Care for Veterinary Technicians*, edited by Battaglia, AM. Philadelphia: Saunders, pp. 305–320.

Brown, SA. 2003. Physiology of the urinary tract. In *Textbook of Small Animal Surgery*, edited by Slatter, DH. Philidelphia: Saunders, pp. 1575–1583.

Christie, BA. 2003. Anatomy of the urinary system. In *Textbook of Small Animal Surgery*, edited by Slatter, DH. Philidelphia: Saunders, pp. 1558–1575.

Dennis, R, Kirberger, R, Wrigley, R, et al. 2001. *Handbook of Small Animal Radiological Differential Diagnosis*. London, UK: Harcourt, p. 186.

DiBartola, SP. 2006. Applied renal physiology. In *Fluid, Electrolyte and Acid Base Disorders in Small Animal Practice*, 3rd ed., edited by Dibartola, SP. St. Louis, MO: WB Saunders, pp. 26–44.

Drobatz, KJ. 2009. Urethral obstruction in cats. In *Kirk's Current Veterinary Therapy XIV*, edited by Bonagura, JD, Twedt, DC. St. Louis, MO: Saunders, pp. 951–954.

Dzyban, LA, Labato, MA. 2000. Peritoneal dialysis: a tool in veterinary critical care. *Journal of Veterinary Emergency Critical Care* 10(2):91–102.

Fischer, JR. 2009. Hemodialysis and peritoneal dialysis. In *Small Animal Critical Care Medicine*, edited by Hopper, K, Silverstein, DC. St. Louis, MO: Saunders Elsevier, pp. 599–603.

Grauer, FG. 2009. Acute renal failure and chronic kidney disease. In *Small Animal Internal Medicine*, edited by Nelson, RW, Couto, CG. St. Louis, MO: Mosby, pp. 645–655.

Labato, MA. 2000. Peritoneal dialysis in emergency and critical care medicine. *Clinical Techniques in Small Animal Practice* 15(3):126–135.

Langston, CE. 2009. Acute renal failure. In *Small Animal Critical Care Medicine*, edited by Hopper, K, Silverstein, DC. St. Louis, MO: Saunders Elsevier, pp. 590–594.

Lee, JA, Drobatz, KJ. 2003. Characterization of the clinical characteristics, electrolytes, acid-base and renal parameters in male cats with urethral obstruction. *Journal of Veterinary Emergency Critical Care* 13(4):227–233.

Marques-Sampaio, BPS, Pereira-Sampaio, MA, Henry, RW, Favorito, LA, Sampaio, FJB. 2007. Dog kidney: anatomical relationships between intrarenal arteries and kidney collecting system. *The Anatomical Record: Advances in Integrative Anatomy and Evolutionary Biology* 290:1017–1022.

Mathews, KA. 2006a. Management of acute renal failure. In *Veterinary Emergency and Critical Care Manual*, 2nd ed., edited by Mathews, KA. Guelph, Ontario, Canada: Lifelearn, pp. 709–722.

Mathews, KA. 2006b. Short term peritoneal dialysis. In *Veterinary Emergency and Critical Care Manual*, 2nd ed., edited by Mathews, KA. Guelph, Ontario, Canada: Lifelearn, pp. 723–726.

Mathews, KA. 2007. Renal and urinary tract emergencies. In *BSAVA Manual of Canine and Feline Emergency and Critical Care*, 2nd ed., edited by King, LG, Boag, A. Gloucester, U.K.: British Small Animal Veterinary Association, pp. 114–129.

Moffat, DB. 1975. *The Mammalian Kidney*. Cambridge: Cambridge University Press.

Rennke, HG, Denker, BM. 2007. *Renal Pathophysiology: The Essentials*. Philadelphia: Lippincott, Williams and Wilkin.

Ross, LA, Labato, MA. 2006. Peritoneal dialysis. In *Fluid, Electrolyte and Acid Base Disorders in Small Animal Practice*, 3rd ed., edited by Dibartola, SP. St. Louis, MO: WB Saunders, pp. 635–649.

Ross, SJ, Osborne, CA, Lulich, JP, et al. 2002. Acute renal failure. In *The ICU Book*, edited by Wingfield, WE, Raffe, MR. Jackson, WY: Teton NewMedia, pp. 298–324.

Smarick, S. 2009a. Urinary catheterization. In *Small Animal Critical Care Medicine*, edited by Hopper, K, Silverstein, DC. St. Louis, MO: Saunders Elsevier, pp. 603–606.

Smarick, S. 2009b. Urine output. In *Small Animal Critical Care Medicine*, edited by Hopper, K, Silverstein, DC. St. Louis, MO: Saunders Elsevier, pp. 865–868.

Waddell, LS, Brown, AJ. 2009. Hemodynamic monitoring. In *Small Animal Critical Care Medicine*, edited by Hopper, K, Silverstein, DC. St. Louis, MO: Saunders Elsevier, pp. 859–864.

Endocrine and Metabolic Emergencies

Angela Randels

Introduction

The endocrine system is composed of a complex network of systems, organs, and glands that work together to regulate the body. The word "endocrine" means "to separate within," referring to the variety of tissues that function as the endocrine system. The endocrine system is responsible for manufacturing hormones that help regulate various functions. The word "hormone" means "to excite"; therefore, it causes an effect on the body. It is imperative to understand the endocrine system and its function in order to fully understand its dysfunction.

There are many parts to the endocrine system. The following serve as the main part of the endocrine system: central nervous system (CNS), thyroid gland, parathyroid gland, adrenal glands, gastrointestinal tract, endocrine pancreas, kidney, gonads, and the placenta (Table 10.1). For the purposes of this discussion, we will focus on the nonreproductive endocrine glands. For the location of these gland, see Figure 10.1.

Endocrine System Anatomy and Physiology

Hormones

Hormones are made by a wide variety of cell types and have effects on a wide variety of tissue types. Hormones directly affect metabolic functions and metabolic rates by either increasing or decreasing specific reactions within the specific cell or cells targeted. Steroids, amino acid derivatives, proteins, smaller peptides, and fatty acid derivatives are all examples of hormones. These chemical messengers act in different ways. Some hormones may act on the very cell that produced them which is called an autocrine process. An example of this is in the case of prostaglandins, which can be secreted into the interstitial fluid and then act on the very cell that secreted it. The paracrine process is when hormones act on cells in the general area of where they are made and do not enter the circulation. Hormones that affect cells that are far away via traveling through the circulatory system are part of an endocrine process. Nerves that produce neurotransmitters that enter the circulation and act as endocrine hormones are termed to be *neuroendocrine* or "neuro-crine agents." See Table 10.2 for examples of hormone types (list is not meant to be inclusive).

What or how much action a hormone exerts on its target cell or cells depends on the following factors:

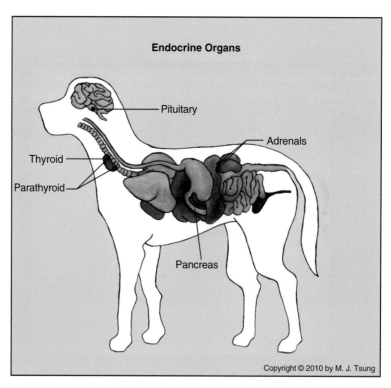

Endocrine Organs

Pituitary

Adrenals

Thyroid

Parathyroid

Pancreas

Copyright © 2010 by M. J. Tsung

Figure 10.1   Schematic drawing of the non-reproductive endocrine organ locations. (Care of Jen Tsung).

Table 10.1   Endocrine gland hormones and functions

Location	Glands	Hormones	Function
Central nervous system	Hypothalamus, posterior and anterior pituitary, pineal gland	Oxytocin, antidiuretic hormone (ADH), melatonin	Salt and water balance, sexual function, growth, skin darkening, lactation, response to stress
Thyroid	Thyroid gland parafollicular cells (calcitonin)	Tetraiodothyronine (T4), triiodothyronine (T3), and reverse T3 (rT3), calcitonin	Increases basal metabolic rate in tissue calcium homeostasis (calcitonin)
Parathyroid	Parathyroid gland	Parathyroid hormone (PTH)	Maintaining levels of calcium and phosphate
Adrenal glands	Outer cortex and inner medulla	Cortex—corticosteroids (cortisol, aldosterone) Inner medulla—catecholamines (epinephrine, norepinephrine)	Glucose homeostasis (cortisol), electrolyte balance (aldosterone), "fight or flight response" (catecholamines)
GI Tract	Entire GI tract	Cholecystokinin (CCK), secretin, gastrin, gastric inhibitory polypeptide (GIP)	GI motility, secretion, digestive action, release of insulin/energy balance
Endocrine pancreas	Islets of Langerhans	Insulin, glucagon, somatostatin	Carbohydrate, protein, and lipid metabolism
Kidney	Kidney	Renin, erythropoietin	Control of blood pressure, erythropoiesis, hydroxylation of vit. D

CHAPTER 10

1. The rate of production and secretion
2. Availability of transport proteins in the plasma
3. Ability of tissues that are targeted to convert the hormone
4. Activity and availability of receptors specific for the hormone on the targeted cells or tissues
5. Breakdown (degradation)
6. Liver and/or kidney excretion

The endocrine system maintains regulatory systems to aid in preventing overproduction or underproduction of hormones. The two most common regulatory systems are known as direct and indirect feedback control. This is primarily regulated by the hypothalamus and pituitary gland. When the level of hormone concentrations exceeds what is needed, this is detected either by the gland producing the hormone or by the

Table 10.2   Neuroendocrine hormones

Hormone Origin	Hormone Name
Amino acid derivatives	Dopamine
	Norepinephrine
	Epinephrine
	Thyroxine
	Triiodothyronine
	Reverse T3
Small peptides	Vasopressin
	Oxytocin
	Somatostatin
	ACTH
	Angiotensins
	Secretin
	Glucagon
Proteins	Calcitonin
	Insulin
	Growth hormone
	Thyroid-stimulating hormone (TSH)
	Prolactin
	Parathyroid hormone
	Erythropoietin
Steroids	Progesterone
	Testosterone
	Estrogens
	Glucocorticoids
	Mineralocorticoids
Fatty acid derivatives	Prostaglandins
	Leukotrines
	Thromboxanes

hypothalamus/pituitary to inhibit further production of this hormone. Hormones may be eliminated from the body by the liver (bile) or kidney's (urine) with or without being metabolized or degraded, either being in an active or inactive form. The detail of production, action, degradation, and elimination of each of these hormones is beyond the scope of this summary.

The dysfunction of one or more parts of the endocrine system can have detrimental metabolic effects. Understanding these various dysfunctions as they present to us in emergency and critical care practice is vital in order to effectively identify and treat these patients.

Dysfunction of the Endocrine Pancreas

Diabetes mellitus (DM), diabetic ketoacidosis (DKA), and insulinoma are all commonly encountered within emergency and critical care (ECC) practice. Early detection and treatment are vital to the outcome in these patients. Knowledge of the disease processes is beneficial in understanding the treatments of these disease states.

Diabetes Mellitus (DM)

The appropriate treatment of nonketotic diabetics, both initially and for long-term maintenance, is vital to minimize complications of DM. This is accomplished through dietary measures, exercise, control of concurrent disease, oral hypoglycemic drugs, and/or insulin treatment. The goals of treatment are to eliminate signs and life-threatening effects of hyperglycemia. While some cases of DM are managed fairly easily, other cases can be at best problematic.

Signalment and history

DM occurs in approximately 1 in 100 to 1 in 500 dogs and cats (Feldman and Nelson 2004). Dogs with diabetes are generally between 4 and 14 years old with a peak incidence in those 7 to 9 years old (Wingfield and Raffe 2002). Female dogs are affected twice as often as males. Diabetes is most common in male neutered cats of any age but most are generally older than 6 years old. In many patients presenting with DKA, the preliminary signs of diabetes (polydipsia [PD], polyuria [PU], polyphagia, and weight loss) have gone unnoticed by the owner. Diabetics may live for up to 6 months with no serious adverse affects. However, once DKA starts, the patient becomes severely ill within only 1–7 days. Concurrent diseases, such as chronic pancreatitis, pneumonia, hyperadrenocorticism (Cushing's disease), urinary tract infection (UTI), or congestive heart failure (CHF) may predispose the patient to developing DKA.

Diabetic types

In veterinary medicine, human nomenclature of diabetic types cannot be applied to dogs and cats with total accuracy. Both Type I and Type II diabetics do seem to occur, however. Type I diabetes results from the destruction of beta cells, which is often immune-mediated, but may be idiopathic. There is generally a progressive and complete loss of insulin secretion. These patients may have a sudden onset of signs and usually require insulin treatment from the onset. Type II diabetes can result from a combination of insulin resistance, dysfunctioning beta cells (producing less insulin), and increase hepatic gluconeogenesis. Insulin secretion may be high, low, or normal, but in any case, is insufficient to overcome the insulin resistance present in the patient. This type of diabetic usually does not become ketoacidotic. They may be either insulin-dependent diabetes mellitus (IDDM) or non-insulin-dependent diabetes melitus (NIDDM). NIDDM may be treated with therapies other than insulin injections, whereas the IDDM patient is dependent on supplemental insulin injections. There is also the presence of secondary diabetes, where the patient develops carbohydrate intolerance secondary to concurrent insulin-resistant disease, such as pregnancy (diestrus), hyperadrenocorticism (Cushing's disease), or acromegaly. This can result in permanent diabetes, and IDDM typically develops. Almost all dogs and 50%–70% of cats are IDDM. Approximately 30%–50% of cats are NIDDM (Type II), which is very uncommon in dogs. Obesity, genetics, islet amyloidosis, and abnormal insulin response are possible causes. Cats with NIDDM often progress to IDDM if not quickly treated due to the effects of glucose toxicity and subsequent pancreatic islet exhaustion, apoptosis, and fibrosis.

Dietary therapy

Dietary therapy should be initiated in all diabetic types. Goals should be to correct obesity, provide caloric stability, and to minimize postprandial blood glucose (BG) concentrations. Typically, the mainstay of diabetic dietary therapy is with a diet high in complex carbohydrates (i.e., fiber). Fiber helps promote weight loss and slows absorption of glucose from the gastrointestinal (GI) tract, which helps reduce the postprandial flux of glucose. Refusal to consume a high-fiber diet is a limiting factor. They should also not be used in thin diabetic dogs or cats. Weight reduction should be gradual, taking at least 2–4 months to reach the desired body weight. Thin patients should be fed a calorie-dense diet until optimum weight is achieved, and then a high-fiber diet should be introduced. Recently, there is evidence that some animals do better on a high-protein diet. This is most likely in cases of carbohydrate intolerance which occurs especially in Type II obese cats. However, there is a lack of evidence indicating either diet leading to increased remission rates. The feeding schedule should enhance the action of insulin, aiding to minimize glucose fluctuations. Typically, dogs and cats are fed twice daily at the time of each insulin injection. If insulin is given only once daily, the second meal should be given 8–10 hours after the first. Some patients require a diet appropriate for treating concurrent disease, such as renal or heart failure. Whenever possible, the dietary considerations for both diseases should be combined. If this is not possible, the more life-threatening disease should be treated with an appropriate dietary therapy.

Oral hypoglycemic drugs

Oral hypoglycemic drugs are generally only attempted for treatment of diabetes only in cats. Ketotic patients are not eligible for use of oral hypoglycemic drugs, and insulin is required in these cases. Only 20%–45% of cats may respond to oral therapy and therefore they are typically a second choice to insulin therapy. But since cats are often Type II diabetics and are therefore NIDDM, a combination of dietary therapy with oral drugs may aid in controlling hyperglycemia, at least for a period of time. In order to consider a cat for oral therapy, they should have normal body weight, no ketonemia present, no history of diabetogenic drug administration, and without underlying diseases, such as pancreatitis. There are several drug options that include sulfonylurea drugs (glipizide, glimepiride); metformin, which decreases hepatic glucose output; acarbose, which inhibits intestinal glucose absorption; troglitazone, which improves peripheral insulin sensitivity; and transition metals such as chromium and vanadium, which may mimic insulin.

Insulin therapy

Insulin therapy is required in all dogs and most cats. Commonly used types are isophane (NPH), protamine zinc (PZI), ultralente (previously available), glargine, or Caninsulin/

Vetsulin (porcine lente). The FDA is eliminating any animal source of insulin available in the human market. Only the veterinary market has beef or pork insulins. The speed of onset and duration of action affect the choice of insulin used (short-acting, intermediate-acting, long-acting). All insulin types are administered SQ, with exception of regular insulin, which can be administered SQ, IM, or IV. Care must be taken to the concentration of the insulin and appropriate syringe size used. Detemir is long-acting insulin, similar to glargine that may be on the horizon in the future.

Intermediate-acting insulin types are Vetsulin and NPH. NPH insulin has onset of action at 0.5–3 hours, with a peak of effect at 2–8 hours, and duration of effect of 4–12 hours. Long-acting insulin types are PZI and glargine. PZI has an onset of action of 1–4 hours, with an average peak effect at 3–12 hours, with duration of effect of 6–24 hours. Glargine is viewed as a "peakless" insulin. Glargine use in newly diagnosed diabetic cats, along with dietary control, can possibly achieve remission in a large percent of cats. Those that do not go into remission are typically experiencing better glycemic control (Fig. 10.2).

Intermediate-acting insulin such as NPH and Vetsulin are the initial insulins of choice for dogs. Because the duration of effect of NPH and Vetsulin is often less than 12 hours, it usually needs to be administered twice daily. Doses generally start at 0.5–1 U/kg 1–2 times daily (Plumb 2005). Long-acting insulins such as PZI or glargine are the initial insulins of choice for diabetic cats. Glargine may be used as once a day or twice a day dosing. Twice daily dosing may result in greater remission rates.

With any initiation of insulin or changes of dose or type of insulin given, an adjustment period of a few days must be given before the patient is rechecked. So, typically, a patient should not be checked more than once weekly. Keep in mind that all patients respond individually. There is not a one-size-fits-all protocol for insulin management. Trial and time are the determining factors to find the protocol that fits the needs of the patient.

Monitoring

Owner observation at home accounts for much of the basis of assessment of diabetics and should begin as soon as the pet returns home. Observation for resolution of PD, PU, and polyphagia are noted. Patients should be examined and BG levels checked weekly. Owners can attempt to monitor for urine glucose at home. The goal should be to have urine free of glucose for most of a 24-hour period. Persistent glucosuria throughout the day and night indicates a problem with control of diabetes, and the patient should be rechecked. The objective in diabetic management is to resolve clinical signs and avoid the complications, often life-threatening, of the disease.

Glucose curves

Evaluation of serial glucose curves during the initial management and periodically throughout the life of the pet in order to assess control of diabetics is considered mandatory. The insulin and feeding protocol of the owner should be followed, and blood should be obtained every 1–2 hours throughout the day, preferably over 24 hours. By doing this, it can be determined if the insulin is being effective, the time of peak effect, and the degree of glucose fluctuation in the given patient. BG should remain >80 mg/dL at all times, ideally between 100–300 mg/dL for the diabetic cat and 100–250 mg/dL for the diabetic dog. Questions used to evaluate the effectiveness of the current therapy used are the following:

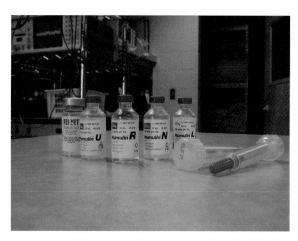

Figure 10.2 Many different types of insulin are available for use with our veterinary patients. The duration of action, syringe type, and route of administration can vary considerably between different insulins.

- Did the insulin effectively lower the BG concentration?
- When is the peak effect?
- How long did it take?
- Did the insulin level drop too low?
- What is the difference between the starting glucose and the lowest measurement?
- Was there rebound hyperglycemia?

There are many problems in obtaining an effective BG curve in the hospital. Stress is generally on top of the list of problems that interfere with results, especially in cats. Inappetence and reproducibility are other factors that are of difficulty in performing BG curves. Due to the above reasons, home monitoring is becoming increasingly favored. With the easy availability of glucose monitoring equipment, owners may be able to obtain full glucose curves at home using an ear prick technique. Despite the challenges of performing a glucose curve, they are still generally considered to be valuable aids in evaluating the effectiveness of insulin therapy. Signs observed at home must be evaluated along with curve results in order to determine the overall picture of whether or not a patient's glucose is being adequately controlled.

Continuous glucose monitoring systems are currently being investigated for use in dogs and cats with promising results. A recent study investigated the use of these systems during treatment of DKA. A strong correlation of BG levels from these sensors and periodic blood sampling was seen (Reineke et al. 2010). Further study will be needed to determine the potential long-term use of these devices.

Fructosamine

Due to the marked stress hyperglycemia response in cats, fructosamine levels are becoming a standard in evaluating control of glucose levels in diabetics and are commonly used to monitor diabetic humans. Fructosamine is formed by glycosylation of serum proteins such as albumin. Fructosamine concentrations are directly related to BG concentrations. The higher the BG concentrations over the past 2–3 weeks, the higher the fructosamine level will be. It is not affected by acute situations, such as stress, as glucose is. Normal serum fructosamine will vary somewhat by lab, but are generally 225–360 μmol/L. Values > 500 μmol/L suggest inadequate control of diabetes. Low fructosamine levels indicated probable periods of hypoglycemia, even if clinical signs are not present. Somogyi phenomenon (see section on "Diabetic Complications") should be suspected if clinical signs of uncontrolled diabetes are present with fructosamine levels of <400 μmol/L. Checking fructosamine levels in the fractious, excitable, or stressed patient is advantageous over glucose curves due to hyperglycemic response to these stresses.

Diabetic Ketoacidosis (DKA)

DKA encompasses a wide range of metabolic and endocrine derangements. DKA is a common endocrine emergency affecting both dogs and cats which can be fatal. The nursing management and care of these patients can be both challenging and consuming. By increasing knowledge of this disease process, potential complications of DKA, patient care, and treatment options, a veterinary nurse can play an invaluable role in the successful outcome in these cases.

Pathophysiology

The endocrine pancreas is composed of cells arranged in groupings known as the Islets of Langerhans. These islets are surrounded by exocrine secreting acinar cells. There are four cell types in the endocrine pancreas which regulate glucose production and utilization. The alpha cells secrete glucagon, beta cells secrete insulin, delta cells secrete somatostatin, and F cells secrete pancreatic polypeptide. In the case of DM, dysfunction of the beta cells results in an absolute or relative deficiency of insulin. All canines and felines in DKA have a relative or absolute deficiency of insulin. If the early signs of diabetes are overlooked by the owners, these patients may progress into DKA. Insulin deficiency, diabetogenic hormone excess (glucagon, cortisol, growth hormone, and catecholamines), fasting, and dehydration are ultimately responsible for the increase in ketogenesis and gluconeogenesis. Concurrent disease processes can play a role in the development of DKA and can make treatment of these patients more challenging.

Insulin deficiency promotes glycogenolysis, gluconeogenesis, lipolysis, proteolysis, and ketogenesis. The liver is stimulated to produce glucose but cells are unable to utilize this glucose due to lack of insulin. Normally, fatty acids are released from adipose tissue, oxidized by the liver, and are formed into triglycerides. However, with the lack of insulin, these fatty acids are converted to a coenzyme A derivative called acyl-CoA, which is further oxidized into acetyl CoA, then into β-hydroxybutyrate, which is further broken down into acetoacetate and acetone. *ß-hydroxybutyrate, acetoacetate*, and *acetone* are known as the three ketone bodies. Ketogenesis is then enhanced by diabetogenic hormone excess. Not only are these hormones insulin antagonistic, but they also provoke acidosis, fluid depletion, and hypotension. Any disease concurrent to DKA, such as pancreatitis or infection, also upregulate diabetic hormone secretion.

Physiologically, DKA is a state of cellular starvation. Normally, the body adapts to short-term starvation by converting free fatty acids to ketones as a safety measure. When the body is glucose-deficient, ketones can be used for an energy source. However, due to the diabetic pet's insulin deficiency, gluconeogenesis and ketogenesis proceed at an elevated rate. This results in an increase of ketones in the blood stream, which eventually overwhelms the buffering system, leading to an increase in hydrogen ion (H^+) concentration, a compensatory decrease in bicarbonate (HCO_3^-), and a lowering of the blood pH. Ketones and glucose begin spilling into the urine, leading to an osmotic diuresis which worsens dehydration and electrolyte imbalances. Nausea and obtundation associated with hyperosmolarity, hyperglycemia, DKA, vomiting, diarrhea, and hyperventilation all contribute to dehydration. Severe dehydration can progress to contraction of the intravascular fluid space (hypovolemia). Pre-renal azotemia, decreased glomerular filtration rate (GFR), and decreased glucose and hydrogen ion secretion are a result. All these lead to a further accumulation of glucose and ketones in the vascular space, worsening the DKA.

Electrolyte abnormalities occur with sodium, potassium, phosphorous, and magnesium. Circulating electrolytes are lost excessively due to increased osmotic renal secretion. To replenish intravascular stores, these electrolytes then move out of the intracellular space into the vascular space, which eventually results in a total body deficit. Sodium and potassium are commonly deficient in these patients and should be monitored regularly. Acid–base assessment should be performed and monitored for improvement, as severe metabolic acidosis is common.

Physical exam and diagnosis

Patients suffering from DKA may present with dehydration, weakness, depression, tachypnea, vomiting, and the smell of acetone on their breath. In cases of severe metabolic acidosis, the patient may exhibit Kussmaul respiration (slow deep breathing pattern). These patients often have an acute onset of abdominal pain and may also have abdominal distension, especially if concurrent pancreatitis or peritonitis is present. Hepatomegaly is common in both dogs and cats with diabetes. Cats may exhibit diabetic neuropathy with plantigrade posture (hocks touch the ground when the cat walks—due to sciatic neuropathy). If DKA is complicated with hyperosmolarity or severe acidosis, the patient may be obtunded or exhibit depressed mentation.

The diagnosis of DKA is based on clinical signs in combination with persistent fasting hyperglycemia, glucosuria, ketonemia, and ketonuria. High levels of BG can be seen due to stress (up to 300–400 mg/dL has been documented in felines). However, the presence or absence of ketones will differentiate stress hyperglycemia from DKA, as ketones will not be present in stress hyperglycemia. Acid–base assessment should be performed in addition to complete blood count (CBC), chemistry profile including amylase and lipase, electrolytes, T4 levels in cats, and urinalysis with culture. A urine culture and sensitivity should be performed on all DKA patients regardless of the presence or absence of pyuria and/or hematuria, because UTIs can be a predisposing factor and are also common due to the immunosuppression of concurrent DM. An electrocardiogram (ECG) should also be routinely performed in these patients to monitor for the cardiac effects of electrolyte derangements.

Clinical abnormalities. A CBC profile can be normal or exhibit derangements such as mild polycythemia (due to dehydration) or leukocytosis. Leukocytosis can be attributed to infection (demonstrated by left shift/toxic changes in neutrophils) or inflammation (i.e., underlying pancreatitis).

Biochemical panels can often demonstrate liver abnormalities caused by hepatic lipidosis, pancreatitis, or extrahepatic biliary obstruction due to severe pancreatitis. Alanine aminotransferase (ALT) and alkaline phosphatase (ALP) are commonly elevated. Increased total bilirubin and icterus are uncommon findings. Diagnosis of primary liver disease requires a biopsy. Blood urea nitrogen (BUN) and creatinine are often elevated due to either primary renal disease or pre-renal azotemia secondary to dehydration and/or hypovolemia. Primary renal failure can occur due to hypoperfusion of the kidney as a result of hypovolemia. In humans, glomerulosclerosis from hyperglycemia has been reported. Hyperlipidemia is often noted due to the increase in triglycerides, cholesterol, lipoproteins, chylomicrons, and free fatty acids. Insulin deficiency prevents activation of lipoprotein lipase, so lipemia results. In humans, this contributes to atherosclerotic vascular disease and coronary artery disease. Pancreatic enzymes (amylase and lipase) are often elevated due to concurrent chronic or acute pancreatitis, chronic inflammation, or renal failure. Pancreatitis is strongly suspected if pancreatic enzyme elevation is accompanied by anorexia, vomiting, positive cPL test results, or supportive radiographic or ultrasonic abnormalities. If renal failure or insufficiency is present, amylase and lipase may be elevated due to decreased renal excretion.

Urinalysis will often reveal glucosuria, ketonuria, proteinuria, bacteriuria, with or without significant pyuria and hematuria. Urine from all DKA patients should be collected by performing aseptic cystocentesis and submitted for culture regardless of presence or absence of pyuria and/or hematuria. Urine strips do not detect β-hydroxybutyrate, but ketoacidosis cannot occur without this acid. Adding a drop or two of hydrogen peroxide to a urine sample that has tested negative for ketones may convert this ketoacid to acetoacetate and acetone, which are detectable on the urine strip. Alternatively, the patient's plasma or serum can be tested on these strips to detect ketonemia. An abstract in the *Journal of Veterinary Emergency and Critical Care* (March 2003, 13[1]) compared plasma ketones with urine ketones, and this practice was found to be clinically useful for confirming ketosis.

Electrolyte abnormalities are very common in pets experiencing DKA. Even if the initial serum levels of sodium, potassium, phosphorous, and magnesium are normal, there is frequently a whole body depletion of these ions from hyperglycemic diuresis. Abnormalities are often diagnosed during treatment, when electrolyte shifting between the intracellular and extracellular spaces can reveal an overall depletion of one or all of these electrolytes.

Treatment

Treatment of a patient with DKA is challenging. The goal should be to rapidly stabilize the patient, but do not expect immediate resolution of the complications that accompany DKA. At best, a patient with DKA will take a minimum of 36–48 hours of treatment in order to normalize their hyperglycemia and acidosis. The slower the recovery process, the better the probability of successful long-term treatment of the patient.

Goals of treatment are to restore and maintain adequate fluid balance and effective circulating volume, provide sufficient amounts of insulin to normalize glucose metabolism, to correct acidosis and electrolyte abnormalities, and to treat any and all underlying or predisposing causes. Strict aseptic technique should be used during all treatments of diabetic patients due to their increased susceptibility to bacterial infection. Gloves should be worn by all personnel handling these patients. All injection ports should be wiped with alcohol before each injection. If possible, the IV line setup should not be disconnected for walks or visitation. Patients experiencing DKA require large amounts of fluids to replenish deficits, keep up with maintenance needs, and replace ongoing losses.

Intravenous fluids should be initiated for at least 4 hours prior to implementing other therapies in order to start correcting fluid imbalances. These patients are best served by a central venous catheter. Not only can large volumes of fluids be delivered through these catheters rapidly, but central venous pressure (CVP) can be monitored to help guide fluid therapy, and blood sampling can be obtained through the same catheter using the three-syringe technique. Proper catheter care of a central line and monitoring is vital to prevent secondary infection (Fig. 10.3).

CVP is the measurement of hydrostatic pressure within the intrathoracic vena cava which is approximately equal to right atrial pressure. CVP gives the practitioner an estimation of both the ability of the heart to pump the fluids given, as well as an assessment if enough fluid is being given or if the patient needs more aggressive fluid resuscitation efforts. CVP should be maintained at adequate levels for perfusion (5–10 cmH$_2$O) in a patient undergoing fluid resuscitation, exercising caution to stay under 10 cmH$_2$O in order to prevent volume overload (Silverstein and Hopper 2009). CVP measurements less than 5 cmH$_2$O, or especially less than 2 cmH$_2$O, are indicative of need of increased fluid resuscitation. CVP measurements should always be performed with the patient in the same recumbency, preferably in the right lateral recumbent position. CVP trends are more meaningful than a single measurement, so they should be repeated frequently during fluid resuscitation.

Urine output should be monitored closely. If the patient is not urinating regularly, it is best to place a urinary catheter with a closed collection system in order to ensure adequate urine production, especially in azotemic patients. A minimum of 1–2 mL/kg/h of urine should be produced while on IV fluid replacement/therapy (Silverstein and Hopper 2009). If urine output is not meeting this minimum, arterial blood pressure (BP) assessment, CVP readings, and blood lactate levels should be checked to see if adequate fluid volume is being supplied. If BP, CVP, and lactate readings are within acceptable parameters, then the use of diuretics, dopamine, or fenoldopam should be considered in order to improve kidney function/excretion.

Other monitoring vital for these patients includes frequent assessment of temperature, mucus membrane color, capillary refill time (CRT), heart rate, pulse rate and character,

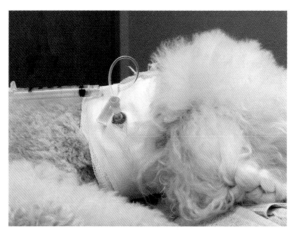

Figure 10.3   A sampling line, such as this jugular catheter, should be placed in DKA patients to avoid repeated, painful, and unnecessary venipuncture.

respirator rate and character, skin turgor, mentation, and BP monitoring. Extra care needs to be taken to keep these patients clean. If the patient is recumbent, it is important to remember to provide adequate bedding and change the position of the patient every 2–4 hours in order to help prevent formation of decubital ulcers and atalectic lungs.

Fluid therapy. The goal of fluid therapy is to reestablish normal fluid balance to ensure adequate hydration, cardiac output, BP, and organ perfusion. Fluid therapy alone can lower plasma glucose concentrations by improving GFR and excretion of excessive glucose. The concentration of diabetogenic hormones is also reduced with fluid administration. It is important to note that, unlike glucose levels, ketone bodies do not decrease with fluid administration alone. Insulin administration is required to rectify this imbalance.

The choice of fluid type is somewhat controversial and should be based on the patient's electrolyte status and acid–base balance. Most patients with DKA are sodium-depleted due to excessive urinary losses, vomiting, and diarrhea. In these cases, 0.9% NaCl is often the best choice initially, even though it is typically described as an "acidifying solution." Supplementation of potassium is often necessary. After 4–6 hours of treatment, electrolyte and acid–base balance should be reassessed. If sodium is >140 mmol/L, then the fluids should be changed to a buffered solution containing less sodium than 0.9% NaCl (DiBartola 2006). In patients with severe acidosis, and/or with mild hyponatremia, an isotonic buffered solution, such as Normosol-R, may be the best choice. Lactated Ringers solution (LRS) contains calcium, which may cause interference if phosphate and/or magnesium supplementation are required. Hypotonic solutions should be used with caution, if at all, due to the potential of excessive free water administration contributing to cerebral edema, and even death. If a DKA patient is also severely hyperosmolar, a hypotonic fluid may be considered. However, since the hyperosmolality is mostly due to hyperglycemia and hypernatremia, and because it typically developed over a prolonged period of time, usually judicious administration of balanced isotonic fluids will lead to the quickest resolution of hyperosmolality. Severe hyperosmolarity should be corrected over a minimum of 24 hours.

The fluid rate is dependent on the degree of dehydration, the presence of shock or hypovolemia, and ongoing losses. If shock is present, treat it aggressively. Shock doses of fluids range from 60–90 mL/kg in canines and 40–60 mL/kg for felines. Boluses should be started incrementally at 20 mL/kg and repeated to effect (Mathews 2006). If shock does not correct with repeated incremental boluses, then colloid administration should be considered. For dehydration deficits, the goal is to replace the deficit, plus meet daily requirements and ongoing losses, over 24–48 hours. Overzealous fluid therapy can lead to fluid overload and pulmonary edema. Inadequate fluid administration can lead to prolonged hyperglycemia and abnormal glucose metabolism, tissue hypoperfusion, hypoxia, continuing pancreatitis, and persistent azotemia. The patient's alertness, heart rate, respiration rate, CRT, pulse pressure, skin turgor, BP, and CVP should all be closely monitored.

Potassium supplementation. Electrolytes should be monitored closely. They should be retested 4–6 hours after treatment is initiated, then a minimum of twice daily thereafter. In severely hypokalemic patients, monitoring may need to be done as frequently as every 2–4 hours for a period of time. Ninety-eight percent of the body's potassium stores are contained in the intracellular compartment. Serum potassium losses are replenished from the intracellular compartment, primarily from muscles. Metabolic acidosis, lack of insulin, and serum hypertonicity contribute to this shift. As insulin is replaced via injection or continuous IV drip, a shift of serum K^+ occurs from the serum into the intracellular space, which reveals the total body deficit. A rapid drop in serum K^+ can have detrimental neurologic and cardiac effects. If serum K^+ is normal, then a minimum of 20 mEq/L potassium should be supplemented. If the K^+ level is unknown, then 40 mEq/L should be supplemented. See Figure 19.4 on potassium supplementation for dosing ranges based on serum K^+ levels in Chapter 19.

ECGs should be monitored for cardiac effects of both hypokalemia and hyperkalemia. Hypokalemia refractory to aggressive supplementation may be due to hypomagnesemia. Potassium supplementation should not be considered in cases with hyperkalemia due to anuric or oliguric renal failure.

Phosphate supplementation. The phosphate ion shifts similarly to potassium. Phosphate levels should be monitored closely after insulin administration begins. Rapid decreases in phosphate levels can occur within 12–24 hours of insulin administration. Severe hypophosphatemia can result in life-threatening hemolytic anemia, as well as weakness, ataxia, and seizures. If the serum phosphate level is <1.5 mg/dL, then phosphate should be supplemented at the rate of 0.1–0.3 mM/kg/h (Wingfield and Raffe 2002). Do *not* use phosphorous supplementation in conjunction with calcium containing fluids! Alternatively, the total potassium supplementation can be split using 50% potassium chloride and 50% potassium phosphate. This should adequately supplement the patient's phosphorous requirements, unless the patient's phosphate levels are very low on entry. Levels should be rechecked at least twice daily. Overzealous phosphate administration can result in iatrogenic hypocalcemia and associated neuromuscular signs, hypernatremia, hypotension, and diffuse tissue calcification. Supplementation of phosphate is not indicated in cases with hypercalcemia, hyperphosphatemia, or oliguria.

Conversely, patients with primary or secondary azotemia often have hyperphosphatemia. These patients should receive oral therapy with aluminum hydroxide when eating to help bind phosphorus from food/GI tract. Anorexic patients need not be given aluminum hydroxide as it will not be helpful.

Bicarbonate therapy. Acid–base evaluation should be an integral part of DKA monitoring. Plasma HCO_3^- or venous TCO_2 along with pH should be evaluated initially, then 4–6 hours after treatment is initiated, then at least twice daily. An arterial or central venous sample will most closely reflect the whole body acid–base status. The use of sodium bicarbonate ($NaHCO_3^-$) administration in the initial treatment of DKA is controversial. Acidosis generally resolves as perfusion improves and ketone bodies are metabolized with insulin administration. Use of a buffered solution, such as Normosol-R or LRS, generally aids metabolic acidosis as well. Guidelines for the use of $NaHCO_3^-$ vary widely. Typically, if the metabolic acidosis is severe after fluid resuscitation, (HCO_3^- or $TCO_2 < 10$ mmol/L or pH < 7.10; Mathews 2006), sodium bicarbonate therapy is recommended. Sodium bicarbonate should *never* be administered to patients suffering respiratory acidosis ($PCO_2 > 45$) unless they can be properly ventilated. Metabolic acidosis should be corrected *slowly*! Bicarbonate administration should take place over 2–6 hours. The base deficit should be calculated (mEq Bicarb = BW (kg) × 0.4 × (12 – patient's bicarb level) × 0.2) (Mathews 2006). If the patient's HCO_3 is unknown, use the number 10 for calculation, or alternatively, the recommendation is to *not* give bicarbonate. The factor of 0.2 provides 20% of the calculated dose to be given over the 2- to 6-hour time frame. After 6 hours, the HCO_3^- or TCO_2 levels should be reevaluated. If the bicarbonate level is >12 mEq, do not give any more supplement. Administration of sodium bicarbonate can result in coronary acidosis, and therefore sudden death. Also, a paradoxical CNS acidosis may occur in pets receiving aggressive sodium bicarbonate therapy, with the cerebrospinal fluid becoming acidotic due to influx of CO_2. Therefore, it is imperative that the patient has been adequately fluid-resuscitated, is able to adequately ventilate itself during administration, as well as the bicarbonate being given over a significant period of time, so as not to overwhelm the blood–brain barrier with rising levels of PCO_2.

Insulin therapy. The backbone of treatment of DKA is fluid therapy and insulin administration. If the patient is severely sick and dehydrated with severe electrolyte and acid–base derangements, it is recommended to administer IV fluid therapy alone for the first few hours of treatment before adding insulin. Regular insulin is chosen for initial treatment of diabetics due to the rapid onset of action and brief duration of effect. Insulin can be administered intramuscularly or intravenously in DKA patients. Intermittent IM technique or intravenous constant rate infusion (CRI) are two commonly used methods. The goal of either therapy is to slowly lower the BG concentration by 50–100 mg/dL/h, resulting in a BG of 200–250 after 8–10 hours.

Intermittent IM Technique: a loading dose of 0.2 U/kg is given IM, then 0.1 U/kg is administered hourly until BG levels lower (Mathews 2006). The preferred site for administration is in the rear legs to diminish likelihood of giving the insulin into adipose tissue. BG levels should be checked every 1–2 hours. After BG < 250 mg/dL, then the insulin is given every 4–6 hours IM at a dose of 0.1–0.4 U/kg (Mathews 2006), based on BG response. The patient is placed on IV supplementation of 2.5%–5% dextrose to maintain a BG between 150 and 300 mg/dL until the patient is stable and eating. Although it seems counterintuitive to administer dextrose to a patient with hyperglycemia, this step is actually vital to achieve metabolic breakdown of the remaining ketone bodies and for resolving acidosis.

Intravenous Insulin CRI: 2 U/kg for canines or 1.1 U/kg for felines of regular insulin is added to 250 mL bag of 0.9% NaCl (Plunkett 2000). The first 50 mL of the mixed solution is run through the IV tubing and discarded due to absorption of the insulin by the plastic administration set. The insulin infusion is then started at 10 mL/h and adjusted as the BG declines. Dextrose must be concurrently supplemented within an intravenous crystalloid as directed by Table 10.3.

The goal again is to maintain the BG level between 150–300 mg/dL until the patient is eating and stable. This is the preferred method for managing DKA in humans, and works effectively in small animals as well. Once the patient is stable and eating, not vomiting, maintaining its fluid balance without the aid of IV fluids, is not acidotic or azotemic, and has no electrolyte abnormalities, then, long-acting insulin is started.

In order for DKA to be successfully managed, it is imperative that any and all concurrent diseases are diagnosed and treated. Bacterial infection, CHF, acute kidney injury (AKI/chronic kidney disease (CKD), Cushing's disease, diestrus, pancreatic, UTI, or other disease must be addressed. Typically, patients are placed on an appropriate, broad-spectrum antibiotic to treat any suspected bacterial infection pending culture results. Typically, hyperglycemia will resolve within approximately 12 hours. Ketosis takes longer; up to 3 days or more, to resolve. Owners must be willing to make the financial expenditures that these patients require in order to recover fully. They must be educated of the long-term commitment and care involved with caring for diabetic patients. Even with

Table 10.3   Insulin-dextrose supplementation guide for treating diabetic ketoacidosis (DKA)

Serum Glucose Level (mg/dL)	Insulin Infusion Rate (mL/h)	Secondary Fluid Type
>250	10	Crystalloid
200–250	7	Crystalloid + 2.5% dextrose
150–200	5	Crystalloid + 2.5% dextrose
100–150	5	Crystalloid + 5% dextrose
<100	Discontinue insulin CRI	Crystalloid + 5% dextrose

appropriate owner dedication, proper diagnosis, and diligent nursing care and monitoring, DKA patients can still be challenging to manage, especially if multiple concurrent problems are present. However, seeing the successful outcome achievable in these patients can be very rewarding.

Diabetic Complications

Iatrogenic hypoglycemia

Hypoglycemia is one of the most common side effects of insulin therapy. It may be symptomatic or asymptomatic as symptoms are dependent both on the rate and magnitude of the decrease of BG levels. Hypoglycemia may occur due to a variety of factors including increasing the dose of insulin, duration of insulin action overlaps into the next insulin dose, strenuous exercise, decreased appetite, anorexia, or vomiting after eating. In some cases, the bottle of insulin was not properly mixed, or was almost empty, allowing a concentrated dose of insulin to be administered. In these cases, profound hypoglycemia occurs before diabetogenic hormone response can be initiated to compensate. Symptomatic signs include lethargy, weakness, ataxia (owner may say the pet is "wobbly" or walking drunk), seizures, coma, and death. Severity of signs is dependent on severity of hypoglycemia and the rate of decrease of BG. Clinically, hypoglycemia is described as a BG level < 60 mg/dL. Signs may become apparent at levels higher or much lower than this. With asymptomatic hypoglycemia, signs are either not present or so subtle that owners do not notice them such as papillary dilation, nervousness, or anxiety. It often will be found incidentally, while checking routine lab work, or if the patient is being seen for another problem, or during a serial BG curve. A low (<350 μmol/L) fructosamine level may also indicate problems with chronic hypoglycemia.

Treatment of hypoglycemia may be as simple as feeding the patient if symptoms are not severe. Owners can administer oral sugar water or Karo syrup at home if the patient's hypoglycemia is more significant. They should note response within 5–10 minutes. If this helps, some of these patients will then eat food and respond accordingly. More severe cases should be brought to the closest emergency facility immediately for treatment, especially if the patient has had a seizure, is recumbent, or comatose. Intravenous dextrose infusion is required in these cases, sometimes for many hours dependent on severity and dose of insulin received. An initial slow IV bolus of 50% dextrose (0.5 g/kg diluted 1:4) (Mathews 2006) should be administered, followed with a CRI of 5% dextrose solution. Sometimes owners will mistake hypoglycemia as signs of hyperglycemia and proceed to administer another dose of insulin prior to bringing them to the hospital. This further complicates the monitoring and length of stay the patient will require. Whenever hypoglycemia occurs, whether corrected at home or in the hospital, a reevaluation of insulin dosages is required. Complications of hypoglycemic events include cerebral edema and neurological effects/abnormalities such as blindness or behavior changes that will typically resolve over a period of weeks or months.

Transient diabetes

Approximately 20% of diabetic cats will have transient diabetes (Feldman and Nelson 2004). They are subclinical until something stresses them, such as systemic inflammation, systemic disease, or administration of an insulin-antagonistic drug. Psychological stress has also been seen as a precursor to onset of symptoms. In these cases, insulin secretion's suppression is reversible. The suppression allows hyperglycemia, however, which further impairs insulin secretion due to glucose toxicity. This impaired response mimics Type I diabetes. These cats are then treated with insulin therapy, which in time decreases the insulin resistance and improves beta cell function, returns insulin secretion, and resolves the IDDM status. All these can happen weeks to months after diagnosis and initiation of treatment. Close attention to monitoring can aid in detecting the resolution of diabetes in these cats prior to the onset of severe or life-threatening hypoglycemia.

Somogyi phenomenon

If asymptomatic hypoglycemia goes on undetected, the rebound release of cortisol and growth hormone result in insulin resistance, which may persist for 24–72 hours after a hypoglycemic event. This is known as the Somogyi phenomenon, which is characterized by episodes of hypoglycemia followed by rebound hyperglycemia. Insulin-induced hyperglycemia should be suspected when there is morning glucosuria of >1 g/dL on urine test strips, with continued PU/ PD, symptoms of hypoglycemia, weight loss, or excessively high insulin doses (nearing 2.2 U/kg). Diagnosis is made most easily by a serial glucose curve demonstrating hypoglycemia (<65 mg/dL) followed by hyperglycemia (>300 mg/dL). The therapy primarily involves reducing the dose of insulin given by 10%–25%. If the patient is on excessively large doses of insulin, the patient should be started over on doses recommended for initial management of a diabetic. The patient should then be reassessed in 3–5 days.

Hyperosmolar coma

Hyperosmolar diabetes, although uncommon, is a syndrome that technicians should be aware of. Hyperosmolar, nonketotic diabetes is exhibited by profound hyperglycemia (BG > 600 mg/dL), along with hyperosmolarity (>350 mOsm/L), extreme dehydration, CNS depression, with a notable absence of ketones or metabolic acidosis. Events leading up to this syndrome often include gastrointestinal abnormalities along with neurologic issues such as weakness that may be progressive, anorexia, vomiting, and lethargy. Examination will reveal profound dehydration, hypothermia, lethargy, extreme depression, and possibly coma. Treatment includes cautious fluid therapy, calculating the patient's dehydration deficit and replacing 80% of this deficit over 12–24 hours. Insulin therapy may begin 2–4 hours after fluid therapy has begun at a lower dosage (1.1 U/kg) (Plunkett 2000).

CHAPTER 10

Insulinoma

Insulinomas are tumors or masses that secrete insulin without regulation, therefore resulting in hypoglycemia. Insulinomas are referred to as an APUDoma. They can form from amine precursor uptake and decarboxylation (APUD) cells found in the body. Types of APUDomas may be somatostatinomas, pheochromocytomas, gastrinomas, and glucagonomas, as well as insulinomas. They generally occur in middle- to older-aged dogs, rarely in cats. Clinical signs are related to the subsequent hypoglycemia occurring due to increased insulin production from the tumor. The test to confirm the presence or absence of an insulinoma is a serum insulin concentration test. Initial treatment involves supplementing dextrose intravenously. Glucocorticoids may be beneficial due to antagonistic effects to insulin, thereby increasing insulin resistance. Exploratory surgery is generally required to locate the tumor, though it may be identified during abdominal ultrasound. Even if ultrasound is performed, surgical intervention is still required to remove the mass. If no tumor be can be identified, a hemipancreatectomy is performed. Postoperative care is as would be for a pancreatitis patient. These patients can be medically managed for several months to a year even without surgery.

Medical management of insulinoma includes several factors. Frequent small meals (3–6 meals per day) consisting of a diet that is high in fat, fiber, and complex carbohydrates should be given. Simple sugars should be avoided. Exercise should be limited. Glucocorticoids are a primary therapy for insulinoma, usually in the form of prednisone at a dose of 2.5 mg/kg q12h (or every 12 hours) (Feldman and Nelson 2004). Other drugs that may be considered are diazoxide, somatostatin therapy, and chemotherapeutic drugs. Diazoxide is a diuretic that works in cases of insulinoma by inhibiting insulin secretion, inhibiting tissue use of glucose, and stimulation of hepatic gluconeogenesis and glycogenolysis. It is expensive and hard to find in the United States. Octreotide is the primary drug used as a somatostatin therapeutic drug—which works by inhibiting both the secretion and synthesis of beta cells—whether they are neoplastic or not.

Streptozocin and alloxan are chemotherapeutic drugs often used in cases of human insulinomas, but their use needs further study in application for small animal medicine.

Dysfunction of the Adrenal Glands

The functions of the adrenal gland are vital for life. Without them life is not possible. When they malfunction, however, they cause a variety of problems that are often hard to identify as well as sometimes being difficult to treat. Hyperadrenocorticism, hypoadrenocorticism, pheochromocytoma, and postoperative complications of adrenalectomy patients are all potential adrenal dysfunctions that can be encountered in ECC practice. Early recognition, diagnosis, and treatment are vital to the positive outcome in these patients. A veterinary technician plays a vital role in the monitoring, care, and aiding in diagnosis of these patients.

Hypoadrenocorticism (Addison's Disease)

Hypoadrenocorticism is notoriously known for being an often overlooked and difficult to diagnose disease. It has been called the "great pretender" and it is reportedly uncommon in dogs and is rare in cats. However, if there is awareness of what to look for and what patients to look for it in, diagnosis can be neither difficult to recognize and diagnose, nor as uncommon as one may think. A veterinary nurse plays a vital role in the monitoring, care, and diagnosis of these patients.

Addison's disease is generally the result of bilateral adrenal atrophy with fibrosis that is thought to be idiopathic in most cases but may have an immune-mediated cause in some cases, or iatrogenic causes (mitotane administration). Inadequate secretion of glucocorticoids and mineralocorticoids by the adrenal cortex are responsible for signs and symptoms of Addison's disease. The primary mineralocorticoid secreted by the adrenal cortex is aldosterone, which promotes renal resorption of sodium and water and excretion of potassium and hydrogen ions. The primary adrenocortical glucocorticoids are cortisol and corticosterone. These are responsible for stimulating appetite, maintaining BG and BP, promoting free water loss through the kidneys, protecting against shock, and helping response to stress. Primary Addison's disease results from destruction of adrenal cortices in which both mineral and glucocorticoids are deficient. Secondary Addison's disease can be the result of natural causes or iatrogenic causes. There is a decreased adrenocorticotropic hormone (ACTH) production from the pituitary gland. Iatrogenic causes are usually the result of prolonged administration of exogenous glucocorticoids. Even otic and ophthalmic preparations can reduce ACTH responsiveness. This suppresses normal pituitary ACTH production which leads to bilateral adrenal atrophy. Ninety percent of adrenal function must be compromised before clinical signs become evident. Secondary disease generally affects only the glucocorticoids being deficient. Although mineralocorticoid deficiency can develop over time, these patients should be monitored every 3–4 months for need of replacement therapy.

Hypoadrenocorticism most often develops in young to middle age female dogs. Breeds that seem to have a higher risk are Standard Poodles, Portuguese Water dogs, Great Danes, Labrador retrievers, Rottweilers, West Highland Terriers, and Wheaten Terriers. Presentation of this disease can vary widely, from intermittent, to chronic, to nonspecific signs, or as an Addisonian crisis. Diagnosis of disease with only glucocorticoids deficiency can be more difficult to recognize without the electrolyte abnormalities that accompany mineralocorticoid deficiency. Signs of Addison's disease can vary widely. Lethargy, anorexia, vomiting, diarrhea, weight loss, weakness, trembling, PU, and PD are all chronic signs in this disease. Animals may also present with acute collapse accompanied by hypovolemic shock known as an Addisonian crisis. These patients will have pale mucus membranes, a slow or increased CRT, and profound weakness. Approximately 1/3 of dogs in crisis will have bradycardia instead of the normal tachycardia associated with hypovolemia. Often, evidence of severe GI hemorrhage is present.

A CBC, chemistry panel, electrolyte analysis, acid–base assessment, and ACTH stimulation test are all necessary for all suspect Addisonians. Classic abnormalities associated with hypoadrenocorticism are hyponatremia, hyperkalemia, hypochloremia, azotemia, and mild to moderate metabolic acidosis. The Na/K ratio will be low (<27:1). If there is collapse with normal sodium and potassium levels, then hypoglycemia or severe GI hemorrhage is likely the cause. Azotemia (BUN up to or over 200 mg/dL) associated with Addison's disease is generally pre-renal in nature, despite a low urine specific gravity (<1.030) due to increased sodium losses. This can be confused with AKI. Hypercalcemia and or hypoglycemia are present in about 30% of cases. There may also be hypochloremia and phosphorus abnormalities. There is often a mild, normocytic, normochromic anemia present which initially may be masked by dehydration. White blood cell counts are generally normal and CBCs will lack the presence of a stress leukogram. A fair amount of dogs will have mild hypoalbuminemia (usually > 2.0 g/dL). ACTH stimulation testing will confirm the presence or absence of the disease. In canines with hypoadrenocorticism, poststimulation values are consistently less than 5.0 μg/mL. Endogenous ACTH concentration testing may be useful to differentiate between primary and secondary hypoadrenocorticism. Samples (plasma) must be drawn and centrifuged immediately, then frozen in plastic tubes. This test is of most value when there is just a glucocorticoid deficiency (secondary Addison's disease). Endogenous ACTH concentrations will be high in patients with secondary/glucocorticoid-only deficiency.

Thoracic radiographs may reveal the presence of microcardia due to hypovolemia. Megaesophagus may also be noted, which resolves with therapy. ECG will have profound changes if hyperkalemia is present. Bradycardia with tall peaked "T" waves, a widening and flattening of the QRS complex, prolonged PR interval, with a decreased P wave amplitude, and increase in duration of the P wave may occur. With increasing severity of hyperkalemia atrial standstill, absence of P waves and deviations of the ST segments can occur. Asystole or ventricular fibrillations are common with severe elevations.

Treatment of an Addisonian crisis involves treating hypotension and hypovolemia, concurrent electrolyte, and acid–base abnormalities, and providing glucocorticoid replacement. Death from hypoadrenocorticism is generally the result of shock with subsequent cardiovascular collapse, not hyperkalemia. Intravenous fluid therapy is first-line treatment in these patients. A short, large bore catheter should be placed and a fluid bolus started. A 0.9% NaCl is generally the initial fluid of choice due to hyperkalemia and hyponatremia present. However, caution should be taken if the patient is profoundly hyponatremic, as rapid rise in sodium may result in detrimental neurological effects. A balanced isotonic crystalloid is an acceptable fluid choice in the majority of Addisonian crises patients. If possible, blood should be collected prior to fluid administration. A typical shock fluid bolus (60–90 mL/kg maximum for a canine, given in 20 mL/kg increments to effect) may be required. The amount given should be determined by degree of dehydration present and response to fluid therapy. If the patient is hypoglycemic, then dextrose may need to be supplemented (2.5%–5% in fluids). If a steroid is needed before completion of an ACTH stimulation test, then dexamethasone sodium phosphate (0.1–2.0 mg/kg IV initially, then 0.05–0.1 mg/kg/12 h) (Mathews 2006) is the drug of choice, as it will not interfere with the test results. If the patient is stable until completion of ACTH-stimulation testing, then prednisolone sodium succinate or methylprednisolone is the glucocorticoid of choice (2–5 mg/kg IV slow) (Mathews 2006). Only use methylprednisolone if mineralocorticoid therapy is not needed. Hydrocortisone sodium succinate (1.25 mg/kg IV initially, then 0.5–1.0 mg/kg IV q8hr—given over 20 minutes) may also be used (Mathews 2006).

The effect of dilution from IV fluid therapy is often sufficient to adequately manage hyperkalemia. If the hyperkalemia is so severe that it is causing life-threatening alterations to heart function/ECG, or remains persistently high, then additional treatments may be required. For life-threatening complications of hyperkalemia, calcium gluconate should be administered (0.5–1.0 mL/kg over 5–10 minutes) (Mathews 2006), as it helps protect the myocardium from the adverse affects of hyperkalemia. An ECG should be continuously monitored during infusion of calcium gluconate. Treatment of the hyperkalemia itself is also required. IV glucose administration is helpful—dosage of 0.7–1.0 g/kg 25%

dextrose over 3–5 minutes (Silverstein and Hopper 2009)—because as glucose enters cells, potassium follows, effectively lowering the serum concentrations. If the patient is normoglycemic or hyperglycemic, insulin can be added to the treatment regimen to aid movement of potassium into cells. A dose of regular insulin (0.5 U/kg IV) can be given. Two grams of dextrose IV should be given for each unit of insulin given (2 g/U) (Silverstein and Hopper 2009) to prevent hypoglycemia. Bicarbonate may be considered, as alkalosis promotes movement of potassium into cells. This step will not be necessary for most hypoadrenal patients. The metabolic acidosis present in these patients is usually mild, and is treated adequately by addressing the underlying problems of hypotension and dehydration (i.e., fluid therapy). If the bicarbonate level or TCO_2 remains less than 12 mEq/L with an extremely low pH after fluid resuscitation, bicarbonate administration can be carefully considered.

Initially hypoadrenal patients should be managed with both glucocorticoids and mineralocorticoid supplementation. Oral prednisone or prednisolone (initially 0.2–0.5 mg/lb/day divided into two doses 12 hours apart) should be continued for 3–4 weeks. Dosages should be tapered by 50% per week until discontinued, or until pet shows signs of glucocorticoid deficiency. Initially, IV fluid therapy normalized mineral values, but for long-term, mineralocorticoids must be administered. There are two options for mineralocorticoid replacement: fludrocortisone acetate (Florinef: 0.015–0.02 mg/kg/day PO) or desoxycorticosterone pivalate (DOCP: 2.2 mg/kg IM or SQ q. 25–30 days) (Mathews 2006). Florinef has both mineral and glucocorticoid action. If the owner is not prohibited by its cost or the commitment to daily medication, then it can be an effective long-term treatment. Initially, Florinef is often used, with the patient transitioning to DOCP for long-term maintenance. Maintenance prednisone dosing may be required in some patients receiving DOCP. Owners should be given a supply of prednisone to keep on hand, being instructed to give as directed during stressful situations with either medication choice (Fig. 10.4).

Patients should be monitored closely. Electrolyte levels should be checked every 4–7 days for the first 1–2 weeks of therapy, then every 3–4 months through the first year, so medication dosages can be adjusted accordingly. The minimum effective dose for any medication should be used.

Prognosis of Addisonian patients is excellent when they are well controlled. The owners need to be educated to the life-long commitment necessary to treat these patients and the follow-up exams and blood work that will be needed on a regular basis. The owners also need to be aware of their pet's increased glucocorticoid needs during stressful situations, and supplement accordingly.

Pheochromocytoma

Pheochromocytomas are tumors that form off of the adrenal medulla, or more specifically, off of the chromaffin cells. These tumors may invade the caudal vena cava, and they release excessive levels of catecholamines that lead to systemic hypertension and cardiac arrhythmias. These tumors are located in the abdomen 90% of the time and rarely metastasize. They are rarely diagnosed before death and are typically found in older patients. They cause very vague and nonspecific signs such as tachypnea, weight loss, restlessness, mydriasis, tachycardia, arrhythmias with pulse deficits, epistaxis, hyperemic skin and mucous membranes, retinal hemorrhages, bounding pulses,

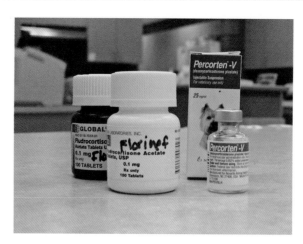

Figure 10.4 Several agents, both oral and injectable, are available for the long term treatment of hypoadrenocorticism.

shock, collapse, syncope, peripheral edema of rear legs, and possible abdominal mass (palpated in ~10%). As diverse as these signs are, they may occur intermittently or continuously. This is due to the often episodic nature of catecholamine release, causing sporadic signs. An abdominal mass may be found by abdominal ultrasound, as 90% of intra-abdominal pheochromocytomas are located on the adrenal glands themselves. Hypertension may or may not be found dependent on its intermittent occurrence. Urine or plasma catecholamines may be tested, but this test is not readily available and is expensive.

Treatment involves adrenalectomy or removal of the mass if located in an alternate area. Stabilization of the patient prior to surgery includes treatment with phenoxybenzamine, starting at a low dose and increasing over several days until hypertension is controlled for at least 7 days prior to surgery. Propranolol or atenolol may be used for control of cardiac arrhythmias with concurrent use of alpha and beta blockers. Phenothiazines should be avoided for anesthesia to aid in preventing hypotension during the surgical procedure. Halothane and thiobarbituates should also not be used due to their potential for causing cathecholamine-induced arrhythmias. The patient must be monitored very closely during surgery and sudden BP changes should be expected. ECG and direct arterial pressures should be monitored throughout surgery. Hypertension may be managed with esmolol or phentolamine. Occurrence of hypotension should be monitored postoperatively and treated with fluid therapy as needed. If adrenalectomy was performed, treatment for hypoadrenocorticism including glucocorticoid supplementation should be started before and immediately after surgery. Preoperative administration of ketoconazole may limit the effects of adrenalectomy.

Critical Illness-Related Corticosteroid Insufficiency (CIRCI)/Relative Adrenal Insufficiency (RAI)

The use of steroids in critical care medicine is always a center of controversy. But it seems, at least in some cases, that the old saying passed down through the decades of "Nothing should die without the benefit of steroids" may not have been so far off the mark!

Previously termed RAI, CIRCI has not always been widely recognized in veterinary medicine (Peyton and Burkett 2009). When a patient becomes severely ill, the hypothalamic–pituitary–adrenal (HPA) axis is stimulated to release ACTH, resulting in a subsequent release of corticosteroid hormones from the adrenal cortex. Cortisol aids the animal's ability to handle the stress of illness and their ability to recover, as adrenal-ectomized animals will quickly succumb if steroids are not replaced. However, in some severely ill patients (sepsis, septic shock), a failure of the adrenals to secrete cortisol seems to occur. This HPA-axis dysfunction is widely recognized and is considered to be a com-monly occurring condition in humans with sepsis or septic shock. The septic shock in these cases will be persistent: refractory to treatment with intravenous fluids (crystalloids or colloids) or pressor (norepinephrine, vasopressin, and dopamine) therapy. This HPA dysfunction appears to be reversible in these cases, with adrenal function returning after recovery.

The best way to confirm the presence of CIRCI in a critical patient is a matter of debate. However, it seems that a standard ACTH stimulation test may be useful. Baseline cortisol levels are subtracted from the stimulated cortisol levels. A difference of <9 µg/dL (<0.25 µmol/L) is consistent with CIRCI.

Treatment consists of replacing physiologic doses of glucocorticoids. In humans, the use of dexamethasone sodium phosphate is not recommended. Hydrocortisone may be given (1.25 mg/kg IV initially, then 0.5–1.0 mg/kg IV) every 8 hours for a maximum dose of 2 mg/kg/d (Mathews 2006). Hypotension will typically respond within a couple of hours after glucocorticoid replacement. It is unknown how CIRCI affects survivability of patients with sepsis/septic shock and if treatment improves the outcome. Treatment of CIRCI does seem to promote improvement in hypotension consistently, and is therefore certainly a consideration in critically ill patients.

Dysfunction of the Thyroid and Parathyroid Gland

Thyroid dysfunction is a common cause of endocrine disease in the cat and dog. Cats typically experience hyperthyroid disease while dogs get to experience hypothyroid states. Parathyroid disease, on the other hand, is a much less common source of endocrine disease. When it occurs, it can manifest itself as hyperparathyroidism or hypoparathyroid-ism. These diseases are not common causes of presentation to the emergency room, however, and therefore are beyond the scope of this text

Conclusion

Clearly, the endocrine system is a wonderfully unique, complex network of systems, organs, and glands all working together to achieve homeostasis in the body. Derangement in one of these or of either production or regulation of their respective hormones can result in life-threatening illness. Familiarity with the endocrine system and how it works is vital for the advanced technician caring for emergent and critical care patients. Though the care of these patients can be arduous, the outcome can be very rewarding!

References

DiBartola, S. 2006. *Fluid and Electrolyte Therapy*, 3rd ed. St. Louis, MO: Saunders.

Feldman & Nelson. 2004. *Canine & Feline Endocrinology and Reproduction*, 3rd ed. St. Louis, MO: Saunders.

Mathews, K. 2006. *Veterinary Emergency and Critical Care Manual*. Guelph, ON: Lifelearn.

Peyton, J, Burkett, JM. 2009. Case report: critical illness related corticosteroid insufficiency in a dog with septic shock. *J Vet Emergency Critical Care* 19(3):262–268.

Plumb, D. 2005. *Veterinary Drug Handbook*, 5th ed. Ames, IA: Blackwell.

Plunkett, S. 2000. *Emergency Procedures for the Small Animal Veterinarian*. St. Louis, MO: Saunders.

Reineke, E, Fletcher, D, King, L, et al. 2010. Accuracy of a continuous glucose monitoring system in dogs and cats with diabetic ketoacidosis. *J Vet Emergency Critical Care* 20(3):303–312.

Silverstein, D, Hopper, K, editors. 2009. *Small Animal Critical Care Medicine*. St. Louis, MO: Saunders Elsevier.

Wingfield, WE, Raffe, MR, editors 2002. *The Veterinary ICU Book*. Jackson Hole, WY: Teton NewMedia.

CHAPTER 10

Hemolymphatic, Immunologic, and Oncology Emergencies

Mary Tefend Campbell

Introduction

The *circulatory system* is made up of two primary components, the blood–vascular system, and the lymphatic system. The blood–vascular system is a closed system composed of the heart, arteries (which distribute blood from the heart to the tissues), veins (which return blood from the tissues to the heart), and capillaries (small thin-walled vessels at which physiological exchange occurs), and the blood. The lymphatic system drains fluids that accumulate in the tissues, which are first collected by lymphatic capillaries, pass into lymphatic vessels, and then empty into the venous system. Disorders of the hematopoietic and lymphoid systems encompass a wide range of diseases. Such diseases may affect the red cells, white cells, or even hemostatic mechanisms. Hemostatic abnormalities typically result in hemorrhage, thrombosis, or disseminated intravascular coagulation (DIC).

Composition of Blood and Hemostasis

The blood itself is a regulatory fluid which acts as a transport system for oxygen, nutrients, waste products of cellular metabolism, hormones, white blood cells (WBCs), and platelets. Blood aids in the regulation of body temperature, regulation of blood pH, and also acts as a defense system via WBCs (e.g., phagocytosis). Blood provides clotting factors and platelet activation when a blood vessel wall is damaged.

The cellular portion of blood is composed of seven types of cells and cell fragments, namely, red blood cells (RBCs) or *erythrocytes*, *platelets* (or thrombocytes), and five kinds of WBCs or *leukocytes*. The cells are suspended in the plasma, or the fluid portion of the blood. *Plasma* makes up from 45% to 78% of a blood sample volume, depending on the species of animal and the size of its RBCs (Colville and Bassert 2002). Plasma is over 90% water, containing proteins such as albumin, globulins, and fibrinogen. Many other substances are also found in plasma, such as oxygen, nitrogen, carbon dioxide, metabolic wastes, electrolytes, lipids, and amino acids.

Red Blood Cells (RBCs)

RBCs, or erythrocytes, carry hemoglobin in the circulation. The process of RBC production (erythropoiesis) begins in the bone marrow, with many other factors necessary to continue RBC development. The process of erythropoiesis depends on the hormone *erythropoietin*, made primarily in the kidneys. The stimulus for erythropoietin synthesis is renal hypoxia, which triggers increased erythropoietin production within minutes to hours. The maximum rate of erythropoietin production is reached within 24 hours after the onset of hypoxia; there may not be a detectable increase in the peripheral RBC count for days. After release from the kidneys, erythropoietin is transported to the bone marrow and (to a lesser degree) the spleen. Here, erythropoietin stimulates the proliferation and maturation of erythroid progenitor cells, which in turn will become erythrocytes. Erythropoietin also facilitates hemoglobin synthesis and stimulates the release of RBCs and reticulocytes into the circulation.

Mature erythrocytes lack a nucleus and have a life span which varies between species (approximately 68 days for the cat, and 110 days for the dog) (Colville and Bassert 2002). As RBCs wear out, they are replaced by young RBCs (called reticulocytes) from the bone marrow. Most aging RBCs are destroyed outside the cardiovascular system by macrophages through a process called *extravascular hemolysis*. Macrophages remove the RBCs from circulation where they are broken down into components that can be recycled or eliminated, particularly in the liver and spleen. Iron from hemoglobin is recovered and reused by red marrow.

The function of the RBC is to carry oxygen to the tissues; the protein *hemoglobin* is responsible for this process. Hemoglobin is composed of two components, heme and globin, produced by the RBC as it matures. Hemoglobin exists in two physiologic states, oxyhemoglobin (hemoglobin carrying oxygen), and deoxyhemoglobin (hemoglobin that has given up its oxygen). Many factors influence the hemoglobin's ability to carry oxygen, including temperature, pH, oxygen, and carbon dioxide levels.

CHAPTER 11

Box 11.1   Formation of a Thrombus in Hemostasis

- Primary hemostasis—Activated platelets form a platelet plug (minutes)
- Secondary hemostasis—Reinforcement of the frail platelet plug with fibrin strands (hours)
- Fibrinolysis—Clot dissolves after vascular wall repair (days)

Platelets

Platelets (thrombocytes) are another blood cell type in the peripheral blood. Production of platelets (thrombopoiesis) is a result of megakaryocytes produced in the bone marrow. As the megakaryocytes develop, they undergo incomplete mitosis (where the nuclei divide but the cytoplasm does not). The megakaryocytes do not leave the bone marrow; they break off into small chunks of cytoplasm and are sent into circulation as platelets. Platelets also help in the maintenance of vascular integrity by attaching to the endothelium of vessels and release endothelial growth factor into endothelial cells.

Hemostasis

Platelets also have a very specific role in hemostasis. *Hemostasis* is a highly advanced, regulated process that keeps blood in a clot-free state while also having the ability to respond rapidly to vascular injury by forming a localized hemostatic plug to prevent blood loss in a damaged blood vessel. The formation and localization of a hemostatic plug is initiated and controlled by elements of the vascular wall, namely platelets, coagulation factors, and the fibrinolytic system. Hemostasis is divided into primary and secondary phases.

Primary hemostasis involves interactions between the vessel wall and the platelets. Primary hemostasis results in the formation of a platelet plug at the site of vascular injury; both platelets and the endothelial cells of the vascular system form a platelet plug, or more specifically, an "unstable" fibrin clot. This platelet plug provides a physical barrier to inhibit further loss of blood, in addition to providing membrane surfaces and binding sites for the assembly of procoagulant enzymes that help promote the formation of thrombin in the process of secondary hemostasis. In primary hemostasis, following platelet adherence, platelets undergo conformational (shape) changes and subsequently release substances that stimulate platelet aggregation. Aggregated platelets constitute the primary hemostatic plug. Defects in primary hemostasis can be due to vascular or platelet disorders (Hackner 2004).

Secondary hemostasis involves the formation of fibrin in and around the primary hemostatic plug. Specifically, secondary hemostasis involves the stabilization and localization of the platelet clot through the generation of thrombin and the activation of the fibrinolytic system, respectively. Thrombin is an essential product of secondary hemostasis. As well as producing fibrin monomers by its action on fibrinogen, thrombin stimulates platelets and endothelial cells to enhance clot formation.

Thrombin is generated through a series of enzymatic reactions known as the *coagulation cascade*. There are two pathways for the activation of the coagulation cascade, an *intrinsic* and an *extrinsic* pathway. The intrinsic pathway is surface-activated, which means it operates strictly with components present in the blood. The extrinsic pathway requires tissue factor for activation (Hackner 2004).

The initiation of the coagulation cascade is primarily through the exposure of tissue factor (TF), a transmembrane glycoprotein not available to the vasculature in health. Tissue factor can, however, be presented to the vascular compartment by any damaged cell. Endothelial cells and activated monocytes are particularly active contributors of tissue factor either through direct injury or through expression of TF initiated by inflammatory mediators. Exposed tissue factor binds to factor VII which forms a thrombin complex that initiates the extrinsic aspect of the coagulation cascade. The small amount of thrombin produced through factor VII activates other clotting factors (from factor XI to factor XIa), which in turn activates even more cofactors (factors V, VIII, and XIII). Through such processes, thrombin formation is maintained.

Calcium (factor IV) is also required for most reactions and is the reason why calcium chelators (e.g., citrate and ethylenediaminetetraacetic acid [EDTA]) are used for blood collection to preserve cells for analysis. All coagulation factors are produced in the liver, with the exception of factor VIII. Vitamin K is required for the formation of factors II, VII, IX, and X (Hackner 2004). Each coagulation factor is converted to its active form by the preceding factor. Coagulation factors are given roman numerals from I to XIII, but the numbering is not sequential.

To summarize, the coagulation cascade consists of a series of enzymatic reactions culminating in cleavage of plasma fibrinogen to form cross-linked fibrin at the site of vessel injury. The coagulation cascade plays three pivotal roles in the formation of fibrin from fibrinogen: (1) the acceleration of fibrin generation, (2) the regulation of the fibrin plug to a size appropriate for the injury, and (3) the localization of the fibrin clot to the site of injury. Defects in secondary hemostasis manifest clinically as hematomas and deep bleeds into joints, tissue, and body cavities.

While a clot is developing, fibrinolytic factors are concurrently activated that serve to remodel and localize the plug so that it does not completely occlude the vasculature. Such a process is part of the *fibrinolytic system*. The fibrinolytic system consists of plasminogen and many other substances that convert plasminogen to its active form, plasmin (Hackner 2004). Plasmin is ultimately responsible for dissolution of the fibrin clot.

Plasmin exists in circulation as the proenzyme plasminogen. Plasminogen is activated primarily by tissue-type plasminogen activator (t-PA) and urokinase-type plasminogen activator (u-PA). The t-PA is produced by endothelial cells and is essential to intravascular fibrinolysis. These factors also participate in the activation of the intrinsic coagulation pathway and in generating inflammatory mediators. Plasmin's cleavage of fibrin releases fibrin degradation products (FDPs) and D-dimers that are used to monitor fibrinolytic activity and are clinical markers for disseminated intravascular coagulation (DIC). FDPs are ultimately removed from circulation by the liver.

To summarize, thrombin and plasmin are two potent, but opposing enzymes. Thrombin "coagulates" and plasmin "degregates." In other words, thrombin affects numerous phases of hemostasis, and plasmin opposes these actions. The effect of thrombin on platelets includes release of platelet granule contents, irreversible platelet aggregation, and platelet consumption which can result in thrombocytopenia. Thrombin activates its opposing enzyme plasmin through activation of plasminogen. Thrombin affects the natural inhibitors of coagulation causing consumption of antithrombin III (ATIII) and protein C, yet more clinical markers used to identify DIC. (Refer to the section on "Clinical Aspects of Specific Hematologic Emergencies.")

White Blood Cells (WBCs)

The WBCs, or leukocytes, can be subdivided into granulocytes (containing large granules in the cytoplasm) and agranulocytes (without granules). The granulocytes consist of neutrophils, eosinophils, and basophils. The agranulocytes are *lymphocytes* (consisting of B cells and T cells) and monocytes. Lymphocytes circulate in the blood and lymph systems, and make their home in the lymphoid organs. WBCs are larger than erythrocytes, have a nucleus, and lack hemoglobin. The function of all WBCs is to defend the body against both infectious disease and foreign materials; the number of WBCs in the blood is often an indicator of disease. WBCs also produce, transport, and distribute antibodies as part of the body's immune response. The life span of WBCs ranges from 13 to 20 days, after which time they are destroyed in the lymphatic system (Moore 2002).

Formation of WBCs occurs in the bone marrow (leukopoiesis); all WBCs arise from a type of cell called a hematopoietic stem cell. WBCs divide by a process of mitosis, forming either more stem cells or WBCs that can differentiate into specific white cell types, such as lymphocytes. (Moore 2002). The type of cell formed is influenced by immune system chemicals known as cytokines and by hormones. WBCs use the peripheral blood to travel from the bone marrow to their site of activity, typically the tissues.

The *neutrophil* is the most numerous WBC in circulation in the dog and cat (Colville and Bassert 2002). Neutrophils are phagocytes, meaning they engulf (phagocytize) microorganisms and unwanted tissue debris. Neutrophils are released into the blood as needed when neutrophils already in circulation leave the bloodstream to enter the tissues to kill microorganisms. Neutrophils and other WBCs leave the blood vessel by squeezing between the cells of the endothelium in a process called *diapedesis*. Neutrophils are attracted to a site of infection by a process called *chemotaxis*; specifically, the neutrophil is attracted by inflammatory chemicals. During ingestion of unwanted microorganisms, the neutrophils increase their metabolism of oxygen to produce substances that are toxic to ingested bacteria.

Eosinophils make up 5% or less of the total WBC count (Colville and Bassert 2002). Named for the red granules in the cytoplasm of mature cells, eosinophils do not stay in the peripheral blood for very long; rather, they migrate into tissues within a few hours. The function of the eosinophil includes the reduction of local allergic and anaphylactic reactions. The granules inside the eosinophil contain anti-inflammatory substances released at the site of the allergic reaction. Eosinophils have minimal phagocytotic and bactericidal functions; however, eosinophils are particularly effective in phagocytosis of pathogenic organisms such as protozoas and some parasitic worms. Eosinophilia can be seen during allergic reactions and in certain parasitic infections such as heartworms or gastrointestinal (GI) parasites.

Basophils, named for the blue granules in the cytoplasm of mature cells, are the WBC seen least often in circulation. Basophil granules contain histamine and heparin. The role of the basophil includes the initiation of inflammation; specifically, eosinophils are attracted to the site of the allergic reaction by eosinophilic chemotactic factors released from basophilic granules. Heparin acts as a localized anticoagulant to keep blood flowing to an area of injury. Basophilia can be associated with an allergic or hypersensitivity reaction.

Monocytes make up 5%–6% of the circulating WBCs in most domestic species (Colville and Bassert 2002). Monocytes mature much faster than neutrophils, stay in the peripheral blood longer, and are the largest WBC in circulation with abundant cytoplasm containing vacuoles of various sizes. Although the monocyte has phagocytotic properties while in the blood, most phagocytosis occurs in the tissues. Consequently, as the monocyte enters the tissues, they are classified as "tissue macrophages." Tissue macrophages are most prevalent in filter organs such as the liver, spleen, lungs, and lymph nodes. Collectively, monocyte and tissue macrophages are known as the *mononuclear phagocyte system (MPS)* (Colville and Bassert 2002). The MPS is responsible for the cleanup of cellular debris left from inflammation and infection, specific antigen destruction by the lymphocytes, and the ingestion of foreign substances through phagocytosis. Monocytes also enter tissues by the process of chemotaxis, and because they have a longer life span than neutrophils, are often associated with chronic infections.

Lymphocytes are the only WBCs without phagocytic capabilities. Lymphocytes are the key element in the production of immunity. Most lymphocytes live in lymphoid tissues and enter the bloodstream for the most part via the lymphatics. There are three different types of lymphocytes, the T cells, B lymphocytes, and natural killer (NK) cells.

T cells are processed in the thymus prior to delivery to the peripheral lymphoid tissue. There are two types of T cells: killer T cells and helper T lymphocytes. T cells are the predominant circulating lymphocyte, accounting for up to 80% of peripheral blood lymphocytes (Tizard 1996). Many T cells continuously circulate through the lymph nodes and the lymphatic circulation. T cells are long-lived cells that survive for an average from 6 months to 10 years.

B lymphocytes (B meaning "bursa equivalent," referring to the bone marrow and other lymphoid tissue thought to be equivalent to a bird organ) are preprogrammed to produce one specific antibody against one specific (foreign) antigen, even if that antigen is one in which there is no history of exposure. When a B lymphocyte recognizes an antigen, they are transformed into a plasma cell that releases antibodies in a process termed humoral immunity. Plasma cells derived from B lymphocytes in response to an antigenic stimulus produce, store, and release antibodies that are known as immunoglobulins. Plasma cells are found in any tissue in the body, but are most common in the lymph nodes and spleen (Colville and Bassert 2002).

NK cells are large, granular lymphocytes found mainly in the secondary lymphoid organs, although a small number can be found in the bone marrow. NK cells have an innate ability to lyse a variety of tumor cells and virally infected cells by responding to lipids and carbohydrates unique to bacterial cell walls and to substances characteristic of tumor cells. NK cells do not have to be activated by a specific antigen and are consequently considered part of the natural (as opposed to adaptive) immune system. NK cells attack abnormal cells largely by osmotic lysis or apoptosis. Their cytokines also activate other cells of the acquired immune system (Ganong 2001).

The Lymphatic System

The *lymphatic system* is a series of thin-walled, endothelium-lined channels that serve as a drainage system for returning interstitial tissue fluid to the blood. The lymphatics also constitute an important pathway for disease dissemination through the transport of bacteria and tumor cells to distant sites.

Lymph is the interstitial fluid that flows into the lymphatic system, formed from the diffusion and filtration of substances that flow through the wall of blood capillaries into the intercellular tissue spaces. Lymph is typically clear, alkaline, contains no RBCs, and has lower protein content than blood. Lymph flows in the lymphatic vessels and bathes tissues in its protective coating. Lymph carries lipids and lipid-soluble vitamins absorbed from the GI tract.

The lymph flows from the interstitial fluid through the lymphatic vessels up to either the thoracic duct or right lymph duct, which terminate in the subclavian veins, where lymph is mixed into the blood. There is no active pump in the lymph system; the lymphatic vessels, like veins, have one-way valves that prevent backflow. Along the lymphatic vessels are *lymph nodes* that serve as filters of the lymphatic fluid. It is in the lymph nodes where antigen is usually presented to the immune system.

The Immune System

The immune system is the body's defense against infectious organisms and foreign substances. Through a series of steps called the *immune response*, the immune system attacks organisms and substances that invade body systems and cause disease.

An immune response is complex and involves several different mechanisms, including trapping and processing an *antigen*, a substance that evokes the immune response. Destruction of the antigen is accomplished by phagocytosis, lysis of foreign cell membranes, inactivation of pathogenic organisms, or agglutination of cells or molecules (Colville and Bassert 2002). The immune system has a means for reacting specifically to each type of antigen, as well as the ability for cells to produce antibiodies against a particular antigen, and can also provide mechanisms wherein cells can retain the memory of the antigen event for appropriate responses in future encounters. Antigens are trapped, processed, and destroyed by several cell types.

Immunity can be classified as either innate, passive, cellular, nonspecific or specific, cellular or humoral. *Innate immunity* is naturally present and is not due to prior sensitization to an antigen (Ganong 2001). Innate immunity (also termed *natural immunity*) is not stimulated by specific antigens, and is generally nonspecific. Innate immunity provides the first line of defense against infection and triggers the slower, but more specific, acquired immune response. Innate immunity is complemented by acquired immunity. *Nonspecific immunity* refers to the tissues and cells (such as the protective barrier of the skin and mucous membranes); a nonspecific immune response is immediate and generalized. Nonspecific immune responses do not initiate a specific type of response against a specific antigen (Colville and Bassert 2002).

Acquired immunity is immunity that develops with exposure to various antigens. The key to acquired immunity is the ability of lymphocytes to produce antibodies that are specific for a particular foreign substance. Specifically, acquired immunity is a system wherein T and B lymphocytes are activated by very specific antigens to form clones of cells that attack foreign proteins and, after an invasion is repelled, persist in small numbers as memory cells so that a second exposure to that same antigen provides a prompt and magnified immune attack. Acquired immunity has two components: *humoral immunity* and *cellular immunity*. The cell killing effects of innate and acquired immunity are mediated by a system of plasma enzymes called the *complement system*.

Humoral immunity is the function of B lymphocytes which produce *immunoglobins* (an antibody) which in turn activates the complement system to attack and neutralize antigens. Distinctively, the B lymphocytes are transformed into plasma cells and produce specific protective proteins called *antibodies*. The processed B lymphocyte has a unique shape that allows it to combine only with an antigen with the corresponding shape. When the specific antigen comes in contact with the antibody, they combine to form the *antigen–antibody complex* that activates the B lymphocytes. Like the T lymphocyte, as a B lymphocyte becomes an activated B lymphocyte, it undergoes many mitotic divisions in order to make numerous clones of itself. The clones transform into plasma cells that will produce more of the specific antibody molecules produced by the B lymphocyte. Humoral immunity is considered the major defense system against bacterial infections.

Cellular immunity is mediated by T lymphocytes and is responsible for delayed allergic reactions and the rejection of transplants of foreign tissue. T lymphocytes have specific antigen receptors on their cell membranes; these receptors are unique for one antigen only. When the T lymphocyte attaches to an antigen, it, too, becomes an activated T lymphocyte that undergoes mitotic divisions to make numerous clones of itself. The cloned, activated T lymphocytes make up three distinct populations of T lymphocytes, namely *killer T lymphocytes*, *helper T cells*, and *suppressor T cells*. Antigenic cells that are attacked by the T lymphocytes are usually viruses or neoplastic in nature (Colville and Bassert 2002).

Natural and acquired immune mechanisms also attack tumors. Once activated, immune cells communicate by means of cytokines. *Cytokines* are hormone-like molecules that are secreted by lymphocytes, macrophages, and endothelial cells. Cytokines kill viruses, bacteria, and activate the complement system (the binding of antibody to its antigen). Certain cytokines can also stimulate hematopoiesis.

Passive immunity is a type of immunity defined by the transfer of antibodies from one individual to another, such as through ingestion of colostrum. Some antibodies are produced by the mother and are passed onto the fetus transplacentally, thereby giving the infant some protective immunity.

Pathophysiology of RBC Disorders

Anemia

Anemia is defined as a reduction of the total circulating red cell mass. In physiologic terms, therefore, anemia can also be defined as a reduction in oxygen carrying capability of the blood. Anemias can be classified on the basis of the appearance of the RBC in the peripheral blood smear or categorized according to the underlying mechanism.

Anemia can be caused by a number of conditions, namely blood loss, blood destruction, or decreased RBC production. Anemia can also be caused by insufficient hemoglobin production, despite adequate RBCs. In this situation, not enough hemoglobin is present to fill each RBC, for instance, when there is a lack of substances needed to synthesize heme or globin (e.g., iron deficiency). Anemia is usually secondary to an underlying disease process and is rarely a primary disease.

Peripheral blood cell morphology can help identify the anemia as either regenerative or non-regenerative. A *regenerative anemia* is one in which the bone marrow responds appropriately to a low packed cell volume (PCV) by increasing red cell production and the release of normal young red cells into circulation (Fig. 11.1).

There are two major categories of regenerative anemias: blood loss anemias and hemolytic anemias. Conversely, a *nonregenerative anemia* is an anemia in which the bone marrow does not respond appropriately to a low PCV and consequently, young red cells are not released in adequate numbers into the circulation. A complete blood count (CBC)

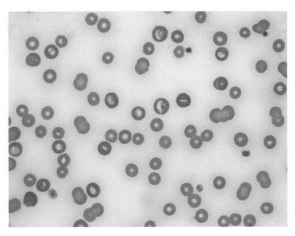

Figure 11.1   Regenerative anemia; peripheral blood cell morphology will show normal young red cells. (Courtesy of Elizabeth Spangler, DVM, PhD, DACVIM, DACVP.)

with a reticulocyte count and blood smear can be helpful in determining whether the anemia is regenerative or non-regenerative. Most cases of non-regenerative anemia have normal RBC indices and are normocytic and normochromic; regenerative anemia typically appears as macrocytic and hypochromic due to the abundance of reticulocytes in circulation.

There are two major categories of nonregenerative anemias. Anemias in which the bone marrow red cell production is not increased or is reduced is termed a hypoproliferative anemia, and those in which there is bone marrow red cell manufacturing but the red cells produced are abnormal and are therefore not released into circulation. Anemias are also classified based on the appearance of RBCs on the peripheral blood smear. Indices evaluated include RBC size (normocytic, microcytic, macrocytic), degree of hemoglobinization as reflected in the color of the red cells (normochromic or hypochromic), and red cell shape.

Clinical signs associated with anemia include pale mucus membranes, weakness, abnormal mentation, increased respiratory effort, abnormal heart rate, heart murmurs, abnormal pulse quality, and abnormal body temperature. Hypoxia associated with severe anemia may cause fatty changes in the liver, myocardium, and kidneys. Acute, severe blood loss may result in hypovolemic shock, as both RBCs and plasma are lost simultaneously. RBC numbers may be normal immediately following acute loss, as the intravascular volume is reestablished by equilibration with extravascular fluids. Hemorrhage into tissues is typically not followed by restoration of the RBC population, as most extravasated erythrocytes are destroyed before they can be reabsorbed. Hemorrhage of RBCs and their components into the abdominal or thoracic cavities are recirculated or reabsorbed.

Regenerative anemia

Regenerative anemia usually is a result of excessive loss of RBCs caused by either loss (hemorrhage) or hemolysis. Normal physiologic response includes enhanced *erythropoiesis* (RBC production) with increased numbers of reticulocytes (young red cells) released into circulation. The bone marrow needs ample time to respond to acute blood loss, typically 2–3 days in cats and 4–5 days in the dog. Chronic external blood loss can trigger a different physiologic response, typically an initial regenerative response to the anemia followed by a progressive deficiency in iron stores. Specifically, as iron becomes unavailable, the hemoglobin cannot be synthesized which will result in poor erythropoeisis. Consequently, the anemia becomes non-regenerative and the red cells appear microcytic.

Acute blood loss into a body cavity will also cause an almost immediate bone marrow response with a leukocytosis and left shift (Coles, 2000). A normocytic, normochromic anemia will surface as a result of hemodilution (as intravascular volume is reestablished by equilibration with extravascular fluids), although this anemia will be regenerative once the bone marrow has had adequate time to respond. Reduction in tissue oxygenation, again as a result of the hemodilution, will result in increased erythropoietin. As the marrow begins to regenerate, changes will occur in the peripheral blood, particularly in the reticulocyte count. Nucleated erythrocytes appear in the peripheral circulation usually within 72–96 hours following acute blood loss (Coles, 2000).

Chronic, progressive anemia institutes compensatory mechanisms such as increased production of RBC 2, 3-diphosphoglycerate (2-3 DPG) which lowers the oxygen–hemoglobin affinity and subsequently enhances oxygen delivery to the tissues. Other physiologic compensatory mechanisms to chronic anemia include increased cardiac output and increased erythropoietin production. Again, chronic anemia will be regenerative until iron stores are depleted by chronic loss (e.g., intestinal bleeding). Chronic, recurring internal hemorrhage (e.g., hemangiosarcoma) does not cause iron deficiency.

Hemolysis is another type of regenerative anemia. Hemolytic anemias are characterized by a marked increase in erythropoiesis within the bone marrow, in an attempt to compensate for loss of RBCs. The premature destruction of the RBCs occurs either within the mononuclear phagocytic cells of the spleen (*extravascular hemolysis*) or within the vascular compartment (*intravascular hemolysis*). Intravascular hemolysis is typically a more severe disease process than extravascular hemolysis, and is manifested by hemoglobinemia, hemoglobinuria, and icterus (jaundice).

Non-regenerative anemia

Non-regenerative anemia occurs when the bone marrow fails to adequately respond to the increased need for RBCs. Bone marrow depression can be caused by several factors, including infectious agents, physical or chemical agents, or secondary reactions associated with a primary disease (termed hypoplastic or aplastic anemias). Most non-regenerative anemias are typically secondary to another disease process.

With bone marrow depression, there is a decrease of erythropoiesis in the marrow usually accompanied by a progressive fall in the total RBC and hemoglobin content. If the bone marrow is severely aplastic (unable to develop new cells), a simultaneous decrease in leukocytes will also be observed. Anemias with bone marrow depression will have an absence of reticulocytes and nucleated erythrocytes in the peripheral circulation. Non-regenerative anemias are often refractory to treatment until the underlying cause of the bone marrow suppression is identified.

There are many causes of non-regenerative anemia (see Table 11.1); categories include primary and secondary failure of erythropoiesis, nuclear maturation defects, hemoglobin synthesis defects, aplastic anemia, and marrow infiltration. In primary failure of erythropoiesis, severe erythroid hypoplasia of the bone marrow occurs. Although uncommon,

Table 11.1 Classification of causes of anemia

- *Acute blood loss*
  - Trauma (intracavitary hemorrhage)
  - Surgical procedures
  - Splenic rupture or torsion
  - Epistaxis
  - Gastrointestinal hemorrhage
- *Chronic blood loss*
  - Gastrointestinal ulcerations or lesions
  - Parasitism
  - Neoplasia
  - Coagulopathies
  - Platelet disorders
- *Hemolysis*
  - Immune-mediated diseases
    - IMHA
    - SLE
    - Drug-induced
    - Neonatal isoerythrolysis
    - Transfusion reaction
  - Parasitic
    - Babesiosis
    - Bartonella
    - Erlichiosis
    - Cytauxzoonosis
  - Toxic
    - Heinz body anemia
    - Zinc, copper
  - Infectious
    - Leptospirosis
    - Clostridia
    - Endotoxemia
  - Intrinsic defects
    - Pyruvate kinase deficiency
    - Phospofructokinase deficiency
    - Hereditary hemolytic anemia
  - Fragmentation
    - DIC
    - Splenic torsion
    - Splenic neoplasia
    - Caval syndrome
- *Impaired red cell production*
  - Primary failure of erythropoiesis
    - Inherited or acquired
    - Immune-mediated
    - Lymphoma
    - Multiple myeloma
    - Drug-induced
  - Secondary failure of erythropoiesis
    - Inflammatory disease
    - Neoplasia
  - Chronic renal disease
  - Chronic liver disease
  - Endocrine diseases

(Continued)

Table 11.1   (*Continued*)

- Aplastic anemia
  - ○ Estrogen-induced
  - ○ Certain antibiotic use
  - ○ Certain NSAID use
  - ○ Certain chemotherapy agents
  - ○ Radiation
  - ○ Infectious diseases
- Bone marrow infiltration
  - ○ Neoplasia
  - ○ Myelofibrosis
  - ○ Osteopetrosis
- Nuclear maturation defects
  - ○ Folate deficiency
  - ○ B-12 deficiency

primary failure is typically immune-mediated, acquired, and may be associated with a number of disease conditions. Diagnosis is made based on a severe, chronic, normocytic, normochromic non-regenerative anemia, with a bone marrow that still has active production of substances such as platelet precursors and WBCs.

Secondary failure of erythropoiesis reveals a bone marrow with normal or mild erythroid hypoplasia; secondary failure includes common diseases such as endocrine disorders (hypothyroidism, hypoadrenocorticism), neoplasia, chronic renal failure, liver insufficiency, and certain inflammatory diseases. With *anemia of inflammatory disease (AID)*, iron metabolism is altered, consequently creating a suppression of erythropoiesis due to iron unavailabilitiy. Altered iron metabolism is a different pathophysiology than iron deficiency and must be differentiated for diagnostic purposes. With AID, total body iron stores are adequate but is sequestered and rendered unavailable.

Chronic inflammatory disease is one of the most common causes of anemia in veterinary patients, occurring with conditions such as infection, trauma (bony or soft tissue), immune-mediated disease, and neoplasia. AID is usually mild to moderate, normocytic, normochromic, and always non-regenerative. In addition, with AID, there may also be decreases in the life span of the RBC.

The pathogenesis of AID is multifactorial. A suspected key mediator is hepcidin, a protein that is produced by the liver in response to inflammatory stimuli (White and Reine 2009). Specifically, interleukin (IL)-6, which is produced early during host defense, induces hepcidin synthesis. Hepcidin inhibits iron export from duodenal enterocytes and macrophages, resulting in decreased iron absorption and the accumulation of iron in macrophages. Consequently, there is a reduction of serum iron level which will ultimately result in decreased iron available for erythropoiesis. Hepcidin is also produced in hypoxic or iron-deficient states.

AID also plays a role in anemia associated with chronic renal failure, although the anemia is primarily associated with ineffective erythropoiesis due to decreased production of erythropoietin by the kidneys, in addition to blood loss and a decreased RBC life span. Certain endocrine disorders can also be associated with anemia, as thyroxine may have negative effects on erythroid colony formation. Anemia found with endocrine abnormalities may also be a physiologic adaptation to decreased oxygen demand.

Aplastic anemia is also a type of non-regenerative anemia, characterized by bone marrow failure. Bone marrow failure can be due to many different agents, namely chemotherapy drugs, certain antibiotics, or infectious agents. Aplastic anemia is characterized by an acellular marrow; neutropenia and thrombocytopenia typically occur before the anemia, as the RBCs have a longer life span in the circulation. *Pure red cell aplasia* is also a type of non-regenerative anemia wherein marrow failure is of erythroid elements only; pure red cell aplasia may be a primary disease or secondary to another disease process such as thymic tumors (thymoma) or leukemia, infection, toxicosis, or renal failure. Pure red cell aplasia is a rare syndrome; primary red cell aplasia is the most common cause in dogs, and secondary red cell aplasia in cats is usually due to feline leukemia.

Other forms of marrow failure include marrow infiltration. *Marrow infiltration* is typically associated with neoplasia, myelofibrosis, or osteopetrosis. In neoplastic diseases (myelophthisis), normal hematopoietic cells are overrun by tumor or fibrosis, causing pancytopenia and subsequent marrow failure. Myelofibrosis (replacement of bone marrow with fibrous connective tissue) may occur as a result of chronic chemotherapy or tumor infiltration. With marrow infiltration, the normal marrow environment is altered, and neoplastic disease processes compete for nutritional factors and produce tumor-related factors that suppress normal hematopoiesis.

Polycythemia

Polycythemia is defined as an abnormally increased PCV, RBC count, and hemoglobin concentration. The consequence of increased red cell mass is an increase in blood viscosity, specifically when the PCV rises above 50%–60% in dogs. Polycythemia increases workload, hinders microcirculation, potentiates thrombosis, creates general tissue hypoxia, and increases the risk of possible neurologic complications.

Polycythemia is either absolute or relative; relative polycythemia refers to a hemoconcentration due to decreased plasma volume such as found in conditions such as dehydration. *Relative polycythemia* occurs as a result of the shifting of body fluids from the vascular space into the interstitial space, inadequate fluid intake, excessive external loss of body fluids, or excessive use of diuretics. Splenic contraction can lead to an increase in circulating RBCs but not in the total number of red cells in dogs.

Absolute polycythemia is caused by an increased total RBC mass, and is divided into primary or secondary polycythemia based on its pathophysiology. Absolute polycythemia is said to be primary when the increase in red cell mass results from an abnormality of the myeloid stem cells, and secondary when the increase in red cells is in response to increased levels of erythropoietin.

Red cell mass is regulated by an endocrine feedback system, with erythropoietin playing a key role in the regulation of the erythrocyte population. Renal hypoxia stimulates renal production of erythropoietin; erythropoietin acts in the bone marrow as a growth factor which results in an increase in circulating RBCs to enhance the oxygen-carrying capability and consequently improve renal oxygenation. Therefore, primary polycythemia (*polycythemia vera*) is erythropoietin independent, whereas secondary polycythemia is dependent on erythropoietin to increase RBC production. Common disorders found with secondary polcythemia include congenital heart defects (e.g., patent ductus arteriosus [PDA]); some renal diseases such as amyloidosis, renal neoplasia, infection, or inflammation may also cause local hypoxia and trigger erythropoietin synthesis and are termed "secondary inappropriate polycythemia."

Hemostasis Abnormalities

Disseminated Intravascular Coagulation (DIC)

DIC is a syndrome in which excessive intravascular coagulation leads to multiple-organ microthrombosis and subsequent multiple organ failure. DIC is a serious, life-threatening complication in both humans and animals. Previously called consumptive coagulopathy or defibrination syndrome, DIC causes a bleeding cascade by the inactivation or inappropriate consumption of platelets and clotting factors secondary to enhanced fibrinolysis. DIC is not a specific disorder; rather, DIC is always secondary to an underlying injury or disease process. DIC can also be associated with a process or disease that induces inflammation or sepsis.

In healthy animals, the normal mechanisms of clot formation and fibrinolysis are well balanced; coagulation and clot formation occur only on demand. With DIC, there is an imbalance between the prothrombotic and antithrombotic activities of the hemostatic system, leading to concurrent excessive clot formation and bleeding. Specifically, there is (1) excessive thrombin generation, (2) activation of systemic fibrin formation, (3) plasmin activation, (4) suppression of normal anticoagulation mechanisms, and (5) delayed fibrin removal as a consequence of impaired fibrinolysis. (Refer to the section on "Composition of Blood and Hemostasis.")

During this excessive intravascular coagulation phase, platelets and coagulation factors are consumed, resulting in thrombocytopenia, impaired thrombocyte function, and depletion and inactivation of coagulation factors (Bruchim et al. 2008).

Pathogenesis of DIC

DIC is a secondary disorder that occurs when a primary disease process initiates *continuous* activation of the coagulation cascade. The delicate balance of prothrombotic and antithrombotic factors that are essential to normal hemostasis are tipped in favor of one process or the other. The patient commonly moves from a hypercoagulable to a hypocoagulable state; patients can die from either thrombotic or hemorrhagic episodes. DIC can occur secondary to a wide variety of disease processes, including endothelial damage (burns, heatstroke, sepsis), platelet activation (viral infections, such as feline infectious peritonitis [FIP]), or a release of tissue "procoagulants" (from trauma, hemolysis, bacterial infections, neoplasia).

As a result of injury or disease, normal primary and secondary hemostatic plugs are formed; if this process is unbalanced, eventual ischemia develops. *Ischemia* leads to excessive intravascular coagulation; subsequently, platelets and coagulation factors are consumed, resulting in thrombocytopenia, thrombocytopathy, and depletion and inactivation of coagulation factors. In an attempt to halt intravascular coagulation, vital proteins (such as *ATIII*) are quickly consumed, exhausting normal anticoagulant activity. Consumption of antithrombin during DIC increases the risk of thrombosis. Three factors, called the *Virchow's triad*, predispose patients to thrombosis: stasis, hypercoagulability, and vessel wall injury (Bruchim et al. 2008).

Thrombomodulin-protein C-protein S is an endothelial-based inhibitor system, which binds thrombin, preventing amplification of procoagulant activity; during DIC, this system is consumed which results in *unopposed* coagulation (Matthews 2006). Unfortunately, the formation of fibrin within the microcirculation can also lead to the development of hemolytic anemia as the RBCs are sheared by these fibrin strands (i.e., fragmented RBCs or schistocytes).

Any disease process that results in capillary stasis, loss of vascular integrity, or hypercoagulability can also disrupt the balance between hemostasis and fibrinolysis and subsequently trigger DIC. Hypercoagulability also occurs in animals that have been exposed to high levels of endogenous or exogenous steroids. Some disorders, such as protein-losing nephropathy, may result in low blood levels of ATIII, triggering a disruption in the regulation of the coagulation system. Once DIC is underway, it follows the same course regardless of the activating agent (s).

Systemic Inflammatory Response Syndrome (SIRS) and DIC

Recent studies have highlighted the importance of the inflammatory mechanism in DIC. The conditions that lead to DIC are the same as those associated with *systemic inflammatory response syndrome (SIRS)*. Any condition that leads to poor perfusion or shock may predispose a patient to stasis of blood, including sepsis, pancreatitis, or immune-mediated diseases such as autoimmune hemolytic anemia. In each of these situations, various inflammatory mediators are activated, all of which can lead to endothelial damage; the endothelial damage is an integral part of SIRS. Once the damage has occurred, activation of the coagulation cascade follows, contributing to the potential development of thrombi.

Capillary leakage also occurs in animals with inflammatory conditions; alterations in the endothelium are due to action of cytokines. Such animals are more predisposed to edema and vasculitis. These patients can become severely hypotensive, especially if there is also a septic process, which can create a life-threatening, hypovolemic situation. (Refer to the section on "Oncology and Immune System Emergencies.")

Inflammation also causes an "upregulation" of procoagulant factors, resulting in increased thrombin generation, systemic fibrin formation, downregulation of natural anticoagulants (e.g., ATIII), and delayed fibrin removal as a consequence of inadequate fibrinolysis (Bruchim et al. 2008). In addition, inflammation tends to lead to an increase in fibrinogen levels (unless there is concurrent fibrinogen consumption). The coagulation cascade is again triggered by inflammation reducing physiologic anticoagulation activity (e.g., ATIII consumption). It has also been discovered that the presence of inflammatory mediators (as well as endotoxin found in sepsis) will reduce the endothelial expression of glycosaminoglycans (e.g., heparin sulfate) that normally augments the activity of anticoagulant ATIII, subsequently impairing endothelial antithrombotic function (Bruchim et al. 2008).

Inflammation is also characterized by activation of cytokine production. The principal mediators are IL-1 and IL-6 and tumor necrosis factor (TNF), which are released from the MPS system. These cytokines stimulate macrophages to express several procoagulants. Increased IL-1 levels have been shown to increase platelet reactivity and thrombogenic potential (Bruchim et al. 2008). (Refer to the section on "Clinical Aspects of Specific Hematologic Emergencies.")

Other Abnormalities of Hemostasis

Acquired coagulation disorders can be caused by liver failure (a *production defect*), or vitamin K deficiency (*activation defect*). As the liver is the primary site of the synthesis of coagulation factors, diseases that cause liver insufficiency or failure will subsequently cause factor deficiency or dysfunction, such as hepatic necrosis, portosystemic shunts, and cholestasis. Liver disease is also associated with vitamin K deficiency due to impaired intrahepatic recycling. Other conditions that can cause a decreased vitamin K absorption in the intestinal tract include infiltrative bowel disease, biliary obstruction, and pancreatic insufficiency. Toxicities such as rodenticide also induce a severe coagulopathy caused by vitamin K deficiency. Moderate to marked deficiencies of all vitamin K-dependent factors will create an active hemorrhagic process.

Inherited factor deficiencies, caused by mutations in genes coded for specific coagulation factors, may also cause severe coagulation disorders. For example, *von Willebrand's disease* is the most common inherited bleeding disorder of dogs. The disease is the result of a deficiency of von Willebrand's factor (vWF), a large, multimeric glycoprotein found in plasma, platelet granules, endothelial cells, and subendothelial connective tissue. vWf is synthesized by the vascular endothelium and megakaryocytes, and is necessary for normal platelet function. Specifically, vWF mediates platelet adhesion to exposed endothelium after vascular injury, in addition to promoting platelet aggregation under high shear conditions, and serves as a carrier for coagulation factor VIII. Dogs with vWF deficiency can have mild bleeding or even life-threatening hemorrhage following injury or surgery. Because von Willebrand's disease (vWD) is a platelet function defect, all coagulation tests (including platelet count) will be normal except those that require functional platelets, such as the buccal mucosal bleeding time (BMBT).

The most common form of vWD is Type I, with notably decreased levels of vWD. It is autosomal dominant and is common in breeds such as Dobermans. Dogs are usually nonclinical until a surgical or trauma event, in which they may experience prolonged bleeding. Hypothyroidism may exacerbate bleeding tendencies in dogs with vWD (Fig. 11.2) (Macintire et al. 2006).

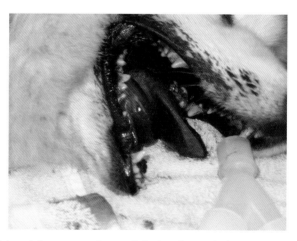

Figure 11.2   Von Willebrand dogs are usually nonclinical until a surgical or trauma event, in which dogs may experience prolonged bleeding.

WBC Disorders

Leukopenia

Leukopenia is defined as an abnormally low WBC count, usually from reduced numbers of neutrophils (*neutropenia*). Neutropenia (agranulocytosis) has serious consequences by predisposing the body to infections. The neutrophil is the predominate granulocyte cell in the marrow, with a high production rate that is modulated under steady state conditions. The production rate can markedly increase in response to inflammation or foreign stimuli.

The neutrophils in the blood are divided into two pools, those in the axial blood flow (circulating pool) and those loosely associated with the walls of blood vessels (marginated pool). Neutrophils spend only a short time in the bloodstream, with a half-life of about 7 hours under normal circumstances (Kociba 2000). This half-life is considerably shorter in inflammatory conditions, as the bloodstream serves as a conduit from the marrow to the site of inflammation.

A reduction in circulating granulocytes occurs if there is reduced or ineffective production of neutrophils or if there is rapid removal of neutrophils from the circulating blood. Ineffective production of neutrophils occurs in the suppression of myeloid stem cells (such as in aplastic anemia) and many types of infiltrative marrow disorders such as *neoplasia* and *granulomatous* diseases. In such conditions, granulocytopenia is almost always accompanied by anemia and thrombocytopenia. Neutropenia can also occur due to the suppression of granulocytic precursors, which can occur as a result of certain chemotherapeutic drugs. When a patient is receiving chemotherapy that suppresses bone marrow production of leukocytes, the point at which the count is lowest is referred to as the *nadir*.

Accelerated destruction of neutrophils can also occur as a result of increased peripheral use (overwhelming bacterial, fungal, or rickettsial infections), or in splenic sequestration secondary to enlargement of the spleen, in which excessive destruction of RBCs and platelets also occurs. Destruction of neutrophils can also take place in certain idiopathic disorders such as systemic lupus erythematosus (SLE), or with exposure to certain drugs (chemotherapeutic agents). The most significant neutropenias are found secondary to cancer treatments, which cause suppression of bone marrow, and in parvovirus infections caused by destruction of hematopoietic precursors in the bone marrow. Suppression secondary to chemotherapy involves erythrocytes and platelets in addition to agranulocytosis. As serious infections tend to occur with chemotherapy, neutropenic patients are treated with broad-spectrum antibiotics at the first sign of infection. Neutrophils are also decreased in the early stages of inflammation, but this neutropenia is typically transient and occurs before the pet is presented for evaluation. Neutrophil counts less than 1000/μL should be closely monitored for signs of sepsis.

Sepsis

Sepsis is defined as the systemic inflammatory response to infection from bacteria or viral, fungal, or protozoal organisms. Sepsis is typically infection with a gram-negative bacteria with subsequent release of endotoxin. Endotoxin is a lipopolysaccharide component of the bacterial cell membrane which plays a key role in the initiation of the inflammatory cascade that leads to SIRS. Presence of endotoxin activates macrophages and causes the release of inflammatory mediators, including TNF and IL-1 (Matthews 2006).

Endotoxin also damages vascular endothelial cells, which contribute to the *continuous* activation of the coagulation cascade, further stimulating the release of cytokines directly from the endothelium. TNF and IL-1 also stimulate the release of other inflammatory mediators. Unfortunately, the effects of these mediators include vasodilation and increased vascular permeability, which again further activates the coagulation cascade. Continuous activation of coagulation cascade results in microvascular thrombosis, resulting in hypoperfusion of tissues, ischemia, and multiple organ dysfunction or failure. In addition, increased vascular permeability causes leakage of fluid into the interstitial space, resulting in decreased intravascular volume and tissue hypoperfusion. Persistent activation of the inflammatory cascade due to ongoing infection will typically result in DIC.

There is now a known link between the hemostatic dysfunction in the pathophysiology of both SIRS and sepsis. SIRS is another clinical manifestation of the patient's response to severe injury, microbial invasion, severe inflammation, or neoplasia. The inflammatory cascades that are activated during SIRS also activate the endothelium. This endothelial activation triggers other cascades including the coagulation cascade which, if left uncontrolled, can lead to DIC.

Clinical consequences of sepsis and SIRS include cardiovascular shock, myocardial dysfunction, coagulation abnormalities, hypotension, acute lung injury, organ failure, and death. Multiple organ dysfunction syndrome (MODS) describes the presence of organ failure, coagulation abnormalities, and cardiovascular derangements that occur due to progression of sepsis and SIRS. Microvascular emboli from coagulation abnormalities, coupled with decreased perfusion due to hypotension, can lead to hepatic and renal failure, cerebral damage, GI ulceration, mucosal sloughing, neurologic insufficiency, and acute lung injury.

Leukocytosis

Leukocytosis is an elevated WBC count and is a common reaction to a variety of inflammatory states. Neutrophilia, or an increase in absolute numbers of circulating neutrophils, is influenced by several factors, including (1) the extravasation rate of cells from the peripheral blood into tissues, (2) the proportion of cells that are marginating (or accumulating) at any one time, (3) the rate of release of cells from the storage pool into circulation, and (4) the size of the myeloid and lymphoid storage cell pools (Kociba 2000). Animals with an inflammatory neutrophilia usually have historical or clinical evidence of septic or nonseptic inflammatory disease such as pyrexia, weight loss, loss of appetite, and specific organ system involvement.

Neutrophils are produced in the bone marrow, released into the blood, circulate briefly, and migrate into tissue spaces and onto epithelial surfaces. Injury or bacterial invasion of tissue causes production and release of *colony-stimulating factors*, which increase proliferation and maturation of neutrophilic progenitor cells in the bone marrow. Other mediators of inflammation stimulate bone marrow release and promote margination and adhesion of neutrophils to vascular endothelium at the site of inflammation.

A *left shift* occurs when there is an increase in immature neutrophils, especially bands (Kociba 2000). A left shift is a sign of inflammatory conditions with release of immature cells in addition to segmented neutrophils from the maturation and storage compartments of the bone marrow. A regenerative left shift refers to a neutrophilic leukocytosis with

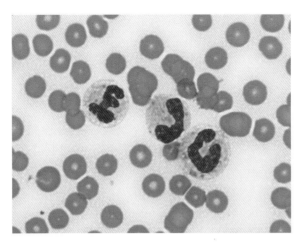

Figure 11.3 Band neutrophils of a dog with a degenerative left shift. (Courtesy of Elizabeth Spangler, DVM, PhD, DACVIM, DACVP.)

an increase in immature neutrophils, but with a larger population of segmented neutrophils. The degree of left shift corresponds with the severity of the inflammation or infection; left shifts are monitored by the absolute concentration of bands in the blood. Severe neutrophilia with a regenerative left shift is not always related to severe infection; neutrophilia can be associated with immune-mediated arthritis.

A *degenerative left shift* refers to a condition wherein the leukocyte count is decreased with a greater concentration of immature neutrophils than segmented neutrophils in the blood (Fig. 11.3).

Degenerative left shifts are associated with severe sepsis and typically have a poor prognosis. In septicemia, damage to endothelial cells in the vascular sinuses of the bone marrow can cause a non-patent barrier that restrains hematopoietic precursors in marrow compartments. Identification of increased nucleated erythrocytes with neutrophils in a left shift is considered a leukoerythroblastic response (Kociba 2000).

Physiologic leukocytosis refers to a mature neutrophilia brought on by epinephrine release, such as with fear, excitement, or strenuous exercise. Physiologic leukocytosis is created by a transient shift of neutrophils from the marginated pool to the circulating pool. The total leukocyte count in the vascular is not changed, so no left shift is observed. Similar shifts from other marginated pools (e.g., lymphocytes) can also occur with the net result of an increased leukocyte concentration, particularly in cats because of the larger size of the marginated pool of both lymphocytes and neutrophils.

Corticosteroids also cause increased mature neutrophils from the bone marrow, regardless of whether it came from either exogenous or endogenous sources (e.g., stress-induced or glucocorticoid administration). Corticosteriods also cause demargination; demargination means that cells in the marginating pool are swept rapidly (within minutes) into the circulation and can double the blood neutrophil count very rapidly (Kociba 2000). Corticosteriods can also decrease tissue migration. Leukocytosis and neutrophilia occur 4–8 hours after administration and return to normal 1–3 days after treatment (Kociba 2000). Lymphopenia, eosinopenia, and monocytosis (dogs) occur concurrently. Pain, traumatic injury, boarding, transport, hospitalization, and other stressful conditions are common causes of what is referred to as a *stress leukogram*.

A neutrophilia of chronic inflammation can also occur with suppuration (e.g., pyometra, abscesses, pyothorax, and pyoderma) and some neoplastic conditions which cause granulocytic hyperplasia that results in severe leukocytosis. Anemia associated with chronic disease may also be present. Hemolytic or hemorrhagic anemias may also have a neutrophilia with a left shift (e.g., dogs with immune-mediated hemolytic anemia). Mature neutrophilia is often found on the leukogram typically 3 hours after acute hemorrhage.

Disorders of the Lymphatic System

The *lymphatics* are specialized endothelium-lined capillaries originating in the interstitium which transport fluid, solutes, and other particles back into the venous system. Lymphatic vessels increase in diameter as lymph flows centrally, passing through either lymph nodes or into lymphatic ducts. The *thoracic duct* is the common duct for all lymph flow, with the exception of the right lymphatic duct. Lymph flow relies on extrinsic (movement of skeletal muscles and organs) and intrinsic (smooth muscle contraction in the lymphatic vessel wall) factors. In addition to the lymphatic system's major function of transport, the lymph system also plays a vital role in host defense by acting as a type of filtering system to prevent the spread of microorganisms and neoplastic cells.

Lymphatic disorders are divided into those of internal organs or those of the peripheral lymphatics. Inflammatory lymphatic disorders (e.g., *lymphangitis* and *lymphadenitis*) are typically secondary to local inflammation, involving the skin, mucous membranes, or the subcutaneous tissues. Lymphangitis can also result from bacterial, fungal, inflammatory, or even adjacent neoplasia. Lymphatics become affected and potentially occluded as they drain inflammatory by-products from the tissues. In lymph nodes, microorganisms are phagocytized and destroyed or inactivated, which may cause the node to become enlarged or obstructed. Pyrexia, anorexia, and a leukocytosis may be present with acute lymphangitis.

Lymphedema occurs as a result of accumulation of fluid in the interstitial space secondary to abnormal lymphatic drainage. Lymphedema is categorized as either primary or secondary, and should not be confused with other types of edema such as circulatory edema or generalized edema associated with hypoproteinemia. *Primary lymphedema* occurs when capillary filtration exceeds the resorptive capacity; the protein-rich fluid causes a high osmotic gradient and exacerbates fluid accumulation. Primary lymphedema refers to an abnormality of the lymphatic vessels or lymph node, wherein *secondary lymphedema* refers to conditions caused by a disease in the lymphatic vessel or lymph node that actually began in a different tissue. Secondary lymphedema is more common than primary lymphedema, occurring as a result of neoplasia, trauma, parasites, or infection.

Differential diagnoses for edema confined to one limb includes inflammation, trauma, vascular obstruction, cellulitis, phlebitis, or A-V fistula. Edema involving both forelimbs include thrombosis of the cranial vena cava or venous invasion by a mediastinal mass. Causes of only bilateral hindlimb edema includes obstruction of a sublumbar lymph node by neoplastic infiltration. If all four limbs are affected, differential diagnoses include hypoproteinemia, congestive heart failure, renal failure, or portal hypertension. Both lymphatic and venous obstruction can occur at the same time, due to the close association of lymphatic and venous structures.

Clinical Aspects of Specific Hematologic Emergencies

Epistaxis

Epistaxis, defined as hemorrhage originating from the nose, is a frequent clinical complaint that can result from intranasal or extranasal (systemic) causes. Signalment and patient history are key in prioritizing the diagnostic plan. Common causes of epistaxis can include immune-mediated thrombocytopenia (ITP), nasal tumors, foreign bodies, nasal trauma, oronasal fistula, rhinitis, platelet disorders (e.g., vWFD), fungal disorders, or coagulopathies such as rodenticide toxicities, and DIC. Diagnostic plans should begin with a detailed history and physical examination.

Patient environment can help identify the cause; outdoor pets are more susceptible than indoor pets to nasal trauma, parasitic and fungal infections, toxicities, and foreign body inhalation (Northrup and Gieger 2004). Environmental factors include fungi, rickettsial organisms, *Leishmania* spp., and *Hepatozoon* spp. Drugs that can inhibit platelet function (aspirin, nonsteroidal anti-inflammatory drugs [NSAIDs]) should also be ruled-out as a cause for epistaxis, as well as chemotherapeutic agents, estrogens, and phenylbutazone, which may cause myelosuppression and thrombocytopenia.

Clinical signs of epistaxis include unilateral or bilateral hemorrhage, in addition to sneezing, stertorous respiration, dysphagia, or halitosis. It is important to note whether the epistaxis is unilateral or bilateral; bilateral epistaxis may occur with intranasal diseases but often indicates systemic causes (e.g., coagulopathies, hypertension, and thrombocytopenia). Acute epistaxis may suggest inhalation of foreign bodies or blunt nasal trauma. Animals with petechia, mucosal bleeding, or fundic hemorrhages are suspicious of a primary hemostasis insufficiency; intracavitary or joint bleeds are suspicious of secondary hemostatic defects. Melena and hematemesis is common with epistaxis as blood from the nasopharynx is swallowed. It is not uncommon for chronic intranasal disease to progress and produce systemic complications that can exacerbate bleeding.

Facial examination is critical in locating any possible signs of trauma, asymmetry, or bony defects that may suggest neoplasia or rhinitis. Ocular examination should include retropulsion (to identify any lesions or globe deviations), a fundic evaluation for chorioretinitis or retinopathy associated with hypertension, and gross inspection of the anterior chamber for evidence of uveitis or hemorrhage. Any ulcerations of the nasal planum can be indicative of aspergillosis or squamous cell carcinoma. Visible polypoid masses extending from the nares are common with rhinosporidiosis, phaeohyphomycosis, and cryptococcosis (Northrup and Gieger 2004).

The mouth should also be visually inspected and palpated for palate deformities or masses; teeth and gum line should be evaluated for presence of any oronasal fistulas or decay. Palpation of regional lymph nodes should be performed; enlargement may suggest infection, inflammation, or neoplasia.

After a complete physical examination and patient history, diagnostics should include an accurate blood pressure, complete blood count (CBC) with platelet count, chemistry profile, urinalysis, a coagulogram, and BMBT to assess platelet function. If hypertension is suspected as a contributing cause of epistaxis, endocrine testing and a search for the primary cause via abdominal and cardiac ultrasonography is recommended.

Radiographs of the nasal cavity and thorax are also recommended pending laboratory and physical examination findings; a computed tomography (CT) or magnetic resonance imaging (MRI) of the nasal cavity, flushing of the nose, cytology of nasal discharge, staining with India ink (for *Cryptococcus* organisms), fungal serology, and nasal biopsy or rhinoscopy are also additional diagnostics that can produce useful information. Nasal cultures are typically not useful because bacterial contaminants are widespread

The CBC is normal in many cases of epistaxis; a regenerative anemia generally indicates a bone marrow response to bleeding and usually occurs within 3–5 days of the blood loss. Chronic epistaxis typically produces a non-regenerative anemia with a secondary iron deficiency. Leukocytosis is not uncommon, typically a result of chronic inflammation or infection. Leukopenia may result from infections, cytotoxic drug administration, immune-mediated disease, or sepsis (Northrup and Gieger 2004). Thrombocytopenia may be caused by increased destruction or consumption, sequestration, or decreased production of platelets. A blood film should be evaluated in any case with thrombocytopenia; dogs and cats should have 10–15 platelets per 100× oil immersion field; spontaneous epistaxis is uncommon unless the platelet count is 30,000/μL or less (Northrup and Gieger 2004). A bone marrow aspirate or core biopsy is indicated in cases of unexplained non-regenerative anemia, thrombocytopenia, or leukopenia. Abnormal buccosal bleeding time (BMBT) should prompt a von Willebrand's titer and evaluation for secondary causes of platelet function defects. In-house coagulation tests, such as partial thromboplastin time (PTT), prothrombin time (PT), and activated clotting time (ACT) should be analyzed, particularly before nasal biopsy or rhinoscopy procedures. A coagulogram should also include fibrinogen, FDPs, and an ATIII concentration if the patient has physical evidence of DIC (petechia, ecchymosis). In addition, as decreased platelet production can result from rickettsial or protozoal infections, laboratory titers should also be evaluated.

Abnormalities in blood chemistries include possible hypoproteinemia, usually as a result of acute blood loss. Hyperglobulinemia may occur secondary to neoplasia or chronic infections. Abdominal ultrasonography may be indicated in some patients with chronic epistaxis; renal, hepatic, or endocrine diseases can cause or exacerbate epistaxis. Thoracic radiographs should be performed, particularly before the use of anesthesia, and especially in geriatric patients, to rule out metastatic neoplasia.

Treatment goals are to first control the bleeding, particularly if severe hemorrhage is present. Treatment includes ice packs, application of digital pressure to the maxillary arteries, and sedation to control hemorrhage and patient anxiety (e.g., acepromazine in the absence of hypotension). Once sedated (or if the patient presents obtunded), blood should be suctioned from the oropharynx to prevent its aspiration. Phenylephrine (10 mg/mL; 0.1 mL in 1 mL of 0.9% NaCl) administered directly into the nares, or dilute (1:100,000) epinephrine-soaked sponges, or tampons packed into the nares may resolve hemorrhage. Neosynephrine spray can also be utilized. If the hemorrhage is refractory, a Foley urinary catheter can be placed through the ventral meatus to the nasopharynx; the balloon is then inflated, and catheter is retracted to the nasal passage (Fig. 11.4).

Local anesthetic can be applied into the nares and packed with Vaseline gauze tape and left in place for 24–48 hours.

Ligation of the external carotid artery on the affected side or both sides may help control bleeding in severe or chronic epistaxis. Severe acute hemorrhage necessitates intravenous fluid therapy and packed RBCs if anemia is severe. Suspected coagulopathies will require transfusions of fresh whole blood or fresh-frozen plasma. *Nursing concerns* include monitoring hemodynamic parameters (heart rate, respiratory rate and effort, pulse quality, blood pressure, body temperature), monitoring bleeding, serial PCV and total solids, monitoring quality of respirations (including auscultation) for potential of aspiration, and patient comfort to minimize hypertension.

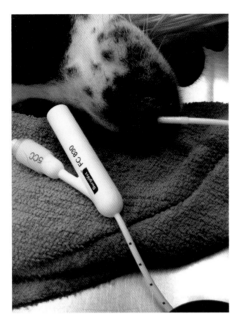

Figure 11.4   If hemorrhage from epistaxis is refractory, a Foley urinary catheter can be placed through the ventral meatus to the nasopharynx; the balloon is then inflated, with catheter retracted up to the nasal passage.

Auto-Immune Hemolytic Anemia

Immune-mediated hemolytic anemia (IMHA) is a pathologic process that causes the premature destruction of RBCs. Considered one of the most common types of anemia in small animals, this abnormal immune response occurs when autoantibodies are produced against the animal's own RBC membrane antigens. In physiologic terms, IMHA is a predominantly Type II hypersensitivity reaction in which anti-RBC antibodies, including IgG, IgM, and IgA, attach directly or indirectly to various components of the RBC membrane, causing extravascular hemolysis, intravascular hemolysis, and intravascular RBC agglutination (Balch and Mackin 2007).

In veterinary medicine, breeds commonly affected with IMHA include Cocker spaniels, miniature poodles, Irish setters, Dobermans, and Old English sheepdogs, with the average age typically from young to middle-age female dogs (Macintire et al. 2006). The mortality rate varies and is generally dependant upon the treatment tactic.

In severe immune reactions, large numbers of antibodies attach to the RBC membrane, which in turn activates the *complement cascade*—a complex series of enzymatic proteins occurring in normal serum that are triggered in a cascade manner by the antibody–antigen complexes, producing cell lysis. In simple terms, the cell membrane is damaged and an influx of extracellular fluid into the RBC causes rupture of the cell while still in circulation, hence the term *intravascular hemolysis*. Consequently, intravascular hemolysis results in the release of free hemoglobin into the bloodstream (hemoglobinemia) and urine (hemoglobinuria). In less severe cases of IMHA with minimal complement-mediated cell-wall damage, antibody attachment causes removal of affected RBCs by the MPS. This MPS-mediated process occurs outside of the circulation and is therefore called *extravascular hemolysis*. In extravascular hemolysis, particular receptors on macrophages in the liver and spleen bind to targeted receptor components on antibodies coating the RBC membrane, resulting in RBC phagocytosis and destruction. Hemoglobinemia and hemoglobinuria do not occur with extravascular hemolysis, as hemoglobin enters the bilirubin metabolic pathway rather than spilling into the circulation (Balch and Mackin 2007).

IMHA may be primary (idiopathic) or secondary to drugs, vaccines, erythroparasites, infectious diseases, or neoplastic disorders. *Primary IMHA* is more common and is considered an autoimmune disorder with no identifiable underlying cause. IMHA occurs in cats less frequently than in dogs; hemolysis in cats with IMHA is complement-mediated and is almost always extravascular (Balch and Mackin 2007). *Secondary IMHA* is caused by an immunologic response to foreign (non-self) antigens associated with normal RBC membranes infected by bacterial, viral, rickettsial, protozoal, or neoplastic pathogens. Vaccine-induced IMHA has been documented in several research studies where patients were within 30 days of vaccination. No particular vaccine was implicated or conclusively linked with IMHA, although it has been theorized that a vaccination may be a nonspecific trigger that either activates the MPS, heightens a low-grade inflammatory condition, or perhaps deregulates the delicate balance of the immune system (Balch and Mackin 2007).

Drugs have also been implicated as causative agents of IMHA (e.g., cephalosporins, penicillins, trimethoprim-sulfa, and NSAIDs). Proposed mechanisms of action include the adhesion of the drug or its breakdown products to the RBC membrane, inducing a complement attack or perhaps cell removal by the MPS, resulting in intravascular hemolysis.

IMHA may also be caused by *alloantibodies* (antibodies produced by one individual that react with antigens in another member of the same species) directed specifically against RBC membrane components. Examples in veterinary medicine include incompatible transfusion reactions and neonatal isoerythrolysis in cats (Refer to Chapter 21 "Transfusion Medicine"). Other causes of non-immune-mediated hemolytic anemia include inherited defects (e.g., pyruvate kinase deficiency found in basenjis), hypophosphatemia (e.g., refeeding syndrome in cats with hepatic lipidosis or diabetic ketoacidosis), and with certain toxin exposure (such as zinc, acetaminophen, napthelene, onion, garlic, and other oxidant agents). Zinc toxicosis typically occurs from ingestion of U.S. pennies minted after 1983. Repeated use of the induction anesthetic agent propofol has been reported to cause a Heinz body anemia in cats.

Another form of IMHA is called *microangiopathic hemolytic anemia*, a condition in which RBCs are physically damaged while in circulation. With microangiopathic hemolytic anemia, the RBCs become injured (fragmented) by an underlying condition, such as splenic torsion, tumors (e.g., hemangiosarcoma), heartworm disease, fibrin clots, vasculitis, liver disease, intravenous catheterization, or by any damaged vessel. Fragmented RBCs are consequently pulled out of circulation by the MPS system. Schistocytes are commonly found on a blood smear. Treatment of microangiopathic hemolytic anemia includes correction of the underlying disease.

Clinical signs associated with IMHA include weakness, lethargy, and poor mentation, pale to icteric mucous membranes, tachycardia, abnormal body temperature, palpable hepatosplenomegaly, and a heart murmur (almost always associated with anemia). Chief complaint of the pet owner is often discolored or "port-wine" colored urine (hemoglobinuria). Laboratory findings include a regenerative anemia, presence of *spherocytes* (small, spherical RBCs with loss of central pallor), leukocytosis, lymphocytosis, hyperbilirubinemia, hyperglobulinemia, and increased liver enzyme values (Fig. 11.5).

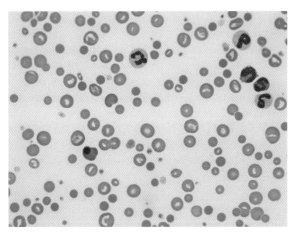

Figure 11.5   Laboratory findings in IMHA include a regenerative anemia, and the presence of spherocytes—small, spherical RBCs. (Courtesy of Elizabeth Spangler, DVM, PhD, DACVIM, DACVP.)

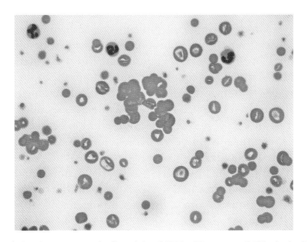

Figure 11.6   RBC agglutination commonly found in IMHA. (Courtesy of Elizabeth Spangler, DVM, PhD, DACVIM, DACVP.)

The diagnosis of IMHA is almost always supported by the presence of spherocytes, RBC agglutination, and a positive Coombs' test (a visual presence of agglutination indicating that antibodies and/or complement proteins are bound to the surface of RBCs). The *Coombs' test* may have some use in diagnosing primary or secondary IMHA, but this test cannot be conducted if severe *agglutination* is present (Fig. 11.6).

Slide agglutination testing can easily be performed to distinguish agglutination from Rouleaux formation. One drop of blood from a capillary tube or anticoagulated blood is placed on a slide with 10 drops of saline; Rouleaux will be dispersed by the saline wherein agglutination yields obvious clumping or flecks ("grains") within the blood. In severe cases of IMHA, agglutionation can be seen within the capillary tube.

Treatment of IMHA first involves therapy for potential underlying conditions that may have triggered the hemolytic process (e.g., doxycycline for rickettsial disease), as well as immunosuppressive doses of glucocorticoids (e.g., prednisolone) and GI protectants (e.g., omeprazole, pantoprazole, misoprostal) to prevent GI bleeding. As IMHA is a hallmark

CHAPTER 11

disease for hypercoagulation and thromboembolism, the use of anticoagulating agents (e.g., heparin, aspirin, dalteparin, enoxaparin, and clopidogrel) is typically warranted. If there is a favorable response (as indicated by a rise in the hematocrit and the reticulocyte count), the glucocorticoid dose is tapered slowly to prevent recurrence of hemolysis once the hematocrit reaches an acceptable, stable number (e.g., PCV of 30%). If glucocorticoid side effects become a problem, other immunosuppressant drugs such as azathioprine, cyclosporine, cyclophoshamide, and mycophenolate, can be given (Macintire et al. 2006). Other treatment therapy for IMHA includes splenectomy, although this practice is now considered a last resort in patients with extravascular hemolysis that have not responded to traditional medical therapy. Splenectomy may not be beneficial as extravascular hemolysis can also occur in the liver.

Complicated cases of IMHA (severe autoagglutination, severe anemia) can involve a combination of immunosuppressive drug therapy in addition to blood transfusion therapy. *Supportive therapy* includes oxygen supplementation (if anemia is severe), intravenous fluids, blood transfusion therapy if anemia severe, and nutritional support. If blood transfusions are indicated, there is a substantial increase in the risk of pulmonary thromboemboli (PTE) and acute renal failure (Macintire 2005). Blood transfusions (typically packed RBCs) are typically not instituted (unless the anemia is severe), with crossmatching procedures recommended, albeit difficult due to hemolysis.

Hemoglobin-based oxygen carrying solutions (HBOCs) can be utilized in lieu of traditional blood products in order to provide an increase in circulating hemoglobin for tissue oxygenation. HBOCs may buy time for immunosuppressant therapy to be effective; HBOCs typically last 24–48 hours at a dosage of 15–30 mL/kg due to the short half-life of these solutions compared with packed RBCs (Macintire et al. 2006). Benefits of HBOCs include the avoided risk of PTE found with traditional blood products, as well as avoiding typical transfusion reactions from donor RBCs. As HBOCs have a higher molecular weight and are considered colloids, volume overload is possible. Nurses should diligently monitor heart rate, central venous pressure (CVP) (if possible), and respiratory effort. The PCV will temporarily drop after use of HBOCs due to the dilutional affect; the only way to monitor these solutions is with a hemoglobinometer. Hemoglobin levels should be kept above 3.5 g/dL (Macintire et al. 2006).

Serial PCV monitoring is important to gauge efficacy of drug therapy or blood product administration. *Nursing concerns* include monitoring for signs of increased respiratory effort, as PTE is a serious potential complication of IMHA. Clinical signs of PTE include acute dyspnea, tachypnea, cyanosis, hypoxemia, and hypothermia (Fig. 11.7).

Physical exam findings of PTE are variable but may include pulmonary crackles, tachypnea, tachycardia, and poor pulse quality. Thoracic radiographic findings are also variable; hypovascular lung regions and/or alveolar infiltrates on dorsoventral or ventrodorsal projections may be seen (Macintire et al. 2006). Right-sided cardiomegaly, pleural effusion, and main pulmonary enlargement may also be found. However, thoracic radiographs may also appear normal despite severe respiratory insufficiency.

Diagnostic tests to confirm PTE include the arterial blood gas (ABG); common findings include decreased PaO_2, increased alveolar–arterial oxygen concentration difference, and decreased $PaCO_2$. However, a normal ABG does not rule out PTE. Pulmonary scintigraphy and pulmonary angiography are the best tests to confirm PTE. Treatment of PTE includes oxygen therapy, anticoagulant therapy (e.g., heparin, low melocular weight heparin [LMWH]), platelet inhibitors, low-dose aspirin, and fibrinoytic drugs such as streptokinase. The goal of anticoagulant therapy such as heparin is to prolong the ACT; the protein ATIII must be present in order for heparin to be effective. Consequently, fresh

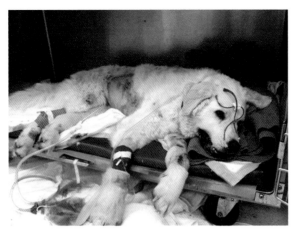

Figure 11.7   Clinical signs of PTE include acute dyspnea, tachypnea, cyanosis, hypoxemia, and hypothermia.

frozen plasma (which contains ATIII) may be necessary if the patient is hypoproteinemic. Anti Xa levels may be monitored if patients are undergoing LMWH therapy. Heparin or warfarin will not dissolve an existing clot, but may help prevent the formation of any additional microthrombi. Dissolution of any existing clots can occur with fibrinolytic drugs such as streptokinase. There are serious complications to anticoagulant and fibrinolytic drugs, specifically hemorrhage; patients should be monitored diligently. The prognosis for patients with severe PTE is generally poor.

Nursing concerns in patients with IMHA include monitoring for signs of respiratory insufficiency, hemorrhage, renal insufficiency, poor nutritional intake, and dehydration. Signs of dehydration should be addressed immediately in patients with agglutination as they are at a higher risk of venous stasis and thrombosis. Central venous catheters should be avoided if possible to decrease the risk of thromboemboli. Hemodynamic monitoring should include blood pressure monitoring, lactate monitoring, pulse oximetry, and the monitoring of urinary output. Electrolyte analysis, blood chemistries, and CBC testing should be performed to ensure that the patient is responding favorably to treatment. As patients with IMHA are on immunosuppressive drug therapy, signs of infection such as any unexplained fever should be addressed immediately. Daily intravenous catheter inspection is recommended for extravasation of fluids; cool limbs or rope-like vessels are suspect for thrombosis, necessitating an immediate catheter change.

Recent treatment options for patients with severe IMHA that have not responded to conventional therapy (or in patients that cannot be treated with glucocorticoids because of GI bleeding or underlying infection) includes the administration of human IgG, reported to be effective in halting immune-mediated destruction of RBCs in dogs. It is thought that IgG binds complement (cell killing), consequently diverting attacks on cellular targets. IgG also is thought to have anti-inflammatory effects, such as inhibiting cytokine release from monocytes, and modulating B and T cell clones, inhibiting cytotoxic T cells, and downregulating antibody production (Macintire 2005). In small animal patients, IgG has also been used to provide passive immunity and for the adjunct treatment of sepsis and other autoimmune diseases such as ITP and SLE. The small size of the IgG molecule allows for unimpeded movement between the vasculature and body tissues; equine IgG has been used in dogs as the cost is significantly less than human IgG and canine IgG is not commercially available (Macintire et al. 2006). The risk of PTE may be increased with the use of IgG; concurrent treatment with LMWH or mini-dose aspirin may be indicated.

Immune Mediated Thrombocytopenia (ITP)

ITP is either primary or secondary; primary ITP is the most common cause of severe thrombocytopenia in dogs. Primary ITP is an idiopathic disease with unknown etiology; platelet life span is significantly decreased and antiplatelet antibodies attach to platelet surfaces and induce destruction by the MPS. Suspected triggers of secondary ITP include neoplasia, infection, drugs, and autoimmune diseases such as IMHA. Thrombopoiesis (the process of thrombocyte generation) is almost always increased in ITP. Hemorrhage is the most common clinical sign, caused by both decreased platelet numbers as well as decreased platelet function. Diagnosis of ITP is based on exclusion; presence of antiplatelet antibodies can be confirmed by enzyme-linked immunosorbent assay (ELISA) or indirect fluorescent antibody (IFA) techniques. ITP usually has a platelet count of less than 30,000 in addition to a low *mean platelet volume (MPV)*. MPV is increased with an active bone marrow response, resulting in the release of immature platelets. Bone marrow analysis shows reduced numbers of megakaryocytes.

Clinical signs of ITP include petechial hemorrhage, ecchymoses hematuria, retinal hemorrhage, and epistaxis. Treatment options include immunosuppressive therapy with glucocorticoids, and doxycycline in areas endemic for rickettsial diseases (Fig. 11.8).

Refractory cases may require a multiple immunosuppressant drug in addition to non-traditional therapy such as intravenous IgG to modulate immune-mediated destruction of platelets (in human medicine, intravenous IgG is considered the treatment of choice for ITP with a 83% success rate and expected response within 48 hours) (Macintire et al. 2006). Intravenous vincristine has also been used in veterinary patients to increase platelet count, which causes megakaryocytic fragmentation and subsequent release of platelets into circulation.

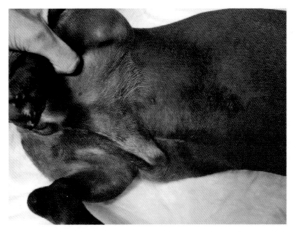

Figure 11.8   Clinical signs of ITP include petechial hemorrhage, ecchymoses, hematuria, retinal hemorrhage, and epistaxis.

Platelet-rich plasma may also be given, although platelet transfusions can be ineffectual, as transfused platelets are quickly destroyed, in addition to the risk of developing platelet alloantibodies enhanced by multiple transfusions. Immunosuppressive therapy is tapered down once the platelet count reaches 200,000 cells/μL (Macintire et al. 2006). Patients with active bleeding should be given fresh whole blood or platelet-rich plasma.

Nursing concerns include monitoring the patient for hemorrhage (hyphema, ecchymosis or petechia, epistaxis), including noting any neurologic signs which may suggest an intracranial bleed. Other nursing aspects in patients with ITP include noting any signs of abnormal perfusion such as abnormal heart rate, abnormal body temperature, cool extremities, decreased urinary output, abnormal blood pressure values, poor mentation, or increased lactate values. Intravenous catheterization or phlebotomy should never be attempted on a large vessel (e.g., jugular vessel). Diligent monitoring during a blood or platelet transfusion should be standard protocol (Refer to Chapter 21, "Transfusion Medicine"). If a bone marrow aspirate is required for diagnostic purposes, constant pressure should be applied to the aspiration site for 5–10 minutes immediately following the procedure.

Other causes of severe thrombocytopenia include increased platelet consumption, destruction induced by drugs, and insufficient production. Drug-induced thrombocytopenia should resolve with discontinuation of the drug in question, unless irreversible myelosuppression has occurred. The hormone estrogen can also induce thrombocytopenia, in addition to aplastic pancytopenia (severe anemia, leucopenia). Thrombocytopenia can also be due to platelet consumption; in contrast to ITP, platelet activation can lead to platelet consumption as platelets adhere to various surfaces, triggering platelet aggregation as found in inflammatory disease processes. Examples include DIC, vasculitis, SIRS, sepsis, and neoplasia.

Platelet sequestration can also be a cause of thrombocytopenia; the spleen, for example, normally contains approximately 30% of the circulating platelets (Gopegui and Feldman 2000), and platelet sequestration is frequently associated with splenomegaly. Canine *Babesia gibsoni* infection is an example of thrombocytopenia-induced splenomegaly. Splenectomy in ITP is not a favorable treatment.

Thrombocytopenia due to neoplasia includes many possible pathogenic processes. Examples include sequestration of platelets in splenic, hepatic, or vascular tumors; decreased platelet production in the bone marrow in estrogen-secreting tumors (Sertoli's cell neoplasia) or as a result of chemotherapy. Thrombocytopenia can also occur with platelet loss in tumor-associated hemorrhage, and immune-mediated destruction of platelets secondary to neoplastic diseases such as mast cell, hemangiosarcoma, nasal adenocarcinoma, and fibrosarcoma (Gopegui and Feldman 2000). Other causes of increased destruction and consumption of platelets include myeloproliferative disorders such as megakaryocytic leukemia. Inherited thrombocytopenias include Chediak–Hegashi syndrome (CHS), an autosomal recessive disease reported in cats and other animals. Other inherited thrombocytopenias are classified as platelet storage pool diseases, wherein platelet aggregation and secretion are impaired.

Disseminated Intravascular Coagulation (DIC)

There are a variety of disorders commonly associated with DIC in dogs and cats. The diagnosis is commonly made based on physical examination, laboratory testing, and the associating underlying disease or injury predisposing the patient to DIC. Neoplasia (primarily hemangiosarcoma), immune-mediated blood diseases, sepsis, SIRS, severe injury, envenomation, heatstroke, liver disease, and endocrine disturbances are the most common disorders associated with DIC.

Clinical signs "classic" of DIC are typically associated with defects in the secondary hemostasis process, such as epistaxis, hematochezia, hematuria, hematemesis, and melena. Large bleeds into deep tissue, joints (hemarthrosis) or body cavities (hemothorax, hemoabdomen) are also highly suspicious for defects in secondary hemostasis. Clinical signs of primary hemostatic dysfunction include small pinpoint hemorrhages (petechiae, ecchymosis), signaling possible platelet dysfunction or loss. Pitting edema is also common, as capillary leakage will occur as a result of low colloid osmotic pressure.

Chronic DIC appears to be common in dogs with chronic disorders or malignancies, as opposed to fulminant DIC found after heatstroke, trauma, acute pancreatitis, envenomation, or certain toxicities. DIC may also present as an acute decompensation of a chronic disease process, such as hemangiosarcoma. Dogs with acute DIC often are brought in because of profuse spontaneous bleeding, or signs secondary to anemia or organ thrombosis (organ failure). Acute DIC is extremely rare in cats. The clinical signs of bleeding indicate both primary and secondary bleeding. Signs of organ failure, such as oliguria or dyspnea, occur as a consequence of obstruction of the microcirculation by thrombi (e.g., PTE).

There is no simple test for diagnosing DIC; however, several hematologic findings help support a presumptive clinical diagnosis of DIC. Such findings include a regenerative hemolytic anemia, hemoglobinemia, red cell fragmentation (schistocytosis), a neutrophilia with a left shift, and thrombocytopenia. Traditionally, declining platelet numbers are the most clinically significant and the most sensitive indicator of DIC. Other laboratory abnormalities associated with DIC include (1) decreased fibrinogen, (2) prolongation of the thrombin time, prolongation of PT, and prolongation of activated partial thromboplastin time (APTT), (3) the production of FDPs, and (4) decreased concentrations of ATIII.

Keep in mind that a severe thrombocytopenia could artificially prolong the ACT, and prolonged PT and PTT are relatively insensitive tests, and clinical signs of bleeding are usually apparent at this time. Declining or decreased ATIII levels is most sensitive and helps to identify impending DIC; unfortunately, measuring ATIII levels are not readily available in most veterinary laboratories. Therefore, thromboelastography (TEG), where available, is a useful modality to evaluate for hypercoagulation and to catch early DIC. Fibrinogen concentrations may be measured to help aid in the diagnosis of DIC, but fibrinogen is an acute phase protein and will be increased in inflammation or dehydration (Bruchim et al. 2008).

Box 11.2   Laboratory Markers of DIC

- Declining platelet numbers
- Decreased fibrinogen
- Prolonged thrombin time
- Prolonged PT
- Prolongation of APTT
- Production of FDPs
- Decreased concentrations of ATII
- Elevated D-dimer concentrations

Other clinical tests used to diagnose DIC include the measurement of FDPs. As aforementioned, hemostasis deals with fibrinolysis; when the fibrin monomers are broken down, FDPs are produced. Large amounts of FDPs suggest increased fibrinolysis, which may be an early indicator of DIC. However, FDP values are often normal in early DIC if the liver is competent to clear them from circulation. In addition, FDPs are not specific in DIC and may be increased following surgery, or in patients with liver or renal failure.

Other developments in the diagnosis of DIC include the *D-dimer*, a very sensitive test that can aid in the recognition of critically ill patients with DIC (and other thromboembolic diseases). D-dimers are breakdown products of plasmin on cross-linked fibrin, thus being more specific in identifying significant activity of both the thrombotic and fibrinolytic processes of the hemostatic system. Elevated D-dimer concentrations suggest DIC or other thrombotic events. However, D-dimers are not specific for DIC and may be increased with other diseases involving thrombosis (e.g., PTE). Other tests for the diagnosis of DIC include TEG, a unique evaluation of the complete process of clot formation and destruction. TEG is currently used in humans for diagnosis of deep vein thrombosis (DVT) and other thrombotic diseases.

The most important *treatment* principle is to remove the stimulus initiating the intravascular clotting process by treatment of the primary disease. Unfortunately, only a few conditions precipitating DIC can be removed, such as a primary hemangiosarcoma (surgical excision), disseminated or metastatic hemangiosarcoma (chemotherapy), sepsis (appropriate antimicrobial treatment), and immune hemolytic anemia in dogs (immunosuppressive treatment). In most other situations (snake bites, trauma, heatstroke, pancreatitis), the cause can rarely be eliminated within a short time, making DIC a life-threatening disease process. Other therapeutics should include the prevention of secondary complications, maintenance of organ perfusion, and improvement of delivery of oxygen (DO_2) to tissues.

Maintaining organ perfusion through aggressive fluid therapy should also be a focus on the treatment of DIC. Fluid therapy should consist of crystalloids and colloid administration to dilute out the clotting and fibrinolytic factors in the circulation, flush out microthrombi from the microcirculation, and maintain patency of the capillary beds in order to provide adequate oxygen exchange. Colloid administration (fresh frozen plasma) will provide coagulation factors consumed by DIC, provide adequate osmotic pressure to retain fluid in the intravascular space, and help prevent capillary leakage. Human serum albumin can also be utilized for severe hypoalbuminemia and low colloid osmotic pressure, but would not provide clotting factors. Crystalloid therapy should be instituted to prevent dehydration and electrolyte disturbances. (*Note*: There is much controversy in the use of synthetic colloids, e.g., hetastarch, a hydroxyethyl starch [HES] solution) in the treatment of DIC and other platelet disorders. Platelet dysfunction in humans due to HES administration has been attributed to decreased platelet adhesion (Jandry 2009). The effects on coagulation secondary to HES solutions are related to alterations in factor VIII (FVIII) and vWF concentration and function. FVIII is a glycoprotein that participates in the intrinsic pathway of coagulation and acts as a cofactor in blood coagulation; decreased concentrations of FVIII have been observed in humans after HES administration, which may account for mildly prolonged coagulation times. Decreases in vWF and FVIII may also occur due to binding with HES molecules. At present, there is no current literature in veterinary medicine to confirm or refute the adverse clinical effects of HES on hemostasis, and the beneficial effects of colloids in resuscitation and therapy are well-known. Use of newer licensed HES solutions with lower molecular weight (e.g., Voluven) has indicated little to no effect on hemostasis and continues to be documented as beneficial to veterinary patients (Jandry 2009).

Nutritional delivery should also be aggressively pursued in the safest physiological route for the treatment of DIC, as early nutrition will improve tissue healing, help maintain adequate protein levels, and provide substrates for energy production and normal homeostatic mechanisms. Enteral nutrition will also provide natural protection of the GI mucosa. *Analgesia* is always essential; opiods are safe and are typically the analgesics of choice (Matthews 2006).

Oxygen therapy is also recommended to improve myocardial function and oxygen delivery to the tissues. *Nursing therapy* should be diligent; specifically, the monitoring of blood pressure, pulse oximetry, urine production, body temperature, and telemetry (or frequent electrocardiograms [ECGs]) to monitor for potential cardiac arrhythmias. CVP monitoring to assess fluid requirements is recommended if a jugular catheter is already in place. Urinary output should be monitored via a closed, sterile indwelling system. Vascular inspection and the monitoring of petechia, ecchymosis, and body weight should be performed daily. (*Note*: Where a central venous catheter is a useful hemodynamic monitoring tool, placement is contraindicated if the patient already has a coagulopathy, respiratory insufficiency, increased intracranial pressure, or if the patient is prone to a thromboembolic event.) Patients with fulminant DIC have a grave prognosis.

Phlebotomy Techniques

Proper sample collection for the coagulation assay is paramount. *Common phlebotomy techniques* such as probing for a vein, drawing blood through a hematoma and excessive back pressure on the syringe while drawing the blood are more than likely to initiate the coagulation cascade and fibrinolytic system. In addition, an excited or aggressive animal may also greatly impact coagulation factor levels and platelet counts through epinephrine-mediated actions. If possible, blood samples for coagulation tests should never be taken through a catheter due to probable contamination with heparin and activation of the coagulation cascade by the catheter surface. Sodium citrate is the anticoagulant of choice for most coagulation profiles; heparin and EDTA anticoagulated samples are unacceptable for coagulation profiles.

Oncology and Immune System Emergencies

Neutropenia and Sepsis

The inciting cause of sepsis is a microorganism in the form of a bacteria, fungus, virus, protozoa, rickettsia, or spirochete. *Sepsis* can occur with any infection in any part of the body. The endogenous response to sepsis includes an acute phase response, activation of the complement and coagulation cascade, and the response of the cytokines and other various factors which triggers a systemic inflammatory response (SIRS) (Matthews 2006). Severe sepsis and subsequent septic shock occurs as sepsis progresses to multiple organ dysfunction and hemodynamic collapse, resulting in hypovolemia, hypotension, and possibly cardiogenic failure. Predisposing factors in sepsis or neutropenia include myelosuppressive chemotherapy, poor nutrition, immune dysfunction, prolonged hospitalization, and severe tissue injury.

In humans, sepsis is the most common cause of death in cancer patients (Ogilvie and Moore 2001). In the dog and cat, neutropenia is typically secondary to malignancy or the myelosuppressive effects of chemotherapy, and is a common predisposing factor for sepsis. The general rule of thumb is that any patient receiving chemotherapy should be considered at risk for the development of chemotherapy-induced neutropenia and sepsis. If a septic event is due to chemotherapy, dose reduction may be necessary for subsequent cancer treatment; prophylactic antibiotic treatment is controversial. As there are many clinical situations that can mimic neutropenia and sepsis which are unrelated to chemotherapy (e.g., SIRS generated by non-microbial stimuli, such as found in trauma, envenomation, acute pancreatitis, heatstroke), complete history and physical examination are critical.

Neutropenia results from impaired granulopoiesis (development of granulocytic WBCs) from overwhelming sepsis wherein tissue demands exceed marrow granulocyte reserve. Neutropenia secondary to chemotherapy most commonly occurs within 5–10 days after administration, although some drugs may cause a later *nadir* (the point at which neutrophil populations in bone marrow are likely to be lowest due to the effects of chemotherapy). Patients with neutrophil counts less than 3000 are at risk for sepsis and are candidates for prophylactic antibiotics. Such patients should have further chemotherapy held until their neutrophil count rises. Concurrent hepatic or renal insufficiency, or preexisting bone marrow disease, may alter the metabolism of the chemotherapeutic agent and increase toxic effects. Although neoplastic cells are the primary target of chemotherapy, normal cells will also be affected. The most commonly affected cell types are the crypt cells of the intestines and cells within the bone marrow (Brugmann and Smith 2008), which is why it is common for some chemotherapeutics to have GI side effects (e.g., inappetence, vomiting, diarrhea). Such side effects are typically mild and rarely require hospitalization. In contrast, neutrophils within the bone marrow can be dramatically affected.

Patients in *septic shock* can have several different clinical presentations. Septic shock is the state of circulatory collapse that occurs secondary to overwhelming sepsis and has a high mortality rate. In the early phase of septic shock, clinical signs can include brick red mucous membranes (due to vasodilation), hyperdynamic or bounding pulses, quick capillary refill time (CRT), tachycardia, and possibly tachypnea. Cats in early septic shock will commonly be hypothermic and potentially bradycardic, presumably from myocardial depressant factors. In addition, because cats tend to hide their clinical signs until late in the disease process, sepsis may be quite advanced when first recognized.

In the later stages of septic shock, clinical signs in both the dog and cat may include poor pulse quality, prolonged CRT, cyanotic or gray mucous membrane color, dehydration, and dull mentation. The systemic effects of septic shock include vasoconstriction leading to multiple organ failure, cardiac dysfunction, increased vascular permeability, liver and renal dysfunction, coagulopathies, and decreased insulin release (Fig. 11.9).

Animals will initially have hyperglycemia, followed by hypoglycemia. Fever may or may not be present; patients with low or nonfunctional neutrophils may not have an inflammatory reaction to induce fever.

Nursing protocols for patients with sepsis (or septic shock) include serial physical examinations with particular emphasis on auscultation; murmurs are suspicious for endocarditis. Muffled heart or lung sounds may indicate a pyothorax; crackles or wheezes are suspicious for pneumonia or acute respiratory distress syndrome (ARDS). In addition,

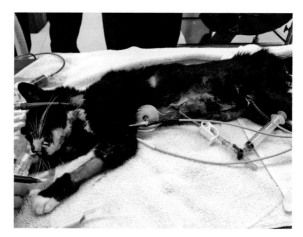

Figure 11.9   The systemic effects of septic shock include vasoconstriction leading to multiple organ failure, cardiac dysfunction, and coagulopathies.

Box 11.3   Clinical Signs of Septic Shock

Early
- Bounding pulse quality
- Rapid or increased CRT
- Tachypnea or hyperpnea
- Red mucous membranes
- Heart murmur
- Abnormal body temperature
- Dehydration

Late
- Poor mentation
- Tachycardia
- Delayed CRT
- Poor pulse quality
- Tachypnea
- Hemorrhagic diarrhea
- Decreased blood pressure
- Hypothermia
- Icterus

---

as fluid therapy is often aggressive during a hypotensive event, auscultation is crucial as patients with inflammatory conditions (SIRS) are more predisposed to pulmonary edema. Oxygen supplementation should be mandatory in all septic shock patients, with vitals recorded every 15 minutes during triage.

Other nursing concerns include monitoring blood glucose levels; hypoglycemic animals should have dextrose added to their intravenous fluids. Strict sterile technique should be performed on all procedures, including routine intravenous injections, in order to minimize exposure to resistant strains of bacteria. Intravascular catheters, urinary catheters, frequent acquisition of blood samples, chest or endotracheal tubes are associated with an increased prevalence of sepsis; handling should always be performed with sterile technique. Nurses should always wear gloves when handling a septic/neutropenic patient, and all catheters should be inspected daily, keeping in mind that the longer a catheter is present, the higher the probability for infection. Nutrition should be addressed early and aggressively, as malnutrition is a serious cause of debilitation and decreased resistance to bacterial infection. Prolonged hospitalization can increase patient morbidity, as the patient is continually exposed to bacterial strains, and should be considered a high risk for nosocomial infection.

The patient should be examined for a septic focus, which may include swollen joints (polyarthritis), neck pain (meningitis), tissue abscesses, or spinal pain (discospondylitis). Blood pressure should be monitored frequently, particularly during the triage phase, keeping in mind that hypotension coupled with hypoproteinemia is suspicious of capillary leakage (SIRS), and judicious fluid management may be required to avoid pulmonary edema. Aliquots of colloids (Hetastarch, human albumin, Oxyglobin® (OPK Biotech, Cambridge, MA), fresh frozen plasma) may be indicated; nurses should monitor respiratory effort and perform frequent auscultation. CVP monitoring is recommended in severe cases if the patient is stable enough for central venous catheterization, or if a jugular catheter is already present, CVP monitoring can immediately assess efficacy of fluid treatment and help determine hemodynamic status. Vasopressors and/or inotropes may be required if hypotension persists after adequate fluid resuscitation (e.g., dopamine, dobutamine, vasopressin or norepinephrine). Such pharmacologic agents are typically used to correct hemodynamically significant hypotension in the absence of hypovolemia. Heart rate and respiratory rate should return to within normal limits after the patient has been rehydrated and the disease process controlled. Temperature should be monitored frequently; fever and hypothermia are common, depending on the severity of the condition. Hypothermia can often indicate deterioration.

Diagnostics include blood work, radiographs, and urine culture and blood cultures when looking for an underlying infection, although cultures may be negative and/or results not available for a significant period of time. *Laboratory findings* include neutropenia (<3000 cells/μL); however, many patients do not show clinical signs until the neutrophil count is significantly low (<1000/μL). A lymphopenia (<1000 cells/μL), anemia (typically normocytic, normochromic non-regenerative), and thrombocytopenia (<150,000/μL) are common findings. Thrombocytopenia may suggest early DIC; however, it is critical to evaluate a blood smear and perform a manual cell differential to determine the accuracy of a CBC and platelet count. Evaluation of RBC and neutrophil morphology will also help identify toxic changes, presence of a left shift or degenerative left shift, or the presence of any intracellular organisms. Biochemical abnormalities include elevated total protein (dehydration or hyperglobulinemia), altered electrolytes (vomiting), elevated bilirubin, azotemia, and hypoglycemia.

The use of broad-spectrum antimicrobials is standard protocol and should be administer as soon as sepsis is first suspected. Antimicrobial selection should favor gram-negative organisms because of the high possibility for bacterial translocation. If resistance is a concern or more gram-negative coverage is needed, aminoglycosides or fluorinated quinolones may be used. Aminoglycosides should be administered after the patient has been fully rehydrated; nurses should monitor urinary output and assess hydration status diligently. Fluorinated quinolones should be diluted 50:50 with saline and given

---

Box 11.4   Nursing Considerations in Sepsis/Septic Shock

- Oxygen supplementation
- Obtain pretreatment blood samples +/– blood cultures
- Sterile IV catheter placement
- Blood glucose monitoring
- Blood pressure monitoring
- Frequent auscultation for arrhythmias, pulmonary edema
- Monitor body temperature
- Monitor heart rate and pulse quality
- Monitor urinary output
- Pain control
- Turn frequently if weak and recumbent
- Sterile handling of patient, catheters
- Monitor IV for extravasation (expect peripheral edema)
- Nutritional delivery
- Monitor integument for signs of DIC (ecchymosis, petechia)

---

intravenously very slowly over a 45–60 minute period, as seizures can occur if given too quickly (Brugmann and Smith 2008). Steroids remain controversial in the treatment of septic shock. Blood samples, including blood cultures when indicated, should be drawn with sterile technique prior to antimicrobial treatment if possible. Antimicrobial therapy should be instituted early and aggressively in the triage phase.

Tumor Lysis Syndrome

Acute tumor lysis syndrome (ATLS) is a rare condition of acute collapse shortly after chemotherapy or radiation administration. ATLS is most often associated with chemotherapy-sensitive tumors such as lymphoma and leukemia, and although exact pathophysiolgoy is unknown, it is suspected that ATLS results from the rapid lysis of tumor cells, which causes the release of intracellular contents into the circulation (Ogilvie 2006). Specifically, there is an acute release of intracellular phosphates and potassium, resulting in clinical signs associated with hypocalcemia, hyperkalemia, and hyperphosphatemia. Death can be imminent; rapid diagnosis and therapy are essential. *Predisposing factors* include sepsis or extensive neoplastic disease that infiltrates the parenchyma of organs (Ogilvie 2006).

Dogs with ATLS present with clinical signs similar to those with neutropenia and septic shock, including pale mucous membranes, slow CRT, vomiting, diarrhea, and cardiovascular collapse. Hyperkalemia is common and will often manifest as bradycardia and diminished P wave amplitude with wide QRS and spiked T waves on ECG, in addition to significant muscle weakness. In the presence of elevated phosphate levels, hypocalcemia can develop as a result of a calcium and phosphate precipitation. Signs of hypocalcemia include anorexia, lethargy, vomiting, pruritus, muscle fasciculations, or seizures. There may also be a release of large amounts of purines, lactate, and uric acid from tumor cells; consequences are that metabolic and excretory capabilities of the kidneys are compromised, commonly resulting in renal failure (Cohen 2003).

There is no gender or age predisposition for the development of ATLS, although middle-aged to geriatric dogs are most commonly affected with lymphoma, which is a common neoplastic disease prone to ATLS. Breed predilection for ATLS is unknown because of a lack of reported cases, although Dalmatians are at an increased risk for hyperuricemia because they lack uricase, which is needed to convert uric acid to allantoin, therefore making them a higher risk for ATLS (Cohen 2003). Other considerations or predispositions to ATLS include renal disease (decreased clearance of uric acid, phosphorous, and potassium), extensive tumor burden, preexisting hypercalcemia, and liver insufficiency (decreased ability to metabolize waste products from tumor cells).

Laboratory findings in ATLS include hyperphosphatemia, hypocalcemia, hyperuricemia, hyperkalemia, azotemia, and metabolic acidosis. Elevated phosphorous is the most common metabolic abnormality; lysis of tumor cells results in the release of phosphorous into both the blood and the urine (triple phosphate crystals can be seen on a urinalysis). Hyocalcemia often accompanies hyperphosphatemia; calcium-phosphate complexes form and can precipitate in the renal tubules, causing renal failure. The release of purines into the circulation results in hyperuricemia; purines are metabolized into uric acid in the liver by the enzyme uricase. Excessive uric acid can lead to precipitation in the renal tubules, also causing renal failure. Consequently, dogs with liver insufficiency, or Dalmatians which lack uricase, may be at an increase risk for ATLS and secondary renal insufficiency. Urate oxidase is used in human patients to decrease uric acid load, which can be beneficial in decreasing hyperuricemia secondary to ATLS. Its use in veterinary medicine is not well documented (Cohen 2003).

Treatment for ATLS begins with prevention. All patients considered at risk should receive prophylactic therapy 12–24 hours before chemotherapy or radiation. Prophylactic therapy is typically fluid diuresis, in addition to intravenous fluids 24–48 hours after treatment. At-risk patients may also require dose reduction in chemotherapy or radiation.

Initial treatment for clinical signs of ATLS includes aggressive intravenous fluids to correct electrolyte disturbances and metabolic acidosis. Fluid types with low potassium content are recommended (0.9% NaCl, Ringer's solution at 4mEq/L potassium, or Normosol® [Hospira, Inc., Lake Forest, IL] at 5mEq/L potassium). If the patient is hypocalcemic, a solution with supplemental calcium is recommended, such as lactated Ringer's solution. Continuous ECG monitoring is crucial to monitor for life-threatening arrhythmias associated with hyperkalemia (cardiac changes can occur with serum potassium levels greater than 6.5mEq/L) or hypocalcemia (tachycardia or prolonged QT intervals). Intravenous calcium supplementation or medication administration should be initiated with any severe hypocalcemia or hyperkalemia, concurrently with diuresis and ECG monitoring (Fig. 11.10).

Restoration of severe metabolic derangements typically takes 24–48 hours. Because the kidneys are the main source of electrolyte secretion, metabolic abnormalities may be exacerbated in patients with renal insufficiency. In addition, as renal failure can be a common sequela of ATLS, useful monitoring tools such as CVP monitoring and placement of a closed urinary catheter is advised. Renal function usually improves with mild renal insufficiency; however, permanent renal damage can occur. The use of any nephrotoxic drugs or anesthesia should be avoided when possible. Cancer therapy should be temporarily discontinued until ATLS is resolved.

Nursing considerations include intense monitoring of the patient's hemodynamic status, such as blood pressure, CVP, urinary output, ECG monitoring, and auscultation. Frequent blood pressure monitoring is important, as alterations can result from various mechanisms during an ATLS episode, such as hypotension in shock. CVP monitoring is

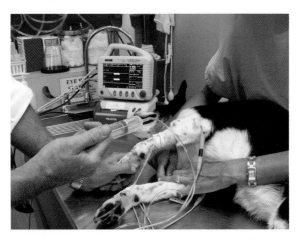

Figure 11.10   Continuous ECG monitoring is crucial during intravenous calcium supplementation with any severe hypocalcemic crisis.

essential to prevent fluid overload during diuresis, as well as serial body weighing (increases in body weight support an increase in body fluid retention; decreases in weight suggest inadequate fluid support). CVP monitoring is also important if there is evidence of renal failure, as well as urinary catheter placement and recording of urinary output every few hours. ECG monitoring is essential, particularly if electrolyte imbalances are severe or calcium is supplemented intravenously. Frequent blood analysis is recommended in order to recheck electrolytes, lactate levels, calcium and phosphorous levels, and renal values. In addition, nurses should ensure adequate nutritional intake, as well as overall patient comfort.

Paraneoplastic Syndrome

Cancer has many affects on the veterinary patient, and often induces clinical signs indirectly related to the primary tumor. Such indirect clinical effects can sometimes be more profound than the consequences of the primary tumor(s); such effects are known as *paraneoplastic syndromes*. Paraneoplastic changes are those that occur in a distant location from the primary tumor and are often the first indication of a neoplastic process. Early identification of such alterations can allow a rapid diagnosis of the primary process, and with treatment of the primary tumor(s), many paraneoplastic symptoms can disappear as tumor remission is achieved.

The most common paraneoplastic syndromes in the dog are thought to be caused by the production of polypeptide hormones, creating endocrine-like effects such as hypercalcemia and hypoglycemia (Ogilvie 2006). Other paraneoplastic effects include, but are not limited to, hematologic manifestations, fever, cachexia, and neurologic symptoms. Initial treatment of the paraneoplastic syndrome itself is often necessary for survival, and complete workups of each condition are often essential to find the underlying cause of abnormal clinical signs.

Hematologic abnormalities are very common with paraneoplastic syndromes; changes in any cell line are possible. Anemia affects approximately 30% of the dogs (Lucas 2009). Several types of anemia are associated with neoplasia; underlying etiology of anemia in cancer of veterinary patients is not fully understood. Anemia can be related to chronic disease, blood loss, immune-mediated hemolysis, chronic chemotherapy, or pure red cell aplasia (Lucas 2009). Anemia of chronic disease is the most common abnormality and results from decreased iron availability, shortened erythrocyte life span, and decreased erythropoiesis.

Anemia of chronic disease is characterized as normocytic and normochromic and non-regenerative; there is no specific treatment although iron supplementation is suggested, in addition to treatment of the primary tumor. In treating iron-deficiency anemia, it is important to identify and address any source of chronic blood loss. Iron replacement therapy can provide sufficient iron to enable hemoglobin synthesis, help correct the anemia, and replenish iron stores. Iron-deficiency anemia does not develop in animals until the body's iron stores have been depleted. If severe GI disease (e.g., hemorrhage, malabsorption) is the cause of the iron deficiency, supplementation may be given parenterally until oral therapy can be tolerated (White and Reine 2009).

Anemia of chronic disease can also be a common side effect of chemotherapy; therefore, a CBC is usually necessary prior to each chemotherapeutic treatment. Anemia is considered a negative prognostic factor for dogs with lymphoma undergoing chemotherapy, as there is an association between moderate anemia and decreased survival time in canine lymphoma (Lucas 2009). Anemia associated with renal insufficiency is usually non-regenerative, with a lack of peripheral reticulocytes and erythroid hypoplasia of the bone marrow. Regardless of the cause of anemia, blood transfusions may be necessary when the PCV becomes dangerously low or if the anemia affects the quality of life. The use of erythropoietin can also be beneficial because it helps to down regulate the factors activated by the hypoxia (Lucas 2009). Chronic hypoxia also contributes to the decreased efficacy of some chemotherapeutic drugs and has the potential to induce the development of acquired drug resistance.

Blood loss can also be observed with bleeding tumors (e.g., hemangiosarcoma). Such anemia is generally microcytic, hypochromic, and can be regenerative or non-regenerative. The treatment of choice is the control of the primary tumor (e.g., splenectomy in splenic hemangiosarcoma). IMHA can also be a paraneoplastic effect and can be diagnosed by the presence of spherocytes. Immune suppression with prednisone alone or in association with another immunosuppressive drug may be necessary. In canine lymphoma, paraneoplastic syndromes can include immune-mediated hemolytic anemia or thrombocytopenia, a process secondary to protein production by malignant lymphocytes. These proteins either bind to or mimic antigens on RBC or platelet membranes, resulting in immune-mediated destruction of RBCs (Chun 2004). Possible causes for thrombocytopenia are decreased platelet life span due to accelerated removal from the circulation, associated with microaggregation stimulated by the tumor. In addition, thrombocytopenia can be caused by the production of antiplatelet antibodies by the tumor, and cross reactivity between tumor antigens and platelet antigens (Lucas 2009). Other CBC abnormalities in paraneoplastic syndrome includes eosinophilia. Eosinophilia is considered a marker for systemic or intestinal mast cell neoplasia.

Abnormal WBC count can also be a paraneoplastic condition. A leukocytosis without obvious infection has been associated with lung, GI, and genitourinary tumors, and lymphoma. Etiology of leukocytosis is thought to be from cytokine production enhancing the production of granulocytes and their release from bone marrow into the peripheral blood (Lucas 2009).

The most common *blood chemistry abnormalities* associated with a paraneoplastic response includes hypercalcemia and hypoglycemia. Hypercalcemia occurs secondary to malignant cell production of a parathyroid hormone-related peptide (PTHrp).

Hypoglycemia is often associated with insulinoma and other tumors such as hepatomas, leiomyomas/leiomyosarcomas, and carcinomas. Patients with hypoglycemia often do not exhibit clinical signs until glucose is very low (<30 mg/dL) due to gradual decline in glucose over time. Diagnosis of hypoglycemia secondary to a neoplastic disease process typically includes abdominal ultrasound to rule out evidence of a mass. Measuring insulin levels are recommended to rule out an insulinoma, as insulinomas are often not visualized on ultrasound or radiographs. *Clinical signs* of hypoglycemia include weakness, disorientation, seizures, coma, and death. Surgical extirpation is the treatment of choice for tumors that produce hypoglycemia.

Hypercalcemia

Hypercalcemia is the most common metabolic emergency seen in veterinary patients with cancer (Matthews 2006). The most common cause of hypercalcemia in dogs is lymphoma, more specifically T cell (Ogilvie 2006). Other disorders associated with hypercalcemia in both the dog and cat include acute and chronic renal failure, vitamin D toxicosis, hypoadrenocorticism, anal gland carcinomas, multiple myeloma, systemic mycoses, and primary hyperparathyroidism (PHP). Hypercalcemia, including its diagnosis and treatment, are discussed further in Chapter 19, "Fluid Therapy, Electrolyte, and Acid–Base Disorders."

Anaphylaxis/Allergic Reactions

Anaphylaxis is a life-threatening, acute allergic reaction caused by drugs, vaccines, food substances, envenomation, insect bites, incompatible blood products, or any ingested foreign material. Clinical signs range in severity from hyperthermia, hypotension, bronchoconstriction, tachypnea, seizures, angioedema, laryngeal and pulmonary edema, to less severe clinical signs of vomiting, diarrhea, urticaria, erythema, and pruritis. Adverse clinical signs can occur within seconds to minutes following intravenous administration but may be delayed for hours with other routes of administration. Chemotherapy-induced anaphylaxis can occur almost immediately after drug administration; common chemotherapy drugs include L-asparaginase and doxorubicin (Ogilvie 2006). Fatal reactions can occur at any time to any drug or stimulating agent, resulting in acute collapse, cardiovascular failure, and/or severe hypotension.

Allergic drug reactions (Type I hypersensitivities) are inflammatory reactions mediated by IgE bound to mast cells and basophils; Type I hypersensitivities are usually unrelated to the drugs' pharmacological effect (Dowling 2004). Clinical signs occur as a result of the release of histamine, serotonin, and chemotactic factors. Although initial exposure to the offending drug usually produces a minimal reaction, subsequent exposures can result in a severe or potentially fatal reaction. Allergic reactions can often be minimized by pretreatment with antihistamines and or corticosteroids. Hypersensitivity reactions can also be treated by simply stopping the drug therapy. Chemotherapy (e.g., L-asparaginase) may be given intramuscularly to reduce the probability of anaphylaxis, or may be given as a slow IV infusion diluted with 0.9% sodium chloride (Fig. 11.11).

Treatment of drug-induced anaphylaxis includes basic triage protocols—ensure a patent airway, provide oxygen (and intubate if needed), and support the patient's cardiovascular system via aggressive crystalloid fluid administration (severe hypotension should

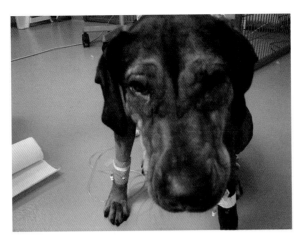

Figure 11.11   Significant facial angioedema in a patient experiencing an allergic reaction. (Courtesy of Thomas Walker DVM, DACVECC.)

be treated with colloids and/or pressor agents). Initiation of drug therapy (antihistamines, corticosteroids, and/or epinephrine in severe cases) should commence immediately. Anaphylaxis patients need continuous monitoring, including frequent auscultation of heart and lung sounds, pulse strength, serial blood pressure monitoring, ECG monitoring, CVP monitoring (if possible), frequent body temperature analysis, and laboratory assessment (blood gases, lactate, electrolytes, CBC, and serum chemistries). GI protectants (H2 blockers) are generally indicated once the patient has been stabilized.

References

Bruchim, Y, et al. 2008. Disseminated intravascular coagulation. *Compendium on Continuing Education for the Practicing Veterinarian* 30(10). Available online.

Brugmann, B, Smith, A. 2008. Neutropenia and sepsis in chemotherapy patients. *Standards of Care: Emergency and Critical Care Medicine* 10(8):1–6.

Chun, R. 2004. *Canine Lymphoma: What is the "Best" Chemotherapy Protocol?* Western Veterinary Conference Proceedings.

Cohen, M. 2003. Acute tumor lysis syndrome. *Standards of Care: Emergency and Critical Care Medicine* 5(8):7–11.

Colville, T, Bassert, J. 2002. *Clinical Anatomy and Physiology for Veterinary Technicians.* St. Louis, MO: Mosby, pp. 194–219.

Dowling, P. 2004. *Adverse Drug Reactions: Recognition and Management.* Western Veterinary Conference Proceedings.

Ganong, WF. 2001. *Review of Medical Physiology*, 20th ed. New York: McGraw-Hill, pp. 556–573.

Gopegui, RR, Feldman, BF. 2000. *Platelets and Von Willebrand's Disease. Textbook of Veterinary Internal Medicine, Ettinger*, Vol. 2, 5th ed. Philadelphia: W.B. Saunders, pp. 1817–1827.

Hackner, S. 2004. *Bleeding Disorders Made Incredibly Simple, Pt.1.* International Veterinary Emergency and Critical Care Symposium Proceedings.

Jandry, K. 2009. *Colloid Effects on Hemostasis*. International Veterinary Emergency and Critical Care Symposium Proceedings.

Kociba, GJ. 2000. *Leukocyte Changes in Disease. Textbook of Veterinary Internal Medicine, Ettinger*, Vol. 2, 5th ed. Philadelphia: W.B. Saunders, pp. 1842–1855.

Lucas, SRR. 2009. *Hematologic Alterations in Neoplasia*. World Small Animal Veterinary Association World Congress Proceedings.

Macintire, D, et al. 2006. *Manual of Small Animal Emergency and Critical Care Medicine*. Ames, IA: Blackwell, pp. 279–295.

Macintire, DK. 2005. *How I Use Immunoglobulins*. International Veterinary Emergency and Critical Care Symposium Proceedings.

Balch, A, Mackin, A. 2007. Canine IMHA: pathophysiology, clinical signs, and diagnosis. *Compendium on Continuing Education for the Practicing Veterinarian* 29(4): 217–224.

Matthews, KA. 2006. *Veterinary Emergency Critical Care Manual*. Guelph, ON: Lifelearn, pp. 627–628, 373–376, 417–421, 588–596.

Moore, E. 2002. *Autoimmune Diseases and Their Environmental Triggers*. Jefferson, NC: McFarland.

Northrup, N, Gieger, T. 2004. Clinical approach to patients with epistaxis. *Compendium on Continuing Education for the Practicing Veterinarian* 26(1):30–43.

Ogilvie, GK. 2006. Neutropenia, sepsis and thrombocytopenia. In *Veterinary Emergency Medicine Secrets*, edited by Wingfield, WE. Philadelphia: Hanley and Belfus, pp. 235–241.

Ogilvie, GK, Moore, AS. 2001. *Managing the Veterinary Cancer Patient*. Philadelphia: Veterinary Learning Systems.

Tizard, I. 1996. *Veterinary Immunology*, 4th ed. Philadelphia: W.B. Saunders, pp. 18–26.

White, C, Reine, N. 2009. Feline nonregenerative anemia: diagnosis and treatment. *Compendium on Continuing Education for the Practicing Veterinarian* 31(5):E1–E12.

CHAPTER 11

Neurological Emergencies

Sally R. Powell

Introduction

Alterations in neurological status are a common presentation in the emergent patient. Many patients with neurological disorders require extended hospital stays and intensive nursing care. Immediate and accurate assessment along with proper treatment is essential to a successful outcome.

The central nervous system (CNS) is a complex system that can be challenging to evaluate and treat. Abnormalities, deficits, and mentation changes that are neurological in origin can be a direct result of primary central nervous disease but can also be secondarily caused by systemic or metabolic disorders.

Increasing the knowledge base of the medical caregivers can only positively affect the patient in the treatment and nursing care they receive. The information in this chapter will cover common neurological disorders affecting the brain and spinal cord. You should gain enhanced knowledge in the areas of pathophysiology, assessment, and treatment of disease process, as well as monitoring and management of these critical patients.

Specific Neurological Emergencies

Traumatic Brain Injury (TBI)

TBI caused by automobile accidents, household accidents (stepped on, fallen on, struck by objects), gunshots, bites, and falls is a relatively common occurrence in small animal emergency medicine. Regardless of the cause, the effects of head trauma are a result of direct tissue injury.

Aggressive treatment aimed at preventing secondary brain injury while stabilizing the major organ systems must be instituted in order to minimize irreversible brain injury or death. Good nursing care and monitoring are essential in decreasing morbidity and mortality in these critically ill patients.

Pathophysiology of TBI

Primary brain injury occurs as a result of direct tissue and vasculature injury from trauma. Damage to the tissue can be in the form of contusions, lacerations, or axonal damage. The vasculature can be affected causing hemorrhage, edema, and a decrease in perfusion to the brain. Little can be done to control the amount of damage that results from primary brain injury. The goal in the treatment of head injury is to prevent the detrimental effects of secondary brain injury.

Secondary brain injury occurs when biochemical pathways, set off by direct tissue injury, hypoxia, and decreased perfusion, act together to perpetuate further brain damage. Secondary brain injury further contributes to an increased intracranial pressure (ICP). Some of the pathophysiological changes that result in neuronal damage include adenosine triphosphate (ATP) depletion, intracellular sodium and calcium accumulation, elevated excitatory neurotransmitters, oxygen free radicals production, unregulated inflammatory mediators, and lactic acidosis.

The most important aspect in controlling secondary brain injury is maintenance of perfusion to the brain and prevention of hypoxemia. Normally, the brain has the ability to regulate changes in pressure and pH within the cranial cavity. Blood flow autoregulation refers to the brain's ability to maintain a normal ICP despite changes in mean arterial blood pressure (MAP). When MAP rises, vasoconstriction occurs in the body; if the MABP falls, vasodilation occurs. Blood flow autoregulation helps prevent increases in ICP when blood pressure is high and assures adequate cerebral blood flow (CBF) in the face of low blood pressure. Patients suffering from TBI can lose the ability to pressure-autoregulate. Therefore, maintaining a normal MAP is essential to assure an adequate CBF.

Chemical changes such as an increase or decrease in pH cause vascular changes in the body. Elevated $PaCO_2$ levels cause vasodilation of the brain's vasculature and decreased $PaCO_2$ levels cause vasoconstriction. Chemical autoregulation refers to the brain's ability to sense changes in pH and regulate blood flow based upon those changes. This helps assure adequate CBF in the face of changes in the pH of the blood.

In order to understand ICP, it is important to understand what makes up the normal contents of the cranial cavity. The cranial cavity consists of brain parenchyma (brain tissue), blood, and cerebrospinal fluid. When brain injury occurs, swelling of the tissue (edema) and changes in the vasculature can cause decreased oxygenation and nutritional support to an organ with extremely high oxygen and nutritional needs. Cerebral perfusion pressure (CPP) determines CBF. The definition of CPP is

$$CPP = MAP - ICP.$$

Changes in ICP and MAP have a direct impact on how much blood is being delivered to brain tissue. Increases in ICP and decreases in MAP can cause a decrease in blood supply, and increases in MAP can cause increases in CBF and ICP. For this reason, it is extremely important to maintain a normal MAP in brain-injured patients. When there is hemorrhage and edema in the intracranial compartment, the result is an increased ICP. The cranial cavity accommodates for the increased volume by shifting fluid in the brain's vasculature and cerebral spinal fluid pathways in an attempt to decrease ICP. This function is called intracranial compliance. The effectiveness of intracranial compliance decreases as ICP increases.

Primary survey and treatment

The primary survey of the TBI patient should focus on stabilization of the patient's major body systems (respiratory, cardiovascular, and central nervous system [CNS]). A patient that presents in hypovolemic shock can often appear depressed or mentally dull. Correction of hypoxia and hypovolemia is the primary goal in the initial resuscitation of the trauma patient.

A decrease in oxygen content of brain tissue is common following TBI. This can occur secondary to cellular swelling and increases in ICP. Decreases in oxygen delivery to all of the tissues in the body may occur when there is trauma to the chest causing pulmonary contusions or pneumothorax or when cardiac output is decreased. Arterial blood gas analysis is a useful tool in evaluating the TBI patient's respiratory status. PaO_2 (partial pressure of oxygen) should be maintained above 90 mmHg, and the $PaCO_2$ should range between 30 and 35 mmHg.

Pulse oximeter readings can be used in the absence of arterial blood gas analysis. Pulse oximeters will measure oxygen saturation of hemoglobin but will not give information about the patient's ventilatory status. When using pulse oximetry, it is important to obtain a good, consistent waveform and keep in mind that these monitors often will not work accurately in patients with poor perfusion and or anemia. Pulse oximeter readings at 95% and above are considered to be normal. It is best to provide oxygen support to the brain-injured patient as they tend to be hypoxic.

Stabilization of the patient's cardiovascular status is paramount in preventing secondary brain injury. Resuscitation choices may be altered in patients with obvious head trauma. Crystalloids are often used in combination with hypertonic saline (7.5%) or hetastarch (6%). The goal of treatment for the brain-injured patient is to restore intravascular volume without exacerbating increases in ICP by over-resuscitating the patient. Both hypertonic saline and hetastarch have been shown to improve MAP without aggravating cerebral edema.

Hypertonic saline requires small volumes to restore intravascular volume and is diluted with hetastarch to a 7.5% solution (1/3 hypertonic saline to 2/3 hetastarch). This solution is given at a dose of 3–5 mL/kg over 10–15 minutes. More judicious doses are used in cats. The return of normal physical parameters (pink mucous membrane [MM], normal capillary refill time [CRT], strong pulse quality with normal pulse rate) is a good indication of euvolemia. MAP should be checked directly or indirectly whenever possible. It is important to maintain patients on a continuous rate infusion of normal isotonic fluids in order to maintain MAP and normal hydration status.

Once euvolemia is accomplished, an initial evaluation of the CNS can be completed and further treatment for cerebral edema may be instituted. In patients that present hypertension and bradycardia (Cushing's reflex), this treatment may be initiated immediately.

Mannitol is an osmotic diuretic and is the most commonly used drug in cases where increased ICP is suspected. The mechanisms of action associated with mannitol are numerous, but the most immediate effect is caused by reflex vasoconstriction. Mannitol thins the blood flowing through the vasculature in the brain, causing the vessels to vasoconstrict. This causes an immediate decrease in ICP by improving CPP at a lower brain blood volume. The osmotic actions of mannitol take effect within 15–30 minutes and will last between 2 and 5 hours.

Because mannitol is a hyperosmolar sugar-alcohol substance, it is given as a bolus slowly over 20 minutes (to avoid irritation of the vessels) at a dose of 1 g/kg. Improvement of clinical signs associated with the administration of mannitol would include positive changes in pupils, mentation, and posture. Additional doses of mannitol may be necessary, with a general rule of no more than 3 doses in a 24-hour period. If no initial response to administration of mannitol is noted, further therapy with mannitol is not recommended.

Secondary survey

When the patient's respiratory and cardiovascular and neurological systems have been addressed and appropriate treatment has been initiated to treat hypoxia, hypovolemia, and cerebral edema, a more thorough assessment of all four major organ systems can be accomplished. The systems include respiratory, cardiovascular, central nervous, and renal. These systems are evaluated and reevaluated in patients that present with any type of acute trauma. Evaluation of skeletal and musculoskeletal systems and assessment of abdominal organs should be performed.

A complete neurological evaluation should include assessment of cranial nerves: menace, fundic, pupil size and reactivity, blink, jaw tone, and gag, along with evaluating the position of the eye (strabismus) and whether there is any eye movement (nystagmus) (Fig. 12.1).

The skull should be palpated for fractures and the ear canals assessed for hemorrhage or cerebral spinal fluid leakage (Fig. 12.2). Evaluation of the patient's level of consciousness and posture may give the most information as to the seriousness of the head injury (Table 12.1).

In the recumbent patient, the head and neck should be elevated approximately 15–30 degrees above the rest of the body. This will facilitate cerebral venous drainage and decrease ICP by reducing intracranial blood volume. Elevating the patient on a board rather than propping the head on a towel will insure proper venous outflow and avoid obstruction of vessels in the neck. It is contraindicated to elevate the head any more than 30 degrees due to the possibility of decreasing CBF.

Monitoring and nursing care of the TBI patient

Monitoring of the TBI patient should include frequent assessment of the CNS and serial evaluations of blood pressure, oxygenation, and ventilatory status. Serial assessment of cranial nerves, brain stem reflexes, level of consciousness, and motor activity will help to determine the degree of damage and response to treatment. Blood pressure can be measured directly or indirectly via Doppler or oscillometric devices. Mean arterial

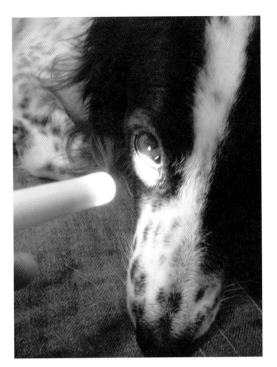

Figure 12.1 A complete neurological evaluation should include assessment of cranial nerves including pupil size and reactivity to light.

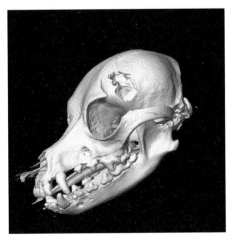

Figure 12.2 The skull should be palpated for fractures and the ear canals assessed for hemorrhage or cerebral spinal fluid leakage. Here a reconstructive computerized tomography (CT) image shows a skull fracture that was detected on skull palpation.

pressure (MAP) should be maintained above 80 mmHg in order to ensure adequate CBF. Oxygenation can be monitored noninvasively via pulse oximetry. Oxygenation and ventilation can be measured by evaluating an arterial blood gas sample. A continuous electrocardiogram (ECG) is ideal to ensure a normal heart rate. Bradycardia with concurrent hypertension (*Cushing's reflex*) is often an indication that the ICP is increasing and aggressive therapy is indicated.

Table 12.1   Level of consciousness assessment

Levels of Consciousness

Alert	Bright and responsive
Depressed	Quiet but responsive
Delirium/dementia	Inappropriate response to stimuli
Obtunded	Decreased alertness with arousable periods
Stuporous	Unresponsive except to painful stimuli
Coma	Unresponsive to any stimuli

Nursing care is fundamental in the treatment and successful recovery of the TBI patient. In the recumbent patient, the head and neck should be elevated approximately 15–30 degrees above the rest of the body. This will facilitate cerebral venous drainage and decrease ICP by reducing intracranial blood volume. Elevating the patient on a board rather than propping the head on a towel will insure proper venous outflow and avoid obstruction of vessels in the neck. It is contraindicated to elevate the head any more than 30 degrees due to the possibility of decreasing CBF. Accessing blood samples via jugular veins should be avoided. Recumbent patients should also be turned every 2–4 hours to prevent atelactasis. Lubrication of the eyes every 4 hours will help prevent corneal drying and ulcers in patients unable to blink.

Serial monitoring of physical parameters (MM color, CRT, pulse rate and quality, temperature, and respiratory rate and effort) and extended database (packed cell volume [PCV], total protein [TP], and blood glucose, Na, K, and blood urea nitrogen [BUN]) provide important information regarding response to treatment or possible deterioration of the patient's status. Patients with altered mentation are often unable to urinate on their own. These patients require serial palpation and emptying of the bladder via expression or urinary catheterization. Clean bedding with adequate padding will prevent pressure sores and urine scald. The outcome of the head trauma patient can be greatly improved by the monitoring and nursing care that the patient receives. Never underestimate your role in the recovery of the head trauma patient.

Cerebrovascular Accident (CVA)

A CVA or stroke is a term used to describe a reduction of blood supply to the brain. Clinical signs vary depending upon which part of the brain is affected, but these patients most commonly present with acute signs of focal, asymmetrical, and nonprogressive brain dysfunction.

Pathophysiology of CVA

There are two causes of CVA recognized in patients: ischemia (obstructive) and hemorrhage (rupture). An ischemic CVA is the consequence of an arterial obstruction, venous thrombosis or embolism, or the occlusion of blood vessels from abnormalities such as vasculitis. In any case, the result is a decrease in blood supply to that part of the brain.

Ischemia, which produces necrosis of neurons and glial elements, results in a focal area of dead tissue called an infarct. A transient ischemic attack (TIA) is a mild form of stroke and presents with an abrupt onset of neurological signs which diminish in less than 24 hours. These types of ischemic CVAs are not well documented but are believed to occur in dogs and cats. Global brain ischemia is a less commonly encountered event as the survival rate from cardiopulmonary arrest is very low. Diseases associated with infarction in dogs and cats include hypothyroidism, idiopathic hyperlipoproteinemia (schnauzers), sepsis, coagulopathy, neoplasia, and heartworm infections.

A hemorrhagic CVA is the result of the rupture of blood vessels within or around the brain. They are classified as epidural, subdural, subarachnoid, intraparenchymal, or intraventricular. Secondary brain injury resulting from cerebral ischemia was previously thought to have occurred due to compression of the region of the brain surrounding the hematoma. However, recent studies indicate that the presence of a hematoma initiates edema and neuronal damage in surrounding parenchyma. Edema is brought on in the early stages by the release and accumulation of osmotically active serum proteins from the clot. Fluid collects in the area around the hematoma and can persist for 5 days to 2 weeks.

Clinical signs and diagnosis

CVA can be categorized by peracute or acute onset of clinical signs. The primary complaint consists of changes in mentation and behavior (aggression, dementia, compulsive circling, stupor, and coma) and/or neurological deficits (proprioception, vision, coordination). The severity of clinical signs is associated with the specific area affected and the type (ischemic or hemorrhagic, global, or focal). Commonly, patients present with acute focal signs that are nonprogressive and asymmetrical. However, progression of clinical signs and neurological deficits can be seen up to 24–72 hours following an infarction. Hemorrhagic CVA can be more progressive in nature, and severity of acute signs is dependent on the size of the lesion. Seizure activity is commonly associated with stroke, especially in hemorrhagic CVA.

Diagnostic testing includes complete blood count, chemistry analysis, thyroid panel, coagulation profile, urinalysis, urine culture, and fecal analysis, which are indicated to rule out underlying disease processes described earlier. The evaluation of cerebrospinal fluid will not confirm a diagnosis of CVA but will help to rule out inflammatory CNS disease.

Computed tomography (CT) and magnetic resonance imaging (MRI) are necessary to differentiate between a CVA and other causes for brain disorders. MRI is more sensitive than CT in early infarction, and CT is very sensitive for acute hemorrhage.

Treatment, monitoring, and prognosis

Treatment goals of CVA are identical to that of a patient experiencing head trauma. The objective of treatment is to maintain normal MAP, ensure adequate CPP, provide oxygen therapy, control seizures, and treat underlying disease processes. Mannitol may be used in the acute phase (0.5 g–1 g/kg) to reduce cerebral edema. Corticosteroids are not shown to provide any beneficial effects.

Thrombolytic agents such as streptokinase and tissue plasminogen activator (TPA) are widely used in human medicine for treatment of nonhemmorhagic CVA. Unfortunately, reperfusion injury is a possible detrimental side effect of using clot-busting agents and

CHAPTER 12

occurs when blood flow is suddenly restored to the limbs. Massive electrolyte disturbances such as hyperkalemia and metabolic acidosis can result. These consequences appear to be especially severe in dogs and cats.

The body is capable of dissolving clots on its own, but this takes time. Vessels in the tissues adjacent to the blocked vessel experience a gradual increase in blood flow, and new vessels form, arising from the embolized vessel. Therefore, because of the high likelihood of severe reperfusion injury, high drug cost, and questionable benefit, many practitioners are reluctant to pursue clot-busting therapy in veterinary patients.

Monitoring and nursing care goals are identical than those of the head trauma patient. Observe changes in neurological, respiratory, cardiovascular, and renal systems.

Prognosis of patients affected by CVA varies depending upon the severity of the clinical signs and the location of the lesion. Most cases will improve over a few days to a few weeks.

Seizure Disorders

A seizure is usually defined as a sudden alteration of behavior due to a temporary change in the electrical functioning of the brain, in particular the outside rim of the brain called the cortex. The type of symptoms and seizures depend on where the abnormal electrical activity takes place in the brain, what its cause is, and such factors as the patient's age and general state of health. Continuous unrelenting seizure activity is referred to as status epilepticus (status) and is a life-threatening condition.

Pathophysiology of seizure activity

Clinically, the etiology of seizures may be broadly categorized into intracranial or extracranial causes. Extracranial causes for seizure activity can be due to metabolic disorders (i.e., hypoglycemia, hypocalcemia, and hypoxia), toxicities and environmental disturbances (i.e., lead, organophosphates, metronidazole, ethylene glycol, heat prostration, and snake envenomation), and nutritional disorders (late-stage thiamine deficiency in cats). Intracranial causes can include neoplasia, congenital, infectious, immune-mediated, traumatic, and vascular disorders.

The seizure activity itself can be further classified into three categories. A generalized seizure is when the electrical discharge in the cerebral cortex is diffuse. These types of seizures are often associated with extracranial causes for seizures. A partial seizure is associated with a focal electrical discharge that only involves one portion of the brain. These seizures are more often linked with intracranial causes for seizures that have caused brain damage and a seizure focus. Finally, a partial with secondary generalized seizure happens when a focal electrical discharge generalizes to the entire cerebral cortex. These, too, are associated with intracranial causes for seizures (Fig. 12.3).

Primary survey and treatment

The primary survey of the seizure patient should focus on stabilization of the patient's major body systems (respiratory, cardiovascular, and CNS). In a patient that is actively convulsing, the aim would be to stabilize the CNS by stopping the seizure.

Placement of an intravenous catheter and collection of blood from the hub of the catheter for evaluation of PCV, total solids, blood glucose, dipstick BUN, serum electrolytes

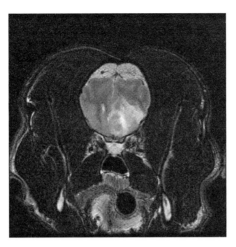

Figure 12.3   One common cause of sudden onset seizures in the older patient is cerebral neoplasia. This case was diagnosed with a brain tumor on MRI.

(particularly calcium and sodium), and osmolality can be performed quickly. If the patient is hypoglycemic (blood glucose less than 60 mg/dL), an intravenous bolus of dextrose (0.5 g/kg of 50% dextrose diluted 1:4 with isotonic fluid) is given first. The bolus may be followed by a constant rate infusion (CRI) of 2.5%–5% dextrose in isotonic crystalloids. The blood glucose should be monitored closely to establish a trend to euglycemia. Hypoglycemia as a cause for seizures is most commonly seen in insulin overdose, insulinoma, or in very young animals with a history of vomiting, anorexia, and diarrhea.

If hypoglycemia is not the cause for the seizure, then diazepam (0.5–1 mg/kg), a gamma-aminobutyric acid (GABA) agonist, is administered intravenously. The effects of diazepam are rapid in onset (less than 1 minute) and relatively short in duration. Diazepam achieves anticonvulsant effects by enhancing GABA activity in the brain. If seizures are not controlled within 30 seconds to 1 minute of administration, then a second intravenous bolus may be necessary.

If seizures are not controlled with the second diazepam bolus, it is unlikely that this drug will be effective. Phenobarbital is often given in conjunction with diazepam. Phenobarbital is a barbiturate as well as an effective anticonvulsant. The onset of action is much slower than diazepam. It may take up to 30 minutes to reach peak effect in the patient's bloodstream. However, its effects may last for hours, while diazepam effects are short in duration (about 30 minutes). The loading dose for phenobarbital (16 mg/kg) is given in divided doses (4 mg/kg) at 30-minute intervals or more to better monitor the level of sedation. The patient may not receive the complete loading dose if the level of sedation is too deep.

While waiting for phenobarbital to reach therapeutic blood levels, it may be necessary to administer second regimen drugs. The administration of Levetiracetam (Keppra®, UCB Pharmaceuticals, Inc., Brussels, Belgium) (20 mg/kg IV every 8 hours), thiopental (10–20 mg/kg), or propofol (1–6 mg/kg slowly to effect) can be used if full seizure activity continues despite diazepam and phenobarbital administration (Fig. 12.4).

Propofol has been shown to control the muscular manifestations of the brain's seizure activity but does little to affect the activity within the brain. If a propofol bolus is effective in halting seizure activity, an intravenous propofol CRI can be initiated (0.1–0.6 mg/kg/minute). Propofol also decreases ICP and brain metabolic activity (Table 12.2).

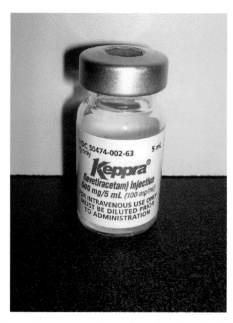

Figure 12.4   Levetiracetam (Keppra) is a newer anticonvulsant that has gained popularity in the last few years.

In all of these second regimen drugs, the patient will be profoundly sedated and may require intubation and possibly ventilation. The patient should be carefully monitored during second regimen drug administration to avoid an overdose. It is also important not to confuse recovery from barbiturate anesthesia (paddling, disorientation, and vocalization, etc.) with another seizure. In the presence of seizure activity, the pupils will usually be dilated. When second regimen drugs fail to control seizure activity, inhalants must be considered.

Obtaining a thorough history from the client is of utmost importance. Acquiring information detailing the type of seizure, duration, onset, and frequency will help determine an active disease process or if the animal has epilepsy.

Epilepsy can be defined differently in the literature. For the purpose of this chapter, epilepsy will be defined as a disorder of recurrent seizures with no underlying disease process. There are two categories of epilepsy, inherited (also known as primary or true) and acquired. Inherited epilepsy is more common in purebred dogs. The first sign of seizure activity commonly begins between 6 months and 3 years of age. Acquired epilepsy is inherited by some type of insult to the brain that causes a seizure focus (prevalent in head trauma cases). The first seizure can occur at any age.

Associated physical examination findings of patients presenting in status or with a history of cluster seizures include hyperthermia, tachycardia, and tachypnea; hyperemic mucous membranes and a less than one second CRT. Cerebral edema and disseminated intravascular coagulation (DIC) are two of the most serious sequelae to unrelenting seizures. Clinical signs of cerebral edema include changes in pupil size or responsiveness to light, dull mentation, seizure activity, and coma. Cerebral edema leads to an increased ICP and can result in herniation of the brain through the foramen magnum. DIC may be manifest by petechiation, ecchymosis, hematemesis, hematuria, and bloody stool (Table 12.3).

Table 12.2   Treatment protocols for cluster seizures or status epilepticus

	Dose	Effects
First line drugs		
Diazepam	0.2–0.5 mg/kg IV or 1 mg/kg rectally; may repeat 2–3 times	Onset within seconds to 3 minutes; good anticonvulsant effects; can be followed by CRI of 0.5–1.0 mg/kg/h in maintenance fluids at 40–60 mL/kg/h (0.9% NACL—wrap bag and line—light sensitive)
Midazolam	0.3 mg/kg IV; may repeat 2–3 times	Onset within seconds to 3 minutes; good anticonvulsant effects; can be followed by CRI of 0.1–0.5 mg/kg/h
Phenobarbital	Loading dose of 16 mg/kg IV divided into 3–4 doses in 30-minute intervals	May take up to 30 minutes before full effects are noted; good anticonvulsant effects
Second line drugs		
Levetiracetam	20 mg/kg IV every 8 hours; single loading dose of 60 mg/kg IV may be given	Rapid onset; may be given with phenobarbital and diazepam/midazolam
Thiopental	10–20 mg/kg IV administered as 2–4 mg/kg boluses to effect	Rapid onset; may not stop seizure activity (when evaluated with an electroencephalograph [EEG], an instrument that measures brain activity); will prevent life-threatening hyperthermia and DIC
Propofol	6–8 mg/kg IV given as 1–2 mg/kg boluses to effect, followed by a continuous rate infusion of 0.1–0.6 mg/kg/min	Rapid onset; has been demonstrated to have GABA agonistic activity in the brain; cerebroprotective by decreasing ICP and brain metabolic activity
Isoflurane anesthesia (last resort)	1%–2% Minimum alveolar concentration (MAC) with ventilatory support if necessary; minimum of 6 hours	Intubation with gas anesthesia can be used as a last resort

Notes: For first line drugs, phenobarbital and diazepam/midazolam may be given concurrently. These doses are based on canines. For second line drugs, information exists that thiopental and propofol abate motor manifestations of seizures but not uncontrolled electrical activity of neurons within the brain based on EEG. Recovery from all of the above drugs can be confused with seizure activity.

Monitoring the seizure patient

Patients that present with cluster seizures or status epilepticus require intense critical care monitoring. Perfusion parameters such as temperature, MM color, CRT, pulse rate and quality, and cranial nerve function should be monitored frequently. These potentially critical patients require routine monitoring of vital signs as well as serial evaluations of lead II ECG and MAP. Hypotension in patients with increased ICP from cerebral edema can be devastating to the brain due to reduced CBF.

Table 12.3   Clinical signs of increasing intracranial pressure

Mild	+/– Anisocoria, depressed LOC, sluggish PLR
Moderate	+/– Anisocoria, obtunded LOC, sluggish PLR, +/– mydriasis
Extensive	Bradycardia, decerbrate posture, myosis, stupor/comatose LOC, $\uparrow$ systolic blood pressure, +/– seizure activity

Adequate ventilation and oxygenation should be assured in all patients, particularly ones that have been heavily sedated. Keen observation of respiratory rate and effort as well as lung auscultation are paramount. These patients may have secondary respiratory problems such as aspiration pneumonia or neurogenic pulmonary edema. Severe depression of ventilatory drive may occur secondary to drug administration and problems with increased ICP. More objective measurements such as serial pulse oximetry and arterial blood gas measurements should be evaluated in patients with suspected respiratory compromise.

Hypoxia to the brain and inadequate ventilation may contribute to cerebral edema and brain damage. In hypoxic patients that can adequately ventilate, oxygen can be delivered via mask, oxygen cage, or through a nasal cannula. Hypoxic patients that cannot ventilate adequately may require mechanical ventilation.

Serial neurological evaluations should be performed in any patient with CNS abnormalities. Observing the level of consciousness and performing cranial nerve examinations are the most helpful methods for monitoring CNS function. A baseline examination done at admission and serial evaluations thereafter will establish trends and effectiveness of therapy.

An altered level of consciousness is a measure of arousal other than normal. Level of consciousness (LOC) is a measurement of a patient's arousability and responsiveness to stimuli from the environment. A dull LOC may be classed as depressed; a patient in this state can be aroused with little difficulty. Patients who are delirious or are suffering from dementia have an abnormal response to their environment. Obtunded patients have a more depressed level of consciousness and cannot be fully aroused but have periods where they are arousable. Those who are not able to be aroused from a sleep-like state and are only responsive to noxious stimuli are said to be stuporous, and a coma is defined as the inability to make any purposeful response. Progression to stupor or coma, or continued seizure activity warrants aggressive treatment.

Basic nursing care should be provided for any patient with altered mentation. Monitoring physical parameters such as temperature, pulse, and respiratory rate and effort, auscultation of lung fields, MAP, serial evaluation of acid–base status, electrolytes, and hydration status (PCV/TS) will help to identify potential serious sequale to seizure activity such as aspiration pneumonia and noncardiogenic pulmonary edema. A patient in lateral recumbency should be turned every 4 hours to prevent atelectasis and pressure sores.

Palpation and complete evacuation of the urinary bladder will help to prevent urinary tract infections and problems with bladder tone in patients unable to void due to abnormal mentation or sedation. Placement of an indwelling urinary catheter should be considered if the bladder is difficult to express. Lubrication of the eyes every 4 hours helps prevent corneal ulcers, and soft padding and removal of collars will help protect the patient during seizure activity. The staff can be protected by placing the intravenous catheter in a peripheral vein in the back leg with a low volume extension set attached to provide easy intravenous access.

Spinal Cord Injury

Spinal cord injury is a frequent emergency presentation in small animal patients. Acute spinal cord lesions may be due to internal or external causes. Internal causes include prolapsed intervertebral disc material, fibrocartilagenous emboli, and fractures secondary to bone diseases like neoplastic or nutritional disorders. External causes of spinal cord injury include fractures, and luxations secondary to traumatic events. Common causes for external trauma include being vehicular trauma, bite wounds, and gunshot wounds.

Fibrocartilagenous Emboli (FCE)

FCE is initiated when a piece of fibrocartilage (intervertebral disc material) enters the spinal artery or vein, causing an infarction (obstruction). The infarction results in necrosis (cell death) in the region affected. Although it is most commonly seen in giant and large breed dogs, some small breed dogs have a predisposition to this disease process (Shetland sheepdogs, miniature schnauzers).

Clinical signs are acute, usually nonpainful, and often follow exercise with some mild trauma. Neurological deficits vary depending upon the area of spine effected but are often asymmetric. Signs may progress over 12–24 hours. A thorough history detailing onset and any progression of clinical signs along with a neurological examination will help localize the lesion. Spinal radiographs will not show any abnormalities and in many cases, an MRI will be normal. Diagnosis is accomplished by ruling out other disease processes that produce similar clinical signs.

Therapy for FCE is centered around supportive care. There is no surgical procedure to repair the infarcted portion of the spinal cord. Healing of the area will take time, and physical therapy can be a critical component to a successful recovery. Management of these patients is similar to that of a patient with intervertebral disc disease (IVDD) which is detailed below.

IVDD

The most common cause of internal trauma to the spinal cord is Hansen Type I IVDD. The intervertebral discs are located between two vertebrae throughout the vertebral column. The function of the disc is to act as a cushion and absorb shock along the spinal column. The disc itself is composed of an outer fibrous material (annulus fibrosus), and a jelly-like inner material (nucleus pulposus). When the annulus fibrosus ruptures, the nucleus pulposus takes the path of least resistance and moves dorsally to impinge on the spinal cord.

Chondrodystrophic breeds of dogs are more likely to suffer from intervertebral disc disease than other breeds. Examples of these breeds include Dachshund, Lhasa Apso, and Basset Hound. In these breeds, the nucleus pulposus degenerates while the annulus

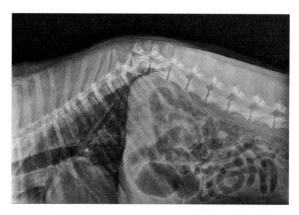

Figure 12.5   A radiograph revealing an obvious spinal fracture in a canine patient.

fibrosus weakens, causing the disc to rupture with minimal stress. The most common location for a disc rupture is at the T13-L1 disc space.

There are several types of forces that are associated with external causes of spinal trauma. Flexion is the first type and usually results in a prolapsed disc. The clinical signs can vary from mild paresis to paralysis and destruction of the spinal cord. Patients involved in automobile accidents often suffer from a combination of compression and flexion forces resulting in a fracture of the ventral portion of the vertebrae. Because these fractures tend to be more stable than many other spinal fractures, the clinical signs can vary. Concurrent flexion and rotation of the spinal column often results in luxation and fracture of the vertebrae. These types of injuries are often very unstable, and careful patient handling is necessary to prevent further injury. Clinical signs are often severe (paralysis) due to the severity of spinal cord damage, although a severe fracture may be present without neurological signs (Fig. 12.5).

To assess the severity of spinal cord lesions, it is necessary to evaluate cord function. In the mildest cases, the patient may experience only back or neck pain but be neurologically intact. The more severely affected animals may have neurological deficits that result from cord dysfunction. Criterion used to evaluate cord function includes conscious proprioception, voluntary motor function, and pain sensation. Because these criteria are always affected progressively, they can be used to judge the severity of the lesion.

Conscious proprioception tests the patient's capacity to recognize the location of the limbs in relation to the rest of his body. Deficits surface as a knuckling of the foot. Voluntary motor is conscious purposeful movement of the limbs. Applying firm pressure to the bones of the digits tests the patient's pain response. When assessing pain, the patient should vocalize or turn to react to the pressure being applied to the bones of the digits. The withdrawal reflex, in which the limb is withdrawn without conscious awareness of pain, is commonly confused for the presence of pain but does not demonstrate the integrity of the spinal cord cranial to the lesion. Pain is the last parameter to be affected. When pain is absent, the lesion is more severe and carries a poorer prognosis.

Imaging spinal cord injuries

Localization of most spinal cord injuries begin with conventional radiographs (spinal radiographs and myelography). Survey radiographs will localize a lesion if the vertebrae

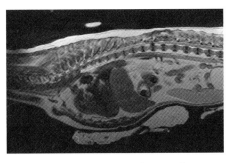

Figure 12.6   An MRI and CT can be invaluable imaging techniques for patients with a neurological disorder. Practices without these tools should consider referral.

or their ligamentous attachments are involved. They do not allow a direct view of the spinal cord. Spinal cord disorders that may not cause a visible change in the vertebrae are FCE, neoplasia of the spinal cord or meninges, intervertebral disc extrusion, and Wobbler's syndrome. Myelography, CT scan, or MRI are required to localize these lesions.

Myelography uses a subarachnoid injection of contrast media to outline the spinal cord. The most commonly used agents are iopamidol (Isovue, Bracco Diagnostics, Milan, Italy) and iohexol (Omnipaque, GE Healthcare, Inc., Princeton, NJ). The study must be performed under general anesthesia, and complications are infrequent, but can include exacerbation of neurological signs, seizures, anaphylaxsis, and death.

CT provides a three-dimensional image of soft tissue structures that cannot be seen on routine radiographic studies. This type of imaging can help to diagnose masses, IVDD, spinal stenosis, and bony proliferations. CT will also identify the invasiveness of a lesion (infection, trauma, neoplasia). This procedure can be costly but is becoming much more widely used in veterinary facilities and prices are coming down.

MRI enables direct visualization of the spinal cord, epidural space, and ligaments of the spine. It is the most sensitive imaging for soft tissue and is the most costly. MRI is, however, becoming very accessible for clients and patients interested in advanced imaging (Fig. 12.6).

Spinal cord injury treatment and management

Treatment of patients with suspected spinal trauma begins with the safe transport and handling of the patient upon arrival. The patient should have a complete physical and neurological examination with attention to stabilizing the respiratory and cardiovascular system when necessary. Analgesics can be used for pain in patients that do not have a compromised respiratory or cardiovascular status. Diazepam can be used in patients that are at risk of injuring themselves by flailing.

Although initial results were promising, no consensus has been met on the beneficial effects of steroids on acute spinal cord injury for either companion animals or humans. If used, methylprednisolone sodium succinate (30 mg/kg IV bolus, followed by two boluses of 15 mg/kg at 2 and 6 hours after the initial bolus) is most commonly prescribed among veterinary neurologists and neurosurgeons. Beneficial effects are demonstrated best when given within 8 hours of spinal cord injury; however, the use of steroid therapy varies between individuals. Dexamethazone has not been demonstrated to be as beneficial as methylprednisolone sodium succinate, and side effects can be more pronounced.

Management of spinal cord injuries may be medical, surgical, or a combination of both. Patients who have milder neurological deficits such as back pain or ataxia with voluntary motor function may be good candidates for conservative treatment. The mainstay of conservative treatment is strict cage rest. Patients with vertebral column fractures that have mild or no neurological deficits may be placed in a back brace to ensure stabilization of the fracture. Many patients will improve with 4–6 weeks of cage rest. The owner is advised to seek further veterinary attention if the neurological status deteriorates.

More severe neurological deficits are a clear indication for surgical intervention such as spinal cord decompression and/or vertebral column stabilization. Surgical intervention is common in patients with deteriorating neurological signs. Patients with surgical cervical spine disorders are treated with various approaches depending upon the location of lesion (ventral slot, fenestration, dorsal laminectomy, dorsolateral hemilaminectomy, or cervical stabilization via dorsal or ventral approach). Surgery of the thoracolumbar spine is treated similarly to cervical spine with the exception of the ventral approach (i.e., dorsal laminectomy, hemilaminectomy, fenestration, or thoracolumbar spinal stabilization via dorsal approach).

Excellent analgesia must also be provided to patients with IVDD regardless of whether cases will be treated medically or surgically. Patients who undergo surgery require aggressive pain management, including the use of mu agonist opioids for a minimum of 24 hours following surgery. Other agents to provide multimodal analgesia (e.g., ketamine, lidocaine, NSAIDs, and gabapentin) are also required.

Monitoring the patient with spinal cord injury

Monitoring of patients suffering from spinal cord trauma consists of serial neurological examinations as well as frequent assessment of routine monitoring parameters. Serial neurological examinations should include assessment of conscious proprioception, voluntary motor function, and pain perception. Assessment of pain perception is not necessary in patients that can purposefully walk. All normal monitoring parameters such as temperature, pulse rate and quality, respiratory rate and effort, and auscultation of lungs and heart are evaluated frequently. Regular turning can help to minimize problems with pressure sores that may occur particularly in quadriplegic or paretic animals. However, manipulation of these patients must be done with extreme care to prevent further damage to the spinal cord.

Monitoring of urine output in patients with spinal cord lesions is important because many animals suffer from bladder dysfunction which can cause urinary retention. A urinary catheter may be placed in these patients or the bladder can be expressed 4–5 times daily to help prevent urinary tract infections. Upper motor neuron bladder (urethral spasms) is a common occurrence of patients suffering from spinal cord trauma. These patients have bladders that are very difficult to express. Medication can be given to decrease urethral spasms and urethral tone.

As always, the recumbent patient presents a special nursing challenge. The complications of long-term recumbency, such as decubital ulcers, can become life-threatening in and of themselves. Nonambulatory patients also benefit greatly from physiotherapy and hydrotherapy. Ambulatory patients require strict confinement and physiotherapy for 2–3 weeks postoperatively. This will maintain joint flexibility. Massage helps to maintain blood flow and relax contracted muscles, tendons, and ligaments. In addition, patient care such as ensuring cleanliness of the patient by bathing in warm water, drying thoroughly, applying medicated baby powder, frequent repositioning, and adequate bedding significantly affect the progress of the patient's recovery. Remember that many of these patients must be hand-fed and offered water. If the patient can sit in a sternal position, make sure that they can reach their food and water.

Clostridium Tetani Infections (Tetanus)

C. tetani infections can develop when spores are introduced into deep, penetrating wounds. *C. tetani* is a gram-positive, anaerobic, spore-forming bacillus. The organisms produce two exotoxins, tetanospasmin and tetanolysin. Tetanospasmin is the toxin that produces marked effects on the grey matter of the brain stem and spinal cord. Neurological deficits result in release of inhibition on motor neurons and a rigidity of muscles (spastic paralysis) all over the head and body. Dogs and cats are more resistant to *C. tetani* infections than horses, but this organism can effect any age, breed, or sex.

Wounds closer to the head are associated with generalized CNS signs than injuries of the extremeties. Generalized muscle stiffness has been observed between 2 and 20 days following the initial wound.

Animals affected walk with a stiff gait and have difficulty standing or lying down. The ears are held erect, forehead is wrinkled, and the lips are drawn up ("risus sardonicus") as a result of facial nerve spasm. Trismus (lockjaw) and dysphagia are a result of spasms of the masticatory and pharyngeal muscles. Rigidity of the extremities gives the patient a "saw horse" stance when placed in a standing position. Noise and tactile stimulation can provoke generalized tonic contraction of all muscles potentially leading to grand mal convulsions.

Tetanus has also been documented to be a complication of ovariohysterectomy, pregnancy, or parturition associated with fetal death. Diagnosis is made by observing the characteristic clinical signs on presentation (Fig. 12.7).

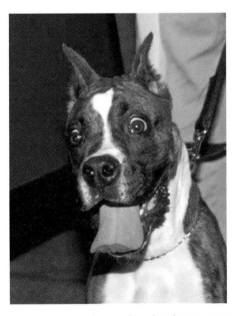

Figure 12.7   A tetanus patient showing risus sardonicus from facial nerve spasm.

CHAPTER 12

Treating a *C. tetani* infection consists of killing the organism, neutralizing the toxin, and controlling the effects of the toxin while providing supportive care. Penicillin G is given intravenously at a dose of 40,000 units/kg initially, followed by intramuscular injections of 20,000 units/kg every 12 hours. Tetanus antitoxin is initially tested in the patient for anaphylaxis at a dose of 0.1–0.2 mL subcutaneously. If no anaphylactic reaction occurs within 30 minutes, a dose of 30,000–100,000 units IV in dogs and 5,000 units IV in cats may be administered for several days depending on the clinical signs. Diazepam and/or methocarbamol may be used to control muscle spasms.

Monitoring of heart rate and rhythm with a continuous ECG is optimal to rule out arrhythmias caused by the effects of the exotoxins on the sympathetic nervous system. The body temperature, respiratory rate and effort, PaO_2, and $PaCO_2$, along with auscultation of lung fields, are closely monitored due to severe muscle spasm and potential inability to ventilate properly. Aspiration pneumonia is also a common occurrence with this disease process.

Providing padding, limited handling, and a quiet, dark environment will help reduce tetanic muscle spasms. Assuring adequate hydration by providing fluid therapy, turning the patient to prevent hydrostatic congestion of lung fields, and monitoring eliminations will help prevent additional problems like urinary tract infections and decubital ulcers.

Vestibular Disease

Vestibular disease is categorized as either peripheral or central in origin. Peripheral vestibular disease means that the problem is associated with the receptor organ in the inner ear or the vestibular nerve. Central vestibular disease refers to disease in the part of the brain that controls balance (brainstem, vestibular nuclei, or cerebellum). Clinical signs of vestibular disease can include head tilt, circling, nystagmus, strabismus, ataxia, falling to one side (side of the lesion), and nausea from motion sickness.

Vestibular diseases can be classified into three major disease processes: idiopathic vestibular disease, inner ear disease, or central vestibular disease. The onset of idiopathic vestibular disease is associated with an acute onset of vestibular signs with severe imbalance, due to its sudden onset and the severe nystagmus. This often results in the rolling described by the owners and can be mistaken for a seizure. The head tilt will be toward the side of dysfunction, and the nystagmus will be horizontal or rotatory with the fast phase away from the head tilt. No other neurological deficits will be noted on physical examination.

The diagnosis of idiopathic vestibular disease is tentatively made by the presence of acute clinical signs in the absence of other physical findings. The signs of idiopathic vestibular will disappear without treatment over time. The nystagmus will usually improve or disappear all together within 3–5 days of the onset. Treatment is typically supportive and includes anti-motion sickness agents (e.g., meclizine) and limiting distress and injury.

Conditions that cause inner ear disease are usually slower in evolution and therefore cause less severe clinical signs than with idiopathic vestibular disease. In addition to the vestibular signs, there are also varying degrees of facial nerve dysfunction and often Horner's syndrome. Signs of facial nerve involvement include paresis or paralysis of the muscles of facial expressions (ear movement, blink, and buccal muscle reaction on palpation).

Inner ear infections are the most common cause of inner ear disease. Bacterial infections make up the majority of inner ear disease and, once diagnosed, are very responsive to treatment with antibiotics. Other causes of inner ear disease may not be treatable, including fungal infections and neoplasia.

Disease of the central vestibular system can be identified by observing additional cranial nerve deficits, proprioceptive deficits and motor deficits. Vertical nystagmus also suggests a central lesion. These clinical signs, in addition to the signs noted above, are an indication of brainstem damage affecting the vestibular nuclei and sensor and motor pathways which course through the vestibular region of the brainstem.

Inflammatory/infectious causes for vestibular diseases in dogs are canine distemper virus, granulomatous meningoencephalitis, toxoplasmosis, neosporidiosis, aspergillosis, cryptococcosis, steroid-responsive meningoencephalitis, Lyme's disease, Rocky Mountain spotted fever, and ehrlichiosis. FeLV, FIP, and cryptococcosis are the most common infectious diseases in the cat. Neoplastic causes for central vestibular disease vary between species but are common in older patients. Dogs are susceptible to any of the primary brain tumors, while only meningiomas are common in cats. Cats that are not eating and stressed can easily develop thiamine deficiency, and this should not be overlooked in treating sick cats with vestibular signs.

Further Reading

Chrisman, CL. 1991. Behavior and personality disorders, seizures, opisthotonos, tetanus, tetany, tremors, myoclonus, and other muscle spasms. In *Problem in Small Animal Neurology*, 2nd ed., 166–203, 307–310.

Clemmons, RM. 2002. Vestibular Disease in Animals, University of Florida.

Cross, R. 2010. Personal communication. April 2010.

DePapp, E. Fibrocartilaginous Embolic Myelopathy. www.PetPlace.com.

Dewey, CW. 2000. Emergency management of the head trauma patient. In *Veterinary Clinics of North America: Small Animal Practice*, Vol. 20, edited by Saunders, WB, Philadelphia.

Dewey, CW. 2003. *Vascular Encephalopathies in the Dog and Cat*, ACVIM Proceedings.

Dewey, CW. 2006. Anticinvulsant therapy in dogs and cats. *Veterinary Clinics of North America: Small Animal Practice* 36:1107–1127.

Fossum, TW. Fundamentals of neurosurgery, surgery of the cervical spine, surgery of the thoracolumbar spine. In *Small Animal Surgery*, 2nd ed., pp. 1192–1301.

Goncalves, R. Seizures and neurological emergencies in the dog and cat. *Irish Veterinary Journal* 62(8):534–540.

Greene, CE. *Infectious Diseases of the Cat and Dog*, 2nd ed. Philadelphia: WB Saunders.

Kube, SA, Olby, NJ. 2008. Managing acute spinal cord injuries. *Compendium on Continuing Education for the Practicing Veterinarian*, 496–506.

Oliver, JE Jr., Lorenz, MD, Kornegay, JN. 1997. *WB Saunders Handbook of Veterinary Neurology*. Philadelphia: WB Saunders.

Platt, SR. *Canine Stroke*, WSAVA 2008 Congress.

Platt, SR. *Cerebrovascular Diseases in Dogs*, WSAVA 2006 Congress.

Plotnick, A. 2006. "Arterial Thromboembolism": A Devastating Disease that Strikes Without Warning. www.manhattancats.com/articles.

Stephenson, RB. 1992. Local control of blood flow. In *Textbook of Veterinary Physiology*, edited by Cunningham, JG. Philadelphia: Saunders WB, pp. 217–219.

Syring, RS, Otto, CM. 2002. *Mechanisms and Management of Head Injury*, IVECCS proceedings.

Trotter, EJ, deLaunta, A. 1990. *Handbook of Veterinary Procedures & Emergency Treatment*, 5th ed., edited by Kirk, RW, Bistner, SI, Ford, RB., pp. 92–97, 145–159.

Vite, CH, Steinberg, SA. 1999. Neurologic emergencies. In *Manual of Canine and Feline Emergency and Critical Care*, pp. 101–115.

Musculoskeletal, Integumentary, and Environmental Emergencies

David Liss

David Liss

Introduction

Emergencies relating to skin, muscle, or bone are numerous. Fractures, bite wounds, and envenomations are quite common in the small animal ER. Technicians working in those settings should be familiar with very important concepts such as wound care, fracture management, and pathophysiology of snake and spider envenomations. Due to the frequency of these disorders, the musculoskeletal and integument emergencies remain an important area for veterinary technicians to be proficient in.

Electrocution/Electrical Cord Injury

Electrical injury is trauma done by electrical energy to tissues. Electrical cord injury mainly results from inadvertent chewing on electrical cords, most often by younger dogs and cats. Rarely, exposure to power lines, or potentially, lightning strikes can cause electrocution. Most standard household outlets supply 120 V energy. Water is an extremely efficient conductor of electricity, so mucous membranes (MMs), such as in the oral cavity, make for low resistance to current flow. The higher the flow, the increased the damage caused by current.

Pathophysiology of Thermal Injury

The pathophysiology of electrical injury is composed of thermal injury to tissues, and cellular pore disruption, termed electroporation. Thermal injury to tissues is caused by an increase in temperature of bodily fluids, causing coagulation and degradation of tissue proteins. The result is tissue necrosis of affected areas. Thermal injury may also be observed in places not originally exposed. Current will arc, or jump across air space, potentially damaging neighboring tissue not initially in proximity of the original current. Cellular pore disruption potentiates the influx of fluid and ions, causing cellular swelling and shrinking, resulting in cell damage and death.

Signalment

Younger animals tend to be those at higher risk for this type of injury. Median age of puppies is reportedly 3.5 months and kittens anywhere from 2 months to 2 years (Silverstein and Hopper 2009). Although there is a year-round risk for patients, holiday time, with festive lights, may be considered a higher risk time period. In addition, any area with multiple cords, such as entertainment systems, should be carefully monitored to prevent this injury.

Initial Presentation

Patients present with a myriad of symptoms and physical exam findings. Thermal burns are common and are usually seen around the mouth, lips, tongue, gums, or oropharynx. They also may be found at other sites, caused by arcing of the electrical current. These may range in severity from mild to severe. Cardiac arrhythmias are common and result from direct thermal and cellular damage to the myocardium. With alternating current (AC current), the most common arrhythmia is ventricular fibrillation, while ventricular tachycardia can also be seen. Asystole is also possible; however, it is usually associated with high current, such as direct current (DC) sources.

These patients may also present with respiratory distress, and often suffer from a specific form of noncardiogenic pulmonary edema, termed neurogenic pulmonary edema. This is a form of pulmonary edema resulting from severe vasoconstriction as a result of sympathetic release from central nervous system (CNS) damage. The resulting vasoconstriction increases the cardiac afterload, decreasing left ventricular stroke volume and increasing pulmonary capillary hydrostatic pressure. This causes fluid to weep into the alveoli and interstitium. This appears radiographically as an alveolar pattern in the caudodorsal lung fields. Respiratory distress from other causes, such as oral/facial edema, or potentially diaphragmatic spasm, may also be found, and should be investigated. CNS injury may be from direct stimulation from the electrical energy as opposed to electroporation, but the latter may still play a part in CNS hypoxia. Patients may present with altered mental status, muscle tremors, seizure activity, or paresis. Burn injuries are also extremely painful and thus analgesic therapy should be instituted as soon as possible. Hypovolemia may result from pulmonary and tissue edema, vasodilation, or impaired cardiac output; however, hypertension may also be a clinical finding resulting from pain or hyperdynamic shock. Gastrointestinal (GI) insult, and potential bacterial translocation, may be from thermal injury to gut tissue and hypomotility resulting from electrical interference. Cataracts also may form several months after the injury, and have been reported in one dog (Silverstein and Hopper 2009).

Laboratory Findings

Initial laboratory findings may represent hypoxemia, respiratory acidosis, metabolic acidosis, hyperlactatemia, hypoalbuminemia, hyperkalemia, myoglobinuria, and hemoglobinuria. Hypoxemia may manifest as a decreased PaO_2 and low $PaO_2:FiO_2$ ratio. Respiratory acidosis may result from hypoventilation. Metabolic acidosis may result from lactic acidosis, caused by decreased tissue perfusion and excessive muscle activity. Hypoalbuminemia may result from burn injury and subsequent fluid third spacing. Hyperkalemia may result from tissue necrosis, as does hemoglobinuria and myoglobinuria.

Treatment

Initial interventions include turning off the electrical source, and then carefully removing the animal from the source. If the patient is in respiratory and cardiac arrest, cardiopulmonary cerebral resuscitation (CPCR) should be initiated.

Once in hospital, the patient should be treated symptomatically. In the event of presentation in cardiac and respiratory arrest, CPCR should be immediately initiated. An immediate ECG may be of benefit to identify the arrest rhythm. Fluid resuscitation should be initiated with patients in hypovolemic shock. Crystalloids and colloids may both be of benefit; however, volumes should be closely monitored as there is a cardiogenic portion to the shock. Because the lung microvasculature is relatively permeable to large molecules, colloids may redistribute across the capillary barrier. They may add to worsening of edema. If colloids are to be used, trial doses are suggested (Silverstein and Hopper 2009). However, hypoproteinemia may benefit from colloidal support to increase colloid oncotic pressure.

Respiratory distress deserves immediate attention. Flow by oxygen should be administered immediately. In the case of total airway obstruction, temporary tracheostomy may be necessary. If a partial obstruction is present, sedation and oxygen supplementation, via cage, nasal insufflation, oxygen hood, or other device, may be satisfactory. Patients with neurogenic pulmonary edema may benefit from furosemide; however, this remains controversial. Alveolar fluid may be highly proteinacious, and therefore unaffected by furosemide, but there is some thought that furosemide may work directly on alveoli, pumping fluid out of airspaces, in addition to its effects at the loop of Henle. Furosemide has the potential to cause or worsen hypovolemia and should be used with caution. Bronchodilators may also be of benefit but again are controversial. With severe refractory hypoxemia, mechanical ventilation may become necessary.

Arrhythmias are treated with antiarrhythmic drugs. Seizure activity may be controlled with appropriate anticonvulsant therapy. Early multimodal pain management should also be instituted early. Early nutrition is also recommended for systemic and local GI effects.

Monitoring recommendations include serial electrolyte and blood gas measurements, constant or serial electrocardiogram (ECG) monitoring, renal function testing (blood urea nitrogen [BUN], creatinine, urine output, and urine-specific gravity), providing evidence not only of renal function, but also of hydration and volume status.

Prognosis

Prognosis of electrical cord injury is reported to be good. Prognosis becomes poor to grave if the patient presents in cardiorespiratory arrest. A study reported the mortality rate to be 39% (Silverstein and Hopper 2009).

High-Rise Syndrome (Gordon 1993)

Pathophysiology

High-rise syndrome is the term for animal injuries sustained from falls of two stories (20 ft) or greater. Most often, this is associated with feline patients; however, dogs are reported to have suffered from injuries as well. Injuries are resultant from vertical deceleration trauma (Pratschke and Kirby 2002).

In feline patients, injuries tend to be more severe up to seven stories. Up until seven stories, the vestibular system "rights" the animal, allowing them to land feet first. This, however, prevents an even distribution of force on impact, leading to severe injuries. Beyond seven stories, terminal velocity is reached, and the feline vestibular system is inactivated. Patients land on their side, more evenly distributing force (Silverstein and Hopper 2009).

Presentation

Injuries tend to be facial, extremity, and thoracic in origin. A study of 119 cats diagnosed with high-rise syndrome revealed 46% of cats had limb fractures, and 34% of cats had thoracic trauma. Fractures of the tibia and femur occurred most often. Pneumothorax and pulmonary contusions were also present in 20% and 13.4% of cats, respectively (Babic et al. 2004) (Fig. 13.1).

Treatment

Initial assessment of the patient includes careful assessment of all bodily systems, with attention to any life-threatening conditions or injuries. Hypovolemia may be treated with

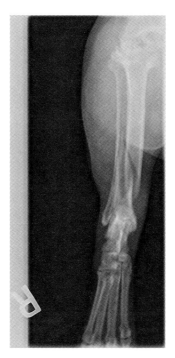

Figure 13.1   Spiral tibia/fibula complete fracture.

fluid resuscitation, including blood products if active hemorrhage is present. Active bleeding should be controlled with direct pressure techniques, or tourniquets as a last resort. Respiratory distress may be the result of pain, pneumothorax, or pulmonary contusions. Careful examination of the respiratory system is necessary to evaluate the extent of damage. Pneumothorax should be treated with immediate thoracocentesis and/or thoracostomy tube placement. Oxygen supplementation should be administered in the face of hypoxemia. Early pain management should be instituted to prevent the development of windup or spinal hypersensitization. Survey radiographs (thoracic and abdominal) were reported to be of immense benefit but should only be performed when patient is stable enough for restraint and positioning.

Prognosis

Prognosis is good with treatment. Survival rates are reported to be 97% and 98% for cats and dogs, respectively (Babic et al. 2004). However, patients with critical injuries may be euthanized, and some reports indicate a higher rate for euthanasia in dogs.

Hypothermia

Hypothermia is commonly encountered in veterinary critical care patients. Anesthetic patients, hypovolemic/hypotensive patients, sick patients, and hypothermia as the result of environmental exposure represent important categories of patients in the emergency and critical care setting. A thorough understanding of classification systems, pathophysiology, and treatment, is essential knowledge for the emergency and critical care technician.

Hypothermia can be defined as a body temperature less than 99°F (<37°C), although it is hard to identify a definite number (Armstrong et al. 2005). It is important to note that hypothermia can only be determined in a patient who can potentially maintain their own body temperature. Thus, hypothermia is a pathologic condition requiring intervention. There are two types of hypothermia, primary and secondary. In addition, two different classification systems have been proposed to identify severity of primary or secondary hypothermia.

Primary hypothermia represents heat loss in the face of normal heat production and encompasses the environmental exposure category. Secondary hypothermia occurs as a result of a disease process, drug administration, or injury causing altered heat production or loss.

Causes

Primary causes of hypothermia are typically defined as environmental exposure to the cold. The patient has normal heat production and loss capacity but is exposed to subnormal temperatures, rendering them unable to keep up with heat loss. Examples include snow and cold water exposure.

Causes of secondary hypothermia are more numerous. The body may intentionally cause some mild hypothermia to conserve metabolic function in key organs, such as the heart and brain (Armstrong et al. 2005). Disease processes can alter thermoregulation and either increase or decrease metabolic rate, leading to increased or decreased heat production. Once heat production is impaired, thermoregulatory ability may be compromised. Depending on the animal's environment, heat loss may predominate, resulting in hypothermia of increasing severity. In addition, heat loss may be increased by vasodilation, caused by toxins, or pharmacological agents such as gas anesthesia, or medications like acepromazine.

Physiologic Results of Hypothermia

When body temperature begins to decrease, signals are sent to the thermoregulatory center in the hypothalamus. Initially, vasoconstriction and piloerection assist with heat loss restriction. As increased heat production is needed, cellular metabolic rates increase, and shivering begins to generate more body heat. The thermoregulatory center's critical set point may also be altered by stressors, including infection, which increases the "set point," and other illness or stressors which decrease it.

During mild and moderate hypothermia, the sympathetic nervous system's activity increases to conserve metabolic function. Heart rate (HR), cardiac output, and mean arterial pressure (MAP) increase. However, as temperature decreases, responsiveness to catecholamines results in a blunted and eventual decreased sympathetic response. Vasodilation, CNS depression, decreased cardiac output, MAP, and respiratory rate may result. Reportedly, when temperature drops below 88°F (31°C) thermoregulation ceases.

Consequences

Consequences of hypothermia are numerous. The cardiovascular, respiratory, neurologic, and immune systems are greatly affected. As temperatures drop, binding of norepinephrine to alpha-1 receptors decreases and limits the amount of sympathetic response (vasoconstriction) in the face of heat loss. In addition to decreased sensitivity of receptors, decreased catecholamine release also occurs. Cardiac function is reported to increase initially, and then decrease. Hypoxemia results due to decreased ventilation (decreased tidal volume, minute ventilation, and respiratory rate), impaired capillary blood flow from increased viscosity, and alveolar hypoventilation.

The respiratory system is at risk from bacterial invasion and pneumonia, edema, and inflammatory mediator damage in the form of acute respiratory distress syndrome (ARDS).

While some hypothermia may be neuroprotective, cerebral blood flow reduces significantly for every 1°C drop in temperature.

Immune system complications include decreased wound healing and increased risk of infection. Coagulation abnormalities are of serious concern but may be potentially missed in clinical practice as coagulation tests are run *in vitro* at body temperatures of 98.6°F (37°C). Thus, coagulation factors regain function as they are warmed. Coagulopathy and thrombopathia are of serious concern in patients at risk for hemorrhage, but fortunately, these are reversible. Platelet function and coagulation factor function return to normal as the patient returns to normothermia.

Perioperative Hypothermia

Hypothermia resulting from anesthesia and surgery is of special concern and constitutes special pathophysiology. Perioperative hypothermia occurs in three phases (Armstrong et al. 2005). The initial phase is a heat loss caused by rapid redistribution of heat from the core to the periphery. This heat redistribution is caused by vasodilation, from anesthetic agents, and resetting of the temperature threshold needed to cause reflex vasoconstriction. The second phase of perioperative hypothermia results from excessive heat loss, not matched by heat production. Heat loss is caused by the patient losing heat on a cold table (conduction), and exposure of bodily fluids and cavities. The last phase occurs after prolonged anesthesia and results in reflex vasoconstriction initiating a plateau in temperature. Continued temperature decreases occur as a result of a decreased sympathetic response.

Rewarming

Therapies for rewarming strongly depend on the severity of the hypothermia and the clinical signs it may be causing.

Passive rewarming

For patients experiencing mild hypothermia (90–99°F), passive rewarming should be instituted. Passive rewarming capitalizes on the patient's own ability to produce some heat. It also prevents further heat loss. Passive rewarming consists mainly of external covers, such as blankets, bubble wrap, or foil (Kirby et al. 2001; Silverstein and Hopper 2009).

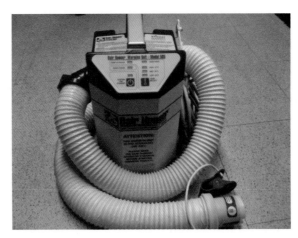

Figure 13.2   This active rewarming device uses forced circulating air to heat the hypothermic postoperative patient.

Active external rewarming

For moderate hypothermia (82–90°F), active external rewarming, which generates heat to the patient, should be utilized. This type of rewarming allows direct transfer of heat from the heat-generating device, such as hot water bottles, heating pads, heat lamps, or forced air warmers, to the patient. These are best used when placed on or near areas with a large blood supply such as the neck or abdomen. Since the patient is in direct contact with the heat-generating device, care must be taken to avoid iatrogenic thermal injury to the patient's skin. Barriers should be placed between the patient and the heat-generating device, if there is concern for burn injury. Heat devices that may cause burn injury include hot water bottles, heating blankets/pads, or heating disks (Fig. 13.2).

Active core rewarming

With severe hypothermia (<82°F), active core rewarming is advised. This includes gaining access to the patient's core, and directly transferring heat to it. Pleural/peritoneal lavage, warmed oxygen delivered intratracheally, warmed IV fluids, warm water bladder lavage, warm enemas, are all examples of active core rewarming. Warmed enemas and bladder lavage, however, may be of little benefit as there is concern as to the limited surface area of these structures. (Silverstein and Hopper 2009).

Consequences of Rewarming

Rewarming is not a benign thing, and the veterinary technician should be ready to antici-pate complications associated with rewarming. After warming therapies are instituted, there may continue to be a decrease in the patient's temperature, known as the "after-drop," and is caused by cold peripheral blood passing into the core.

Second, rewarming shock is a phenomenon that patients may experience as a result of rewarming. Rewarming shock is characterized by vasodilation as a result of applied heat. This vasodilation has the potential to negatively impact organ perfusion and oxygen delivery to tissues during the rewarming period. In addition, patients undergo an extensive metabolic requirement once rewarming is begun, drawing from crucial cellular stores of metabolites. This phenomenon is important to keep in mind when rewarming patients with significant hypothermia and disease. Constantly reassess the patient's vital signs and perfusion parameters, to ensure adequate tissue and organ perfusion.

Patients experiencing trauma and concurrent hypothermia represent a particularly important subgroup. There is a high correlation between hypothermia and mortality among human trauma patients (Kirby et al. 2001). Recommendations for rewarming include actively rewarming to 98.5°F (37°C), replacing intravascular volume, if indicated, and then using passive methods to have the patient slowly return to normothermia. However, when using aggressive surface rewarming, the patient's core (thoracic and abdominal cavities) should receive the bulk of the heat support. This allows warmed blood to move to the periphery and avoid peripheral vasodilation as a result of applied heat.

Hypothermia, as a result of exposure to the elements, is widely known as a medical emergency. However, secondary hypothermia, as a result of hypovolemia, shock, anesthesia, pharmacological agents, or illness, represents serious concern as well. Electrolytes, blood gases, arterial blood pressure, perfusion parameters, urinary output, and mental status should be constantly monitored during the rewarming phase. The critical care veterinary technician is essential in assessing and intervening in the treatment of hypothermic patients.

Hyperthermia

Hyperthermia is the increase in a patient's core body temperature beyond the expected physiologic normals. Fever is a special category of hyperthermic patients for which the temperature regulatory center in the hypothalamus' critical set point has been increased to a higher level as the result of an endogenous or exogenous pyrogen (Silverstein and Hopper 2009).

Fever

Hyperthermia represents an elevated core body temperature above accepted reference ranges for that particular species (Silverstein and Hopper 2009). Fever corresponds to the specific patient population that has had its thermoregulatory set point increased to meet some physiologic demand.

Differing from hyperthermia as a result of heat stroke, fever patients have had their hypothalamic thermoregulatory center's set point altered as a result of a pyrogen, and thus are still able to dissipate heat. True fever is a response of the body to invasion or injury, from pathogenic or nonpathogenic molecules that have the ability to induce fever, known as pyrogens.

Most pyrogens are pathogenic; however, some pharmacologic agents, and sterile tissue inflammation and necrosis, may also cause fever. Exogenous pyrogens have the ability to release endogenous pyrogens, which act directly on the thermoregulatory center. Among these, interleukin (IL)-1, IL-6, and tumor necrosis factor (TNF)-α are the most important fever-producing cytokines (Silverstein and Hopper 2009). Exogenous pyrogens include pathogens such as bacteria or bacterial products (lipopolysaccharide, endotoxin), fungi, viruses, rickettsiae, and protozoa. In addition, soluble antigen–antibody complexes, bile acids, a few pharmacological agents (colchicine, tetracycline, levamisole), tissue inflammation/necrosis, and neoplasia may induce fever (Silverstein and Hopper 2009).

Fever development in the ICU

Fever development in an intensive care unit (ICU) patient warrants immediate concern. Cause of the fever must be investigated, and can include infectious and noninfectious (inflammatory) culprits. Infectious or inflammatory causes may be connected with invasive devices such as intravenous catheters, urinary catheters, chest catheters, nasal oxygen cannulas, feeding tubes, or any other implanted device. These may be colonized with microbes, or may be causing sterile tissue irritation.

Development of abscesses or "bedsores" may be another cause. Nonreadily apparent causes of fever of infectious nature may include urinary tract infections, CNS infections, pneumonia or respiratory infections, or joint infections. A thorough evaluation of all bodily systems is warranted.

Noninfectious causes may be inflammation related to invasive devices, such as phlebitis from an intravenous catheter, aspiration pneumonitis, transfusion reactions, postoperative inflammation, pancreatitis, hepatitis, cholecystitis, ARDS, and neoplasia or paraneoplastic processes.

Nosocomial infection is of great concern and thus, any patient with immunosuppression should be handled very carefully according to hospital protocol.

Heatstroke

Heatstroke is a commonly used term to describe severe hyperthermia, where the ability to dissipate heat is surpassed by the surrounding environment's temperature. Heatstroke is mainly experienced in dogs and can be the result of overexertion, physiologic reduction of heat dissipation, or unfortunate circumstance such as being locked in a car on a hot day. Examples of overexertion include hiking without proper water stores or without acclimatization. Examples of physiologic predisposition include brachycephalic patients, who have a reduced ability to lose heat through their respiratory tract. However the offense occurred, these patients present in severely critical condition and require immediate intervention and constant monitoring.

Pathophysiology of Heatstroke

Heatstroke is defined as a core body temperature >104°F (40°C), CNS dysfunction, such as coma, seizures, obtundation, and organ dysfunction (Silverstein and Hopper 2009). It is most often reported in the summer months, more commonly in states with high humidity. Although the definition includes a temperature of 104°F or greater, it is not uncommon for a patient to present with temperatures >108°F (42°C). At these temperatures, brain damage may occur, along with cellular destruction and necrosis.

As referenced above, heat is dissipated by four mechanisms: conduction, convection, radiation, and evaporation. The main method of heat dissipation, as opposed to heat loss as in hypothermic animals, is panting. This allows large amounts of convective and evaporative losses via the respiratory tract. Some evaporation and radiation occurs as well, as animals sweat through their foot pads. Animals will also seek cooler environments, such as tile floors, to lose heat via conduction.

As body temperature increases, significant peripheral vasodilation occurs, with some constriction of renal and splanchnic vessels, delivering a larger amount of cardiac output to the cutaneous vessels for heat dissipation. Panting is an initial response in dogs and results from stimulation of the panting center. As dehydration occurs, less water is available for evaporative losses, reducing the amount of heat dissipation. Tachycardia, increased cardiac output, and minute ventilation occur to maximize heat loss.

Predisposing Factors

Predisposing factors are numerous but do represent significant concern for patients exposed to high temperatures. Brachycephalic dogs, and those with laryngeal paralysis, or tracheal collapse, have a reduced ability to lose heat via their ventilatory efforts. Obesity and cardiovascular disease also represent serious concern and represent a decent amount of the domesticated canine population. In addition to endogenous concerns, exogenous ones such as lack of water sources, confinement, and increased humidity, which reduce evaporative losses, raise the risk of severe damage from heatstroke.

Presentation

Patients exposed to high temperatures represent the classic presentation for heatstroke. A less common presentation includes exertional heatstroke, consisting of improper acclimatization or exercise. These patients will be at great risk for multiple organ dysfunction syndrome (MODS), resulting from systemic inflammatory response syndrome (SIRS), shock, and disseminated intravascular coagulation (DIC). Cytotoxicity from thermal damage, endotoxemia from bacterial translocation, activation of the DIC, and hypovolemic shock all contribute to the development of MODS.

Patients presenting with possible heatstroke may have a history of environmental exposure or recent exercise. These patients present hyperthermic, >104°F (40°C), but also may present hypothermic <100°F (37.8°C). They are often depressed, obtunded, comatose, or seizuring. They may be panting, orthopneic, dyspneic, and hyperemic. They will usually have tacky MMs and a greatly prolonged capillary refill time (CRT). They may also have weak or bounding pulses, with tachycardia and/or bradycardia, depending on their shock state. They may have petechiae or ecchymoses on their skin, often found when clipping fur for IV catheter placement, or prolonged bleeding at venipuncture sites.

If the GI barrier has been compromised, hematochezia or melena, representing intestinal hypoperfusion and bleeding, may or may not be evident at admission, but may develop in hospital. Laboratory findings indicate an elevated packed cell volume (PCV) and total solids (TS), alanine aminotransferase, bilirubin, azotemia, and creatine kinase. Hypoglycemia is also common.

Cytotoxicity results from extreme temperatures applied to cells and results in damage and rupture. Temperature ranges for damage include 107–109°F (42–43°C) for non-gut cells, and as low as 102–104°F (39–40°C) for gut cells (Johnson et al. 2006). Patients experiencing heat stroke also experience an initial increase in cardiac output and significant reduction in peripheral systemic vascular resistance as an attempt to reduce core temperature. As blood pooling occurs, effective circulating volume is reduced, and eventually, cardiac output falls. Coagulation abnormalities are also common, including the development of DIC, and/or widespread fibrinolysis and thrombosis. These patients will usually have elevated coagulation times (prothrombin time, activated partial thromboplastin time, and/or activated clotting time), thrombocytopenia, and elevated fibrinolytic parameters, such as D-dimers, fibrin degradation products (FDPs), thrombin, and antithrombin levels. This may be resultant from direct thermal activation of the clotting cascade, and/or thermal endothelial damage.

Initial Treatment

In the treatment of these patients, rapid assessment should occur prior to or in conjunction with treatment. Their airway, breathing, and circulatory parameters should be briefly assessed. The reported mainstays of treatment are rapid evaporative cooling, volume replacement, and management of secondary complications (Johnson et al. 2006).

Cooling Measures

Cooling involves using room temperature water, and exposure to air, or potentially a fan. This not only utilizes evaporative cooling but also convective losses as well. The use of ice or ice baths is not recommended. Ice will cause cutaneous vasoconstriction, shivering, and patient discomfort. Core cooling techniques such as gastric, urinary, or peritoneal, or rectal enemas or lavage have been reported but may cause rebound hypothermia.

Recommendations to stop cooling efforts, to prevent secondary hypothermia, remain at 103.5–104°F (39.7–40°C). Room temperature crystalloid fluids will greatly assist with volume expansion and heat loss. Constant monitoring of perfusion parameters (HR, mental status, extremity temperature, MM, CRT, lactate, blood pH, urine output, and blood pressure) will help guide volume expansion. Colloids may be used as needed to assist with volume expansion. If patients are coagulopathic, the administration of fresh frozen plasma will help replenish clotting factors. Hypoglycemia may be addressed with dextrose supplementation.

Complications of Heatstroke

Secondary complications of heatstroke are numerous. Acute renal failure, azotemia, and oliguria/anuria, may result from hypotensive renal damage, or direct thermal injury to nephrons. If urine output is less than 1 mL/kg/h, treatment of oliguria/anuria should ensue. In these cases, where fluid/pharmacological therapy is not sufficient at restoring urine output, peritoneal/hemodialysis may be indicated.

GI complications represent mucosal sloughing and ulcer formation. Gastro-protectants, such as sucralfate, H_2 blockers, and proton pump inhibitors, should be considered in these patients. As endotoxemia results from disruption of the GI mucosal barrier and bacterial translocation, broad-spectrum antibiotics should be considered if hematochezia is present (Silverstein and Hopper 2009).

CNS disturbances may result from hypoglycemia, cerebral edema, and potentially cerebral cellular damage. Cerebral edema can be managed with head elevation, Mannitol administration, after normovolemia, and avoidance of jugular vein distension. Normoglycemia should be maintained for adequate CNS function.

As with any critical illness, the respiratory tract is susceptible to damage from inflammatory mediators, bacteremia, or potentially thermal injury. Monitoring of respiratory rate and character, peripheral oxygen saturation, and arterial or venous blood gases will help guide therapy. Hypovolemia, inflammatory mediator release, and thermal injury all may cause direct myocardial injury, resulting in cardiac arrhythmias and heart failure.

HR, ECG monitoring, auscultation, arterial blood pressure, and central venous pressure (CVP) may all help evaluate the cardiovascular system. Arrhythmias may be treated with appropriate antiarrhythmic therapy. Refractory hypotension may necessitate the need for inotropic or vasopressor therapy.

Heatstroke is a serious condition, with a guarded prognosis. Negative prognostic indicators include refractory hypoglycemia, coma or hypothermia on presentation, acute renal failure, evidence of DIC, refractory hypotension, or development of ARDS. Prevention is extremely important, as this condition is often a result of uneducated or experienced pet owners, or unfortunate and potentially preventable circumstance.

Snake/Spider Envenomation

Snake Envenomation

Snake envenomation is a complex medical emergency often encountered by emergency hospitals in endemic areas. Spider bites, to a lesser extent, also represent serious emergencies, and the critical care technician must be ready to evaluate and treat these patients.

Snake identification

Various venomous snakes have different physiological effects and must be identified for rapid treatment to ensue. Pit vipers, the Crotalidae family, are the main group of venomous snakes in the United States and encompass the rattlesnakes, *Crotalus* and *Sistrurus* spp., and the copperheads and water mocassins, *Agkistrodon* spp. Rattlesnakes are found throughout the United States whereas copperheads and water moccasins are found in eastern and central United States (Silverstein and Hopper 2009).

Contrary to popular belief, venom is not "more" toxic in the summer months, but rather, snakes become more aggressive and release more venom. Pit vipers have a curious ability to control the amount of venom they inject. This is dependent on the situation they perceive. They may strike defensively, which may often contain no venom, and be deemed "dry bites," or may strike aggressively and inject a dose of venom. The most dangerous bites are those while the snake is dying, where the entire venom load may be injected.

Severity of illness is usually associated with venom load, and rate of venom uptake. Rattlesnakes have the most pungent venom of the other pit vipers, and bites encouraging rapid venom uptake may be more severe. Several species and subspecies of rattlesnake exist, with some subspecies' venom mimicking the Mojave's neurotoxins.

Venom is 90% water and 10% enzymes and proteins, which function to immobilize the prey and digest its tissues. Although only 10% of the venom is proteinaceous, each protein and enzyme may have a specific detrimental function and also may act synergistically with other proteins.

Predisposing factors

Because of the complex physiology of envenomations, many predisposing factors exist, and patients range in clinical signs and severity. Species, body mass, location of bite, excitement after bite, concurrent medications (e.g., nonsteroidal anti-inflammatory drugs [NSAIDs]), may make victims more susceptible to venom. Cats are apparently more resistant to venom than dogs, yet cats are often more critical patients, from their desire to antagonize the snake and induce offensive bites, and their tendency to hide after trauma, making transit time to the veterinary hospital prolonged.

Presentation

Patients presenting for possible snake bite envenomation may or may not have local evidence. Fang marks, up to 6, may be present but give no indication of whether a venomous bite was given (Silverstein and Hopper 2009). In addition, severe swelling, and hair, may cover an area, making fang marks hard to locate.

Clinical signs range from local swelling, discharge, and pain, to severe hypotension, thrombocytopenia, petechiae and ecchymoses, coagulation abnormalities, cardiac arrhythmias, echinocytosis, and potentially seizure activity and obtundation or coma. Hypotension may result from blood pooling or third spacing of fluid from swelling at the bite site. Coagulopathies are common and most often are resultant from blocking or deactivating of various coagulation factors. Thrombocytopenia may also develop.

Echinocytosis

Echinocystosis is a cytologic finding of red blood cells, characterized by an irregular shape, and multiple blunt projections distorting the cell surface (Fig. 13.3).

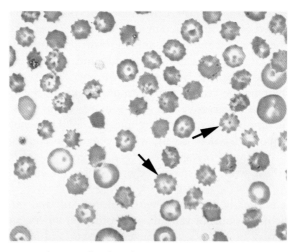

Figure 13.3   Echinocytosis is indicative of rattlesnake envenomation. However, a negative finding on a blood smear does not rule it out. (Courtesy of Thrall's Veterinary Hematology & Clinical Chemistry, with permission from Wiley-Blackwell.)

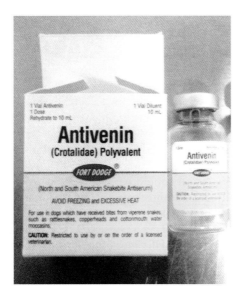

Figure 13.4   Remember to never shake antivenin when reconstituting. Always add diluents slowly, and let sit until it is rehydrated.

CHAPTER 13

According to a 1997 study, venom from *Crotalus atrox* induced echinocytosis, and the amount of projections increased with increasing venom concentrations (Brown et al. 1997). In addition, a retrospective study in 1994 revealed that 89% of dogs revealed some form of echinocytosis after rattlesnake envenomation (Brown et al. 1994). Theories of the pathophysiology of this phenomenon include venom-mediated ATP depletion, cation depletion (Na^+ and K^+), and potentially calcium-mediated PLA_2 activity. PLA_2 is an enzyme that converts lecithin to lysolecithin, a known echinocytic agent (Brown et al. 1997). Echinocytosis will not show up in "dry bites," and local tissue damage may still be evident with a nonvenomous attack (Fig. 13.4).

Treatment

Antivenin. Antivenin is the only proven specific therapy for envenomation. Amazingly, antivenin can stop and reverse detrimental physiological phenomena such as coagulation defects, cardiac and neurological effects, and tissue necrosis. There are several types of venom that exist. The first is the commonly used Fort Dodge brand of polyvalent equine-origin antivenin. This covers the Crotalidae family. Horses are inoculated with venoms from the eastern and western diamondback rattlesnakes, the South American rattlesnake, and the Fer-De-Lance. It contains not only high amounts of antibodies but also equine proteins, including albumin. Therefore, it carries a significant risk of hypersensitivity reaction.

It is recommended to administer antivenin slowly, over the course of 30 minutes, and provide constant monitoring of all vital signs and patient condition (Silverstein and Hopper 2009). The infusion should be started very slowly initially, and the rate increased every few minutes if the patient shows no sign of reaction. If the patient shows no sign of reaction several minutes into the infusion, the rate may be increased to the final rate, infusing the solution over the remaining time. Patients undergoing antivenin administration should be monitored for signs of a hypersensitivity reaction and if observed, administration of diphenhydramine is indicated. Premedication with diphenhydramine before administration of antivenin will potentially alleviate symptoms of a reaction but will not actually prevent a reaction from happening.

Reconstitution of antivenin can prove challenging. It can take some time after the addition of diluent for it to be fully reconstituted. Warming the vial to body temperature may speed this process. It is not recommended to shake the vial, as it may destroy fragile proteins. The antivenin vial should be diluted prior to administration. Further dilution in 100–250 mL of crystalloid fluids is recommended. If fluid overload is a concern, the volume and rate of administration should be adjusted.

Antivenin is most effective if administered within the first 4 hours of envenomation, according to the package insert. However, it can be administered as long as there is venom in the bloodstream and may reverse some coagulation defects, or cardiac arrhythmias, but tissue damage will most likely be irreversible (Silverstein and Hopper 2009).

Antivenin is highly efficient at reversing coagulation defects of the primary and secondary hemostatic systems. Thrombocytopenias are potentially reversible with antivenin administration, as well as coagulation factor defects. Continued coagulopathic signs should be treated with additional antivenin.

A novel antivenin, named CroFab, is approved only for human use but combines western and eastern rattlesnake, cottonmouth/water moccasin, and Mojave rattlesnake venom. These are injected into sheep, and the antibodies are collected. There are successful reports of use in dogs and cats, yet the product still contains risk of allergic reaction, and is extremely expensive.

Neurotoxic envenomation

Several species of snakes contain neurotoxins instead of the more common hemotoxin venom. These species include the Mojave rattlesnake and the coral snake. Mojave snakes are of the genus *Crotalus* and species *scutulatus*. Mojave rattlesnakes are found in the southwest United States and may be hard to differentiate from other rattlesnakes with hemotoxic venom. They possess a similar diamond pattern to other *Crotalus* species (Clark et al. 1997).

Coral snakes are found in Arizona, New Mexico, Texas, and Florida. They are of the genus *Micruroides* and comprise two different species. They are multicolored, with black, yellow, and red bands. If the yellow bands touch the red bands, they are poisonous coral snakes. Rather a rare envenomation, coral snakes cause little pain at the bite site, but their venom is mainly neurotoxic.

The toxins are chemically similar to nondepolarizing neuromuscular blocking agents and cause paralysis and CNS depression. Clinical signs include muscle fasciculations, spasms, paralysis, and respiratory failure. There are some reports of hemolytic anemia, but that mechanism is poorly understood.

Treatment consists of supporting clinical signs, and potentially supporting ventilation if necessary. Coral snake antivenin exists and is manufactured by Wyeth laboratories. It appears, however, that Wyeth has discontinued its manufacturing of this antivenin (Silverstein and Hopper 2009).

Spider Envenomation

Spider identification: black widow spider

Five species of black widow spiders exist in the United States. The female is the gender with the poison glands, and the younger females, characterized by a blurred red/brown hourglass on their abdomen, can potentially deliver a full venom load in a single bite. Older females have a more distinct and red hourglass on their abdomen. Dogs are reported to be more resistant to venom but seem to have more severe signs of reaction (Silverstein and Hopper 2009).

Venom characteristics: black widow spider

Black widow venom is unique in that it causes no tissue trauma at injection site; therefore, no pain occurs, making it hard to diagnose. There may be a slightly red small area at the site of the bite, but patients with excessive hair may prove to be difficult to locate a bite source. The black widow venom is a potent neurotoxin that initially stimulates secretion of neurotransmitters such as acetylcholine and norepinephrine, and then inhibits their reuptake.

Clinical signs: black widow spider

Clinical signs vary, but most often seem to consist of muscle cramping or spasm initially, along with tachycardia and hypertension. Respiratory failure may also occur. Diagnosis relies entirely on clinical signs; therefore, rapid administration of antivenin is necessary for survival.

Antivenin: black widow spider

Similar to snake antivenin, this must be reconstituted and may take some time. It also carries the potential for hypersensitivity reaction and therefore should be diluted in 100 mL of 0.9% NaCl and administered slowly. Observing closely for hyperemia of the ear pinna is recommended. If a reaction is noted, the infusion must be stopped and diphenhydramine administered (Silverstein and Hopper 2009).

Treatment: black widow spider

Treatment for muscle fasciculations seems to be better controlled with benzodiazepine medications instead of muscle relaxants. In addition, hypertensive crises may occur and may need emergency treatment. Prognosis is uncertain in veterinary medicine, but at the minimum, several days of recovery may be necessary.

Spider identification: brown recluse spider

Brown recluse spiders are found in many states in the United States but primarily reside in the southern states including Georgia to Texas, Wisconsin, and the West. The venomous spiders have a violin-shaped icon on their dorsum. They are highly reclusive and nocturnal. They have not been shown to be aggressive and only bite in defense (Silverstein and Hopper 2009). Male spiders inject half the venom load of females, and larger spiders may be able to deliver higher amounts of venom.

Venom characteristics: brown recluse spider

The venom is highly toxic to tissues by interfering with leukocytes and causing dermonecrosis. (Silverstein and Hopper 2009). It also affects the coagulation system by clogging local capillaries and causing decreased tissue perfusion, thereby inciting necrosis. Systemically, it initiates an inflammatory response and depletes various clotting factors.

Diagnosis is potentially made from the shape and character of the bite wound. It has a classic "bull's eye" appearance with a red ring of edema surrounding a pale or dark ischemic and necrotic central area. Other clinical signs can vary from hemoglobinemia or hemoglobinuria, hemolytic anemia, fever, joint pain, vomiting, collapse, and erythema.

Treatment: brown recluse spider

Treatment consists of managing local and systemic signs. There is no antivenin available to neutralize the toxin. Dapsone, a leukocyte inhibitor, seems to be effective at halting necrosis at the bite site. The wound itself is then allowed to heal by second intention (Silverstein and Hopper 2009). Systemic signs, such as inflammatory response or hemolysis, may be treated with fluids, anti-inflammatory, analgesic, and antipyretic medications. Reportedly, glucocorticoids may be of benefit in treating red cell destruction. Coagulopathies may be treated as needed with blood product transfusions.

Burn Injury

Thermal burn injuries are considered uncommon in veterinary medicine. However, they can have devastating systemic effects and thus a veterinary ICU must be ready to address these critical patients. Burns may occur as a result of fire damage, radiation therapy, electric heating blankets or pads, heat lamps or hot water bottles, scalding with heated liquid, chemical burns, burns from electric cords, and automobile equipment. Burn injuries consist of highly intensive wound care and management of systemic sequelae.

Classification

Current terminology for burn injuries consist of classifying burns as superficial, partial thickness, or full thickness burns. Superficial burns consist of thermal damage to the epidermis. These burns will show signs of pain, redness, and inflammation. Some edema may be present. Blistering will most likely not be present. These burns are previously classified at "first-degree" burns.

Partial thickness burns include the epidermis and some of the dermis, the upper plexus, and potentially middle plexus. If only the top layer of the dermis is affected, the small vessels will be destroyed and plasma fluid will leak. Hair will still be present, or potentially singed, as the follicles are still present. If the partial thickness burn is

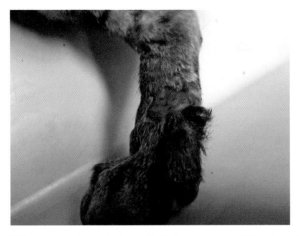

Figure 13.5   A partial thickness burn. Note the loss of hair, but presence of blood supply.

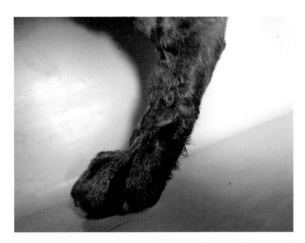

Figure 13.6   This is a cleaned burn 2 days after injury. Notice alopecia but no eschar. This burn has been bandaged for 2 days.

deeper, hair loss will be evident, and skin may be discolored from yellow to brown, as opposed to red. These burns are previously classified at "second-degree" burns (Figs. 13.5 and 13.6).

Full thickness burns have surpassed the epidermis and dermal layers. These burns penetrate into the hypodermis, also called the subcutaneous tissue, and can possibly involve deep structures like muscles, bones, and tendons. The skin is often described as "leathery" or may have a dark, blackened appearance. Because nerve tissue is also often involved, the area lacks sensation, and often no pain will be generated from loss of local nociceptors. These burns are previously classified at "third-degree" burns.

When skin is badly burned, most often deep partial thickness or full thickness burns, it may form an eschar. An eschar is a deep layer of tissue sloughed by the burn. It often looks like a burnt, dark, crusty layer of skin, and often can be removed and will contain discharge underneath. It typically takes 7–10 days to develop.

% TBSA for Burn Injuries–Feline

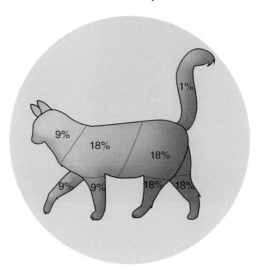

Katherine Sitseri ©

Figure 13.7   Diagram outlining the different body surface areas of various major anatomical parts of the feline patient. (Courtesy of Katherine Sitseri.)

Burn Scoring Systems

Burn scoring systems are widely utilized in human medicine. A standardized system has yet to be developed in veterinary medicine, but an adaptation of the "Rule of 9s" from human medicine can be extended to dogs and cats. Because of their varying surface area, this system is not precise but can give the clinician an estimation of the total body surface area, or TBSA, affected by the burns (Pavletic and Trout 2006).

The Rule of 9s states that a section of the body is given either 1%, 9%, or 18% of the TBSA, and if the burn affects that area, can be summed to give the total TBSA affected by the burns. Head/neck, and each forelimb is counted as 9%, each rear limb is counted as 18%, the thorax and abdomen are counted as 18% each, and the tail as 1%. So, head/neck = 9, 2 forelimbs = 18, 2 hind limbs = 36, and thorax and abdomen = 36. Thus, 36 + 36 + 18 + 9 + 1 = 100% TBSA (Silverstein and Hopper 2009; Pavletic and Trout 2006). If greater than 20% of TBSA is affected, the patient may be in serious crisis. Patients with greater than 20% of TBSA affected may exhibit serious fluid and electrolyte imbalances, anemia, and increased likelihood of infection and sepsis (Figs. 13.7 and 13.8).

Treatment

Burn injuries require intensive wound management in addition to the systemic complications they may cause. First step in evaluating a burn patient, after they are deemed hemodynamically stable, is to evaluate the areas burned, the TBSA affected, and the severity of the burn. Analgesic medications should be administered early as well. Quick cursory scoring of burn depth can include assessing for pain (presence means less than

% TBSA for Burn Injuries–Canine

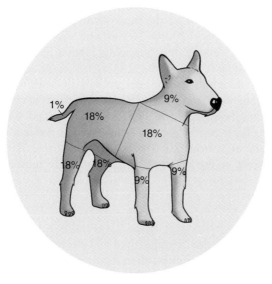

Katherine Sitseri ©

Figure 13.8   Diagram outlining the different body surface areas of various major anatomical parts of the canine patient. (Courtesy of Katherine Sitseri.)

full thickness), assessing epilation (if hair pulls out usually deep partial thickness or full thickness), and general color of skin (superficial burns tend to be red, partial thickness deep red to yellow and discolored, and full thickness often darker, with areas of eschar). If the patient presents quickly to the veterinary hospital, cold water on the affected limb will help relieve some heat from the skin by conduction. However, care must be taken to not further damage the skin with frigid water, and not to cause iatrogenic secondary hypothermia if cooling large amounts of body surface area.

Wound Care

Wound care for the burn patient will depend on the severity of the burn. For superficial burns, lavage and topical agents and bandages may possibly be the only therapy needed. After a few days, if there are any other injuries present, the treatment plan can be reassessed. Partial thickness and full thickness burns usually require debridement.

Several options exist for topical agents on a burn wound. Aloe vera has been shown to have anti-thromboxane effects which can prevent progression of a burn. It should not be used on full thickness burns (Silverstein and Hopper 2009). Silver sulfadiazine remains the mainstay in topical treatment of burn injuries. It should be applied to a burn wound when the fur has been clipped from the area and the site of injury is free of necrotic debris. For lavage prior to application, a 1:40 dilution of chlorhexidine or a 1:9 dilution of povidone-iodine solution may be used.

Once the skin is clean, liberal application with ointment, and then covering with a sterile nonadherent dressing is recommended. Silver sulfadiazine possesses bacteriocidal activity against gram-positive and gram-negative bacteria, as well as Candida yeast, a common opportunistic pathogen. If the burn injury is in an anatomical location unable to be bandaged, management of the injury with just silver sulfadiazine cream is an option (Silverstein and Hopper 2009). Newer options for wound healing involve sugar and honey application. These will be discussed further in the wound section of this chapter.

Superficial and partial thickness burns heal potentially within 2–3 weeks of initial injury with proper management, and assuming no infection develops (Silverstein and Hopper 2009). The eschar layer, necrotic skin that has bonded with newer skin, may thicken and harden. This layer can be gently trimmed off as needed. Full thickness burns heal quite slowly (Pavletic and Trout 2006). Because they are so damaged, they run the risk of developing infection, severe scarring, and potential disfigurement.

Fluid Therapy

Systemic complications of burn injury include fluid and electrolyte abnormalities, systemic infection, and intense pain. Fluid and electrolyte requirements are extremely high in burn patients. Because of capillary damage and permeability, intense loss of fluids, proteins, and red cells can occur at the burn site. Patients with severe losses may present in hypovolemic shock, and appropriate fluid resuscitation should take place. Balanced crystalloid electrolyte solutions are appropriate for management of hypovolemia and electrolyte replacement. Serial PCV/TS and electrolyte measurements should be monitored.

Fluid therapy requirements have been described as $1–4\,mL/kg \times TBSA\,\%$. Because plasma proteins are also lost, a synthetic colloid may be necessary to maintain appropriate colloid oncotic pressure. Electrolyte derangements usually involve sodium and potassium and can range from hypernatremia and hyponatremia, and hyper and hypokalemia. Acidemia, both metabolic and respiratory, may also be present. Azotemia and oliguria may be clinical findings from hypovolemia or renal dysfunction. Because burns evoke a systemic inflammatory response, the burn patient should be monitored for SIRS, DIC, and MODS syndromes.

Monitoring

These patients should be closely monitored and potentially could benefit from CVP and urine output monitoring. Patients with burn injury should be kept in an isolated area. Hospital personnel should use non-sterile gloves and be as clean as possible when dealing with these patients. Using other infection control procedures such as gowns, gloves, and face masks can be utilized as necessary. Nosocomial infection is a huge concern, as their primary defense mechanism has been altered.

Nutrition is also of great concern in burn patients. A recent chapter on nutrition highlighted that "…the importance of adequate nutrition cannot be overemphasized in assisting with the healing of burn wounds…" (Silverstein and Hopper 2009). Nutrition should be provided in whatever form necessary, enteral or parenteral, and should be high calorie and high protein, for energy and repair.

Empirical antibiotic therapy is not recommended in burn patients, unless they are already potentially septic, have pneumonia, or are immunocompromised. Bacterial colonization and proliferation at the burn site is common but is usually managed with topical modalities. These patients should be identified as high risk for development of infection, and hospital personnel should be aware of this.

Patient comfort and emotional support can also be a large part of the nursing care of a burn patient. Systemic analgesia should be administered on a regular basis. Recumbent patients should receive adequate bedding and proper eye and mouth care. Prevention and prompt cleaning of soil is important and passive range of motion exercises can be beneficial in healing.

In addition, any burn injury should be thought of as having caused damage to the respiratory tract, from smoke or flames, until proven otherwise. Therefore, vigilant monitoring of the respiratory system should be instituted. In addition, because of systemic response to burn injury, patients are at risk for acute lung injury (ALI) or ARDS. Systemic infection can result in pneumonia. Aggressive fluid therapy can result in fluid overload and subsequent pulmonary edema. Monitoring of respiratory tract through regular respiration rate and character assessment, thoracic radiographs, pulse oximetry, and blood gas analysis may be necessary.

In addition to respiratory side effects, corneal ulcers may be present in a patient presented for burns, who was exposed to smoke. A careful ocular exam should also be performed in order to diagnose potential ulceration.

Wounds

Wounds and wound care are more than likely a daily part of the critical care technician's duties. Knowledge of wound types, healing, and methods of closure are crucial for the experienced veterinary technician's essential role in patient care.

Classification

Wounds are classified in many ways. First, a classification system by level of contamination has been developed. Wounds may be either clean, clean contaminated, contaminated, or dirty wounds. Clean wounds represent those that have happened under clean conditions. An example would be a surgical incision, which has been aseptically prepared and draped, and sterile instruments used to make the wound. This wound can be considered to have very minimal pathogenic contamination, if any at all.

Clean contaminated wounds are those in which some contamination of a clean wound has occurred. Mostly these can be described as wounds in the process of surgery, GI resection, and anastomosis, for example, where some mild contamination of a sterile field has occurred, but this can be corrected and the wound returned to a clean state.

Contaminated wounds represent wounds with a serious degree of contamination from either non-sterile bodily fluids or potentially the environment. These wounds are considered newer, (presentation to hospital is not delayed), and will either be contaminated with dirt or soil, saliva, or represents a surgical wound with a break in asepsis, such as GI perforation and rupture.

Finally, dirty or infected wounds are older wounds with obvious signs of infection. These wounds should contain at least 10^5 organisms/g of tissue. An example of a dirty wound would be a cat bite abscess. A dirty/infected wound is typically converted to a clean contaminated wound via debridement and irrigation.

Wound Types

Several types of wounds exist. Abrasions, lacerations, burns, puncture wounds, and degloving injuries represent the major wound types.

Abrasions are considered to be partial-thickness wounds where the epidermis has been sheared off, exposing the under layers of the dermis and subcutaneous tissue. They are often associated with minimal bleeding and develop a negligible amount of fluid accumulation.

Lacerations are considered wounds with sharp edges, often in a somewhat straight line. These are considered to cause minimal tissue trauma, as their surface area is quite small. If any tissue is torn away, it is a special type of laceration called an avulsion. Lacerations may be superficial or deep, depending on how many layers of tissue or deep structures (muscles, tendons) they affect.

Burn injuries are wounds caused by thermal exposure. As described above, they may be superficial, partial thickness, or full thickness.

Puncture wounds are often described by a small skin opening, under which extensive tissue trauma may exist. Puncture wounds are often considered contaminated, as the foreign object (tooth, bullet, arrow, etc.) often drags bacteria with it into the subcutaneous space.

Degloving injuries are characterized as extensive amounts of tissue, tendon, and muscle being torn from a limb from some traumatic event. They may also exist where the outermost layer of skin is intact but the underlying fascia, muscles, and blood supply have been compromised (Bassert and McCurnin 2002) (Fig. 13.9).

Wound Healing

Wound healing is described in four phases: inflammatory, debridement, repair, and maturation. The inflammatory phase is the immediate phase, occurring within 5 days of injury. During this phase, after initial bleeding from vascular trauma, local vasoconstriction and platelet aggregation prevent excessive hemorrhage. Shortly after bleeding stops, some

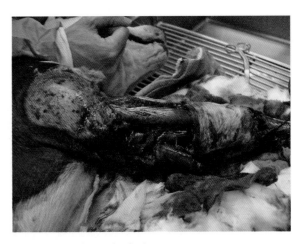

Figure 13.9   A severe degloving wound in a dog limb.

vasodilation occurs, which allows clotting factors and fibrinogen to enter the wound and begin to form a clot. This process also signals neutrophils, monocytes, fibroblasts, and endothelial cells to enter into the wound. In addition to cells, inflammatory mediators such as cytokines, histamines, leukotrienes, complement, and growth factor also start to exude into the wound, beginning the local inflammatory response.

The debridement phase occurs in parallel to the inflammatory phase. As white blood cells, namely neutrophils, enter the wound, any foreign debris is removed via phagocytosis. After neutrophils, monocytes enter the wound and develop into macrophages aiding in the removal of foreign material and pathogens. They also signal fibroblasts to begin entering the wound.

The repair phase, or proliferative phase, begins several days after the injury and may last several weeks (Silverstein and Hopper 2009). There are several parts to this stage, including angiogenesis, formation of granulation tissue, and epithelialization. Angiogenesis, or growth of blood vessels from existing ones, allows blood supply to return to the affected area. As collagen is also being synthesized for tissue repair, granulation tissue forms as new capillaries start to perfuse the new tissue. Granulation tissue forms a bed that allows epithelialization to happen. Epithelialization represents the development of a new skin layer over the existing, healing wound.

After the repair phase is complete, several weeks after injury, the maturation phase begins. During this phase, collagen is deposited at the wound site, and the wound begins to contract, although the tissue is never as strong as the original.

Initial Treatment

In managing patients with wounds, it is recommended to use exam gloves to assess their injuries (Silverstein and Hopper 2009). If any excessive bleeding is occurring, direct pressure should be applied. If bleeding occurs through direct pressure, a pressure tourniquet, inflated to 200 mmHg, may be used for 1 hour (Silverstein and Hopper 2009). Beyond this, surgical intervention is required. Keeping a new wound covered and moist are important in order to prevent nosocomial infection and dessication. A sterile water-soluble lubricant such as K-Y Jelly may be applied to the wound, and sterile saline-soaked gauze sponges may be used to cover the wound while a light bandage is applied. It is important to always note what structures are present under the wound's surface, as traumatic wounds may affect important internal structures.

The steps in wound management are assessing the location and type of wound, debriding and lavaging the wound if necessary, deciding on closure of the wound, and protection of the wound with a bandage if necessary. When debriding a wound, sterile lubricating jelly should be applied, which will minimize any continued contamination of a wound. Fur should be clipped in a wide margin, and the skin should be scrubbed with a dilute chlorhexidine (0.05%), or povidone-iodine (1%) solution, around, but not on the surface, of the wound, as these chemicals can inhibit wound healing. The wound should be debrided under sterile surgical conditions and any necrotic tissue removed. To make a chlorhexidine or povidone-iodine dilution, add 1 part 2% chlorhexidine to 40 parts sterile solution, or 1 part 10% povidone-iodine to 9 parts sterile solution (Silverstein and Hopper 2009).

If wounds are heavily contaminated, such as those with road rash, a water faucet nozzle with tap water may be effective in removing gross debris before sterile lavage needs to be performed (Silverstein and Hopper 2009). Wound lavage is typically done with a syringe, 3-way stopcock, and 18-gauge needle or catheter, attached to a fluid bag. Reportedly, Lactated Ringer's solution is less toxic to fibroblasts and thus should be used if available (Silverstein and Hopper 2009). Decent pressure, 7–8 psi, can be generated using this method (Bassert and McCurnin 2002).

Wound Closure

Types of closure

Wound closure has several types. Primary closure represents a method of healing where the tissue heals by first intention, or appositional healing. In this method, the wound is sutured together shortly after trauma, and healing occurs as fresh edges are in contact with each other. Wounds with clean edges should only be sutured within 6–8 hours of initial injury, termed the golden period, where pathogens have not yet reached the 10^5 organisms/g tissue (Bassert and McCurnin 2002).

Delayed primary closure represents primary, or appositional, closure occurring after 6–8 hours, but before 3–5 days after initial injury, which is before a granulation layer may form. Delayed primary closure is reserved for mild to moderately contaminated wounds, which have undergone debridement, and will wait for closure until a granulation bed forms.

Secondary closure of wounds represents wounds that are considered quite contaminated, or even dirty, and are closed sometime after 5 days of initial injury. Often, accumulated granulation tissue must be trimmed before closure.

Second intention healing refers to healing by contraction and epithelialization. This method may be used for large wounds, unable to be sutured, and requires intensive bandaging and long-term management (Fig. 13.10).

A newer approach to wounds has been the use of sugar and honey in wound healing and repair. Several studies and publications have been addressed on this topic. Recently, an article by Mathews and Binnington (2002a,b) described a procedure and indications for sugar and honey with regard to wound therapy. Honey is reported to be bacteriocidal

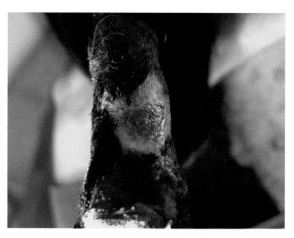

Figure 13.10   A wound healing by second intention. Notice the extent of the wound and the presence of a granulation bed in the center. Redness indicates fresh tissue and blood supply. The perimeter has started to form a scar.

as well as effective in decreasing tissue edema, attracting macrophages, digesting necrotic tissue; it is also a nutrient source for tissue, and is a protective layer for the development of a granulation bed. It is antibacterial due to its high osmolarity, acidity, and levels of H_2O_2 (Mathews and Binnington 2002a).

Wound management with honey results in chemical debridement and thus, there is no need for surgical debridement of wounds. Sterile sponges soaked in honey may be applied to burns or cumbersome wounds not easily closed or managed. These may be then covered with an outer bandage. Sugar has similar attributes. Wounds packed with sugar paste will heal in similar fashion to the ones treated with honey (Mathews and Binnington 2002b). There was some concern that honey may be painful, so in one patient, sugar was used over honey, and the painful sensation seemed to subside (Mathews and Binnington 2002a).

Nursing Care

Nursing care for patients with wounds and bandages includes pain management, recumbent patient care, bandage care, nutrition, appropriate antimicrobial therapy, fluid therapy, and tender loving care (TLC). Patients having experienced a wound or traumatic injury are often in pain. Regular pain scoring and assessments need to be performed to ensure adequate analgesic medications are administered. If patients are suffering from fractures or paresis, they may be recumbent and require proper padding and prevention or prompt cleaning of any soil. Patients need their bandages kept clean and dry, observed for any limb swelling, slipping, or strike through. In addition, these patients need adequate nutrition to ensure proper wound closure and mobilization of the immune system.

Feeding tubes, enteral nutrition, and parenteral nutrition may be necessary to support the body in time of stress. Patients with infections require appropriate antibiotic therapy, and prompt administration of medications, along with knowledge of mechanism of action and side effects, is crucial. Patients in hospital may also require fluid therapy and monitoring for electrolyte changes, or fluid overload require diligent nursing.

Finally, these patients require love and attention to support their emotional needs and to alleviate their physiologic stress.

Fractures

Fractures are another unfortunate consequence of trauma. The location of the fracture, degree of tissue trauma, nearby anatomy and degree of pain are all important parts of fracture patient assessment. The force applied to the bone determines the type of fracture line that may exist. Depending on the location of the fracture, different modalities (splints, bandages, slings) may be appropriate.

Classification of Fractures

Classification of fractures is based on several aspects. Variation of displacement of the bone and stability, location, direction, and number of fracture lines, reducibility, open or non-open, completeness, and involvement of other musculoskeletal structures such as tendons and ligaments, make up the various schemes to classify fractures (Fossum et al. 2007). Fractures can occur at various points of anatomy of a bone, including the articular surface, metaphysis, physis, and diaphysis (Fossum et al. 2007) (Fig.13.11).

Transverse fractures have a fracture line perpendicular to the long axis of a bone. Oblique fractures have their fracture line at an angle to the long axis. Spiral fractures have a spiral fracture line that rotates approximately 360 degrees around the bone, usually at an angle to the long axis. Comminuted fractures represent fractures that have multiple broken fragments, representing several fracture lines. Physeal fractures have their own scoring system, the Salter–Harris system.

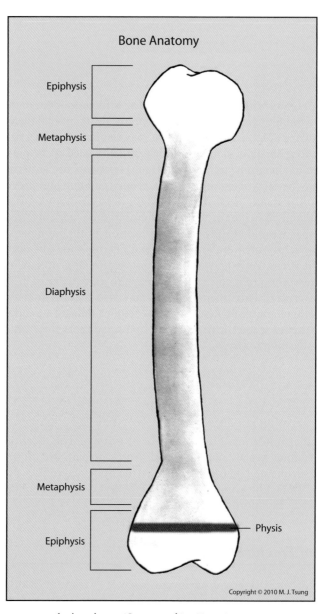

Figure 13.11   Gross anatomy of a long bone. (Courtesy of Jen Tsung.)

Avulsion fractures are fractures that involve tendons or ligaments near the fracture site. Greenstick fractures are best described as one splintered fragment of bone, where the fracture is incomplete and the fractured bone is able to stabilize the cortex of the bone.

Open fractures have a specific classification system. An open fracture is a fracture with an associated wound. First-degree open fractures are when the broken bone penetrates the skin from the inside. There is a small skin wound, and there is a moderate degree of tissue trauma and contusion. Second-degree open fractures are fractures that have happened as a result of a wound from the outside. There is a greater degree of tissue trauma and a higher risk of contamination due to the foreign debris from skin contact with the environment. Third-degree open fractures are reserved for patients who suffer severe trauma from high velocity impact, such as gunshot injury, or high-rise syndrome (Schwartz and Moore 2002) (Fig. 13.12).

Initial treatment of fractures, especially open fractures, follow a similar approach to managing wound. Assessment of the wound, followed by debridement, must occur. The wounds should be covered with sterile wet-dry bandages. Surgical repair, if indicated, should take place as soon as possible. In the interim, temporary fixation of a fracture is accomplished with splinting and bandaging. Extremity fractures, such as of the radius/ulna, are often secured with a caudal splint, or spoon splint. Injuries to tarsus, humerus, or tibia are often secured using a lateral splint. Spica splints may also be used. Shoulder, stifle, humerus, and femur fractures are often not immobilized. These may be left until surgical correction can occur, with cage confinement and analgesic therapy commencing until surgery.

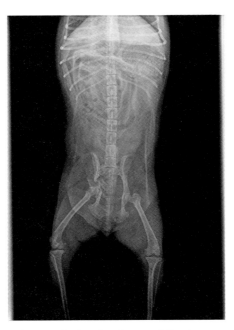

Figure 13.12 This patient has suffered multiple pelvic fractures following trauma. Remember that pelvic fractures cause tremendous pain, can cause trauma to caudal intra-abdominal structures such as blood vessels and the bladder, and can require long-term nursing care.

CHAPTER 13

Nursing Care

Patients with fractures require dedicated nursing care. Fractures are considered extremely painful and regular, and vigilant pain scoring and assessment are necessary to ensure adequate analgesia. Patients with fractures may have bandages in place and require bandage care in addition to proper padding. Fractures require similar nursing recommendations as patients with wounds. Nutrition, pain control, bandage and wound care, and recumbent care are all extremely important in successful patient outcome.

References

Armstrong, S, et al. 2005. Perioperative hypothermia. *Journal of Veterinary Emergency and Critical Care* 15(1):32–27.

Babic, T, et al. 2004. Feline high-rise syndrome: 119 cases (1998–2001). *Journal of Feline Medicine and Surgery* 6(5):305–312.

Bassert, JM, McCurnin, DM. 2002. *Clinical Textbook for Veterinary Technicians*, 5th ed. Philadelphia: Saunders Elsevier.

Brown, DE, et al. 1994. Echinocytosis associated with rattlesnake envenomation in dogs. *Veterinary Pathology* 31(6):654–657.

Brown, RF, et al. 1997. Mechanisms of echinocytosis induced by *Crotalus atrox* venom. *Veterinary Pathology* 34:442–449.

Clark, RF, et al. 1997. Successful treatment of crotalid-induced neurotoxicity with a new polyspecific crotalid Fab antivenom. *Annals of Emergency Medicine* 30(1):54–57.

Fossum, T, et al. 2007. *Small Animal Surgery*, 3rd ed. St. Louis, MO: Mosby Elsevier.

Gordon, LE, et al. 1993. High-rise syndrome in dogs: 81 cases (1985–1991). *Journal of American Veterinary Medical Association* 202(1):118–122.

Johnson, SI, et al. 2006. Heatstroke in small animal medicine: a clinical practice review. *Journal of Veterinary Emergency and Critical Care* 16(2):112–119.

Kirby, R, et al. 2001. Hypothermia in critically ill dogs and cats. *Compendium on Continuing Education for the Practicing Veterinarian* 23(6):506–521.

Mathews, KA, Binnington, AG. 2002a Wound management using honey. *Compendium on Continuing Education for the Practicing Veterinarian* 24(1):53–60.

Mathews, KA, Binnington, AG. 2002b Wound management using sugar. *Standards of Care: Emergency and Critical Care Medicine* 4:6–9.

Pavletic, MM, Trout, NJ. 2006. Bullet, bite, and burn wounds in dogs and cats. *Veterinary Clinics Small Animal Practice* 36:873–893.

Pratschke, KM, Kirby, BM. 2002. High rise syndrome with impalement in three cats. *Journal of Small Animal Practice* 43:261–264.

Schwarz, DJ, Moore, KW. 2002. Emergency stabilization of long bone fractures. *Standards of Care: Emergency and Critical Care Medicine* 4(2):1–p5.

Silverstein, DC, Hopper, K. 2009. *Small Animal Critical Care Medicine*. St. Louis, MO: Elsevier Saunders.

Toxicological Emergencies

Christopher L. Norkus

Introduction

In 2008, the American Society for the Prevention of Cruelty to Animals ASPCA Animal Poison Control Center (APCC) in Urbana, Illinois, reported handling more than 140,000 cases of pets exposed to toxic substances. Many of these cases and many other unreported cases are seen and treated each year in emergency rooms and critical care facilities across the country. Clinical signs of toxicity can involve essentially any body system. Therefore, toxicity should always be considered as a potential differential whenever a patient presents with an illness of unknown cause. As with many realms of veterinary medicine, veterinary technicians play a crucial role in the triage, stabilization, detoxification, diagnosis, and ongoing care of these patients.

General Principles of Toxicology

Toxins can gain entrance into the body predominantly through four routes: ingestion, inhalation, injection, or topical exposure (including contact with mucous membranes, skin, or eyes). By far, ingestion remains the most common means of toxicity for dogs and cats. Whenever a patient is believed to have encountered a toxin, it should be brought to the hospital and examined promptly. With the goal of limiting toxic absorption and progression of toxicity, time is of the essence, and owners should not be instructed to treat animals at home aside from the most basic care.

Technicians advising owners over the phone on pre-hospital care should instruct the animal to first be removed from the source of the toxin, if applicable, to prevent further exposure. In cases of topical or inhaled exposure, owners must protect themselves from accidental toxicity by wearing gloves, mask protection, and additional protective clothing before handling the animal. Stable patients that have had topical exposure can be washed in a mild dishwashing detergent (e.g., Dawn, Procter & Gamble Cincinnati, OH) before being brought to the hospital. Owners should be told to handle dogs and cats under the influence of a toxin with care as some patients will show abnormal behavior that could result in unexpected injury to the owner. Any container or package that the toxin was in, including a sample of the suspected toxin if available, should also be brought to the veterinary hospital. Vomit, feces, and urine produced after the animal's exposure should also be collected and brought in for potential laboratory analysis (Fig. 14.1).

With there being tens of thousands of agents that can potentially cause toxicity in dogs and cats, this chapter is by no means an inclusive guide. Whenever faced with an unfamiliar toxicity, the reader is highly encouraged to contact the ASPCA APCC 24 hours a day, 365 days a year at (888) 426–4435.

Initial Assessment and Stabilization

Patients presenting with toxicity can arrive in various clinical states ranging from essentially normal to comatose. Like any patient presenting to the emergency room, a brief chief complaint is determined and an initial assessment is made which includes a rapid

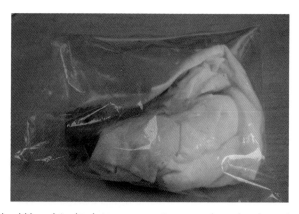

Figure 14.1   Clients should be advised to bring any container or package that the toxin was in to the hospital. (Courtesy of Thomas Walker, DVM, DACVECC.)

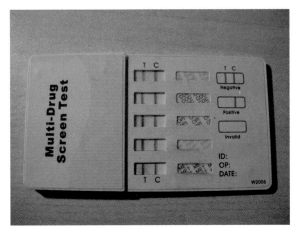

Figure 14.2 Commercial illegal drug test kits are available to screen for many toxins at one time.

evaluation of airway, breathing, and circulation. Life-saving stabilization is begun as necessary, including cardiopulmonary cerebral resuscitation (CPCR), intubation, ventilation, intravenous catheter placement and intravenous fluids, oxygen administration, seizure control, and emergency drug therapy. Laboratory samples are next collected, and monitoring techniques are employed to assess the patient's present status and aid in the diagnosis phase. A secondary evaluation is then performed and will include a more detailed physical exam and a full patient history from the owners.

Diagnosis

In many incidences of toxicity, a specific inciting cause is not identified. Many toxins do not have pathognomonic signs (e.g., CNS excitement with seizures) or laboratory findings. In some incidences, though, in-house test kits (e.g., ethylene glycol [EG], illegal drug panels) and specific laboratory chemical analysis (e.g., lead) may be utilized to identify a toxic substance. Specific tests and laboratory findings are discussed within each specific toxicosis later in this chapter. In general, diagnosis of toxicity is most commonly made based on the history, patient signs, and treatment response (Fig. 14.2).

Decontamination

The main goal of the decontamination phase is to prevent initial absorption or further absorption of a toxin. The specific form of decontamination will depend on the route of toxic exposure. Cases that have been exposed to toxins topically should be bathed immediately in a mild hand or dishwashing detergent. Dawn is an excellent choice. It is important to use ample detergent and water to ensure that the toxin is not just being dispersed to a larger surface area but rather removed from the patient. Protective gloves, clothing, mask, and glasses should be worn by staff to prevent their contamination. Patients with ocular exposure should have their eyes flushed with copious amount of warm water or 0.9% saline for a minimum of 15 minutes.

When a toxin is ingested, the method of decontamination will depend on the individual toxin. In general, corrosive substances (e.g., bleach), strong acids, and strong bases should be treated with rapid dilution of the toxin by administration of milk or water. In such cases, emesis is avoided because the individual substance could cause significant damage to the esophagus leading to esophagitis, strictures, or perforation if vomiting occurred.

When not contraindicated, emesis remains one of the mainstay decontamination procedures for toxic ingestion. The use of emetics should not be indiscriminant, however. Emetics are contraindicated in rodents or rabbits as these species may have weak stomach walls and are unable to vomit. The induction of emesis is also contraindicated in patients that are comatose, seizuring, severely depressed, dyspneic, hypoxic, or lack normal swallowing reflexes. The use of emetics after ingestion of strychnine or other central nervous system (CNS) stimulants may precipitate seizures.

Vomiting generally removes between 40% and 60% of stomach contents and can therefore dramatically decrease what amount of toxin remains in the body. Several emetics are available for use. Two mechanisms of action are recognized for emetics: stimulation of the chemoreceptor trigger zone (CRTZ) or direct gastric irritation. When emetics are used, they are most effective when they are administered shortly after toxin ingestion and when food is already present in the stomach. Therefore, sometimes feeding a patient who is reluctant to vomit after it has received an emetic in a small meal may successfully result in vomiting. The most common emetics used in veterinary practice are apomorphine, xylazine, and hydrogen peroxide.

Apomorphine

Apomorphine is used primarily as an emetic in dogs and is considered the emetic of choice by many clinicians. It can, however, also be utilized in cats. Apomorphine acts as a D1 and D2 dopaminergic agonist to stimulate receptors in the CRTZ, thus inducing vomiting. The drug can cause either CNS depression or stimulation but more frequently results in a stimulatory effects. Some cats may become overly stimulated with the administration of the drug and therefore, its use is controversial and another agent such xylazine may be preferred. Apomorphine is available in a soluble tablet for use in either the conjunctival sack or via the injectable route after solubilizing the tablets in at least 1–2 mL of sterile water for injection or 0.9% sodium chloride. After sufficient vomiting occurs, the conjunctiva should be rinsed free of unabsorbed apomorphine. A dopaminergic antagonist such as metoclopramide can be used to reverse refractory vomiting, and naloxone can be utilized to reverse the drug's CNS depressive effect if it occurs. Acepromazine and other dopaminergic antagonists may negate the effect of apomorphine. Apomorphine may be administered in dogs and cats at 0.04 mg/kg IV or 0.08 mg/kg IM, SQ, or via the conjunctival sac (Plumb 2005) (Fig. 14.3).

Xylazine

Xylazine is an alpha-2 adrenergic agonist that has profound sedative and analgesic qualities. In the cat, it is a popular and highly effective emetic. The agent is not commonly used in the dog. A dose of 0.4 mg/kg IM, SQ is recommended (Plumb 2005). Important side effects may include bradycardia, cardiac arrhythmias, respiratory depression, and sedation. The agent can be quickly reversed with yohimbine or atipamazole if necessary.

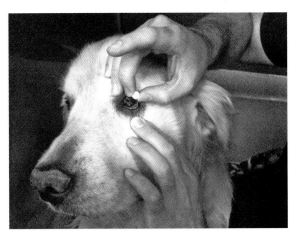

Figure 14.3　Apomorphine can be administration into the conjunctival sac, intravenously, or intramuscularly. (Courtesy of David Liss, RVT, VTS [Emergency & Critical Care].)

Hydrogen Peroxide

Three percent hydrogen peroxide (H_2O_2) causes vomiting by direct gastric irritation. It is an excellent choice for owners to use in dogs as a pre-hospital care because it is cheap and is often readily available. Unfortunately, the product's ability to produce emesis can be unreliable. In addition, it has been known to cause refractory vomiting and eshopagitis in cats and therefore is not recommend as a first choice agent for that species. A dose of 1–2 mL/kg PO has been proposed (Plunkett 2001).

Gastric Lavage

Gastric lavage is a technique used predominantly when the induction of emesis is contra-indicated or when a large dose of toxin has been ingested. Its use is most effective when performed less than 4 hours after toxic ingestion. The patient is lightly anesthetized (e.g., an opioid and a benzodiazepine) and intubated with a cuffed endotracheal tube to mini-mize the risk of aspiration. A large-bore stomach tube is premeasured from the tip of the nose to the last rib, and a marker is placed to indicate the correct length. The tube is then lubricated and gently introduced via the oropharynx to the stomach. Large amounts of warm water are then administered through the tube and then are allowed to siphon back into a collection bucket. The received stomach contents should be reserved for potential chemical analysis. Activated charcoal may then be administered into the stomach. The tube is then tightly kinked at the patient end before removal from the mouth to help minimize the risk of aspiration. Because of the risk of esophageal damage previously described, gastric lavage is generally avoided with caustic substances (Fig. 14.4).

Activated Charcoal

Activated charcoal is an extremely porous form of carbon that, having a large surface area, acts as an effective absorbent. As a result, activated charcoal binds to many toxins and will therefore prevent absorption in the gastrointestinal tract. Unfortunately, some toxins such as ethanol, methanol, bleach, and xylitol do not effectively bind to activated

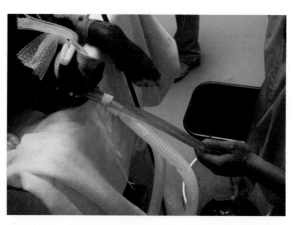

Figure 14.4   Gastric lavage should not be an overlooked form of decontamination. (Courtesy of Thomas Walker, DVM, DACVECC.)

charcoal and therefore, its use is ineffective in such cases. Activated charcoal is available commercially as a suspension (Toxiban, Lloyd, Inc., Shenandoah, IA), tablet, and powder. A dose of 2–5 g/kg (5–10 mL/kg PO) q2-6hs is suggested (Plunkett 2001). Administering charcoal suspension by a red rubber feeding tube attached to a 60-cc oral syringe and slowly dribbling it into the side of the pet's mouth is typically very well tolerated.

Due to the potential for enterohepatic recirculation of some toxins, administration of activated charcoal may need to be repeated. Some suspension products are also available with the cathartic sorbital. Cathartics accelerate defecation and therefore help to eliminate the toxin once they are bound to charcoal. Sodium sulfate is occasionally used as a stand-alone agent. Cathartics should be avoided in patients with or at risk of having diarrhea and should typically only be given once.

Treatment

In many incidences, patients may present after toxicity has already occurred. Depending on the toxin, decontamination may or may not be beneficial at this point. In general, treatment for toxicity is supportive care. Supportive care may range from observation in hospital to seizure control or assisted ventilation. Unfortunately, many toxins do not have specific antidotes or treatment. Exceptions to this statement are discussed later in this chapter under individual toxicities.

Most toxins are biotransformed in the liver and excreted through the kidneys. Therefore, as an effort to support organ perfusion and promote diuresis, intravenous fluids are nearly always advocated. After the initial stabilization and replacement of fluid deficits, fluid rates generally will be set at or above maintenance rates (40–66 mL/kg/day) to ensure a minimum urine output of 2–4 mL/kg/h.

Ion Trapping

Most drugs are weak acids (e.g., aspirin, acetaminophen, warfarin, ibuprofen) or weak bases (e.g., amphetamines, ephedrine, strychnine, diphenhydramine). Ion trapping is a technique used to increase the excretion rate of toxicity-causing drugs. Drugs typically are unable to pass through cell membranes unless they are in a nonionized state. Drugs that are weak acids are absorbed well when placed into an acidic environment as they will be in a nonionized form. Likewise, drugs that are weak bases are absorbed best when placed into an alkaline environment. By modifying the pH of a surrounding environment, we can therefore potentially modify ionization, trap a drug, and prevent its absorption. In clinical practice, the technique of ion trapping is most often utilized for drugs that are readily reabsorbed in the kidney's nephron or bladder. In such cases, by changing the pH of the urine, urinary alkalinizers (e.g., sodium bicarbonate) increase elimination of weak acids and urine acidifier (e.g., ammonium chloride) increase elimination of weak bases. A dose for ammonium chloride is 100–200 mg/kg/day PO divided q8-12h in the dog and 20 mg/kg PO q12h in the cat (Plunkett 2001).

Intravenous Lipid Therapy

Perhaps the most exciting advance in recent years to treating drug toxicities in veterinary patients is the use of intravenous lipid therapy (e.g., 20% Liposyn). Pharmaceuticals and other toxins that are highly lipid-soluble appear to bind well to lipid infusions that are inexpensive and commonly available for total parenteral nutrition (TPN). Although experience in dogs and cats is still limited, such therapy appears to reverse the signs of toxicity and has already shown to be a highly effective therapy in cases of bupivacaine and moxidectin toxicity (Crandell and Weinberg 2009). It appears to also have potential benefit in pyrethrin toxicity, marijuana, and many other drugs. When using an emulsion of 20% soybean oil in water, the ASPCA APCC has suggested bolus dose of 1.5–4 mL/kg (Fernandez et al. 2011) followed by a constant rate infusion (CRI) of 0.25 mL/kg/min for 30–60 minutes. They report this dose can be repeated in 6–8 hours if the patient is not lipemic and is still symptomatic. Further investigation into this treatment modality is necessary.

Specific Toxicities

Acetaminophen (Tylenol)

Acetaminophen is a common over-the-counter household analgesic and antipyretic. It is available in tablets, capsules, liquids, and in several preparations with other drugs. A dose of as little as 50 mg/kg is toxic to the cat. Cats become poisoned through oral ingestion, generally by accidental administration by owners. Toxicity is due to lethal synthesis of acetaminophen into a toxic metabolite that alters glutathione concentrations in both hepatic and red blood cells. Hepatic and erythrocyte damage occurs, including the development of methemoglobinemia. Dogs may develop hepatic necrosis at doses of 150 mg/kg (Plunkett 2001). Keratoconjunctiva sicca (KCS) has also been reported in the dog following acetaminophen toxicity (Mariani and Fulton 2001).

Clinical signs in cats occur rapidly, generally within 2 hours of ingestion. Anorexia, vomiting, salivation, lethargy, weakness, brown or cyanotic mucous membranes, dyspnea, chocolate-colored urine and blood, along with facial and paw edema may be observed. Death occurs rapidly within 18–36 hours. Prognosis is guarded to poor in cats. Diagnosis is typically made by history and clinical signs. Laboratory findings include methemoglobinemia, Heinz body anemia, elevations to alanine aminotransferase (ALT),

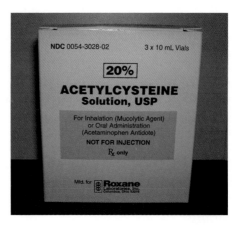

Figure 14.5   Acetaminophen Toxicity Antidote. (Courtesy of Thomas Walker, DVM, DACVECC.)

alkaline phosphatase (ALKP), and bilirubin concentration. Metabolic acidosis may also be observed.

If ingestion was recent, initial treatment includes the induction of emesis, gastric lavage, and the administration of activated charcoal. *N*-acetylcystine at 140 mg/kg PO or IV as a loading dose and then 70 mg/kg q6h for seven treatments acts as an antidote (Plunkett 2001). For intravenous administration, the drug is diluted to a 5% concentration in D5W and administered slowly over 15–30 minutes. Additional treatment includes ascorbic acid (vitamin C) 30 mg/kg PO or SQ q6h to treat the methemoglobinemia and cimetidine 5–10 mg/kg q6-8h IV, IM to act as a P450 enzyme inhibitor and reduce the amount of metabolized acetaminophen by the liver. (Plunkett 2001). Intravenous fluids, oxygen therapy, and transfusions with whole blood, hemoglobin oxygen-carrying solutions (HBOCs), or packed red blood cells (pRBCs) may be necessary. Due to the very fragile nature of cats with severe methemoglobinemia, they should be handled quietly and calmly to minimize stress and potential death (Fig. 14.5).

Amitraz

Amitraz (Preventic [Virbac Corporation, Fort Worth, TX], Mitaban [Pharmacia & Upjohn, Inc., Bridgewater, NJ], etc.) is an alpha-1 and 2 adrenergic agonist that is predominantly used in tick/flea colors and for the treatment of demodicosis in small animals. Cats are highly sensitive to its toxic effects. Toxicity from amitraz can occur either through the oral or dermal route and results from excessive alpha-2 adrenergic stimulation. Toxicity can potentially cause CNS sedation, bradycardia, polyuria, pale mucous membranes, hypothermia, vomiting, and respiratory depression. Diagnosis is made via history and clinical signs and is supported by hyperglycemia on serum chemistry. Oral decontamination can include emesis, gastric lavage, and activated charcoal. The toxicity is specifically treated with an alpha-2 adrenergic antagonist such as yohimbine or atipamazole. Intravenous fluids may be used to support organ perfusion and blood pressure. Atropine should be avoided even in the face of bradycardia as it is likely to produce significant hypertension. Prognosis is generally fair.

Anticoagulant Rodenticides

Numerous anticoagulant rodenticides are available on the market as rat and mice poison. These agents work by antagonizing vitamin K epoxide reductase, thereby preventing the activation of clotting factors II, VII, IX, and X. The depletion of these factors slows all coagulation pathways, eventually leading to cogaulopathy, hemorrhage, and death.

Dogs and cats are usually poisoned by direct ingestion, malicious poisoning, or ingestion of a poisoned rodent. Dogs are most sensitive to anticoagulant rodenticide toxicity and it is uncommon to see toxicity in cats. The toxic dose varies with agent, species, age, preexisting disease conditions (hepatic or renal disease), and concurrent drug use (aspirin, phenylbutazone, sulfonamides, etc.). First-generation rodenticides can depress clotting factors for approximately 7–10 days while second-generation rodenticide can depress clotting factors for 3–4 weeks. Clinical signs occur several days after ingestion and include lethargy, vomiting, weakness, pallor, melena, epistaxsis, hematemesis, hematuria, gingival bleeding, prolonged bleeding from wounds or venipuncture sites, dyspnea, sclerotic and conjunctival hemorrhage, lameness, joint swelling, brushings, and hematomas. Acute death may result from hemorrhage into the pleural cavity, abdomen, pericardial sac, or mediastinum. Rodenticide toxicity should always be considered a differential whenever there is evidence of bleeding or coagulopathy.

At a minimum, patients should have a packed cell volume (PCV), total protein (TP), complete blood count (CBC), platelet estimate, prothrombin time (PT), and activated partial thromboplastin time (aPTT) evaluated. Due to the short half-life of factor 7, a prolonged PT is the most sensitive indication of early toxicity. When time allows, fibrinogen, fibrin degradation products (FDPs), and a proteins induced by vitamin K antagonism (PIVKA) test can be run to support the diagnosis. A minimum database including a chemistry panel and urinalysis should also be obtained. Diagnosis is based on history of exposure to the toxin, clinical signs, prolonged bleeding times, and response to therapy.

Treatment includes induction of emesis and administration of activated charcoal. Gastric lavage can be considered in cases of massive ingestion. Vitamin K1 (phytonadione) is the specific antidote of choice and should be administered as a loading at 2.5–5 mg/kg SQ and followed by 2.5–5 mg/kg PO q24h for 14–21 days (Plunkett 2001). Second-generation or unknown sources should be treated with the higher dose range for the full 21 days. Oral administration is the preferred route of administration and higher fat meals help increase vitamin K1 absorption. In general, a PT and aPTT should be rechecked 48 hours after discontinuing drug therapy.

The intravenous route of vitamin K1 is typically avoided because of concern of anaphylaxis. In human medicine, studies have suggested this is of low incidence, however. In one veterinary report, effective reversal of prolonged clotting times in the cat was achieved by intravenous vitamin K (Reezigit 2007). In this particular case, a slow intravenous bolus diluted 1:1 with saline was administered over 30 minutes and was felt to outweigh the risk of anaphylaxis. No anaphylaxis was observed.

In the acute management phase, it is critical to understand that vitamin K administration will not restore new clotting factors for 12–24 hours. Therefore, patients often need to receive whole blood transfusions or fresh frozen plasma when they are in need of immediate clotting factors or oxygen delivery. Failure to recognize this may prove to be a fatal mistake.

Patients should also have their clinical signs treated as they occur. This may include oxygen therapy, thoracocentesis, and intravenous fluid therapy. Thoracocentesis is only advocated for patients having significant respiratory impairment and, in an emergency, red cells aspirated from a body cavity can be quickly autotransfused back into the patient

---

Box 14.1   Common Anticoagulant Rodenticides

- First Generation (Warfarin, Coumarin, and Coumatetralyl)
- 1,3-Indandiones (Pindone, Chlorophacinone, Diphacinone)
- Second Generation (Brodifacoum, Bromadiolone, Flocoumafen, Difethialone, Difenacoum)

---

as a short-term solution while steps are made to restore clotting factors with plasma or whole blood.

Avermectin (Ivermectin, Moxidectin, Milbemycin, Selamectin)

Avermectins are antiparasitc agents that are commonly used in large and small animal species. Their mode of action is via gamma aminobutyric acid (GABA) agonism. A toxic dose of ivermectin in puppies and kittens is >300 mcg/kg, cats >500 mcg/kg, and >2000 mcg/kg in dogs (Plunkett 2001). Some dog breeds with genetic MDR1 mutations, such as collies, Australian shepherds, Shetland sheepdogs, and old English sheepdogs, may show toxicity at doses as low as 100 mcg/kg (Plunkett 2001). Clinical signs generally include ataxia, behavioral disturbances, depression, hypersalivation, seizures, mydriasis, muscle tremors, recumbency, coma, and death. Plasma, liver, fat, and brain analysis may identify avermectin toxicity through chemical analysis. Otherwise, the diagnosis is generally made on history of exposure and clinical signs.

The prognosis varies with the species, breed, and age of the patient, the product, and the dose. Decontamination should include the induction of emesis, gastric lavage, and activated charcoal. Seizures should be controlled with anticonvulsant medication, however, because benzodiazepines also stimulate the GABA receptor; thus, their use is controversial. More recently, some have advocated that benzodiazepines may actually be helpful by displacing avermectins from GABA receptor sites. Intravenous lipid administration has been successfully used in the dog to rapidly treat moxidectin toxicity, and may prove beneficial with other avermectins (Crandell and Weinberg 2009). Picrotoxin has been discussed in the literature as a treatment option but is not considered standard treatment at this time. Hospitalization for symptomatic and supportive care, including intravenous fluid to maintain perfusion, hydration, and diuresis, is indicated. The recovery period may be prolonged.

Bleach and Household Cleaners

Household bleach (sodium hypochlorite) is a mild to moderate irritant. The incidence of gastrointestinal burns is low (Plunkett 2001). Clinical signs include hypersalivation, vomiting, and abdominal pain. Treatment includes oral administration of milk or water to dilute the bleach. Emesis and gastric lavage are contraindicated. Symptomatic care for gastroenteritis is instituted.

Nonionic detergents (alkyl ethoxylate, alkyl phenoxy polyethoxy ethanols, and polyethylene glycol stearate) and anionic detergents (alkysodium suldate, alkusodium sulfonates, linear alkylbenzene lauryl sulfate, and tetrapropylene benzene sulfonate) are found in hand dishwashing detergents, shampoos, and laundry detergents. Nonionic detergents typically cause minimal toxicity. Aside from electric dishwashing detergents, anionic detergents are considered slightly to moderately toxic (Plunkett 2001). They may cause vomiting, diarrhea, corrosive stomatitis, esophagitis, contact dermatitis, and keratitis. Treatment includes oral administration of milk or water for dilution. Emesis and gastric lavage are contraindicated. Activated charcoal should be administered. If contact with skin, mucous membranes, or eyes occurred, they should be lavaged extensively. Patients should be treated supportively for vomiting, diarrhea, and corrosive injury.

Cationic detergents (benzalkonium chloride, benzethonium chloride, alkyldimethyl 3.4-dichlorobenzene, and cetylpyridinium chloride) are found in fabric softeners and sanitizers. Clinical signs include corrosive burns to the mouth, pharynx, and esophagus, depression, hypersalivation, vomiting, hematemesis, seizures, shock, and coma. Emesis and gastric lavage are contraindicated if the concentration of cationic detergent ingested is greater than 7.5% (Plunkett 2001). Treatment includes oral administration of milk or water for dilution and administration of activated charcoal. Patients should be treated supportively.

Bromethalin

Bromethalin is a blue-green-colored general use pesticide that results in acute toxicity of dogs and cats. The toxin works by the uncoupling of oxidative phosphorylation in the CNS and liver mitochondria, thereby causing a decrease in adenosine triphosphate (ATP) production. Such a decrease in ATP causes a decrease in Na/K ATPase activity, which results in lost ability to maintain the osmotic gradient and membrane potential in the cell. This results in Na influx into brain cells, consequently causing cerebral edema and loss of function.

Clinical signs include muscle tremors, hyperthermia, seizures, forelimb extensor rigidity (Schiff–Sherrington-like posture), ataxia, vomiting, respiratory paralysis, and death. Chemical analysis may confirm bromethalin in tissues, but diagnostic values are not well established and analysis is not commonly available in clinical laboratories. Therefore, diagnosis is generally based on history and clinical signs.

Early recognition and treatment is paramount to patient survival. Aggressive decontamination is warranted by inducing emesis, gastric lavage, and activated charcoal administration. Charcoal administration is recommended for up to three consecutive days to reduce enterohepatic recirculation. Once clinical signs have developed, treatment

CHAPTER 14

Box 14.2   Common Bromethalin Trade Names

- Fastrac
- Talpirid
- Vengeance
- Hot Shot
- Assault
- Mouse Killer
- Trouce
- Sudden Death

Box 14.3   Common Carbamates

- Carbaryl
- Aldricarb ("tres pasitos")
- Methiocarb
- Propoxus
- Methomyl
- Bendiocarb
- Carbofuran
- Dimetlan
- Isolan
- Oxamyl
- Mexacarbate

---

is symptomatic and supportive. Therapy generally includes intravenous fluids, halting seizures with benzodiazepines and or barbiturates, and decreasing cerebral edema with hypertonic saline or intravenous mannitol, and perhaps furosemide and/or corticosteroids. To minimize worsening existing cerebral edema, nursing staff should also avoid the use of jugular veins for intravenous catheterization and venipunture, elevate the front end of the patient if recumbent by 10–30 degrees, and avoid compression of the neck and jugular veins. Prognosis is guarded to grave as death may occur following the ingestion of even a small amount of bromethalin. Patients should be hospitalized for 72 h for observation regardless of whether signs occur or not.

Carbamates

Carbamates cause a nearly identical toxicity to organophosphates with the exception that they cause reversible inhibition of cholinesterase activity. As a result, the clinical signs are the same as organophosphate toxicity; however, these are usually less severe and shorter in duration. These products are commonly found in dusts, sprays, shampoos, and flea and tick collars. Pralidoxime chloride is not used for the treatment of carbamate. Atropine 0.2–0.5 mg/kg IV, IM, SQ (Plumb 2005) and support care is typically all that is required for successful recovery.

Chocolate and Methylxanthines

Methylxanthines include caffeine, theobromine, and theophylline. Methylxanthines are found in caffeinated sodas, chocolate, cocoa beans, cocoa bean hulls, caffeine, and tea. In chocolate, the active ingredient theobromine is toxic to both dogs and cats in doses of starting at 100 mg/kg (Plunkett 2001). Milk chocolate contains 45–60 mg/oz, semisweet or dark chocolate contains 130–185 mg/oz, and unsweetened (baking) chocolate contains 400–450 mg/oz of theobromine (Plunkett 2001). Methylxanthine toxicity causes adenosine receptor blockage and increases in cyclic adenosine monophosphate (cyclic AMP or cAMP). The result is an increased calcium concentration within the cell which leads to increased muscular contractility.

Clinical signs include vomiting, diarrhea, hyperactivity, restlessness, urination, ataxia, muscle tremors, cardiac arrhythmias (often ventricular), hyperthermia, seizures, coma, and sudden death. Clinical signs typically begin within 1–4 hours following ingestion. Diagnosis is based on patient history and clinical signs. Patients usually recover with aggressive therapy; however, if a large amount is ingested and allowed to be absorbed, toxicity can be fatal.

Patients should be hospitalized for treatment and observation. Decontamination for chocolate and methylxanthine toxicity includes inducing emesis, gastric lavage, and activated charcoal. Initial therapy includes intravenous fluids along with anticonvulsants such as diazepam 0.5–2 mg/kg IV as necessary to control muscle tremors and seizures (Plunkett 2001). Patients should be monitored by blood pressure and continuous electrocardiogram, and hypertension and cardiac arrhythmias should be treated as needed. A urinary catheter and closed collection system should also be considered because methylxanthines can be reabsorbed from the urinary bladder and perpetuate toxicity. Antiemetics and gastric protectants may help neutralize gastrointestinal irritation and vomiting. Methylxanthines can have a long half-life and may required prolonged treatment lasting up to 72 hours.

Cholecalciferol

Numerous commercial rodenticides contain cholecalciferol rather than anticoagulants. Cholecalciferol is metabolized to 25-hydroxyvitamin D in the liver, which is then converted by the kidney to active vitamin D3 (1,25-dihydroxyvitamin D). Vitamin D3 promotes the body's retention of calcium, and this leads to potentially fatal hypercalcemia and tissue mineralization of blood vessels, kidneys, and lungs. Dogs and cats are exposed to cholecalciferol via ingestion of direct ingestion, malicious poisoning, or ingestion of a poisoned rodent. Clinical signs occur in dogs following ingestion of 0.5–3 mg/kg (Plunkett 2001). Cats, however, are more sensitive to toxicosis and require even less of a dose. The prognosis is guarded to poor. Death often occurs within 2–5 days following the onset of clinical signs.

Clinical signs occur generally 12–36 hours after ingestion. They include lethargy, polyuria, polydipsia, constipation, anorexia, vomiting, hypertension, and seizures. Renal failure may already be observed as could petechia, hematemesis, hemorrhagic diarrhea, and cardiac arrhythmias. Serum biochemical profiles reveal hypercalcemia (>11.5 mg/dL), hyperphosphatemia, and azotemia. Hyperphosphatemia may occur early in the progression of toxicosis and may be an early indicator of cholecalciferol ingestion. Patients are typically at risk for tissue mineralization and subsequent renal tubular injury when the calcium phosphorous product is over 60 (Ca × P).

Presumptive diagnosis is made based upon history, clinical signs, and supporting serum chemistry findings. Initial treatment includes inducing vomiting, gastric lavage, and

---

Box 14.4   Common Cholecalciferol Rodenticide Trade Names

- Ortho Mouse-B-Gone
- Rat-B-Gone
- Quintox
- Rampage
- Hyperkil and many others

activated charcoal. Intravenous fluids are begun to maintain renal perfusion, hydration, and promote diuresis and calciuresis. Fluid rates can initially be as high as 120–180 mL/kg/day. Over other balanced crystalloids, 0.9% sodium chloride is selected (e.g., Lactated Ringer's solution) because it does not contain calcium. Numerous drug options exist to reduce and prevent the impending hypercalcemia. Furosemide 4–5 mg/kg IV q12h initially will produce rapid calciuresis and can be followed by oral therapy (Plunkett 2001). Prednisone 2–4 mg/kg PO q12 can also be selected (Plunkett 2001). Calcitonin 4–6 IU/kg SQ q2-12h and intravenous pamidronate, 1.3–2 mg/kg IV over 2 hours in 150 mL 0.9% NaCl, a biphosphonate, can be selected for severe hypercalcemia. Another bisphosphonate, clodronate at 4 mg/kg IV in 150 mL 0.9% NaCl slowly may also be another useful therapy (Plumb 2005; Ulutas et al. 2006). Electrolytes, blood urea nitrogen (BUN), and creatinine must be monitored regularly during treatment. A low calcium diet and oral therapy with furosemide and prednisone are continued typically for up to 4 weeks.

Ethylene Glycol (EG)

EG is found in automobile antifreeze, rust removers, film processing solutions, and solvents. Because of its sweat color it is a frequent source of poisoning in dogs and cats. EG is often bright green in color. A toxic dose is as little as 4 mL/kg in the dog and 1.5 mL/kg in the cat (Plunkett 2001). Once ingested, EG is metabolized by the liver to glycoaldehyde, glycolic acid, glyoxalic acid, and oxalic acid. Oxalic acid forms insoluble calcium oxalate crystals which precipitate in the renal tubules, ultimately resulting in acute renal failure and severe metabolic acidosis.

Patients typically present in two potential phases. The initial phase (Stage 1) is marked by mild depression, ataxia, polyuria, polydipsia, vomiting, anorexia, hypothermia, and potentially, seizures. Patients appear intoxicated. Cats may present depressed and with elevation of the third eyelids. This phase may occur up to 12 hours post ingestion. Phase 2 begins between 12–24 hours post ingestion and initially only include cardiorespiratory signs such as tachycardia and tachypnea. These signs are then followed by more severe depression, vomiting, azotemia, isothenuria, and eventually, oliguric renal failure by 24–72 hours post ingestion (Thrall et al. 1998).

Presumptive diagnosis often can be made based upon history and clinical signs. Fluorescence of the oral cavity, vomitus, or urine using a Wood's lamp may be detected and can give early clues to EG ingestion. Laboratory findings include an unexplained metabolic acidosis with a severely increased anion gap. Serum osmolality is increased and an increased osmalar gap is present. Hyperglycemia, hypocalcemia, hyperphosphatemia, and azotemia are noted on serum biochemical profiles. Hyperkalemia may be noted if anuria is present. Urinalysis may show evidence of glucosuria, renal tubular casts, isothenuria, and calcium oxalate crytalluria (often monohydrates). Calcium oxalate crystals will form with 5 hours of ingestion in the dog and 3 hours within the cat. A hyperechoic renal cortex and medulla, referred to as the "Halo Sign," may also be observed with ultrasound (Fig. 14.6).

Several in-house EG test kits are available for confirmation of the diagnosis; however, they are often not reliable. False positives may occur in patients who received activated charcoal or drugs containing propylene glycol (e.g., diazepam). False negatives may occur in cats or when testing patients 18 hours or more following ingestion (Plunkett 2001). In cats, such kits are less sensitive, and negative results must be evaluated along with clinical signs, supporting labwork, and history (Acierno et al. 2008). Ethanol, methanol,

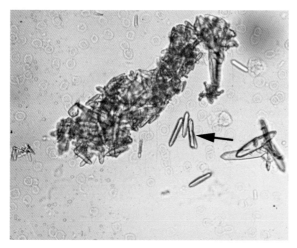

Figure 14.6 Calcium Oxylate crystaluria, especially the monohydrate form, is supportive of ethylene glycol intoxication. (Reprinted with permission from Thrall's *Veterinary Hematology and Clinical Chemistry*, 2006, Blackwell Publishing).

or isopropyl alcohol will not interfere with test results. Another option for testing is to have the blood analyzed for a quantitative level of EG at a local human hospital. Prognosis is grave for patients exhibiting clinical signs or who are azotemic upon arrival. Cats treated within 3 hours and dogs within 6 hours of ingestion have a guarded prognosis.

Initially, midazolam or propofol can be used if necessary to control seizures. Patients with confirmed or suspected EG toxicity must be treated immediately. Fomeprazole or 4-methylprazole (4-MP) is an alcohol dehydogenase inhibitor that directly competes with EG for alcohol hydrogenase, thereby preventing EG metabolism and allowing it to be excreted unchanged. Having minimal side effects, 4-MP is currently the drug of choice for dogs and is also safe and effective in cats at higher doses if given within 3 hours of ingestion (Connally et al. 1996, 2010; Plumb 2005). For dogs, an initial loading dose of 20 mg/kg IV is given. The drug is then repeated at 15 mg/kg IV at 12 and 24 hours after initiation of therapy. A 5 mg/kg IV is then given at 36 hours after beginning therapy. If the patient has not recovered or still has a positive EG test, additional 5 mg/kg IV doses may be given (Connally et al. 1996). Cats are treated initially with 125 mg/kg slow IV and are followed by 31.25 mg/kg at 12, 24, and 36 hours (Connally et al. 2002, 2010) (Fig. 14.7).

When 4-MP is unavailable, ethanol can also be used to compete for alcohol dehydrogenase and therefore act as an antidose for EG toxicity. However, treatment with ethanol often causes significant CNS depression, hypothermia, increases plasma osmolality, and can easily result in death if overdosed. It appears to be less effective than fomepizole in cats as well (Connally et al. 2010). A loading dose of 600 mg/kg IV (7% ethanol) is followed by a 7% ethanol CRI at 100–200 mg/kg/h (Plunkett 2001).

After treatment has begun with either 4-MP or ethanol, patients who present within 4 hours of ingestion should be decontaminated by inducing emesis, gastric lavage, and administration of activate charcoal. Cats and dogs should next be treated with aggressive intravenous fluid therapy to support renal perfusion and institute diuresis. Especially if the patient becomes anuric or oliguric, peritoneal dialysis may be necessary to remove EG and its metabolites from the body. Sodium bicarbonate may be required in patients with severe metabolic acidosis. Lastly, hemodyalysis is also another highly effective option at practices that have such technology.

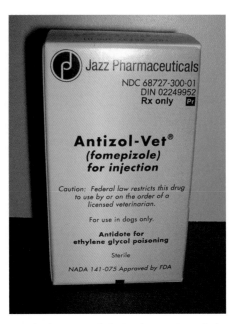

Figure 14.7   Fomepizole is currently the agent of choice for treating ethylene glycol toxicity. (Courtesy of Thomas Walker, DVM, DACVECC.)

Lead

Lead is a potential toxicity of young dogs and cats because of their indiscriminant eating habits. Common sources of acute or chronic lead toxicity include old paint, batteries, pipes, fishing sinkers, shotgun pellets, linoleum, putty, golf balls, lubricants, and insulation. Lead toxicity results in nervous tissue demyelination and interference with GABA, cholinergic function, and heme synthesis. Clinical signs therefore involve the gastrointestinal and nervous systems and initially include vomiting, abdominal pain, diarrhea, anorexia, and constipation. Neurological signs include anxiety, odd behavioral changes, seizures, ataxia, head pressing, polyneuropathy, opisthotonos, mydriasis, and blindness. These findings are often the result of cerebral edema. Prognosis is favorable for patients who undergo chelation therapy.

Diagnosis for lead toxicity begins with a supporting history and clinical signs. On hemogram, abnormal findings may include large numbers of nucleated red blood cells (NRBCs) without evidence of severe anemia, anisocytosis, polychromasia, poikilocytosis, target cells, hypochromasia, and potentially, basophilic stippling (Plunkett 2001). Evidence of basophilic stippling in the small animal is highly suggestive of lead toxicity and makes red blood cells look similar to a chocolate chip cookies. Additionally, lead toxicity can be diagnosed via blood or urine lead levels. A blood lead level of 0.3–0.5 ppm indicates lead poisoning if supporting clinical hematological signs exist. Blood levels of 0.6 ppm or greater are diagnostic. Urine lead levels of 0.75 ppm or greater support lead poisoning (Plunkett 2001).

If lead is still present in the gastrointestinal tract, induction of emesis or endoscopy is recommended. Activated charcoal is not beneficial. Intravenous fluids and thiamine supplementation at 1–2 mg/kg q24h IM, PO should be intuited (Plunkett 2001). Lead should then be removed from blood and body tissues by the administration of a chelating agent. Calcium ethylenediaminetetraacetic acid (EDTA) as 25 mg/kg SQ q4h or 50 mg/kg q12h for 2–5 days is the treatment of choice (Plunkett 2001). Other chelating options include D-penicillamine, dimercaprol (BAL), and succimer (DMSA). In addition to chelating therapy, supportive treatment should include treatment of seizures, cerebral edema, and gastrointestinal signs. Owners with animals suffering from lead toxicity should be advised about the potential for human toxicity if the pet and humans share the same living environment.

Lilies

Several members of the Liliaceae family, including easter lilies (*Lilium longiflorum*), stargazer lilies, asiatic lilies, oriental lilies, tiger lilies (*Lilium tigrinum*), rubrum or Japanese showy lilies (*Lilium speciosum* and *Lilium lancifolium*), and various day lilies (*Hemerocallis* species) have been shown to cause renal tubular injury, acute renal failure, and death in cats (Hall 1992; Gulledge et al. 1997; Volmer 1999; Brady and Janovitz 2000). All parts of these plants, including the flowers, have been shown to cause clinical signs. Consumption of even one leaf can cause fatal toxicity (Volmer 1999) (Fig. 14.8).

Clinical signs may appear within 2 hours following plant ingestion and may initially include vomiting, lethargy, and anorexia. Patients may then appear to recover. Over the next 1–3 days, polyuria, polydipsia, glucosuria, azotemia, and hyperphosphatemia are observed. The creatinine concentration is often elevated disproportionally to the BUN concentration (Volmer 1999; Richardson 2002). Immediate decontamination is performed by inducing vomiting and administering activated charcoal if ingestion was recent. Aggressive fluid diuresis should be continued for a minimum of 48 hours. Supportive care is provided for acute renal failure. Cats who become oliguric or anuric have a worse prognosis and may require peritoneal dialysis for survival (Volmer 1999; Hall 2001; Richardson 2002).

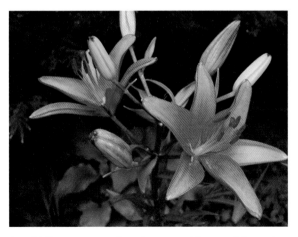

Figure 14.8 Many species of Lilies are extremely toxic to cats. All parts of these plants, including the flowers, have been shown to cause clinical signs, and consumption of as little as one leaf can be fatal. (Courtesy of Linda Leighton, PhD.)

CHAPTER 14

Metaldyhyde (Snail Bait)

Metaldyhyde is a molluscicide (snail/slug killer) that is highly palatable to dogs and cats. Toxicity therefore results from ingestion. Metaldyhyde's mechanism of action is unknown but may act by decreasing brain GABA, serotonin, and norepinephrine, resulting in convulsions. A toxic dose in dogs has been reported to be 100 mg/kg and is suspected to be similar for cats (Plunkett 2001). The agent causes a rapid onset of severe signs that include seizures, hypersalivation, incoordination, muscle fasciculations, metabolic acidosis, and tachycardia. Significant hyperthermia is an important finding (>108 F). Many patients will also be highly sensitive to light and sound. As the toxicity progresses, initial CNS stimulation becomes CNS depression, bradycardia, and respiratory failure. Liver damage may also occur 3–5 days following exposure.

Diagnosis is predominantly based on history and clinical signs. An odor of acetaldehyde, resembling formaldehyde, may be noted on the patient's breath or within the stomach contents. Treatment initially includes decontamination with emesis, gastric lavage, and activated charcoal. Supportive care, including fluid therapy, patient cooling, muscle relaxants such as methocarbamol, and anticonvulsants such as diazepam, midazolam, and barbiturates are necessary to control hyperthermia and CNS stimulation. In general, prognosis with supportive care is excellent (Firth 1992).

Naphthalene (Mothballs)

Mothballs contain either toxic naphthalene or inert paradichlorobenzene. Naphthalene causes acute oxidative hemolytic anemia, Heinz bodies, and occasionally methemoglobinemia. Cats are most sensitive to the toxic effects of naphthalene. Patients who have ingested mothballs will often have a characteristic "mothball" odor to their breath. Clinical signs include gastrointestinal upset, vomiting, lethargy, weakness, collapse, icterus, or brown-colored mucous membranes. Whenever a patient ingests a mothball of unknown type, a remaining mothball can be placed into a cup of warm water that has had three heaping tablespoons of table salt vigorously dissolved within. Naphthalene mothballs float and paradichlorobenzene mothballs sink (DeClementi 2005).

Initial treatment includes emesis, gastric lavage if emesis was unsuccessful, and activated charcoal administration. Patients that are already exhibiting clinical signs should be started on intravenous fluid diuresis in order to minimize the risk of hemoglobin-induced renal nephrosis secondary to red blood cell (RBC) hemolysis. Vomiting can be controlled with antiemetics such as miropitant, ondansetron, dolasetron, and metoclopramide. The addition of a gastrointestinal protectant (e.g., H_2 blockers, sucralfate Carafate, proton pump inhibitors) may also be indicated if gastrointestinal signs persist. Blood transfusion with either whole blood, HBOC, or packed red cells may be needed in patients with anemia or severe methemoglobinemia. If methemoglobinemia is present, then it should additionally be treated with either ascorbic acid (vitamin C) 20 mg/kg PO, IM, or SC up to every 6 hours or methylene blue 1.5 mg/kg slowly IV as a 1% solution (Plunkett 2001). Patients should be monitored closely for renal and hepatic failure.

Nonsteroidal Anti-Inflammatory Drugs (NSAIDs)

NSAIDs (ibuprofen, aspirin, naproxen, ketoprofen, carprofen, meloxicam, deracoxib, firocoxib, piroxicam, etc.) are a common source of toxicity in dogs and cats. They have analgesic, antipyretic, and anti-inflammatory properties and are available over the counter and via prescription in pill, capsule, liquid, and injectable form. Pets typically become exposed to NSAIDs by owner administration, by self-ingestion, or through accidental iatrogenic overdose. Concurrent administration of corticosteroids and NSAID administration together or the use of an NSAID in a hypotensive or dehydrated patient are two common causes of iatrogenic toxicity. In general, cats are more sensitive to NSAID toxicity than dogs.

NSAIDs work by inhibiting cyclooxygenase and therefore prostaglandin production. Inhibition of gastric prostaglandin synthesis can result in gastroenteritis or gastrointestinal ulceration, and inhibition of renal prostaglandin synthesis results in renal toxicity. Some NSAIDs have also been associated with CNS signs such as seizures and coma at higher doses. The more common drugs that can cause such a CNS effect include carprofen, ibuprofen, deracoxib, naproxen, etodolac, meloxicam, and indomethacin (Villar et al. 1998; Roder 2004). Additionally, carprofen may additionally cause an idiosyncratic hepatic toxicosis in Labrador retrievers.

Clinical signs usually develop within 4–6 hours (Plunkett 2001). Depression, anorexia, vomiting, hematemesis, melena, ataxia, seizures, and acute renal failure may follow. Diagnosis is made predominantly based on history and clinical signs. Serum biochemical profiles may reveal azotemia and increased hepatic enzymes. Heinz body anemia may occur in the cat. On laboratory analysis, metabolic acidosis and prolonged bleeding times may also be observed. Additionally, asprin may also cause an increased anion gap. Prognosis of NSAID toxicity depends on the drug and amount ingested; however, usually if treatment is started before severe clinical signs are observed, then prognosis is favorable.

Patients presenting in cardiovascular shock, which could occur with gastrointestinal perforation, should initially be managed with aggressive fluid resuscitation and oxygen support. Anticonvulsants may be necessary if seizures are present. If drug exposure was recent, decontamination by inducing emesis, gastric lavage, and activated charcoal administration should be performed. Due to enterohepatic recirculation, patients will benefit from repeated doses of activated charcoal with many NSAIDs.

Intravenous fluids are initiated to rehydrate patients, induce diuresis, and support organ perfusion. Dogs and cats should be continued for a minimum of 48 hours on intravenous fluids, during which time urine output should also be monitored closely. Normal urine production should be more than 2–4 mL/kg/h in the adequately hydrated dog and cat while on intravenous fluids. As some NSAIDs (e.g., aspirin) are weak acids, ion trapping by urine alkalinization with sodium bicarbonate may increase urinary excretion and be of benefit. To prevent gastrointestinal ulceration, combinations of Carafate, H_2 blockers (e.g., ranitidine, famotidine), proton pump inhibitors (e.g., omeprazole, pantoprazole), and prostaglandins (e.g., misoprostol) are selected. Acute renal or hepatic failure should be treated supportively. All nephrotoxic and hepatotoxic drugs should be discontinued. Peritoneal dialysis may be required.

Organophosphates

Organophosphates are regularly found in pet sprays, dips, kennel sprays, powders, yard sprays, and as systemics. Toxicity may result after one of these preparations is applied to a patient's skin or if the animal ingests the product. Organophosphates are readily absorbed from the skin and gastrointestinal tract and cause acute irreversible inhibition of cholinersterase activity. As a result, acetylcholine is not able to be broken down effectively, and the abundance of acetylcholine interferes with autonomic nervous system

---

Box 14.5   Common Organophosphates

- Chlorpyrifos
- Coumaphos
- Diazinon
- Fenthion
- Malathion
- Methyl parathion
- Temephos
- Diclorvos
- Chlorfenvinphos
- Cythioate
- Dioxathion
- Disulfoton
- Parathion
- Phosdrin
- Runnel
- Trichlorfon
- Vaponnac

---

function. The toxic dosage varies upon the compound involved, the species of the patient, and amount of exposure.

Clinical signs associated with organophosphate toxicity include parasympathomimetic effects (mucarinic stimulation) such as salivation, lacrimation, vomiting, diarrhea, miosis, and bradycardia. As the toxicity progresses, nicotinic stimulation occurs and is followed finally by nicotinic blockade. As signs progress, muscle twitching, seizures, respiratory depression, coma, and death occur. Diagnosis is made based on the history and patient signs.

Treatment for organophosphate toxicity first includes washing the dog or cat in a mild detergent if topic exposure has occurred and administration of activated charcoal if oral ingestion has occurred. Atropine 0.2–0.5 mg/kg IV, IM, SQ (Plunkett 2001) is utilized as a parasympatholytic agent to combat the mucarinic signs of the toxicity and may need to be repeated. In less severe cases, atropine, along with supportive care, may be the only required treatment. Pralioxime chloride (2-PAM chloride) specifically reactivates the cholinesterase that has been inhibited and may be necessary in some patients. A dosage of 10–50 mg/kg IM, SQ, IV over 15 minutes q8-12h (Plunkett 2001) is used until clinical signs of the toxicity are no longer observed. The use of acepromazine and other pheno-thiazine derivatives are contraindicated in patients with organophosphate toxicity. The prognosis is usually guarded to poor depending on severity of signs.

Pyrethrins/Pyrethroids

Pyrethrins are derived from the *Chrysanthemum cinerariaefolium* plant and are frequently used in a wide variety of products for flea and tick control. Pyrethroids are synthetically derived (e.g., resmethrin, allethrin, and permethrin). Their route of toxicity can be either topic or oral ingestion. Cats and birds are especially sensitive to acute toxicity. The oral

---

Box 14.6   Common Pyrethrin/Pyrethroids

- Bifenthrin
- Rallethrin
- Fenvalerate
- Permethrin
- Permethrin
- Pyrethrin
- Resmethrin
- Sumethrin
- Cypermethrin
- Deltamethrin

---

toxic dose of several common pyrethrins varies from 100–2000 mg/kg. When used correctly, pyrethrins are seldom toxic in dogs as there is a wide safety margin (Richardson 2000).

Pyrethrins work by delaying sodium channel closing, resulting in repetitive nerve firing. Pyrethroids also act as antagonists of GABA and glutamic acid. The result is systemic tremors, hypersalivation, hyperthermia, vomiting, diarrhea, dehydration, hyperexcitability, or CNS depression. Most cases are mild and response to treatment, but toxicity can progress to seizures. A presumptive diagnosis is made based on the history and patient signs.

Initial treatment includes decontamination by bathing the animal in a mild soap for topical exposures. Emesis and activated charcoal are recommended for ingestion. Intravenous fluids are instituted if the patient has vomiting, diarrhea, dehydration, or is experiencing hyperthermia. Boluses of the skeletal muscle relaxant diazepam (0. 5–2 mg/kg IV) or a diazepam CRI may be necessary to control seizure activity. Methocarbamol at 55–220 mg/kg IV, not to exceed 330 mg/kg/day (Plumb 2005), or guaifenesin are both highly effective in treating associated muscle tremors. While atropine is not antidotal, it may occasionally be used to help control diarrhea and salivation at a preanesthetic dose. Intravenous lipids may prove to be of additional usefulness in the treatment of these cases. The prognosis for pyrethrin/pyrethroid toxicity is generally good.

Raisins and Grapes

Recently, raisins and grapes, when eaten in quantity, have been identified as potential causes of acute renal failure in dogs (Gwaltney-Brant et al. 2001; Mazzaferro et al. 2004; Porterpan 2005). Some anecdotal evidence suggests cats may also be affected. The pathogenesis for kidney failure following consumption of grapes and raisins remains unclear. Additionally, the amount of grapes or raisins that may cause renal failure is not exactly known. Some patients appear to be able to tolerate large doses while in others as little as 0.7 oz/kg of grapes and 0.11 oz/kg raisins have caused toxicity. Toxicity should be considered as a differential in any case of acute renal failure in the dog. Presently, a presumptive diagnosis is made based upon history and clinical signs. Prognosis with early decontamination is good; however, if acute renal failure occurs, the prognosis is guarded at best.

Proposed treatment for recent ingestion of grapes or raisins includes the induction of emesis and activated charcoal administration (Gwaltney-Brant 2001; Porterpan 2005). Patients should then be hospitalized, placed on intravenous fluid diuresis for 48 h, and monitored for azotemia (Gwaltney-Brant 2001; Porterpan 2005). No specific treatment or antidote currently has been identified, and supportive care should be provided.

Strychnine

Strychnine is a restricted use pesticide that antagonizes glycine, the inhibitory spinal cord neural transmitter, resulting in excitation of the spinal reflexes and striated muscles. Although uncommon, dogs and cats become poisoned by accidently ingesting strychnine containing rodenticide or by being poisoned with food laced with strychnine. Baits containing strychnine often contain a purple, red, or green dye. Toxic dosages are 0.75 mg/kg in the dog and 2.0 mg/kg in the cat (Plunkett 2001).

Toxic signs begin within minutes after consumption and progress usually over 1–2 hours after onset of signs. Clinical signs include initial anxiousness and muscle tremors, followed by collapse, seizures, extensor rigidity, apnea, and death. Animals with strychnine toxicity are extremely sensitive to external stimuli, and this may be a clue as to the cause of the toxicity if it is not already known. Dramatic hyperthermia is also frequently observed. Diagnosis is predominantly not only made by history and clinical signs, but can also be confirmed via laboratory analysis of stomach contents, urine, or liver.

Emesis may be initially considered for treatment; however, vomiting may result in increased seizure activity. Therefore, gastric lavage and activated charcoal is primarily recommended to prevent further absorption. Intravenous fluids are instituted to combat the hyperthermia and support perfusion. Anticonvulsant agents and anesthetics such as diazepam, midazolam, propofol, and pentobarbital will likely be necessary to control seizure and muscle activity. Methocarbamol may also be beneficial. Ion trapping with IV or oral ammonium chloride may acidify urine and enhance urinary strychnine excretion. Avoid stimulation by sound and light. Patients should be kept sedated in a quiet, darkened room. Depending on the dosage ingested, prognosis ranges from guarded to poor. Patients surviving the first 48 hours usually make a full recovery.

Xylitol

Xylitol is a sugar substitute that is commonly found in chewing gum and artificial sweeteners. In dogs, xylitol toxicity results in the secretion of insulin, thereby potentially causing severe acute hypoglycemia, ataxia, collapse, and seizures. Because of insulin release driving potassium into cells, hypokalemia can also be observed. Xylitol can additionally cause a delayed hepatic necrosis and death approximately 72 hours after initial recovery (Dunayer 2004; Todd and Powell 2007). Dogs who do not initially present with hypoglycemia are still at risk for hepatic injury. The exact toxic dose is not elucidated at this time but has been as little as one or two pieces of gum (2–4 g xylitol) in a 10 kg dog. Cats do not appear to be sensitive to xylitol's toxic effects. Prognosis is not fully identified at this time.

Initial decontamination includes the induction of emesis. Activated charcoal is unnecessary because it is not effective at binding xylitol (Cope 2004). Intravenous fluid support is instituted to maintain hydration, maximize hepatic perfusion, and help prevent disseminated intravascular coagulation (DIC). Blood glucose must be monitored regularly and will likely require supplementation with intravenous dextrose bolus and CRIs. Electrolytes and liver enzymes should be monitored carefully. S-Adenosylmethionine, ursodeoxycholic acid, silymarin, and vitamin E may be of benefit in minimizing hepatic injury.

Zinc

Zinc toxicity most commonly occurs after the ingestion of pennies made after the year 1983. Zinc toxicity results in acute hemolysis, possibly due to oxidative injury. A toxic dosage is 0.7–1 g/kg (Plunkett 2001). Patients may present with anorexia, vomiting, CNS depression, weakness and lethargy, diarrhea, pale mucous membranes, and icterus. Additionally, laboratory findings may include an inflammatory leukogram, regenerative anemia, spherocytosis, renal failure from tubular injury by hemoglobinuria, and increased levels of serum zinc. The prognosis is variable.

Treatment includes decontamination by induction of emesis or endoscopy to remove foreign bodies in the gastrointestinal tract. Exploratory surgery may be necessary if the source of the zinc toxicity was not able to be removed via less invasive means. Intravenous fluids should be started to maintain perfusion, hydration, diuresis, and to limit the potential for DIC. Supportive therapy for vomiting and diarrhea may be necessary. Patients may require transfusions with blood products or HBOCs. Rarely, chelation therapy is required with calcium EDTA or D-penicillamine. Urine output and the progression of renal failure should be observed and treated as appropriate.

References

Acierno, MJ, Serra, VF, Johnson, ME, Mitchell, MA. 2008. Preliminary validation of a point-of-care ethylene glycol test for cats. *J Vet Emerg Crit Care* 18(5):477–479.

Brady, MA, Janovitz, EB. 2000. Nephrotoxicosis in a cat following ingestion of Asiatic hybrid lily (*Lilium* sp.). *J Vet Diagn Invest* 12:566–569.

Connally, HE, Thrall, MA, Forney, SD, et al. 1996. Safety and efficacy of 4-methylpyrazole for treatment of suspected or confirmed ethylene glycol intoxication in dogs—107 cases (1983–1995). *J Am Vet Med Assoc* 209(11):1880–1883.

Connally, HE, Thrall, MA, Hamar, DW. 2002. Safety and efficacy of high dose fomeprazole as therapy for ethylene glycol intoxication in cats [Abstract]. *J Vet Emerg Crit Care* 12:191.

Connaly, HE, Thral, MA, Hamar, D. 2010. Safety and efficacy of high-dose fomepizole compared with ethanol as therapy for ethylene glycol intoxication in cats. *J Vet Emerg Crit Care* 20(2):191–206.

Cope, RB. 2004. A screening study of xylitol binding *in vitro* to activated charcoal. *Vet Hum Toxicol* 46:336–7.

Crandell, DE, Weinberg, GL. 2009. Moxidectin toxicosis in a puppy successfully treated with intravenous lipids. *J Vet Emerg Crit Care* 19(2):181–186.

DeClementi, C. 2005. Moth repellent toxicosis. *Vet Med* 100(1):167–181.

Dunayer, EK. 2004. Hypoglycemia following canine ingestion of xylitol-containing gum. *Vet Hum Toxicol* 46(2):87–88.

Fernandez, A, Lee, J, Rahilly, L, et al. 2011. The use of intravenous lipid emulsion as an antidote in veterinary toxicology. *J Vet Emerg Crit Care* 21(4):309–320.

CHAPTER 14

Firth, A. 1992. Treatment of snail bait toxicity in dogs: retrospective study of 56 cases. *J Vet Emerg Crit Care* 2(1):25–30.

Gulledge, L, Boos, D, Wachsstock, R. 1997. Acute renal failure in a cat secondary to tiger lily (*Lilium tigrinum*) toxicity. *Feline Pract* 25(5–6):38–39.

Gwaltney-Brant, S, Holding, JK, Donaldson, CW, Eubig, PA, Khan, SA. 2001. Renal failure associated with ingestion of grapes or raisins in dogs. *J Am Vet Med Assoc* 218(10):1555–1556.

Hall, JO. 1992. Nephrotoxicity of Easter lily (*Lilium longiflorum*) when ingested by the cat [Abstract]. *J Vet Intern Med* 6:121.

Hall, JO. 2001. Lily nephrotoxicity. In *Consultations in Feline Internal Medicine*, 4th ed., edited by August, JR. Philadelphia: WB Saunders, pp. 308–310.

Mariani, C, Fulton, R. 2001. Atypical reaction to acetaminophen intoxication in a dog. *J Vet Emerg Crit Care* 11(2):123–126.

Mazzaferro, EM, Eugbig, PA, Hackett, TB, et al. 2004. Acute renal failure associated with raisin or grape ingestion in 4 dogs. *J Vet Emerg Crit Care* 14(3):203–212.

Plumb, DC. 2005. *Plumb's Veterinary Drug Handbook*, 5th ed. Ames, IA: Blackwell.

Plunkett, SJ. 2001. *Emergency Procedure for the Small Animal Veterinarian*, 2nd ed. Philadelphia: W.B. Saunders.

Porterpan, B. 2005. Raisins and grapes: potentially lethal treats for dogs. *Vet Med* 100(5):346–350.

Reezigit, BJ. 2007. Effective reversal of prolonged clotting times with intravenous vitamin K in a warfarin intoxicated cat. *Abstract* IVECCS.

Richardson, J. 2000. Permethrin spot-on toxicoses in cats. *J Vet Emerg Crit Care* 10(2):103–106.

Richardson, JA. 2002. Lily toxicoses in cats. *Stand Care Emerg Crit Care* 4(4):5–8.

Roder, JD. 2004. Analgesics. In *Clinical Veterinary Toxicology*, edited by Plumlee, KH. St. Louis, MO: Mosby, pp. 282–284.

Thrall, MA, Connally, HE, Dial, SM, Grauer, GF. 1998. Advances in therapy for antifreeze poisoning. *Calif Vet* 52(6):18–22.

Todd, JM, Powell, L. 2007. Xylitol intoxication associated with fulminant hepatic failure in a dog. *J Vet Emerg Crit Care* 17(3):286–289.

Ulutas, B, Voyvoda, H, Pasa, S, Alingan, MK. 2006. Codronate treatment of vitamin D-induced hypercalcemia in dogs. *J Vet Emerg Crit Care* 16(2):141–145.

Villar, D, Buck, WB, Gonzalez, JM. 1998. Ibuprofen, aspirin, and acetaminophen toxicosis and treatment in dogs and cats. *Vet Hum Toxicol* 40:156–161.

Volmer, PA. 1999. Easter lily toxicosis in cats. *Vet Med* 94:331.

Reproductive Emergencies

Jaime Maher

Introduction

There are several reproductive emergencies that can present themselves in small animal veterinary medicine. In most instances, spaying or neutering the pet early on can avoid these emergency situations. Castration and ovariohysterectomy are sometimes part of the treatment once disease presents.

Emergencies involving the reproductive system are unique in that each disease is specific only to its related sex. In females, many of the emergencies we see are directly associated with heat cycles or pregnancy. In males, reproductive emergencies can arise at any time. In all of the following emergencies, triage and patient history are paramount in successful diagnosis and treatment (Table 15.1).

Table 15.1   Common reproductive emergencies

Female emergencies	Male emergencies
Pyometra	Paraphimosis
Metritis	Prostatic infection and abscess
Eclampsia	
Mastitis	
Dystocia	
Uterine torsion	
Uterine prolapse	

Female Emergencies

Pyometra

Pyometra is a bacterial infection in the uterus associated directly with the estrus cycle. While this disease can occur at any age, it is most represented in middle-aged intact females, with incidence increasing with age (Hopper 2003). It is important to understand the estrus cycle and role of the hormones estrogen and progesterone as related to pyometra. *Proestrus* is the first phase in the cycle. Estrogen increases in preparation for ovulation and breeding, and the uterine lining becomes thickened. The second stage, *estrus*, is what we think of when we say an animal is in "heat." Estrogen is now at its peak, ovulation is about to occur, and the animal is ready for breeding (Colville 2002). The only exceptions to this are the species which are induced ovulators, such as cats. These species do not reach ovulation until mating occurs. Because of this, the estrus phase may be prolonged until the process starts over again. Following estrus, the female will enter *metestrus* and then *diestrus*. Estrogen levels fall while progesterone rises. Fluid can accumulate in the uterus during these last phases due to uterine inactivity and the increase in mucous production. If fertilization of the ovum has occurred, progesterone will remain high to keep the uterus calm and inactive for the duration of the pregnancy. If pregnancy has not occurred, progesterone will decline and the estrus cycle will begin again (Colville 2002).

Pyometra generally develops within 3 months post estrus. During proestrus and estrus, the cervix is open, allowing for normal vaginal flora and possibly perineal or fecal bacteria to ascend into the uterus. Following the estrus phase, the cervix closes, essentially locking in bacteria and allowing proliferation if the uterus is unable to rid the bacteria using its own defenses. The release of progesterone from the ovaries during certain phases of the estrus cycle leads to decreased uterine contractions, increased glandular secretions, and promotes development of endometrium (mucous lining of the uterus). This ultimately leads to an environment ideal for bacterial growth. *Escherichia coli* is the most common organism isolated from an infected uterus (Hopper 2003).

With progesterone being the key trigger, the development of cystic endometrial hyperplasia (CEH) often leads to pyometra in middle-aged and older patients. These patients have had repeat exposure to progesterone and estrogen through their heat cycles and over time develop a uterus that is more susceptible to infection. CEH can occur with estrogen or progesterone exogenous treatments as well, leaving the patient more likely to develop pyometra (Raffe et al. 2003).

Pyometra is classified as either open or closed as indicated by the cervix. When the cervix is open, clinical signs with an open pyometra will include a purulent vaginal discharge as infected fluid drains from the uterus. This is most often the presenting complaint of the client bringing the patient to the hospital. When the cervix is closed, clinical signs in a closed pyometra may be more difficult to observe. This may delay the client in seeking veterinary care and the disease can progress with more profound clinical signs. Untreated pyometra can lead to septic peritonitis and systemic inflammatory response syndrome (SIRS) as the uterus continues to fill with septic fluid and then perforate (Fransson and Ragle 2003) or leak into the peritoneal cavity. Clinical signs associated with either classification include lethargy, polydipsia/polyuria, decreased appetite, and gastrointestinal signs such as vomiting and/or diarrhea (Ostwald 2001; Hopper 2003). In the absence of purulent vaginal discharge, these varied symptoms could indicate a number of illnesses. Advanced cases can present with symptoms consistent with septic shock. Quick diagnosis is essential in successful treatment and successful patient outcome.

Triage and client communication are key to assessing whether the patient is intact and has recently come out of estrus. Physical exam findings may include tachycardia, either pale or brick red mucous membranes, and distended and painful abdomen (more often with closed pyometra). A complete blood count (CBC) and serum chemistry should be performed. The CBC may be unremarkable, although in many cases there is an initial neutrophilia with left shift (Raffe et al. 2003). In patients who are in a state of septic shock, there can be evidence of neutropenia with toxic neutrophils. Elevated blood urea nitrogen (BUN) may be present in the serum chemistry, likely due to prerenal causes. This can be differentiated from renal azotemia by evaluating dehydration and urine-specific gravity. A urine-specific gravity greater than 1.030 in the presence of azotemia and dehydration indicates prerenal disease (Hopper 2003).

Abdominal radiographs and/or an abdominal ultrasound should be performed. Radiography in a closed pyometra will often reveal a large fluid-filled uterus. In an open pyometra, much of the fluid may be draining, preventing helpful diagnostic images. In cases involving septic peritonitis, loss of abdominal details suggestive of free fluid can be visualized in the abdomen. Oftentimes, the patient will have a concurrent urinary tract infection secondary to bacteria from vaginal discharge; therefore, a urinalysis should be performed as well (Fransson and Ragle 2003). Cystocentesis without the aid of ultrasound is contraindicated, as the needle may penetrate the enlarged, fluid-filled uterus (Hopper 2003).

Initial treatment includes aggressive fluid resuscitation with crystalloids to correct dehydration and acid–base and electrolyte derangements. Broad-spectrum antibiotics should be started. In both open and closed pyometra, surgical removal of the uterus as soon as the patient is stable remains the best treatment following emergency medical intervention. A culture and sensitivity of the uterine exudate should be obtained during surgery. Antibiotics can be altered if necessary once sensitivity results are available.

Once initial stabilization has been accomplished, the patient can be prepared for surgery. Patients may be more of an anesthetic risk, especially in cases with septic peritonitis. Premedication drugs and induction agent are chosen based on the patient's clinical status. Blood pressure should be monitored and maintained carefully. Crystalloids should

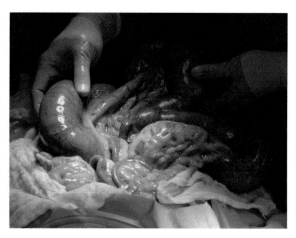

Figure 15.1   Pus filled uterus in a closed pyometra.

be administered during anesthesia at the surgical rate of 10 mL/kg/h or greater. Keep in mind that although initial stabilization efforts have taken place at this point, the patient may require continued resuscitation during surgery with additional crystalloid boluses and/or addition of a colloid (Fig. 15.1).

Following ovariohysterectomy, patients generally recover well. The exception may be those cases involving septic peritonitis or SIRS. These patients will often remain in the intensive care unit (ICU) for several days receiving supportive treatment for their condition. Cases with septic peritonitis will often have a closed-suction drain placed during surgery. In some severe cases, it may be necessary to maintain the patient with an open abdomen, which will increase the duration of stay in the ICU and require daily anesthesia to flush the abdomen, change bandages, and finally, close the abdomen (Fransson and Ragle 2003). More intense monitoring and daily blood work are required for these cases based on typical protocols for critical patients.

Although it is the best proven treatment, surgery is not the only option for treating pyometra. Open pyometra can be treated with medical management in some young, very stable cases where the client wishes to maintain the patient's breeding potential. In this case, a patient being medically treated should be bred during the next estrus to avoid subsequent pyometra (Hopper 2003; Raffe et al. 2003). The current recommended treatment is prostaglandin F2α (PGF2α)—a drug which stimulates uterine contraction, relaxes the cervix, and forces exudate from the uterus. Natural prostaglandins have been recommended, as synthetic versions have been linked with more severe side effects (Fransson and Ragle 2003; Hopper 2003). PGF2α is administered subcutaneously once daily in increasing doses for 5–7 days. If unsuccessful, a second course of treatment may be necessary. Experimentally, PGF2α has been instilled intravaginally with some success (Fransson and Ragle 2003). Due to the many side effects, prolonged treatment, and questionable efficacy, medical therapy is often discouraged. The most extreme consequence is that the uterus may perforate while waiting for medical treatments to work (Raffe et al. 2003). PGF2α can take 48 hours to begin working, and therefore is not the treatment of choice in critically ill patients or those with a closed pyometra. The side effects associated with PGF2α include hypersalivation, vomiting, defecation, panting, and restlessness. Side effects are usually seen immediately following injection and often resolve within an hour after treatment (Ostwald 2001; Raffe et al. 2003). Patients should be monitored closely during this time and supportive care provided as needed. Antibiotics should be continued as well as fluid therapy if indicated. The uterus should be evaluated by abdominal ultrasound every 2–3 days to determine if the treatment is successful and to look for signs of peritonitis. Vaginal discharge should gradually decrease over 2 weeks. It is important to remember that patients with CEH will always be predisposed to pyometra even with successful medical management (Raffe et al. 2003).

Metritis

Like pyometra, metritis (also called endometritis) is also an infection of the uterus, although this occurs postpartum when the progesterone levels are low (Raffe et al. 2003). Clinical signs may not only be similar to pyometra (lethargy, decreased appetite, purulent vaginal discharge), but may also include decreased milk production and aversion to young. Animals have a normal postpartum vaginal discharge called lochia. This discharge should not be odorous. If it is malodorous, metritis should be suspected. Certain factors may predispose a patient to developing metritis, such as dystocia, retained fetus, contamination during medical intervention for dystocia, and septic mastitis (Baker and Davidson 2008). If treatment is delayed, signs of sepsis can occur as with pyometra.

Diagnosis is typically based on clinical signs along with abdominal ultrasound. Ultrasound may show a large, fluid-filled uterus that is not undergoing normal involution (Baker and Davidson 2008). Ultrasound will also show if there is a retained fetus or placenta, evidence of peritonitis, or a uterine torsion—all of which may require surgical intervention. CBC and serum chemistry should be evaluated. Slight anemia can be normal in pregnancy. The recent postpartum patient may still be slightly anemic; however, this should be monitored throughout treatment (Baker and Davidson 2008).

One difference in treating metritis versus pyometra is that metritis often responds well to medical therapy due to the decrease in progesterone production. Broad-spectrum antibiotics may be started as long as they are safe for nursing neonates. Amoxicillin-clavulanic acid (Clavamox, Pfizer Animal Health Madison, NJ)) or cephalexin are both safe options. The patient may be treated as an outpatient as long as she continues to improve and her young continue to nurse and thrive. Prostaglandin F2α may be administered as with pyometra to assist the uterus in draining, although the patient will need to be monitored for side effects (Baker and Davidson 2008). If the patient is critically ill or septic, she should be hospitalized for intravenous fluid and antibiotic therapy along with closer monitoring. Ovariohysterectomy may be required once the patient is stable if medical management is not successful. If the patient requires more intensive care in the hospital or requires antibiotics or other medication contraindicated in neonates, the young will need to be hand-fed and closely monitored. The client should be educated in hand rearing unless the neonates are to stay in the ICU.

Patients with metritis often show improvement after 24 hours of medical treatment (Baker and Davidson 2008). Mastitis should be treated concurrently if present. Abdominal ultrasound should be repeated as with medical treatment of pyometra to evaluate uterine size and treatment success.

Mastitis

Mastitis, a disease that occurs in lactating females, is simply defined as inflammation of the mammary gland. One or several mammary glands may be involved, and

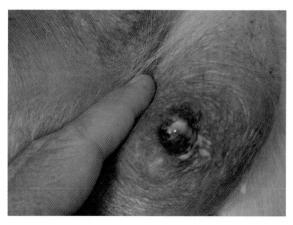

Figure 15.2   Septic milk expressed from a swollen, hot, and painful nipple. (Courtesy of Thomas Walker, DVM, DACVECC.)

the inflammation can be septic or non-septic (Hopper 2003). Patients can present with lethargy, fever, anorexia, firm or painful affected mammary glands, and reluctance to nurse. Mastitis can often be treated on an outpatient basis. Clients must be informed of the importance of maintaining a clean environment for the dam and her young and instructed to evaluate and clean mammary glands daily. In the hospital and at home, good hygiene should be practiced around the dam after parturition and while nursing.

Non-septic mastitis is called galactostasis, or impaction of milk (Hopper 2003). This occurs without infection, and is often when young are not nursing from all mammary glands. Gentle manipulation and encouraging young to nurse from different glands can help relieve the impaction. Warm compresses can also promote milk flow and alleviate pain. Recovery is usually quick, pending rapid intervention and excellent client compliance.

Septic mastitis may reveal discolored and thickened milk from the affected gland(s) and can lead to cellulitis and abscessed glands (Davidson 2008). These cases require broad-spectrum antibiotic choices safe for nursing neonates. All drugs given to a dam have the potential to be transmitted to the nursing young via milk. Amoxicillin-calvulanic acid and cephalexin are both safe, broad-spectrum choices. Chloramphenicol, aminoglycosides, and tetracyclines should be avoided for the safety of the neonates (Boothe and Bucheler 2001). *E. coli*, streptococci, and staphylococci are common organisms discovered in septic mastitis (Hopper 2003) (Figs. 15.2 and 15.3).

A culture and sensitivity may be performed on a sample of milk from an affected gland and antibiotics adjusted accordingly. If abscessed, the affected gland(s) should be surgically drained and flushed. If severe, the tissue may become necrotic, requiring daily treatment as an open wound or ultimately mastectomy (Hopper 2003; Davidson 2008). As with any infected or septic wound, SIRS can occur even with adequate monitoring and intervention. Metritis may occur concurrently in cases of septicemia (Baker and Davidson 2008). Critically ill patients will carry a worsened prognosis. If the case is severe, neonates should not be allowed to nurse and should be hand-fed.

In either case of mastitis, nursing or hand-fed neonates must be closely monitored by the client to ensure adequate weight gain. Neonates should gain 10% body weight per day (Davidson 2008). Analgesia may be provided for the dam; however, nursing neonates should be monitored for sedation from narcotics. If neonatal sedation becomes too

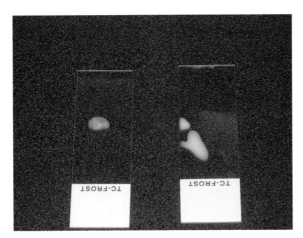

Figure 15.3   Two slides demonstrating mastitis (left) versus normal milk (right). (Courtesy of Thomas Walker, DVM, DACVECC.)

extreme, reversal agents can be administered (Davidson 2008). Topical antibacterial agents and analgesics should be avoided due to neonatal ingestion during nursing.

Dystocia

Dystocia is the inability or difficulty in passing a fetus through the birth canal from the uterus. This is a common emergency in small animal veterinary medicine, and occurs far more often in dogs than in cats. The conformation, size, and shape varieties in dogs play a role in the rate of occurrence. Small breed dogs with large heads, such as Boston terriers, Bulldogs, Scottish terriers, and Chihuahuas have a substantially increased occurrence rate (Hackett 2003; Macintyre 2006; McMillan and Serrano 2009).

Most cases of dystocia are maternal in origin. This means that the reason for the difficult birth is related in some way to the mother. Breed factors, uterine inertia (primary or secondary), or obstruction due to a narrow pelvis, pelvic trauma, uterine torsion, or prolapse are all maternal factors that can cause dystocia. Fetal causes of dystocia include fetal positioning, fetal size (too big), malformed, or dead fetuses (Brourman et al. 2007; McMillan and Serrano 2009). It is important to remember that a breech presentation is not abnormal in dogs and cats and typically is not a cause for concern.

It is important to understand gestation times and normal stages of labor so that one may better communicate with the client during either the initial phone call or during triage. The client may not know exactly when copulation occurred unless the pet was intentionally bred, and therefore he or she may not know the gestation time of the pet or what stage of labor that the pet is in. The normal gestation period in canines can range from 58–72 days (average 64–65 days). In cats, the range is 63–65 days (Hackett 2003; Brourman et al. 2007).

Labor is divided into three stages. *Stage 1* involves changes that often go unnoticed to the client. The pet may be restless and exhibit signs of nesting. During this time, the uterus begins to contract, the cervix dilates, and temperature starts to drop. Decline in temperature coincides with the decline in progesterone. This is usually the last physical sign to take place before Stage 2 begins, with the temperature falling to 97–99 degrees. Stage 1 usually lasts 6–12 hours, but may last up to 24 hours. The behavioral changes often begin first and can be prolonged, so the actual duration of Stage 1 labor may last up to 48 hours. *Stage 2* involves what most people consider true labor. Strong contractions begin, and a clear vaginal discharge will be noticed prior to the delivery of each fetus. The expulsion of the first puppy or kitten occurs within 2–4 hours of the initiation of Stage 2. Stage 2 can last 12–24 hours in dogs and up to 36 hours in cats, with up to an hour between the birth of each puppy or kitten. *Stage 3* involves the passing of the placenta. This often happens along with Stage 2, as placenta will be passed after each fetus. If multiple fetuses are passed within a short amount of time, the placentas will follow together (Reiss 2001a; Hackett 2003; Brourman et al. 2007).

Concern for dystocia should arise with any of the following: no signs of Stage 2 labor 24 hours after the dam's temperature drops, brownish-green (uteroverdin) or bloody vaginal discharge without the presence of a fetus, more than 4 hours after Stage 2 labor has begun with no signs of a fetus, more than 2 hours between delivery of fetuses without contractions, or strong contractions for more than 30 minutes without producing a fetus (Reiss 2001a; Hackett 2003; McMillan and Serrano 2009). The client should be instructed to bring the pet to the emergency room if any of these indications are present.

Upon arrival to the emergency room, the patient should be kept calm and quiet during physical examination. Additional stress to the pet can further complicate the dystocia and put the fetuses at risk. It is important to know the cause of dystocia soon after the patient arrives in the emergency room in order to provide appropriate treatment. A vaginal examination should be performed to see if there is a trapped fetus in the birth canal. Vaginal exams should be performed wearing sterile gloves and ample sterile lubricant. If there is a puppy or kitten lodged in the birth canal, gentle manipulation may help. One should be cautioned that even with gentle manipulation, cervical or limb dislocation can occur. Abdominal radiographs should be taken to assess fetal size and position and to see if there is narrowing of the pelvis. Radiographs are also used to check for the presence of intrafetal gas, indicating fetal death (Macintyre 2006; Ryan and Wagner 2006; Brourman et al. 2007) (Fig. 15.4).

Ultrasound can be used to detect fetal heartbeats and movement, aiding in determining viability of the fetuses. If fetal distress is a concern and/or there is evidence of fetal obstruction, a cesarean section should be performed. Fetal distress can be identified by

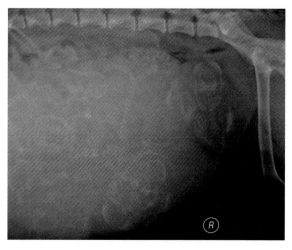

Figure 15.4   A lateral radiograph confirms the presence of several fetuses.

decreased fetal movement and fetal heart rate. Heart rates below 150 bpm indicate fetal distress. Heart rates below 100 bpm indicate severe fetal distress. In general, a normal fetal heart rate is approximately twice that of the dam or queen.

At some point during the physical examination and radiographs, blood should be collected to measure packed cell volume, total protein, serum and ionized calcium, and blood glucose. If there is no evidence of obstruction, uterine inertia is suspected. Uterine inertia occurs when the uterus is unable to push the fetus into the birth canal due to poor myometrial contractions. It can be caused by any number of factors, including exhaustion, stretching of the uterus from large or prior litters, calcium or glucose deficiencies, or other systemic disease. Small or single fetus litters are said to increase the risk of primary uterine inertia by allowing one or few fetuses to become too large to deliver or by preventing enough hormonal stimulation from the fetuses to initiate parturition (Brourman et al. 2007). Primary uterine inertia is suspected when Stage 2 labor never seems to begin. The strong abdominal contractions that characterize the initiation of Stage 2 do not occur or are too weak to notice. Secondary uterine inertia occurs when normal Stage 2 labor begins with strong contractions, but then the contractions stop. There has been an obstruction or a large fetus so that uterine contractions have become ineffective. The uterus essentially exhausts itself, and further contractions become too weak (Reiss 2001a; McMillan and Serrano 2009).

In cases of dystocia involving uterine inertia where obstruction has been ruled out, oxytocin can be administered to stimulate uterine contractions. The patient's hydration should be addressed and electrolyte abnormalities and calcium and glucose deficiencies should be corrected prior to oxytocin administration. There is a wide dose range for oxytocin; however, the typical dose is 1–2 IU/kg IM or SQ for dogs and 2–5 IU/kg IM or SQ for cats. The dose may be repeated if no progress is seen after 30 minutes. Since exogenous treatment with oxytocin relies in part on the flow of extracellular calcium into the cells of the myometrium, 10% calcium gluconate is sometimes given prior to the second dose of oxytocin even in the presence of normal serum calcium. This will aid in increasing the strength of the contractions, working concurrently with the oxytocin (Hackett 2003; Brourman et al. 2007; McMillan and Serrano 2009). If there is still no effect after the second dose, a cesarean section should be performed in a timely manner. Oxytocin should not be overdosed. Overdose can cause tetanic uterine contractions which are not useful and can impair blood flow to placentas (Reiss 2001a).

When it has been decided that a cesarean section will be performed, many members of the emergency team will be needed to ensure safe delivery and resuscitation of the neonates, as well as a safe surgery and recovery for the dam. The time from induction of the dam to delivery of the fetuses should be minimized. All necessary equipment for anesthesia and neonate care should be ready prior to surgery. These include: warmed incubator, warm towels, hemostats, suture and scissors for clamping and cutting umbilical cords, naloxone, and small face masks for providing oxygen supplementation or ventilation to neonates.

Many anesthetic protocols have been described for cesarean sections. Premedication remains a topic of debate and often is dependent on the state of the dam. Any drugs given to the dam prior to delivery have the potential to adversely affect the neonates by transplacental transmission. If the dam is relatively calm and relaxed, premedication for sedation purposes is not required. Excessive maternal stress and agitation, however, are good indicators for providing some preoperative medication. Reversible agent should be used, and low doses should be used, taking care to base the dose on the dam's reduced body weight.

Short-acting opioids are preferred because they are reversible and offer both sedation and analgesia. While they can cause fetal bradycardia and respiratory depression, these effects are typically dose-dependant and can be reversed once the fetuses are delivered. If premedication is warranted, a low dose of butorphanol (IM or IV) or fentanyl (IV) is usually sufficient to facilitate induction.

Acepromazine is associated with hypotension and requires hepatic metabolism (which is immature in the fetuses); it is therefore not recommended if it can be helped. Acepromazine is not reversible and is long lasting. While caution should be used, in an overly excited or stressed patient, very low doses of acepromazine have been recommended to reduce anxiety (0.01–0.02 mg/kg) (Ryan and Wagner 2006).

Alpha-2 agonists, such as dexmedetomidine and xylazine, are not recommended in cesarean sections. Although they are reversible, alpha-2s carry significant cardiovascular risks to the fetuses.

Keep in mind that when used, premedication allows for the use of less induction agent and reduced inhalant. If analgesia is not provided with premedication or is no longer effective, a dose of a longer lasting opioid such as buprenorphine or hydromorphone can be administered once all of the fetuses have been delivered. Buprenorphine usually provides sufficient analgesia postoperatively.

An anticholinergic is sometimes administered preoperatively to the dam to prevent bradycardia and subsequent hypotension after induction. Glycopyrrolate is a large molecule that does not readily cross the placenta. Atropine does cross the placenta and because of its rapid onset is usually given in emergency situations to treat significant bradycardia once it occurs. When used, atropine will increase the heart rate of both mother and fetuses, improving cardiac output (Ryan and Wagner 2006). Glycopyrrolate is usually the drug of choice in treating maternal bradycardia. While some clinicians opt to give it as part of the premedication cocktail, glycopyrrolate is not often necessary and is best reserved for cases experiencing opioid-induced bradycardia that is reducing cardiac output.

The use of an epidural provides excellent analgesia, significantly reduces the amount of inhalant anesthesia required, and does not negatively affect the fetuses. Sedation is required to administer epidural analgesia and, depending on the status of the patient, may not be able to be performed in a timely manner.

If the patient will allow, the abdomen should be clipped and prepped for surgery prior to induction. Induction can then take place in the operating room. The dam should be preoxygenated prior to and during induction to prevent maternal hypoxia. Greater oxygen demands, decreased lung volume, and decreased functional residual capacity predispose the dam to hypoxia after induction, which then leads to fetal hypoxia. Propofol (4–6 mg/kg) is the usual induction agent of choice in pregnant animals because, although it does cross the placenta, it is short-acting and does not appear to decrease neonate vigor. Etomidate is an induction agent typically reserved for the critically ill dam. Its use is often immediately preceded by a benzodiazepine to reduce excitement. The addition of a benzodiazepine carries a small risk to the fetuses in that prolonged sedation can decrease neonatal vigor (Moon-Massat and Erb 2002). Etomidate may not completely cross the placental barrier, and it has been shown that fetal absorption decreases quickly (Ryan and Wagner 2006). The use of barbiturates, although short-acting, is contraindicated due to their association with decreased neonatal vigor and increased mortality (Jutkowitz 2005). Another induction choice currently available in the United Kingdom is alfaxalone (Alfaxan, Vétoquinol S A, Lure Cedex, France). Alfaxalone is an injectable neurosteroid anesthetic that has recently been altered to provide safe anesthetic induction

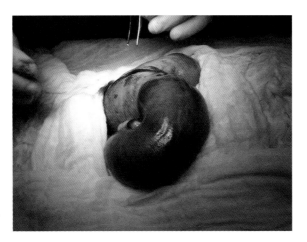

Figure 15.5   Two puppies in the uterus during a C-section.

or maintenance. Its effects are similar to that of propofol (Ambros et al. 2008). Inhalant induction via face mask is not recommended for patients undergoing cesarean section. Mask induction adds further stress to the patient and environmental pollution to the anesthetist.

Once induced, intubation should take place quickly, as pregnant females are more prone to esophageal reflux (Brourman et al. 2007; Ryan and Wagner 2006).

Maintaining the patient on a propofol constant rate infusion (CRI) until the fetuses are delivered or providing general anesthesia with an inhalant are both accepted methods of anesthetizing the pregnant animal. If available, alfaxalone could alternatively be used as a CRI to maintain adequate anesthesia. Minimum alveolar concentration (MAC) is greatly reduced in the pregnant female (MAC of isoflurane is reduced by up to 40%), reducing the amount of anesthesia required by the patient (Ryan and Wagner 2006). An incisional line block using a local anesthetic (lidocaine or bupivicaine, 2 mg/kg and 1.5 mg/kg, respectively) can provide additional analgesia—another tool in allowing reduction of inhalant anesthesia. As mentioned, an opioid can then be administered once the puppies or kittens have been removed. Care should be taken to monitor the dam's heart rate, blood pressure, and ventilation. She should not be hyperventilated as this can decrease uterine blood flow (Fig. 15.5).

Once the surgeon has gained access to the uterus, the fetuses can be delivered in a few different ways. The client will have given instructions as to whether he or she would prefer the patient to have an ovariohysterectomy at the time of surgery. The uterus can be removed along with the fetuses (en-bloc ovariohysterectomy) and handed to a technician. The neonates can then be removed from the uterus and resuscitated by veterinary staff waiting to accept them. With this method, the veterinary staff will need to clamp and cut each umbilical cord and remove each placenta. Another method involves the surgeon removing each puppy or kitten (having clamped and cut each umbilicus) and handing each to a technician standing by. The uterus can then either be removed by ovariohysterectomy, or sutured and closed.

When resuscitating puppies and kittens, any residual membranes and mucous should be suctioned from the mouth using a bulb syringe (mechanical suction is not recommended). Respiration will likely be depressed due to inhalant anesthesia and use of opioids. Vigorous warm rubbing of the neonate can help stimulate respiration. Swinging the

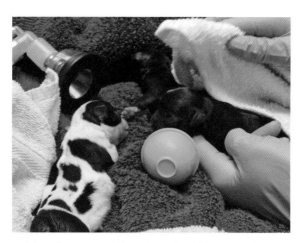

Figure 15.6   Upon removal from the uterus, each newborn should be wrapped in a warm dry towel and gently rubbed to stimulate breathing.

neonate to clear secretions and stimulate respiration is not recommended and can cause severe cerebral trauma and remove pulmonary surfactant. If opioids have been used preoperatively and the neonate is sedate or respiratory depressed, one drop of naloxone can be administered sublingually (Brourman et al. 2007; McMillan and Serrano 2009). Oxygen can be provided via face mask until the neonate is responsive, with assisted ventilation provided if needed. The use of doxapram to stimulate respiration has been controversial and is not indicated as an initial tool in resuscitating neonates. It is known to increase cerebral oxygen demand while decreasing cerebral blood flow (Brourman et al. 2007; McMillan and Serrano 2009). Once the neonates are showing signs of increased vigor, they should be placed in a warmed incubator until they can be introduced to the mother. Introduction should take place after the dam has recovered from anesthesia (Fig. 15.6).

Uterine Torsion

Uterine torsion, although a relatively uncommon phenomenon in small animals, can mimic either pyometra or dystocia. A painful and distended abdomen is often among the presenting clinical signs. As with other emergency presentations, initial stabilization should take place either before or while diagnostics are being performed.

Abdominal ultrasound proves to be the most useful imaging tool in diagnosing disorders of the uterus. In addition to evaluating the uterus, it will confirm the presence or absence of live fetuses. If the animal is pregnant, the uterine torsion will be contributing to dystocia. In the absence of pregnancy, abdominal ultrasound may reveal images similar to pyometra (dilated, fluid-filled uterine horns). Pyometra may be present concurrently with uterine torsion if the tissue becomes necrotic (Pacchiana and Stanley 2008).

Uterine torsion occurs more often late in pregnancy. The cause is not certain although it is believed that fetal activity, a uterus that is stretched thin from previous pregnancies, or simply overactivity by the dam, can play a role. Since occurring so infrequently, uterine torsion is not often documented. One case presentation reports a cat with concurrent pyometra and uterine torsion. After initial stabilization, an ovariohysterectomy was performed (Pacchiana and Stanley 2008). Ovariohysterectomy is the treatment of choice for uterine torsion. It is important to note that since the uterus is being removed, it is not only unnecessary but contraindicated to derotate the torsion. Derotating a diseased uterus or uterine horn can result in the release of free radicals and endotoxins into the patient's circulation (Pacchiana and Stanley 2008). Prognosis is generally good depending on the patient's initial clinical status.

Uterine Prolapse

Patients with uterine prolapse will present with a mass-like substance in the vagina. Uterine prolapse most often occurs during parturition or shortly after, as the cervix is open (Hopper 2003). Either one or both uterine horns are susceptible to prolapse. Fetuses may remain viable if they are in the intact horn. Immediate action is necessary to determine the presence of viable fetuses and prevent systemic infection from the contaminated uterus (Hopper 2003). Under sedation or anesthesia, the prolapsed portion of uterus should be cleaned with 0.9% saline and lubricated using sterile water-based lubricant. The uterus may then be able to be gently reduced manually. Hyperosmotic agents such as 50% dextrose may be used to reduce tissue edema. If the cervix extends too far to easily reduce the uterus, a longer, sterile, blunt instrument may be used (Hopper 2003). Oxytocin should be administered at 5–10 U intramuscularly following successful reduction. This assists in involution of the uterus (Hopper 2003). If unable to reduce or if the uterus is severely damaged, surgical intervention may be necessary, including possible ovariohysterectomy.

Eclampsia

Eclampsia in veterinary medicine is an emergency associated with hypocalcemia in the pregnant or postpartum patient. Eclampsia is most common in small and toy breed dogs, although it can occur in many species (Freshman 2003). Incidentally, in small animals, eclampsia differs from that in human medicine, where it is a disorder initiated by hypertension in pregnant women.

During pregnancy, calcium is depleted by the growing fetuses. The body's calcium stores continue to be exhausted during lactation, especially if the mother is experiencing decreased appetite or poor nutrition (Dye 2001). Large litters may predispose the dam to developing eclampsia. Animals treated with calcium supplements during pregnancy also have an increased risk of developing eclampsia postpartum due to the reduction of parathyroid hormone secretion when serum calcium level is high (Dye 2001; Freshman 2003; Davidson 2009). Because excess calcium can be present in some foods as well, care should be taken when choosing a diet and should be appropriate for pregnant or lactating animals.

Eclampsia usually occurs either late in gestation or within a few weeks of whelping. In cases of dystocia maternal in origin, it is important to measure ionized calcium levels. Hypocalcemia and concurrent hypoglycemia may contribute to uterine inertia. Correcting hypocalcemia and hypoglycemia are often part of the medical treatment of dystocia to help increase the strength of weak uterine contractions (McMillan and Serrano 2009).

Hypocalcemia can cause nerve fibers to fire spontaneously. This causes muscular contractions and can lead to tonic-clonic, or whole-body grand mal seizures (Dye 2001).

Patients presenting with eclampsia are often lethargic, ataxic, have a stiff gait, and/or have muscle rigidity or tremors (Dye 2001; Freshman 2003). Severe cases can present with seizures. Presenting symptoms along with a current or recent history of pregnancy should lead to a working diagnosis of eclampsia. Diagnosis can be confirmed by analyzing ionized and serum calcium levels. Patients experiencing eclampsia will typically have serum calcium levels <7 mg/dL (9–11 mg/dL) (Dye 2001; Freshman 2003). Treatment, however, is first begun based on clinical signs followed by ionized calcium <0.6 mmol/L (1–1.25 mmol/L). Therefore, serum calcium may be normal in some patients (Freshman 2003). In addition to the initial signs, physical exam findings can include hyperthermia (due to muscle spasms), tachycardia, and/or tachypnea.

The young should be removed from the dam and hand-fed until she is stable. The standard treatment for eclampsia involves intravenous administration of 10% calcium gluconate (Dye 2001; Freshman 2003). Dose ranges from 50–150 mg/kg or 0.5–1.5 mL/kg infused slowly over 20–30 minutes (Plumb 1999). This is given to effect while monitoring electrocardiogram (ECG). Hypocalcemia can cause a prolonged Q-T interval (Freshman 2003). Bradycardia and shortening of Q-T interval can result if calcium is given too rapidly. If this occurs, stop infusing temporarily until normal rate and rhythm return (Dye 2001). Patients typically respond to treatment quickly, within 15–20 minutes. Additional calcium gluconate can be administered at the same initial dose subcutaneously (diluted 50:50 with 0.9% NaCl) every 6–8 hours until the patient is stable and calcium levels are normal (Freshman 2003).

If the patient is experiencing grand mal seizures, diazepam may be administered IV at 0.5–1 mg/kg concurrently with calcium therapy (Freshman 2003; Plumb 1999). In severe cases where seizures may continue, cerebral edema may ensue. Corticosteroids are contraindicated in treatment of cerebral edema with hypocalcemia as they increase renal calcium excretion, which in turn will decrease calcium absorption (Dye 2001; Freshman 2003).

Once the patient is able to eat, calcium may be supplemented orally at a dose of 10–30 mg/kg three times daily (Davidson 2009; Freshman 2003). This is usually given in the form of calcium carbonate (Tums®, GlaxoSmithKline, Stafford Springs, CT). Tums® must be given with caution as different types can vary in calcium content. A typical 500 mg Tums® tablet will contain 200 mg of calcium (Davidson 2009). Serum calcium levels should be monitored daily during treatment until normal. Longer monitoring may be necessary if neonates continue to nurse.

Male Reproductive Emergencies

Paraphimosis

Paraphimosis is a condition, more common in dogs than in cats, in which the penis is unable to retract into the prepuce. It can be present with or without penile strangulation and entrapment. In either case, the patient may present agitated and in pain, trying to lick or bite at the penis. On presentation, the penis may be dry due to exposure and loss of natural lubrication. The penis is also prone to injury and to collecting debris while exposed.

In paraphimosis with entrapment and strangulation, the penis becomes enlarged and swollen to the point it is unable to retract into the prepuce. It is often associated with erection or coitus. Hair surrounding the prepuce (preputial hair) can become wrapped around the base of an extruded penis preventing retraction and causing strangulation. This causes increased swelling and edema, and the strangulation can compromise venous blood flow (Pavletic 2005). This condition can be exceptionally painful as swelling continues. Sedation is usually necessary to provide even initial treatment. If untreated, urethral obstruction can occur. The penis can also eventually become necrotic requiring amputation (Pavletic 2005; Reis 2001b).

Paraphimosis without entrapment does not usually present with the same acutely painful symptoms of entrapment and strangulation. These cases may be more chronic in nature, with the penis extruding intermittently. The preputial opening may be small, and when an extruded penis attempts to retract, the penis will turn the skin inward. If the orifice does not allow retraction, the turned-in skin can lead to entrapment and further complicate the paraphimosis. This differs from phimosis, where the preputial opening is small enough that it does not easily allow extrusion of the penis (Pavletic 2005). In other cases, paraphimosis may be due to an irregularity in the relationship between penile and preputial length (Pavletic 2005).

Treatment for paraphimosis involves retracting the penis back into its normal position in the prepuce. In cases without entrapment, this may be fairly simple and performed manually using a water-soluble lubricant. Hyperosmolar solutions such as 50% dextrose can be used to reduce tissue edema. Analgesia and anti-inflammatory drugs are also likely necessary. The exposed penis should first be cleaned thoroughly prior to replacement. Clients can be instructed on how to examine their pet's prepuce at home, instill topical antibiotic ointment, and retract the penis into the prepuce if necessary. If conservative treatment fails, surgical correction may be necessary. If the paraphimosis is caused by a narrowed preputial opening, a small V-shaped incision can be made on the dorsal aspect of the prepuce to enlarge the orifice (Pavletic 2005). In cases where the length of the prepuce is inappropriate for the penis, preputial advancement can be performed to lengthen the prepuce using incisions cranial to the prepuce (Pavletic 2005). Alternatively, phallopexy can be performed to surgically secure the dorsal penis to the prepuce (Papazoglou 2004).

In cases of paraphimosis with entrapment and strangulation, the penis is often too swollen to simply be manually retracted into the prepuce. As mentioned, sedation or general anesthesia may be required for full examination and initial treatment. Adequate analgesia must be provided as well as IV fluid therapy during anesthesia. The penis should still be cleaned and lubricated before any attempt at replacement is made. If the swelling is severe enough and penile necrosis is a growing concern, an incision can be made in the prepuce to relieve the tension (Pavletic 2005). Any hair or debris causing the strangulation should be removed or cut. The patient should be evaluated for its ability to urinate, with a sterile urinary catheter being placed if warranted. Cold compresses may help to alleviate swelling enough to allow for retraction into the prepuce. If the swelling does not improve, 50% dextrose can be applied directly to the penis. The hyperosmotic solution will help decrease the edema. Subsequent applications may be necessary every few hours (Pavletic 2005). The patient should wear an Elizabethan collar to avoid licking and self-trauma. A recheck should be performed in the few days following treatment to ensure the penis is remaining in place and assess viability of penile tissue. Necrosis may not be evident during initial treatment. As with cases not involving entrapment and strangulation, owners should also be instructed to evaluate their pet at home.

The Prostate: Acute Prostatitis and Prostatic Abscesses

The canine prostate is an accessory sex organ that surrounds the urethra. Unlike in felines, where prostate disease is rare, the canine prostate is a common source of pathology in the adult, intact male. Benign prostatic hyperplasia (BPH) is a common condition involving older, intact male dogs (as well as humans) in which the prostate becomes enlarged due to hormonal changes (Wallace 2001). This rarely causes symptoms; however it can lead to difficulty with urination and defecation. The size and shape changes along with hormone imbalances associated with BPH can predispose the prostate to bacterial infections. Castration drastically reduces prostate size and can alleviate symptoms in these patients. Castration is often a treatment recommendation in all cases with prostatic diseases.

The prostate can be palpated during a digital rectal examination. The normal prostate sits in the pelvic canal at the pelvic floor, and is smooth and non-painful. An enlarged prostate gland with or without clinical signs may indicate BPH (Wallace 2001).

Prostatic ducts connect the prostate and urethra. Ascending infection is considered the route of bacterial transmission into the prostate. The most commonly isolated bacteria is *E. coli*, although many different organisms have been identified (Freitag et al. 2007). Patients with prostatic disorders typically arrive to the emergency room with signs of urinary tract infection: hematuria, difficulty urinating, tenesmus, urethral discharge, stiff or wide gait, and painful caudal abdomen. Pain may be elicited on digital rectal examination. Polyuria and polydipsia may be described due to the release of endotoxins from *E. coli* interfering with synthesis of antidiuretic hormone (Lane and Matwichuk 2001). This phenomenon is also associated with pyometra.

Although presumed prostatitis is diagnosed based on clinical signs and physical examination, a urine sample should be collected via cystocentesis or sterile urinary catheter. Urinalysis will often reveal bacteriuria, and a urine culture and sensitivity should be performed. Serum chemistry and CBC may be unremarkable unless the patient is exhibiting signs of systemic illness. Radiographic imaging often will reveal an enlarged prostate, and ultrasound will show a hypoechoic prostate with irregular texture (Wallace 2001). An abscess in an enclosed capsule may be appreciated on ultrasound as well as any peritonitis. Pending sensitivity results, long-term antibiotic therapy (4–6 weeks) should be started using antibiotics shown to penetrate the blood–prostate barrier well. Trimethoprim-sulfamethoxazole and enrofloxacin are examples of good antibiotic choices for infections of the prostate (Wallace 2001). Again, castration as part of the treatment protocol will greatly reduce the size of the prostate and decrease prostatic secretions.

Prostatitis, in some cases, can lead to development of an abscess. Patients experiencing a prostatic abscess may present more critically ill than those with bacterial prostatitis. They will show signs of systemic illness including fever, painful abdomen or splinting of the abdomen, and lethargy. A prostatic abscess is prone to rupture, leading to septic peritonitis. These cases require emergency medical and surgical intervention. If septic peritonitis is present, emergency surgery may be indicated to flush the abdomen and place drains. If peritonitis is not present, the abscess should be surgically drained after initial stabilization has taken place. Various surgical techniques have been described as methods of treating prostatic abscesses, and the method will depend on the severity of disease and response to treatment. Prostatic omentalization has been described as the method of choice in cases requiring surgical intervention. Once the abscess has been surgically drained, omentum is inserted and secured into the cavity (Freitag et al. 2007). This promotes healing, blood flow, and drainage of secretions.

An alternate method described involves ultrasound-guided percutaneous drainage of the abscess (Boland et al. 2003). This is the method most often used in treating prostatic abscesses in humans. The risk of percutaneous drainage is that septic fluid from the abscess may leak into the abdomen causing peritonitis. This can be avoided by draining the abscess completely and by maintaining suction on the syringe as the needle is withdrawn (Boland et al. 2003). In some cases, subsequent drainage treatments may be necessary. Antibiotic therapy is still essential, and follow-up examinations are necessary to monitor improvement. Patients undergoing this form of treatment often require far less hospitalization and expense than other surgical interventions (Boland et al. 2003). Castration is recommended following drainage of the abscess.

Prostatic carcinoma, while rare, can present with any of the symptoms described above involving infections of the prostate. Upon rectal examination, the prostate will feel more nodular and irregular in shape than with bacterial infections (Freitag et al. 2007). Abdominal radiographs or ultrasound may reveal mineralization of the prostate, which is described as a nearly definitive indication of neoplasia in the castrated male (Bradbury et al. 2009).

References

Ambros, B, Duke-Novakovski, T, Pasloske, KS. 2008. Comparison of the anesthetic efficacy & cardiopulmonary effects of constant rate infusion of alfaxalone-2-hydroxypropyl-beta-cyclodextrin and propofol. *American Journal of Veterinary Research* 69(11):1391–1398.

Baker, T, Davidson, A. 2008. Acute metritis. *Standards Care: Emergency Critical Care Medicine* 10(11).

Boland, L, Gregory, S, Hardie, R, et al. 2003. Ultrasound-guided percutaneous drainage as the primary treatment for prostatic abscesses and cysts in dogs. *Journal of the American Animal Hospital Association* 39:151–159.

Boothe, D, Bucheler, J. 2001. Drug and blood component therapy and neonatal isoerythrolysis. In *Veterinary Pediatrics: Dogs and Cats from Birth to Six Months*, 3rd ed., edited by Hoskins, JD. Philadelphia: W.B. Saunders, pp. 35–56.

Bradbury, C, Pollard, R, Westropp, J. 2009. Relationship between prostatomegaly, prostatic mineralization, and cytologic diagnosis. *Veterinary Radiology Ultrasound* 50(2):167–171.

Brourman, J, Gendler, A, Graf, K. 2007. Canine dystocia: medical and surgical management. *Compendium Continuing Education for Practicing Veterinarian* 29(9).

Colville, T. 2002. The reproductive system. In *Clinical Anatomy and Physiology for Veterinary Technicians*, edited by Bassert, J, Colville, T. St. Louis, MO: Mosby, pp. 318–343.

Davidson, A. 2008. Mastitis. *Standards Care: Emergency Critical Care Medicine* 10(1).

Davidson, A. 2009. *Postpartum Disorders in the Bitch and Queen*. Proceedings: Western Veterinary Conference.

Dye, T. 2001. Eclampsia. In *Veterinary Emergency Medicine Secrets*, 2nd ed., edited by Wingfield, W, Wise, L. Philadelphia: Hanley & Belfus, pp. 368–370.

Fransson, B, Ragle, C. 2003. Canine pyometra: an update on pathogenesis and treatment. *Compendium Continuing Education for Practicing Veterinarian* 25(8):602–612.

Freitag, T, Jerram, R, Walker, A, et al. 2007. Surgical management of common canine prostatic conditions. *Compendium Continuing Education for Practicing Veterinarian* 29(11).

Freshman, J. 2003. Eclampsia in dogs. *Standards Care: Emergency Critical Care Medicine* 5.4:1–5.

Hackett, T. 2003. *Dystocia: Push or Pull?* Proceedings: 9th International Veterinary Emergency & Critical Care Symposium.

Hopper, K. 2003. *Pyometra, Mastitis and Uterine Prolapse*. Proceedings: 9th International Veterinary Emergency & Critical Care Symposium.

Jutkowitz, A. 2005. Reproductive emergencies. *Veterinary Clinics of North America: Small Animal Practice* 35(2):397–420.

Lane, I, Matwichuk, C. 2001. Acute bacterial prostatitis and prostatic abscesses. In *Veterinary Emergency Medicine Secrets*, 2nd ed., edited by Wingfield, W, Lane, I. Philadelphia: Hanley & Belfus, pp. 377–379.

Macintyre, D. 2006. *Reproductive Emergencies*. Proceedings: Atlantic Coast Veterinary Conference.

McMillan, M, Serrano, S. 2009. Dystocia. *Standards Care: Emergency Critical Care Medicine* 11(1).

Moon-Massat, PF, Erb, H. 2002. Perioperative factors associated with puppy vigor after delivery by cesarean section. *Journal of the American Animal Hospital Association* 38(Jan/Feb):90–96.

Ostwald, D. 2001. Pyometritis. In *Veterinary Emergency Medicine Secrets*, 2nd ed., edited by Wingfield, W, Wise, L. Philadelphia: Hanley & Belfus, pp. 364–366.

Pacchiana, P, Stanley, S. 2008. Uterine torsion and metabolic abnormalities in a cat with a pyometra. *The Canadian Veterinary Journal* 49:398–400.

Papazoglou, L. 2004. *Diseases and Surgery of the Canine Penis and Prepuce*. Proceedings: 29th World Congress of the World Small Animal Veterinary Association.

Pavletic, M. 2005. Management of canine paraphimosis. *Standards Care: Emergency Critical Care Medicine* September:6–10.

Plumb, D. 1999. *Veterinary Drug Handbook*, 3rd ed. Ames, IA: Iowa State University.

Raffe, M, Roberts, J, Marks, S. 2003. Canine pyometra. *Standards Care: Emergency Critical Care Medicine* May:5–9.

Reiss, A. 2001a. Dystocia. In *Veterinary Emergency Medicine Secrets*, 2nd ed., edited by Wingfield, W, Wise, L. Philadelphia: Hanley & Belfus, pp. 370–374.

Reiss, A. 2001b. Paraphimosis. In *Veterinary Emergency Medicine Secrets*, 2nd ed., edited by Wingfield, W, Wise, L. Philadelphia: Hanley & Belfus, pp. 366–368.

Ryan, S, Wagner, A. 2006. An in-depth look: cesarean section in dogs: anesthetic management. *Compendium Continuing Education for Practicing Veterinarian* 28(1):44–56.

Wallace, M. 2001. *Diagnosis and Medical Management of Canine Prostatic Disease*. Proceedings: Atlantic Coast Veterinary Conference.

Ocular Emergencies

Jonathan A. Esmond

CHAPTER 16

Introduction

In small animal veterinary medicine, ophthalmology cases are often an underappreciated emergency by the owner as well as the veterinary support staff. In reality though, it is one of the most emergent of situations, if sight is to be preserved. Therefore, these cases should be quickly and accurately assessed and treated by the clinician. It is the veterinary technician's responsibility to recognize these situations, begin proactively caring for the pet, while having the veterinarian examine the patient within a reasonable amount of time. Referral to a board-certified ophthalmologist is recommended in many of the cases.

355

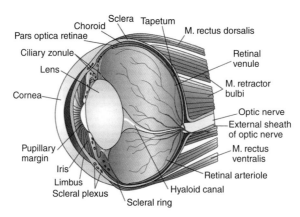

Figure 16.1   Ocular and Periocular anatomy. (This image was published in *Small Animal Surgery*, 3rd ed., Fossum et al., ocular and periocular anatomy, p. 262, Copyright Mosby Elsevier 2007.)

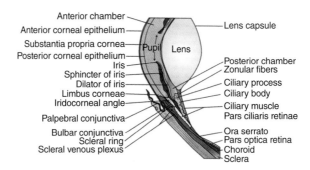

Figure 16.2   Ocular and Periocular anatomy. (This image was published in *Small Animal Surgery*, 3rd ed., Fossum et al., ocular and periocular anatomy, p. 262, Copyright Mosby Elsevier 2007.)

Anatomy and Physiology of the Eye

The eye is composed of many structures that are inherently dependent on one another. Therefore, ocular emergencies may affect one or multiple structures simultaneously. The eye is an intricate and delicate organ whose job it is to focus and direct light onto the retina resulting in vision (Figs. 16.1 and 16.2).

The Globe

The eyeball itself, or globe, is composed of three layers. The fibrous tunic includes the sclera, cornea, limbus, and area cribosa. The fibrous tunic and nervous tunic surround the vascular tunic (uvea) which is composed of the choroid, ciliary body, and the iris. The nervous tunic includes the photoreceptor layers and the fundus, which can be viewed with an ophthalmoscope. These vital structures are protected by the orbit.

The orbit is a circular bony structure that gives support to the globe and its supporting anatomy. The anterior portion of the orbit is open, leaving enough space for the globe to move rostrally in the event of trauma or a particular disease process. The orbit is composed of several different bones and is layered by the periorbita. The orbital ligament,

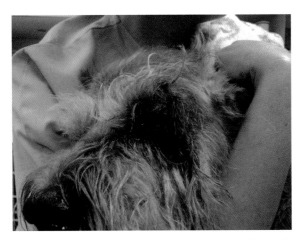

Figure 16.3 Patients with eye injuries should have an E-collar placed to help minimize the risk of self-injury.

as well as connective tissues, adhere to the orbit as well as seven striated extraocular muscles. The third, fourth, and sixth cranial nerves along with the extraocular muscles control movement of the globe within the orbit, allowing nearly 240 degrees of vision in the dog and cat versus the 200 degrees seen in human vision. This is due to the eyes being located more laterally within the skull.

The extraocular muscles consist of the dorsal (m. rectus dorsalis), ventral (m. rectus ventralis), and lateral (m. rectus lateralis) muscles as well as the medial rectus muscle (m. rectus medialis), the dorsal oblique (m. obliquus ventralis), and the retractor bulbi muscle (m. retractor bulbi). These muscles may be damaged in the event of a traumatic proptosis inhibiting the normal movement and vision of the eye (Frandson et al. 2003) (Fig. 16.3).

If one was able to move forward through the structures of eye posterior to anterior you would come in contact with these major structures: the retina, vascular tunic which is composed of the ciliary body, iris, and choroid. The lens and sclera are followed by the ciliary zonules, limbus, and cornea.

The Ciliary Body

The ciliary body is the caudal portion of the iris in which aqueous humor is produced by the ciliary epithelium. Passive ultrafiltration and active secretion of carbonic anhydrase within the ciliary epithelium produces a fluid know as the aqueous humor, which helps distends the eye and is directly affected by mean arterial pressure. The aqueous humor is anterior to the lens but flows around the ciliary body, or more correctly, from the ciliary body through the pupil, exiting through the trabecular meshwork. Eighty percent exits in this fashion. The remaining 20% exits through uveoscleral pathway. Intraocular pressure (IOP) is influenced by inflammation, or lack thereof, in the anterior uvea. The obstruction of this outflow tract through the trabecular meshwork will increase IOP. Posterior to the lens lies the vitreous chamber. This accounts for 75% of the globe and is filled with a jelly-like substance called the vitreous body. This material is acellular and provides shape to the globe.

The Iris and Pupil

Within the center of the iris lies the pupil. The iris is the pigmented portion of the eye surrounding the pupil. It divides anterior and posterior portions of the eye, keeping the aqueous filled anterior portion separated from the posterior (between lens and iris) portions. The iris controls the size of the pupil, dilating or contracting, to allow more or less light in to reach the photoreceptor cells of the retina. The constriction of the pupil is controlled by the parasympathetic nervous system. Dilation is controlled by sympathetic nerves. *Mydriasis* refers to dilation of pupils while *miosis* refers to the constriction of pupils. *Anisocoria* refers to irregularity in pupil's size such that one pupil is constricted while the other is dilated. These pupil changes all give clues as to a patient's progress during serial neurologic exams and allow clinicians to assess severity of damage to different parts of the brain in traumatic brain injury (TBI).

The Choroid

At the most posterior portion of the vascular tunic (uvea) is the choroid. It is exceptionally vascular and provides nourishment to the outer layers of the retina. It has many layers, one being the tapetum lucidum which controls the reflection of light, allowing more light to reach photoreceptors. This increases vision in times of low light. In some animals, this has led to their superior night vision. Humans lack a tapetum lucidum accounting for the lack of "eye shine." Eye shine can be observed at night if a light source is shown upon an animal's eyes (Frandson et al. 2003).

The Lens

The lens is fixed and anchored by zonules, small fibers connecting to the ciliary body. These zonules control the movement and shape of the lens allowing for change in its optics. It is clear with no vascular structures and receives its nutrition from the aqueous humor through diffusion. In some disease processes, the lens can become detached from the zonules and be free floating such as seen in sudden acquired retinal detachment.

The Retina

The retina is the photoreceptor of the eye. It has nine layers. The different cells of the retina perform different processes. Photoreceptors connect to bipolar cells which then connect to ganglion cells within the inner plexiform. Axons of the ganglion form the nerve fiber layer joining to the optic nerve. Amacrine cells are interneurons and along with horizontal cells have internal connections to ganglion cells.

The Cornea

The cornea is more refractory than the lens. Its shape is very important in allowing light to reach the retina. It is collagenous, clear, smooth, and avascular, and is the most anterior portion of the fibrous tunic and eye. It has three layers consisting of surface epithelium, collagenous stroma, and Descemet's membrane. Being avascular, it obtains oxygen and nutrition through diffusion from aqueous humor and the precorneal tear film. In ocular emergencies, it is one of the most often damaged portions of the eye but also one of the most regenerative. Descemet's membrane is relatively elastic, resisting damage in trauma. If a laceration or wound reaches this membrane and is full thickness, it is referred to as a *descemetocele*. Damage to the cornea can mean loss of vision if not corrected as soon as possible.

The Lacrimal System

The lacrimal system provides lubrication, nutrition, and protection to the outer surfaces of the eye. It is composed of several glands that secrete mucous and tears. The lacrimal gland contributes the largest percentage of tears. It lies dorsolateral in the orbit. The remaining tears and mucous are produced within glands of the conjunctiva and are part of the ocular adnexa and third eyelid. The glands and muscles make up the ocular adnexa. The conjunctiva is the mucous membrane lining the anterior portion of the eyelid and eyeball. Its many mucous-producing glands lubricate the eye. In the author's experience, one of the most common presenting complaints, in regard to the eye, are disorders of the conjunctiva (conjunctivitis).

The third eyelid, or nictitating membrane, protects the cornea. It lies ventromedial and is composed of firm cartilage. The third eyelid found in our domestic species is not found in humans. Swelling, inflammation, and prolapse of the third eyelid are commonly referred to as "cherry eye."

The palpebrae (eyelids) protect and smooth the tear film. They contain many sweat and sebaceous glands along the margin, called meibomian glands. Along with the third eyelid glands they comprise the majority of the tear film.

Common Ocular Emergencies

Ocular emergencies come in many shapes and sizes. It is important for the clinician as well as the veterinary technician to become familiar with the appearance that different ocular emergencies may take (Table 16.1).

Ocular Trauma and Traumatic Proptosis

One of the most common and most traumatic of ocular injuries, for pets as well as for the owner, is the traumatic proptosis (Fig. 16.4). Proptosis is where the globe actually moves rostrally out of the orbit. It is most often seen in small brachycephalic breeds, and often occurs due to bite wounds, being hit by a car or some other type of trauma to the head. Proptosis is usually unilateral. It does not take much for the globe to become prolapsed and sometimes proptosis may occur even from simple patient restraint. Even a minor scuffle, with a bite to the face and a tooth in just the right place, can push the globe forward. Tearing of nerves and muscles are common. Of the muscles, the medial rectus muscle is the most common to be damaged.

Upon ocular examination, common findings in mild proptosis may include mild exophthalmos, conjunctiva inflammation, mild corneal damage, and normal or slightly decreased pupillary light response (PLR). In more severe cases, the exophthalmos is more pronounced, there is obvious tearing of ocular muscles and the optic nerve, hyphema is present, severe drying and dessication of ocular structures exist, corneal laceration or

Table 16.1   Ocular disorders and etiologies

Globe		
	Exophthalmos	Orbital fractures, retrobulbar space-occupying lesions (e.g., neoplasia, abscess, zygomatic mucocele), traumatic proptosis
	Enophthalmos	Horner's syndrome, loss of retrobulbar fat, orbital fracture, temporal muscle atrophy
	Small globe	Globe rupture, microphthalmos
	Enlarged glove	Glaucoma, neoplasia
Eyelids		
	Alopecia	Bacterial pyoderma, immune-mediated disease, mycoses, parasitic infection, seborrhea
	Swelling/masses	Abscess, allergy, neoplasia, trauma
	Shape of palpebral fissure	Coloboma, ectropion, entropion, laceration, Horner's syndrome
Third eyelid (membrana nictitans)		
	Prominence	Dysautonomia, Horner's syndrome, sedation, retrobulbar lesion, systemic disease (e.g., tetanus)
	Distortion	Prolapse
	Masses	Lymphoid follicles, neoplasia, plasma cell infiltration
Conjunctiva/sclera		
	Redness	Conjunctivitis, episcleritis, episcleral congestion, hemorrhage
	Swelling	Allergy, conjunctivitis, diffuse neoplasia
	Masses	Cyst, neoplasia, nodular episcleritis
Cornea		
	Opacity	Cellular infiltration (white/gray), edema (white/blue), pigmentation (black), scarring (blue/gray), vascularization (red)
	Masses	Dermoid, granulation tissue, inclusion cyst, abscess, infiltrative neoplasia
	Vascularization	Superficial and deep keratitis, healing ulcer, eosinophilic keratitis, herpes infection, immune-mediated disease, sequestrum, trauma
	Infiltration	Melting ulcer, lipidosis, neoplasia
	Change in contour	Abscess, laceration, descemetocele, inclusion cyst, iris prolapsed, bullous keratopathy
Anterior chamber		
	Turbidity	Lipid-laden aqueous, uveitis (hypopyon, hyphema)
	Masses	Foreign body, lens luxation, neoplasia, cyst
	Hyphema	Chronic glaucoma, congenital, hypertension, neoplasia, retinal detachment, trauma, uveitits

Table 16.1   (*Continued*)

Iris	
Discoloration	Chronic uveitis
Masses	Neoplasia, uveal cyst
Strands	Persistent papillary membrane, synechiae
Pupil	
Dilated	Coloboma, dysautonomia, glaucoma, iris atrophy, oculomotor nerve lesion, optic nerve lesion, retinopathy, drugs, anxiety, pain
Constricted	Uveitis, Horner's syndrome, drugs
Lens	
Opacification	Cataract, uveitis, nuclear sclerosis, persistent pupillary membrane
Position	Luxation, subluxation
Posterior segment	
Leukocoria (white pupil)	Cataract, intraocular foreign body, neoplasia, retinal detachment, abscess

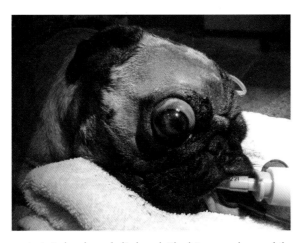

Figure 16.4   A severe proptosis in brachycephalic breed. The bite wound caused the majority of extraocular muscles to be torn along with the optic nerve. Enucleation was recommended, though at the owner's request, a proptosis reduction with tarsorrhaphy was performed.

globe rupture is present, and severe pain is evident. Patients may have concurrent systemic shock or head trauma from their disease process.

Medical and Surgical Treatment

If severe damage to the globe exists, enucleation is often the treatment of choice. If the medial rectus muscle was torn, lateral strabismus of the eye post surgery will exist. In only the most mild of exophthalmos is surgery not necessary. Reduction may even be attempted digitally with success. If reduction requires general anesthesia, it must be attempted as soon as systemic circulation has been stabilized. Lubrication of the eye in interim is vital. Anesthesia is never attempted until the patient is stabilized cardiovascularly first.

Analgesia is always warranted in cases of proptosis. For moderate to severe pain, pure mu agonists are generally recommended. Morphine, hydromorphone, and fentanyl are desirable. For mild to moderate pain, a partial agonist such as buprenorphine, or the oral agent tramadol are both very effective. A careful clip and scrub of the surgical site is important to obtain a sterile surgical field and reduce iatrogenic harm to an already damaged globe. A tarsorrhaphy is the act of suturing together the upper and lower eyelid in an attempt to bring the palpebral tissues together. This is done to give time for swelling to resolve and for tissues to heal. A tarsorrhaphy can be attempted to correct ocular proptosis when the optic nerve and extraocular muscles are not completely avulsed. After replacing and repositioning the globe, sutures are placed. A horizontal mattress, continuous, or simple interrupted suture pattern may be used to pull together palpebral tissue. Placing a blade handle on the globe while pulling up on the sutures will generally "pop" the globe back into place. Sutures are left in place for at least 3 weeks to allow for reduction in swelling and inflammation and to guard against proptosis recurring.

Medical management consists of topical and systemic antibiotics. Topical triple antibiotics (BNP) are applied between tarsorrhaphy sutures. Topical atropine 1% ophthalmic solution is applied predominantly for analgesia if a miotic pupil is present or if uveitis exists. Atropine will dilate the pupil causing myosis and relieve muscle spasms of the iris and ciliary body. Generally, its use is for a short period of time (two to three treatments). If no corneal laceration or ulceration is present, topical corticosteroids (e.g., prednisolone 1%, dexamethasone 0.1%) may be used for their anti-inflammatory affects. Systemic nonsteroidal anti-inflammatory drugs (NSAIDs) (e.g., carprofen, meloxicam) in addition to opioids are used for multimodal analgesia. Systemic NSAIDS are useful to reduce inflammation and to control pain but have contraindications in some patients (see Chapter 18, "Clinical Care Pharmacology"). Meloxicam at 0.2 mg/kg for a loading dose followed by 0.1 mg/kg daily or carprofen at 2.2 mg/kg q12h are well tolerated in conjunction with tramadol at 2–5 mg/kg every 8 hours to provide excellent oral analgesia for most canine cases when they leave the hospital (Plumb 2005). Systemic antibiotics (broad spectrum) such as enrofloxacin and amoxicillin clavulanic acid are good choices (Plumb 2005).

Enucleation is recommended if the optic nerve is damaged, multiple ocular muscles are torn, and/or globe rupture or puncture has occurred (resulting in loss of aqueous fluid).

Hyphema

Hyphema refers to blood collecting in the anterior chamber of the globe. Some of the causes include coagulopathy, hypertension, trauma, and neoplasia. Collection of blood in the anterior chamber can lead to glaucoma due to fibrin collection not allowing drainage of aqueous humor (Fig. 16.5).

Upon examination, the anterior chamber may be filled with fresh red blood. If blood is old, it may be clotted, taking on a dark appearance. Ocular structures may be difficult to locate. IOP may vary depending on severity of trauma. An ultrasound of the eye may be needed for a definitive diagnosis if not already obvious. If not related to trauma, a coagulation profile (e.g., prothrombin [PT], partial thromboplastin time [PTT]) should

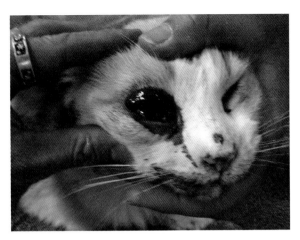

Figure 16.5   Dog attack resulting in severe conjunctival inflammation, third eyelid prolapse, and hyphema. Atropine 1% ophthalmic solution was applied to dilate pupils and reduce pain associated with muscular spasms of the ciliary body and iris. Triple antibiotic was also applied.

be performed, including a manual platelet count. The prognosis for hyphema varies greatly depending on the exact etiology or severity of trauma. In the event of severe systemic disease or neoplasia, loss of vision is possible. Treatment consists of topical corticosteroids if no corneal ulcer is present as well as atropine 1% topical instilled 2–4 times daily until pupil can be seen. Surgical intervention is rare especially if an elevated IOP exists. Irrigation is possibly advantageous through intracameral injections using fibrinolytic agents such as tissue plasminogen activator (tPA). This is an enzyme used to break down clots (Macintire et al. 2005).

Anterior Uveitis

The definition of anterior uveitis is inflammation of the iris and ciliary body. A search for the cause may be revealed (see Table 16.2) through a thorough examination including tonometry. IOP in uveitis will generate a low IOP differentiating it from glaucoma. Acute uveitis is generally very painful resulting in muscular spasms of the iris and ciliary body. Clinical signs include, but are not limited to, blepharospasm, enophthalmos, photophobia, extrusion of third eyelid, hyperemia of sclera and conjunctiva, aqueous flare, and miosis (Macintire et al. 2005).

Chronic uveitis may not be as painful as an acute case but results in clinical signs associated with the chronicity of the process. These signs include keratic precipitates on cornea, neovascularization of the iris, pigment changes of iris, adhesions between the iris and lens/cornea, and iris bombe.

Treatment for uveitis lies in controlling pain and inflammation while treating the underlying disease process. Corticosterioids and NSAIDS are useful systemically and/or topically.

Mydriatic cycloplegics may be used to dilate the pupil and relieve muscle spasms of the iris and ciliary body. Atropine sulfate and tropicamide are the most commonly used agents. Tropicamide is useful clinically for fundascopic examinations due to its rapid onset and short duration of action. The likelihood of synechiae (scar) formation is reduced

Table 16.2   Common causes of uveitis

Ocular	Lens luxation
	Trauma
	Neoplasia
Fungal	Blastomycosis
	Cryptococcosis
	Coccidioidomycosis
	Candidiasis
	Histoplasmosis
	Blastomyces
Rickettsial	*Rickettsia rickettsii*
	Ehrlichiosis
Bacterial	Systemic sepsis
	Brucellosis
	Leptospirosis
	Borellia burgdorferi
Viral	Feline (feline infectious peritonitis [FIP], feline leukemia virus, feline immudodeficiency virus [FIV], herpesvirus, rabies)
	Canine (Adenovirus, Distemper, Rabies)
Other	Immune mediated
	Hypertension (systemic)
	Idiopathic
	Hyperviscosity syndrome
	Protozoal (toxoplasmosis)
	Parasitic (ocular larva migrans)

as well. Close monitoring by the family veterinarian after leaving the emergency room is required to prevent relapse of symptoms (Wingfield and Raffe 2002).

Acute Glaucoma

Glaucoma is defined as an IOP greater than 25 mmHg in one or both eyes. Acute glaucoma is very painful and can result in a permanent loss of vision very rapidly. The increased IOP damages retinal ganglion cells as well as the optic nerve (Macintire et al. 2005). It is a true ocular emergency that requires immediate attention. Referral to a specialist is recommended after patient stabilization.

The causes of acute glaucoma may be primary or secondary. Primary causes may be breed related (English and American Cocker spaniels, Siberian husky, Toy, and Miniature poodles, and Bassetts. Secondary causes of glaucoma may be related to disease processes such as neoplasia, anterior lens luxation, severe uveitis, iris bombe, pre-iridial fibrovascular membrane, large number or iridial cysts, or high cellular debris (Macintire et al. 2005).

The treatment and management of glaucoma consists of reducing IOP as soon as possible, thereby preventing loss of vision and reducing pain. In severe cases where all else has failed, enucleation may be recommended.

Systemic use of mannitol at 0.5–1 mg/kg over 20 minutes is often the agent of choice to reduce IOPs quickly within the emergency room (Plumb 2005). If necessary, repeating this dose in 12 hours maybe warranted. Topical treatment consists of carbonic anhydrase inhibitors (CAIs). CAIs catalyze carbonic acid (carbon dioxide and water), eventually resulting in the elimination of carbon dioxide through the respiratory system. By inhibiting the enzyme carbonic anhydrase (which is essential in the formation of aqueous humor), IOP is hopefully reduced. Of the CAIs, dorzalomide 2% and brinzolamide 1% are applied three times daily. Oral CAIs are not recommended at this time.

Beta blockers timolol maleate 0.5%, levobunolol 0.25%–0.5%, and betataxolol 0.25% are useful for maintenance therapy as is the prostaglandin analogue latanoprost applied once daily. Topically, latanoprost acts to increase the outflow of aqueous drainage in the dog. If just one eye is initially affected, prophylactic treatment is an option using timolol 0.5% (1 drop BID) in the other eye (Macintire et al. 2005).

Surgical techniques are available but results can be unpredictable. The drainage procedures involve placement of implants to increase the aqueous outflow. Development of scar tissue can greatly hinder this technique and in some cases completely occlude drainage outflow. Cyclodestructive techniques involve the use of cryotherapy (transcleral), laser therapy, and chemical ablation (Peiffer and Peterson-Jones 2001).

Ocular Foreign Bodies

Ocular foreign bodies can result in penetration of the cornea or even deep puncture to the level of the lens resulting in damage severe enough to result in loss of the eye.

Corneal foreign bodies often consist of foxtails, wood, glass, metal, or other outdoor material. Often, these types of foreign bodies are found embedded within the conjunctiva or under the third eyelid causing pain and erosion of the cornea. In general, these cases require sedation and topical anesthesia or general anesthesia. In some cases, the foreign body may be difficult to find. Treatment consists of removing the foreign body followed by generous irrigation of wound. Topical antibiotics, a triple antibiotic (BNP) or gentamicin solution, and occasionally for pain, a topical anesthetic, can be applied by the owner. In most cases, a systemic anti-inflammatory is sufficient, such as carprofen or meloxicam, along with tramadol orally. To identify specific erosions or ulcerations, a fluorescein stain can be applied. The use of corticosteroids are contraindicated topically. An Elizabethan collar must be sent home to reduce self-inflicted trauma to the healing wound (Macintire et al. 2005).

Lacerations of the Palpebrae

Lacerations to the eyelid often involve altercations between pets. In many cases, they involve polytrauma and in some cases, the trauma is severe. Treatment consists of

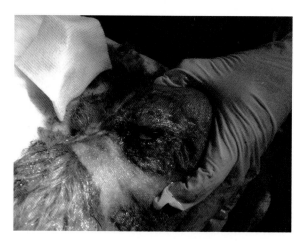

Figure 16.6 Markedly severe eyelid bite wounds requiring general anesthesia and laceration repair. A careful clip, scrub, and flush of wounds was performed by the attending technician.

stabilizing the patient's cardiac and respiratory functions prior to anesthesia (see Chapter 2, "Shock and Initial Stabilization"). Preoperative fluid resuscitation is likely to be indicated and in moderate to severe systemic disturbances, colloid therapy may be initiated. Analgesia should be instituted for the patient's comfort, to treat shock, and to balance anesthesia. Specific analgesics include the partial mu agonist buprenorphine (0.01–0.03 mg/kg), pure mu agonists hydromorphone (0.1–0.2 mg/kg), and fentanyl (3–6 mcg/kg/h) as a constant rate infusion (Plumb 2005). General anesthesia is recommended to repair eyelid lacerations. Working close to the eye requires some skill, and movement by the patient should be avoided so margins can be well aligned. Clipping and cleaning wounds by the technician should be performed carefully, with a steady hand, to avoid iatrogenic harm to the cornea. Lacerations involving the medial canthus should be approached cautiously preferably by a board certified ophthalmologist. The lacrimal duct resides here and care should be taken to avoid damage to it. Postoperative treatment should consist of a broad-spectrum antibiotic, systemic as well as topical, along with an Elizabethan collar to prevent self-mutilation of healing wound (Fig. 16.6) (Macintire et al. 2005).

Anterior Lens Luxation

Lens luxation can result in permanent loss of vision and is a result of many disease processes from glaucoma to trauma. Treatment, as in glaucoma, is to treat the underlying disorder while correcting the high IOP. Lens luxation is a result of loss of the ciliary zonule attachments. The reflective tapetum can be seen along with margins of the lens upon ocular examination. A flutter-type movement when the eye changes position can also be appreciated. Movement of the lens anterior is emergent while posterior is not considered so.

An examination by the clinician with tonometry to rule out glaucoma should be initiated. There are several ways to measure IOP today including the Shiotz tonometer, tonopen, and tonovet. The Shiotz tonometer and tonopen require the use of a topical anesthetic to the eye. The Tonovet (Icare, Helsinki, Finland) is a more recent option in veterinary medicine for measurement of IOP and does not require anesthesia of the globe.

The Shiotiz tonometer requires some skill and correct positioning of the patient and the globe. It is more uncomfortable for the patient but has a long history of use and has been proven to be accurate if used correctly.

Congenital defects are one of the more numerous reasons behind lens subluxation and luxation. In the middle years of life, these defects are more apt to present themselves and are predisposed in the German shepherd, border collie, and terriers. Clinically, upon examination, signs of luxation are blepharospasm, epiphora, corneal edema, acute blindness, and episcleral injection.

A temporary reduction of the lens luxation may be attempted by dilating the pupil with parasympatholytics (mydriatic cycloplegics) such as tropicamide or atropine. By tipping the nose of the patient up, movement of the lens into the posterior chamber may be possible. Constriction then of the pupil must be attempted using cholinergic agonists such as pilocarpine. Under general anesthesia, this is most easily done. In dorso ventral recumbency, the cornea is pushed (giving mannitol to soften the eye may be helpful), moving the lens behind the iris as it constricts. This procedure is only temporary, and surgery is often necessary. Intracapsular lens extraction is possible though long-term success is poor. Enucleation is recommended if acute glaucoma presents itself (Macintire et al. 2005).

Sudden Acquired Retinal Degeneration (SARD)

SARD is seen in middle age and older dogs. Dachshunds and miniature schnauzers may be predisposed but can occur in any breed. Polyuria, polydipsia, and polyphagia may precede vision loss. The vision loss associated with SARD is permanent. There is some data to say that hyperadrenocorticism may have something to do with SARD though no definitive proof exists (Macintire et al. 2005). There is no treatment for SARDS. Owners must become accustomed to living with a pet that has lost vision. Quality of life can still be quite high as long as some simple rules are followed by the owner.

Progressive Retinal Atropy (PRA)

PRA is often seen as acute loss of vision by the owner, but in reality, the loss of vision has been in development over a period of years. This congential photoreceptor dysplasia is seen in many breeds including the malamute, Belgian Shepherd, collie, greyhound, Irish setter, elkhound, and miniature schnauzer. A late onset of PRA is seen from an abnormal photoreceptor that developed poorly, early, and has slowly progressed over the pet's lifetime. Breeds predisposed to this are the Akita, English cocker spaniel, Labrador retriever, miniature long-haired dachshund, miniature poodle, Samoyed, Swiss hound, and Tibetan terrier.

Retinal Detachment

Retinal detachment seen in the emergency room is often the result of systemic hypertension and often is not be noticed by the owner until it occurs bilaterally resulting in acute blindness. Any cause of hypertension (e.g., chronic renal failure, heart disease) may predispose patients. Amlodipine is often used initially to treat hypertension in the cat and enalapril is often initially selected in the dog. In the hypertensive crisis, agents such as nitroprusside may be selected to rapidly lower arterial blood pressure. Amazingly retinal reattachment may occur once the underlying problems have been treated successfully (Macintire et al. 2005).

Conjunctivitis

Conjunctivitis is very common in the dog and cat. It is defined simply as inflammation of the conjunctiva. Reasons for this inflammation are many. In the cat, the cause is often viral, (calicivirus, herpesvirus, mycoplasma) or bacterial (chlamydia). Clinical signs of inflammation are often noted, ocular discharge, hyperemia, and chemosis are common. Common reasons for conjunctivitis in the dog are trauma, third eyelid prolapse, allergies, or systemic disease. Again, treatment lies in alleviating the underlying problem whether viral, bacterial, or allergic. A topical triple antibiotic (BNP) is used in dogs. A corticosteroid containing triple antibiotic may be used if no corneal ulceration is present. In the cat, if bacterial, oxytetracycline or erythromycin may be used (Macintire et al. 2005). As in most viral cases, antiviral medications may not be effective. Time, patience, and treatment of any secondary bacterial infections are the most effective treatment for viral infection.

References

Frandson, RD, Wilke, WL, Fails, AD. 2003. Senses organs. In *Anatomy and Physiology of Farm Animals*, Vol. 1, 6th ed., edited by Troy, D. Baltimore, MD: Philadelphia: Lippincott, Williams & Wilkins, pp. 178–184.

Macintire, D, Drobatz, KJ, Haskins, SC, et al. 2005. Ocular emergencies. In *Manual of Small Animal Emergency and Critical Care Medicine*, Vol. 1, 1st ed., edited by Troy, D. Baltimore, MD; Philadelphia: Lippincott, Williams & Wilkins, pp. 353–372.

Peiffer, RL, Jr., Peterson-Jones, SM. 2001. *Small Animal Ophthalmology: A Problem-Oriented Approach*. London: Saunders Elsevier Limited.

Plumb, DC. 2005. *Plumbs Veterinary Drug Handbook*, 5th ed. Ames, IA: Blackwell.

Wingfield, WE, Raffe, MR. 2002. Ocular manifestations of systemic disease. In *The Veterinary ICU Book*, Vol. 1, 1st ed., edited by Cann, CC. Jackson, WY: Teton New Media.

Special Species and Avian Emergencies

Kimm Wuestenberg

Introduction

In recent years, there has been an increasing number of special species making their way into human homes as family pets. Today "special species" is a phrase commonly used to describe pet birds, small mammals, and reptiles. As these critters fall ill, their owners seek veterinary expertise for their pet's care. Although many practices do not routinely treat exotic species, it is important for veterinary personnel to become familiar with proper treatment of up-and-coming popular exotic pets, including proper transporting, handling, and husbandry (Provencio 2003; Samples and Murphy 2004; Avila-Guevara 2009). Encountering exotic patients can be challenging for veterinary personnel, especially when it is in an emergency situation. This chapter will primarily focus on some of the most common special species, their common disease, their species differences, and their condition and treatment (Fig. 17.1).

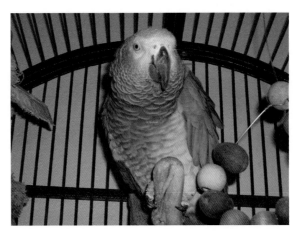

Figure 17.1 In recent years there has been an increasing number of special species making their way into human homes as family pets therefore it is important for veterinary paraprofessionals to become familiar with their treatment.

Triage and History Taking

Fortunately, many general small animal medicine practices can be applied to exotic species. It is important, however, to keep an open mind by remembering they are not dogs or cats (Hoenisch 1997). For the most part, the primary survey and triage is the same as would be for dogs and cats. Many procedures, therapeutics, anatomical structures, and physiological processes of special species are similar to cats and dogs, making it relatively simple to obtain vital signs, perform diagnostics, administer therapy, and recognize trends associated with disease pathophysiology.

Since most exotic pets are smaller than cats and dogs, it is important to have access to smaller medical supplies such as a pediatric stethoscope, small-gauged needles and catheters, rodent mouth speculums, and small endotracheal tubes. Proper housing items such as an incubator, an aquarium, an ultraviolet light, or a perch are important to have as well in the event an exotic pet requires long-term hospitalization.

Obtaining a history is an essential part of the secondary survey and full physical examination. Many conditions of exotic pets are a result of inadequate husbandry. Exotic pet owners should be asked about the type of habitat the pet is kept in, including temperature, humidity and light, the size of the enclosure, substrate within the housing, material the enclosure is made of, and the number of housed mates kept within the enclosure. Nutritional information should be obtained including primary diet, treats, and other components such as vitamins and supplements. Food storage should be confirmed as well since improper storage can lead to the growth of microorganisms or the breakdown of nutrients. The sanitation routine should be discussed including the frequency of substrate changing, cleaning of exercise wheels or branches, and the type of disinfectant used for cleaning. Technicians should also question owners about patient hygiene, say, for example, the frequency of dust baths for chinchillas or the availability of gnawing aids for rabbits (Table 17.1).

Table 17.1   Special species parameters

Species	Heart Rate (bpm)	Respiratory Rate (Breaths per Minute)	Temperature (Fahrenheit)	Blood Pressure (Systolic)	Weight
Chinchilla	200–350	45–80	100.5–102.5		450–800 g
Degu	270	120	97–100.9		170–300 g
Ferret	180–250	30–36	100–103.5	140–164	500 g–2.5 kg
Gerbil	250–500	85–160	98.6–102.2		45–130 g
Guinea pig	230–380	50–130	101.5–103	>100	700–1200 g
Hamster	250–500	40–110	101–103		85–150 g
Hedgehog	190–320	60–220	95–98		250–1200 g
Rabbit	130–325	30–60	101–103	70–170	2–6 kg
Mouse	325–780	60–220	98–100	125	20–60 g
Pot-bellied pig	70–80	13–18	101.5		100–250 lbs
Rat	250–500	70–140	99.5–101.5	121	250–520 g
Sugar glider	200–300	16–40	96.5–98		100–160 g

CHAPTER 17

Ferrets

Ferrets are very social animals, quickly forming bonds with both owners and other pets in the household. They are generally easy to handle, but may resist and struggle during certain procedures such as blood collection and intravenous catheter placement. Ferrets can be scruffed in a manner similar to cats. Care should be taken to monitor the patient's stress level if they resist handling. Intact male ferrets tend to be more aggressive than altered ferrets (Fig. 17.2).

Blood volume for ferrets is approximately 50–60 mL/kg. Veterinary technicians can easily perform blood collection via the jugular, lateral saphenous, cephalic, and lateral tail veins. Because of their short gastrointestinal (GI) transit time, fasting before anesthesia requires only 3–4 hours. Prolonged fasting can result in hypoglycemia, prolonged anesthetic recovery, and acid–base disturbances.

Intravenous catheter placement in ferrets is quite similar to that of the cat. The lateral saphenous, cephalic, and jugular veins are easily accessible. It may be beneficial to puncture the skin at the placement site with a needle prior to attempting catheterization. A 22- to 24-gauge catheter works well for most cases. Intraosseous catheterization can be performed within the femur, tibia, and humorous.

Ferrets have a blood volume of 50–60 mL/kg (Lichtenberger 2007). Ferrets in shock can be volume-resuscitated initially with a 10–15 mL/kg bolus with or without a 5 mL/kg hetastarch bolus over 5–10 minutes (Lichtenberger 2007). Similar to dogs and cats, these initial volume resuscitation doses may need to be repeated. Ferrets can also be put on a hetastarch CRI at 0.8 mL/kr/h. Oxyglobin (OPK Biotech, Cambridge, MA) can be administered in 2 mL/kg boluses over 10–15 minutes and given by CRI at 0.2–0.4 mL/kg/h

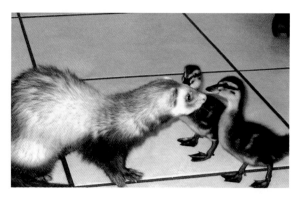

Figure 17.2 Ferrets are very social and friendly animals, quickly forming bonds with both owners and other pets in the household.

(Lichtenberger 2007). Replacement fluid therapy is calculated like other mammals by deficit (L) = % dehydrated × body weight (kg) × 1000.

Excellent sedative combinations for ferrets include midazolam combined with hydromorphone, morphine, or butorphanol. Similarly to cats, the local anesthetic benzocaine (e.g., Cetacaine Spray, Cetylite Industries, Inc., Pennsauken, NJ) will result in methemoglobinemia and Heinz body anemia. As a result, the agent should be avoided in ferrets.

Ferrets are commonly seen in the emergency setting due to GI conditions. Ferrets have a carnivorous GI system and short GI transit time. They have a strong vagal reflex, which can be stimulated during cervical manipulation (e.g., care should be given when drawing blood from jugular veins), and lack a cecum. Ferrets are affected by irritable bowel disease (IBD), megaesophagus, and are susceptible to intestinal obstruction, often from either foreign bodies or due to a trichobezoar. Other causes of GI symptoms include helicobacter induced gastritis, enzootic catarrhal enteritis (coronavirus), and neoplasia. Helicobacter can cause GI ulceration with subsequent hemorrhage, resulting in melena and anemia, bruxism, ptyalism, anorexia, and chronic weight loss. Ferrets are also susceptible to hepatic lipidosis and cholangiohepatitis.

Insulinoma, pancreatic islet cell neoplasia causing excess insulin production, often results in hypoglycemia. Clinical presentation is similar to that of small animal clinical signs in that ferrets will often appear weak or obtunded, may exhibit ptyalism, panting or appear anxious. Additionally, weakness in the hind limbs or pelvic limb ataxia may also be present. Seizures can occur with profound hypoglycemia.

Respiratory symptoms in the ferret may be due to cardiac disease, respiratory disease or neoplasia. Ferrets are affected by restrictive, dilatative, and hypertrophic cardiomyopathy in addition to valvular and electrical conductivity disorders. Although ferrets are susceptible, the only domestic species to be susceptible to human influenza, the most common respiratory emergencies are related to thoracic trauma or neoplasia, such as lymphoma (Hoefer 2001a,b,c,d,e). Pleural effusion and pneumothorax can be managed similar to small animals by performing therapeutic thoracocentesis or placement of a chest tube. Ferrets are also susceptible to canine distemper (fatal in ferrets), feline panleukopenia, aspiration pneumonia, and *Pasturella multocida* and *Clostridium botulinum* infections.

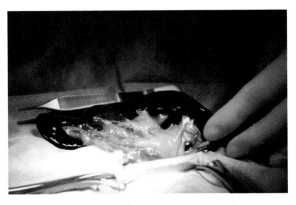

Figure 17.3   Splenomegaly in a ferret seen here during an exploratory celiotomy.

Urolithiasis affects both male and female ferrets. Clinical signs and symptoms include stranguria, hematuria, vomiting, lethargy, anorexia, and swollen, painful abdomen. Males are more commonly affected by urethral obstructions. Anesthesia is usually required to pass a urinary catheter in the male ferret due to the anatomical ("J") shape of the os penis (Ballard and Cheek 2003).

Anemia can be caused by prolonged estrus, GI hemorrhage, trauma, or ruptured neoplastic masses. Splenomegaly is commonly seen in adult ferrets, usually caused by extramedullary hematopoiesis (EMH); however, nodular tumors such as lymphosarcoma or rarely hemangiosarcoma can also occur (Hoefer 2001a,b,c,d,e). Ferrets lack sweat glands leaving them susceptible to heat exhaustion. Rabies, although rare among ferrets because they are usually not permitted to roam freely outdoors, is possible for ferrets to contract and transmit. Distemper and rabies vaccinations are required in ferrets (Fig. 17.3).

Rabbits

Rabbits are very gentle animals and usually are easy to handle. Rabbits should not be restrained by their ears, but rather supported with one hand under the body while the other cradles the body. It is important to handle rabbits carefully, making slow and gentle movements so as not to startle or cause stress to the rabbit.

Rabbits are at high risk for suffering from spinal fractures, especially when handled incorrectly. Unfortunately, iatrogenic insult is the leading cause of spinal fractures in this species. This is because the lumbar spine of the rabbit is surrounded by powerful muscles which may cause damage to the spine if excessive force or inadequate support is used during handling. If a rabbit is struggling during handling, the restrainer should immediately release the rabbit instead of using force. A towel may be wrapped around a rabbit to calm them down and minimize the risk of self-induced injury (Thompson and Martin 2002; Ballard and Cheek 2003). Additionally, as the lumbar spine is fragile, it may also easily fracture if the rabbit suffers from trauma or a fall while at home. Clinical signs of spinal trauma include ataxia, uncontrolled urination or defection, and hind end paresis or paralysis.

Rabbits are monogastric hindgut fermentors (non-ruminant herbivores) that require high fiber diets. In addition, rabbits lack the ability to vomit. Clinically, these traits are significant as rabbits therefore do not need to be fasted prior to anesthesia. Dysbiosis of the gut can result with poor antibiotic selection. Drugs that selectively kill gram-positive bacteria can lead to diarrhea, inappetence, and even death. Poor choices for antibiotics in rabbits include oral penicillins lincomycins, amoxicillin and ampicillin, cephalosporins, clindamycin, and erythromycin. A simple way to remember these drugs is by the acronym "PLACE." Acceptable choices include enrofloxacin, sulfonamides, chloramphenicol, azithromycin, and parenteral penicillins. Interestingly, rabbits produce unique granulomatous abscesses that are typically impenetrable for most antibiotics and require surgical excision.

Rabbits have a blood volume of 50–60 mL/kg (Lichtenberger 2007). Rabbits in shock can be volume-resuscitated initially with a 10–15 mL/kg bolus with or without a 5 mL/kg hetastarch bolus over 5–10 minutes (Lichtenberger 2007). Similar to dogs and cats, these initial volume resuscitation doses may need to be repeated. Replacement fluid therapy is calculated like other mammals by deficit (L) = % dehydrated × body weight (kg) × 1000.

Rabbits are susceptible to heat exhaustion. Those housed in temperatures over 85°F, kept in a crowded or stressful environment and those suffering from obesity are at risk for heat exhaustion. Clinical signs include panting, ptyalism, lethargy or weakness, and seizure activity.

Urolithiasis in rabbits is commonly caused by calcium carbonate and triple phosphate crystals. Urolithiasis may be due to dietary, metabolic, or hereditary influences. Clinical signs are generally limited to gross hematuria. Treatment generally involves cystotomy and dietary changes. Normal rabbit urine may have a cloudy appearance or may have yellow, brown, or red coloration.

"Snuffles," a bacterial upper respiratory disease complex that may include *Pasturella multocida, Bordatella bronchiseptica, Staphylococcus aureus, Moraxella catarrhalis, Francisella paratuberculosis*, and others, is very common occurrence in rabbits. There are a variety of clinical manifestations, ranging from upper and lower respiratory infections to ocular, genital, dermal, and aural infections. Transmission is typically direct contact of nasal secretions, but aerosol transmission may occur. Asymptomatic rabbits may be carriers so proper hygiene when handling multiple rabbits is imperative. Viral diseases have not yet been identified in rabbits.

Rabbits (and rodents) require nail trims. When nails become overgrown, they can be torn or injured when caught in cages or housing materials. Common blood collection sites include the marginal ear, central ear, jugular, cephalic, and saphenous veins.

Small Rodents

All rodents have hypsodontal teeth, meaning they continuously grow, leaving them at risk for malocclusions. When overgrowth ensues (either due to hereditary abnormalities, inappropriate diet, or dental disease), the teeth can cause damage to the mouth itself, prevent the ability to eat and even grow in a manner that entraps the tongue to the roof of the mouth (Nugent-Deal 2005).

Box 17.1   Helpful Tips

- Rodents have large incisors and a prominent tongue which makes visualization of the arytenoids and thus endotracheal intubation challenging. In addition, the mouth narrowly opens. A 16- or 18-gauge intravenous catheter may be used as an endotracheal tube.
- If a bird's beak or oropharynx has suffered trauma, an air sac can be cannulated to establish an airway.
- Pulse oximetry can be obtained in small rodents by using the rear foot.
- Most reptiles require intramuscular injections to be given in the triceps due to their renal-portal system.
- It can be difficult to draw blood from an exotic pet. A small needle (25–27 g) can be placed in the vein while a hematocrit tube collects the blood from the hub of the needle.
- A hiding turtle may come out of its shell when placed in shallow, lukewarm water.
- Lizards should never be picked up or restrained by their tail due to the ability of tail autotomy.
- An exotic formulary should always be referenced to prevent pharmaceutical toxicosis in exotic animals.

Guinea Pigs (Cavy)

Guinea pigs are generally calm and usually do not bite, thus requiring light restraint when examined. They can be held by placing one hand under the thorax and the other supporting the hind end (Nugent-Deal 2005). Guinea pigs have a short neck with little skin, so restraint via "scruffing" is not recommended.

The guinea pig has a blood volume of 7 mL/100 g. One can safely collect between 0.5 and 0.7 mL/100 g in a healthy guinea pig. Blood collection is commonly performed via the lateral saphenous, lingual, marginal ear, or dorsal penis vein.

Guinea pigs are also susceptible to heat exhaustion, particularly in temperatures above 85°F and humidity levels above 70%. Other factors may contribute to heat exhaustion, including obesity, crowding, inadequate ventilation, and shade. Guinea pigs suffering from heat exhaustion typically present with weakness, decreased mental status, ptyalism, and panting. Seizures and death may also occur with heat exhaustion.

Scorbutitis is caused by a vitamin C deficiency and is often referred to as a condition known as "scurvy." Guinea pigs cannot synthesize vitamin C, thus requiring a dietary supplement. Most guinea pig diets contain vitamin C; however, improper food storage and handling may reduce the amount of vitamin C in the formula. Guinea pigs with scurvy will present with pain, primarily of the joints and ribs. There may be accompanying edema, anorexia, and decreased activity level and ambulation. In addition, bone and dental development may be deficient. Vitamin C also plays a role in the coagulation cascade, thus bleeding may be a presenting complaint. Sick guinea pigs should receive ascorbic acid (vitamin C) supplementation whenever in hospital. A dose of 10 mg/kg IM every 72 hours has been proposed (Plunkett 2001).

Cervical lymphadenitis, or "lumps," usually occurs when food has injured the mouth or penetrated the skin near the submandibular lymph nodes while eating. Bacteria, predominantly *Streptococcus zooepidemicus*, are then transferred from the site to the lymph node, which causes painful abscesses under the mandible. These abscesses may rupture. Torticollis may be seen if the inner ear is involved. Respiratory involvement results in ocular and nasal discharge, dyspnea, and potentially, cyanosis. Septicemia, hematuria, and hemoglobinuria may also be seen. Draining, lavage, and support care with antibiotics is required for treatment.

Guinea pigs with inadequate diet, husbandry, or environmental stress are at risk for bacteria invading the reparatory system, causing infection and potentially pneumonia. Clinical signs are similar to small animal with nasal and ocular discharge, sneezing, coughing, loss of appetite, lethargy, and labored breathing. If an inner ear infection is involved, ataxia and vestibular signs may be present. Type of bacteria which contribute to respiratory disease of guinea pigs includes *Klebsiella, Bordetella bronchiseptica, Pseudomonas aeruginosa, Staphylococcus* species, and *Streptococcus* species. The disease may be acute or chronic. Treatment is often rewarding or unsuccessful.

Dystocia in guinea pigs most commonly results from pelvic anatomical changes which occur if females are not bred at a young age. The pelvic symphysis will fuse in female guinea pigs not bred by 6 months of age. Guinea pigs bred for the first time over 7 months of age will inevitably suffer from dystocia due to the inability of the pelvis symphysis to widen for parturition (Hoefer 2001a,b,c,d,e). Cesarean section is generally required in this situation. Like other species, fetal size and position can play a role in dystocia. Other contributors to dystocia include uterine inertia, uterine prolapse, metabolic disturbances, and toxemia. Treatment involves oxytocin injections (0.2–0.3 U/kg IM), assisted vaginal delivery, or emergency cesarean section (Plunkett 2001).

Pregnancy toxemia in guinea pigs often results in acute death. Obesity and inadequate diet may contribute to toxemia and ketosis in the pregnant sow. This condition is more commonly seen in stressed, heavily pregnant sows that are 56 days or more into gestation and are carrying 3 or more fetuses. Clinical signs include lethargy, dyspnea, anorexia, and death. Clinical pathology findings include hypoglycemia, hyperkalemia, elevated hepatic enzymes, hyperlipidemia, ketonemia, anemia, thrombocytopenia, and proteinuria. Although the prognosis is poor, treatment with intravenous fluids, dextrose supplementation, systemic antibiotics, and possible corticosteroids should be tried.

Mice and Rats

While rats are generally very friendly and social creatures, mice tend to be easily frightened and are more prone to bite (Nugent-Deal 2005). A nervous rat or mouse can be gently scruffed if needed during the physical exam. If needed, the head can be gently placed between the thumb and forefinger. Grasping by the base of the tail may be used as an initial means of capture and restraint until the scruff can be handled.

Many pet owners will find red or red-brown spots in the cage or food dishes and fear their pet is bleeding. The discoloration is referred to as "red tearing" or chromodacryorrhea, which can also be seen at the nostril and eye, as it is a normal naso-ocular secretion. The secretions are most often produced in response to stress.

Respiratory infection causing sneezing, coughing, ataxia, chromodacryorrhea and labored breathing in rats and mice may be caused by *Mycoplasma* spp., *Pasteurella pneumotropica, Streptococcus pneumoniae, Corynebacterium*, Sendai virus, and others. Severe respiratory infection and pneumonia can result in dyspnea and death. Supportive care and antibiotics are indicated.

Neoplasia is common in both rats and mice. Large overgrown tumors and subsequent ulceration are a common cause of presentation to the emergency room. As there are both benign and malignant tumors which affect mice and rats, surgical removal and histopathology is indicated for definitive diagnosis and prognosis.

Common venipuncture sites in the rat or mouse include the orbital sinus, facial, saphenous, or the tail vein. Whole blood samples should be placed into ethylenediaminetetraacetic acid (EDTA) containing tubes rather than heparin. Like rabbits and other rodents, rats and mice do not require fasting before anesthesia (Table 17.2).

Table 17.2   Venous access options

Species	Cephalic	Saphenous	Femoral	Jugular	Intraosseous	Other
Avian				Yes	Tibia and tarsus (non-pneumatic)	Basilic (wing vein) medial metatarsal
Chelonians			Yes	Yes	Tibia, plastrocarapace bridge	Brachial, dorsal tail, subcarapacial
Chinchilla	Yes	Yes	Yes	Yes	Yes	
Degu	Possible	Possible	Possible	Yes	Yes	
Ferret	Yes	Yes	Yes	Yes	Yes	Cranial vena cava
Fish						Caudal vertebral vein
Gerbil	Possible	Possible	Possible	Yes	Yes	Lateral tail vein
Guinea pig	Yes	Yes	Yes	Yes	Yes	Cranial vena cava
Hamster	Possible	Possible	Possible	Yes	Yes	
Hedgehog		Yes		Yes	Yes	Cranial vena cava
Lizards	Possible			Yes	Tibial crest	Ventral tail vein
Rabbit	Yes	Yes	Possible	Yes	Yes	Auricular, cranial vena cava
Mouse	Possible	Possible	Possible	Yes	Yes	Lateral tail vein
Pot-bellied pig	Yes	Yes	Yes	Yes	Neonate	
Rat	Possible	Possible	Possible		Yes	Lateral tail vein
Snakes				Yes		Ventral tail vein, palatine vessels
Sugar glider	Possible	Possible	Possible	Yes	Yes	

Hamsters

Hamsters can be handled and restrained in a similar manner as rats and mice. Like mice, they tend to be easily frightened and may bite. Blood collection in hamsters is tough because of their small size. Additionally, unlike rats and mice, hamsters do not possess a tail vein as a potential venipuncture site. Alternative sites include the orbital venous sinus, jugular, and lateral marginal vein of the tarsus.

Proliferative ileitis, or "wet tail," is most often seen in young, newly weaned hamsters but can affect hamsters of any age (Ballard and Cheek 2003). It is currently thought to be caused by a bacterium, *Lawsonia intracellularis*. Symptoms include liquid diarrhea, with or without blood, lethargy, anorexia, and dehydration. In severe cases, rectal prolapsing may be seen. Proliferative ileitis is the most serious intestinal disease of hamsters due to the rapid dehydration in which death may occur in 48 hours if left untreated. Fluid resuscitation, including crystalloids and colloids and antibiotics is warranted. The prognosis is guarded.

Bladder stone formation is relatively common in hamsters. Symptoms are similar to small animals with stranguria, hematuria, and pollakiuria exhibited. Additionally, anorexia, lethargy, and polydipsia may be noted with urolithiasis. Treatment is similar to that of the dog or cat.

Wounds and abscesses when seen are usually caused by fighting. Alternatively, abscesses of the cheek pouches may occur due to food penetration. Standard wound care such as draining the abscess and antibiotic therapy is generally implemented.

Gerbils

Gerbils are social animals and live in groups in the wild. They are well adapted for dessert living and are omnivorous. Gerbils tend to be friendly, clean, quiet, and curious pets. They rarely bite and can be easily handled which lend themselves nicely to be children's pets.

When presented to the veterinary hospital, gerbils should not be grasped distal to the base of the tail as loss of the skin of the tail may easily occur. Blood collection is best performed via the lateral saphenous vein although the tail vein can also be used. Less than 10% of body weight can be obtained for blood collection (e.g., 0.3 mL in an adult hamster).

Conditions affecting gerbils include Tyzzer's disease (*Clostridium piliforme* infection), aminoglycoside toxicosis, chronic interstitial glomerulonephritis, and diabetes mellitus. Tyzzer's disease is an acute, often fatal, hepatoenteric disease. Symptoms of *C. piliforme* infection include lethargy, weight loss, diarrhea, rough hair coat, and death. Treatment to date has been unrewarding. Aminoglycosides are toxic to gerbils. Antibiotic ointments containing aminoglycosides should be avoided as they may cause death.

More than 50% of gerbils may also be affected by idiopathic epilepsy. Seizure activity which ranges from pinna fasciculations to severe mycolonic convulsions can be seen as early as 2–3 months of age. The seizures persist and increase with severity until approximately 6 months of age. Seizures may be stimulated by handling or stress. In genetically predisposed gerbils (primarily in-bred), frequent handling at a young age (during the first 3 weeks of life) can help suppress the seizure response. Anticonvulsants are not therapeutically used in epileptic gerbils because the medication side effects can be more harmful than the seizures, which rarely prove to be harmful. The frequency of seizure tends to decrease with age (Table 17.3).

Table 17.3   Baseline laboratory values

Species	Packed Cell Volume (%)	Total Protein (g/dL)	Blood Glucose (mg/dL)
Avian	35–55	3.0–6.0	200–500
Chelonians	22–35	3.3–5.5	40–120
Ferret	43–55	5.5–7.6	80–120
Guinea pig	37–48	4.7–6.4	60–180
Lizards	22–35	3.3–5.5	40–140
Rabbit	35–50	5.4–7.3	80–150
Rodents	33–50	4.5–6.5	60–125
Snakes	26–42	3.3–5.5	40–100

Chinchillas

Chinchillas are generally friendly and are easy to handle. When frightened or startled, they may bark or urinate at a threatening object. Chinchillas exhibit a defense mechanism called "fur slip" which cause their fur to release, or fall out, when grasped in a stressful situation (Nugent-Deal 2005). To prevent this from occurring in a clinical setting, restraint should be limited to cupping one hand in front and one hand behind the chinchilla. Care should be taken to ensure the chinchilla does not jump out of the restraint. Alternatively, the chinchilla can be picked up by the base of the tail if necessary.

Chinchillas suffer from a variety of GI disorders, from diarrhea to constipation. The most pressing conditions include gastric ulceration and gastric tympany, or bloat. Gastric ulcers are generally due to an inappropriate diet and are more commonly seen in young chinchillas. Gastric tympany occurs from dietary changes or polyphagia but may also be related to hypocalcemia in nursing females. Gastric decompression via orogastric tube placement or gastrocentesis is usually required to relieve the distension and promote cardiovascular perfusion.

Other conditions affecting chinchillas include heat exhaustion, paraphimosis, and respiratory disease, primarily caused by *Bordetella bronchiseptica*, *Pasturellosis*, *Pseudomonas*, and *Streptoccocus* species.

Birds

Birds are well-known for their ability to hide their illness so well that by the time they present for medical attention, they are often in a critically ill state. Therefore, the sick bird is always an emergency. Interestingly, birds show similar disease signs regardless of the disease cause. General indicators of illness include "sick bird signs" (SBS) and include resting on the bottom of the cage, decreased or selective appetite, a change in quantity or quality of droppings, squinting and ruffled or dirty feathers, inactivity and increased sleeping, decreased vocalization, and discharges and excessive sneezing. Additionally,

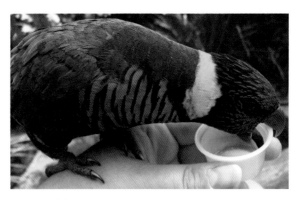

Figure 17.4   General indicators of illness in birds include "Sick Bird Signs" (SBS). This bird does not displace SBS signs.

birds will fluff their feathers to conserve heat and energy (Palmer-Holtry 2004a,b) (Fig. 17.4).

Birds are often seen in an emergency setting as a result of trauma, hemorrhage from a broken blood feather, beak, or nail, egg binding, and toxicosis. The initial triage and examination of the bird is a visual assessment. Birds can easily become stressed or fractious in a veterinary setting leading to injury, either of the patient or veterinary personnel. Birds should be assessed for mental alertness or level of consciousness, behavior, and activity level. The visual inspection includes the head (eyes, nares, beak, etc.), the uropygial gland and quality of feathers and skin, the cloaca and feces if possible, and lastly, the plantar surface of the feet for signs of pododermatitis.

Once a visual inspection has been performed, a physical examination can begin if the patients' stress level allows. The physical examination, including palpation and auscultation, should be quickly performed, taking breaks as necessary when indicated by the patients' demeanor. Birds should continuously be assessed throughout handling with the physical exam or procedures, ceasing in the event of distress or anxiety. Patients who are showing signs of respiratory distress should be placed in warmed oxygen cages immediately. If the patient is suffering from anxiety, inhalation anesthesia (isoflurane or sevoflurane) can be delivered via face mask and intubated if necessary (Table 17.4).

Puncture wounds and lacerations should be cleaned, flushed, and sutured as necessary. In general, puncture wounds specifically should be left open to drain and heal by second intension. Cat or dog bites are always considered an emergency whether or not the skin appears broken. Wounds require quick attention, with aggressive antibiotic therapy to prevent bacteremia and sepsis. Head trauma, beak trauma, and fractures can be managed in a similar manner as in small animals. Fractures should be splinted once the patient has stabilized and until surgical correction can be performed (if required). Fractured blood feathers can result in massive hemorrhage and should be carefully removed from the follicle. After plucking of the affective feather, gentle pressure may be applied for 1–2 minutes for hemostasis. Occasionally, placement of a suture is required to stop the hemorrhaging. If severe, fluid therapy and blood transfusion may be required.

It is important to keep the sternum free from bandages so the avian patient does not asphyxiate. Fractures in the distal wing may be bandaged using a figure-eight pattern, and proximal wing using a figure-eight pattern, attaching to the birds' body as long as

Table 17.4   Avian parameters based on weight

Weight	Resting Heart Rate (bpm)	Resting Respiratory Rate
25 g	274 beats per minute	60–70 breaths per minute
100–500 g	147–206	20–52
1–10 kg	79–127	17–32
100 kg	49	15–20
150 kg	45	6–10

respiration is not compromised (Ballard and Cheek 2003). Distal leg fractures can be stabilized with a Robert Jones bandage, where a spica splint may be used for the proximal leg (femoral fractures). Since birds have some pneumatic bones, a fracture may be accompanied by subcutaneous emphysema.

Trauma resulting in internal hemorrhaging may be detected by observation of bruising or distension of the abdomen. Clinical signs of hypovolemia or hypotension include generalized pallor of skin, pale mucous membranes, prolonged capillary refill time, tachycardia, tachypnea or dyspnea, and a decreased level of consciousness. Intravenous or intraosseous fluid therapy is imperative to restore homeostasis. Colloids, including (avian) blood products including heterologous and homologous blood, can be administered.

Egg binding and dystocia can occur due to many influences including (but not limited to) husbandry, infection, obesity, and trauma. These birds may present resting on the bottom of the cage, may have dyspnea or labored breathing, straining, abdominal distension, as well as a recent history of egg-laying. Additionally, leg lameness or paralysis may be present if nerve pressure has occurred. Cloacal prolapse may be observed; however, it is important to recognize that uterine or egg rupture can also occur with birds suffering from dystocia, possibly resulting in peritonitis. Radiographs may be beneficial in confirming the condition. Once the bird has been stabilized, attempts to remove the egg can be made. Various techniques can be used, including the use of medications to promote uterine contractions (oxytocin, prostaglandin gels, dextrose, calcium, etc., depending on cause), lubricating the vent, collapsing the egg using a needle and syringe (ovocentesis), expelling the egg using digital pressure, and surgical removal of the egg. Egg binding is more common in the smaller bird species such as parakeets, cockatiels, lovebirds, canaries, and finches.

Toxicosis may occur as a result of exposure to common household products. Birds are sensitive to inhalation toxicosis due to their air sacs and physiology. Toxicosis may also occur due to dermal exposure and ingestion. Like small animals, acids, alkalis, alcohols, bleaches, detergents, and oils may be problematic to birds (McKnight 2004). However, unlike small animals, birds can be affected by fumes such as polytetraflouethylene which may be found on coffee pots, cookware and utensils, heat lamps, and portable heaters. Ingestion of heavy metals (e.g., lead) are a common cause of neurological symptoms, anemia, and death. Other sources of toxicity in birds include ingestion of plants or certain foods such as some avocados, salt, and chocolate (Ballard and Cheek 2003).

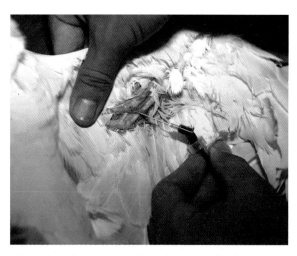

Figure 17.5   Blood bring drawn from the wing vein of a bird. (Reprinted with permission from Thrall's *Veterinary Hematology and Clinical Chemistry*, Blackwell Publishing.)

Aside from the commonly seen avian emergencies, birds also suffer from many respiratory, digestive, integumentary ailments, as well as self-mutilating behavioral problems. Birds presenting with respiratory symptoms should have the upper respiratory system evaluated for signs of a foreign body, parasites, sinusitis, or signs of infection. Lower respiratory signs may be associated with pneumonia, air sacculitis, granuloma, or allergies. Digestive problems range from vomiting or diarrhea to crop stasis ("sour crop"), crop burns, cloacal prolapse, and parasitism.

General treatment for critically ill birds is somewhat universal. In general, sick birds benefit from broad spectrum bactericidal antibiotics, warmed subcutaneous, intravenous or intraosseous fluids, and oxygen if the bird is in shock or respiratory distress. Additionally, birds can be placed in an incubator warmed to 85–90°F, unless the bird has head trauma or hyperthermia, in which case the incubator should be set cooler at 75°F. When stabilized, birds should be offered fresh food or tube-fed.

The daily maintenance fluid requirement for birds is 50 mL/kg/day. Warmed fluids should be administered. Subcutaneous fluids can be administered at 5–10 mL/kg in the axilla, lateral flank areas, or in the intrascapular area. Intravenous fluid boluses of 10 mL/kg can be given over 5–10 minutes to birds in shock. Popular venipuncture intravenous catheterization sites include the right jugular vein or at the medial elbow into the basilica (wing) veins. Intraosseous catheters can be placed into the ulna or tibiotarsus. The average blood volume for birds is 6–12 mL/100 g body weight. Most birds can withstand a 10%–30% loss (Fig. 17.5).

Reptiles

Reptiles commonly kept as pets include those in the chelonia family (turtles and tortoises), serpentes (snakes, pythons, and boas), and squamata (iguanas and lizards). Reptiles can be tamed and oftentimes are easily handled. Gloves should be worn for protection when handling a difficult reptile (Fig. 17.6).

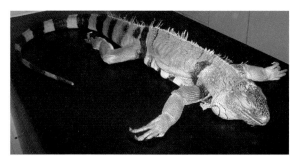

Figure 17.6   Gloves should be worn for protection when handling a difficult reptile.

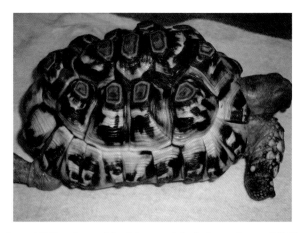

Figure 17.7   A chelonian exhibiting "pyramiding" from metabolic bone disease (MBD).

Metabolic bone disease (MBD) is one of the most common conditions seen in captive reptiles and in many cases, it is caused by poor husbandry. It occurs when there is an imbalance in the calcium to phosphorous ratio. Dietary components such as calcium, vitamin D or protein deficiency, and too much phosphorus can contribute to MBD. Additionally, the inability to metabolize or absorb calcium or vitamin D can lead to MBD, often a result of inadequate light sources (e.g., not providing UVB light sources) or habitat temperature (reptiles are ectothermic). Liver disease, kidney disease, and thyroid or para-thyroid conditions are all possible causes and contributors to MBD. Rodent-fed snakes usually do not suffer from MBD. Clinical signs include lethargy, anorexia, a soft or swollen jaw, tail, or limbs and in severe cases, pathological fractures of the jaw or extremi-ties. Chelonians may exhibit softening of the shell or gross deformities such as "pyramid-ing" (Provencio 2003). Radiographs may confirm MBD and may also be beneficial in monitoring the progress of therapeutics. Treatment begins with correction of husbandry and treating underlying or concurrent conditions (Fig. 17.7).

Traumas can occur due to numerous causes, including dog or cat bites, vehicle impact, and habitat flaws such as thermal injury or lacerations and fighting among cage mates. Snakes fed live prey are at risk for trauma and developing secondary infections from bite wounds received during the feeding. Abscesses can also occur due to bite or puncture wounds. Additionally, reptiles may become injured by being dropped when handled or stepped on.

Other conditions affecting reptiles include respiratory, ocular and digestive disorders, and parasitic infections. Poor husbandry such as improper diet, lighting, humidity, and sanitation can lead to numerous problems ranging from blister disease to oral bacterial infections ("mouth rot"). Desert tortoises have been known to develop bladder stones and diabetes mellitus. Iguanas can suffer from rear leg paralysis when there is a vitamin B or mineral deficiency. Like birds, reptiles can suffer from egg binding.

Venipuncture for most reptiles is usually a blind technique. No more than 0.5–0.8 mL/100 g of body weight should be collected in blood volume. EDTA causes lysis of red blood cells in some species (e.g., sea turtles and other chelonians) and therefore, lithium and sodium heparin are usually good anticoagulants of choice (Fig. 17.8).

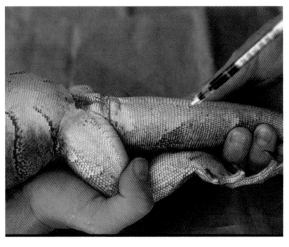

Figure 17.8   Venipuncture for most reptiles is usually a blind technique. (Reprinted with permission from Thrall's *Veterinary Hematology and Clinical Chemistry*, Blackwell Publishing.)

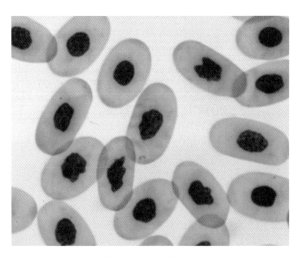

Figure 17.9   Because reptiles have nucleated red blood cells, manual complete blood counts should be performed as automated cell counts are not accurate. (Reprinted with permission from Thrall's *Veterinary Hematology and Clinical Chemistry*, Blackwell Publishing.)

For turtles and tortoises, the jugular, coccygeal, brachial, subcarapacial, and interdigital veins may all be selected for blood draw. In snakes, the caudal (ventral tail) vein is often selected, with puncture caudal to the cloaca, 25%–50% down the tail, at a 45–60 degree angle on the ventral midline. The caudal tail vein, ventral abdominal vein, and jugular vein are selected sites for lizards. Because reptiles have nucleated red blood cells, manual complete blood counts should be performed as automated cell counts are not accurate (Fig. 17.9).

References

Avila-Guevara, R. 2009. Optimum nutrition for iguanas. *The National Association Veterinary Technicians America Journal*, 8–31.

Ballard, B, Cheek, R. 2003. *Exotic Animal Medicine for the Veterinary Technician.* Hoboken, NJ: Wiley-Blackwell.

Hoefer, H. 2001a. *Thoracic Disease in the Ferret.* Atlantic Coast Veterinary Conference.

Hoefer, H. 2001b. *Clinical Techniques in Ferrets.* Atlantic Coast Veterinary Conference.

Hoefer, H. 2001c. *Rabbit Respiratory Disease.* Atlantic Coast Veterinary Conference.

Hoefer, H. 2001d. *Common Problems in Guinea Pigs.* Atlantic Coast Veterinary Conference.

Hoefer, H. 2001e. *Clinical Approach to the Chinchilla.* Atlantic Coast Veterinary Conference.

Hoenisch, J. 1997. Ferret facts. *Veterinary Technician Complete Journal for Veterinary Hospital Staff* 18(11):753–758.

Lichtenberger, M. 2007. Emergency and critical care. *Veterinary Clinics of North America: Exotic Animal Practice* 10(2):275–292.

McKnight, K. 2004. Toxicology brief: cleaning products- exposures in birds. *Veterinary Technician Complete Journal for Veterinary Hospital Staff* 25(5):332–334.

Nugent-Deal, J. 2005. Basic techniques in rodent medicine. *Veterinary Technician Complete Journal for Veterinary Hospital Staff* 26(11):768–780.

Palmer-Holtry, K. 2004a. Avian physical examination: the detailed (in-depth) exam. *Veterinary Technician Complete Journal for Veterinary Hospital Staff* 25(5):316–328.

Palmer-Holtry, K. 2004b. Avian physical examination: preliminary procedures. *Veterinary Technician Complete Journal for Veterinary Hospital Staff* 25(5):305–314.

Plunkett, SJ. 2001. *Emergency Procedure for the Small Animal Veterinarian*, 2nd ed. Philadelphia: W.B. Saunders.

Provencio, S. 2003. Exotic animal husbandry: the nature of the beast. *Veterinary Technician Complete Journal for Veterinary Hospital Staff* 24(2):90–100.

Samples, O, Murphy, K. 2004. Emergency care of rabbits: a clinical challenge. *Veterinary Technician Complete Journal for Veterinary Hospital Staff* 25(5):336–340.

Thompson, S, Martin, A. 2002. Rabbit and ferret wellness more than vaccinations. *The National Association Veterinary Technicians America Journal*, 41–46.

Section 3

Select Emergency/Critical Care Topics
and Therapies

Critical Care Pharmacology

David Liss

Introduction

Clinical pharmacology seems to be a weak point for the majority of veterinary technicians. Knowledge of broad categories, such as antibiotics and anti-inflammatories, seem to be commonplace, but additional knowledge of drug delivery, absorption, metabolism, and excretion can be lacking. This chapter will focus on drugs used in an emergency setting, focusing on acute conditions. A strong foundation of pharmacology is extremely important to ensure drug reactions are minimized, appropriate therapy is instituted, and appropriate drug mechanisms are utilized. All of these answers will be found within this expansive chapter on emergency and critical care pharmacology.

Pharmacokinetics

Pharmacokinetics are what the body does to a given drug. The absorption of drugs is mitigated by many factors including the route of administration, the makeup of the drug, and the metabolic state of the body. Drugs enter the body in a variety of routes but ultimately reside in the extracellular space. For them to exert their effects, they often must pass through the cellular membrane and affect cellular processes. Drugs move into the intracellular space by a variety of mechanisms including passive diffusion, facilitated diffusion, and active transport. Because cell membranes are hydrophobic and lipophilic, the composition of a drug with regard to these characteristics determines its ability to pass through the cell membrane. Nonpolar, nonionized, lipophilic drugs (hydrophobic) will pass through the easiest, with ionic substances (hydrophilic, lipophobic) being the least able to traverse the discriminating cell membrane.

Drug Delivery Routes

Route of administration is also an important factor in drug uptake. Parenteral routes include those where the drug is introduced in a route other than the gastrointestinal (GI) tract. Examples of parenteral administration include subcutaneous (SC), intramuscular (IM), intravenous (IV), intra-articular, intraosseous, intraperitoneal, intratracheal, and intraocular. Enteral administration is drug delivery via the gut. The majority of enteral administration is per os; however, with the advent of GI tubes, administration can be done directly into the esophagus, stomach, or jejunum. They can also be given colonically or rectally. Topical administration of drugs also remains an important category of drug administration route. However, topical medications are seldom used in critical care.

The quickest route, with regard to drug uptake, is the IV route. In this method, the drug is delivered directly to the extracellular fluid, bypassing any additional tissue. Because drugs must pass through tissues and capillary membranes to be delivered into the extracellular, intravascular space, the solubility of a drug, as well as its molecular size affect its ability to be absorbed in routes other than IV. The IM and SC routes will take longer for the drug to be systemically absorbed but can still provide some rapid delivery, with the IM being quicker than SC (Fig. 18.1).

Benefits of parenteral administration are mainly the speed at which a drug is absorbed. Rapid administration means quicker effects. In addition, IV titration allows for cessation of administration of a drug, should side effects be witnessed. However, concerns with parenteral administration are numerous. Drugs administered by this route have the ability to cause pain and irritation at the injection site depending on their osmolality and chemical makeup. Perivascular injection also represents serious tissue injury concerns and IV injections invariably require more skill. With the IM and SC routes, the injection cannot be stopped once given; however, with an IV titration, the injection can be stopped if adverse effects are noticed.

Enteral administration is a less invasive way to administer drugs but can be the most unpredictable in terms of absorption time. Many factors work against a drug and its absorption. If the gastric mucosa is irritated, emesis may occur. Motility also affects drug absorption by determining the transit time a drug takes from stomach to intestine. In

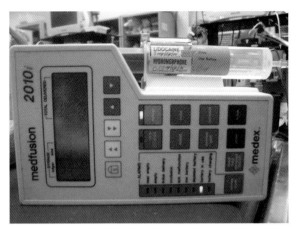

Figure 18.1 Syringe pumps are probably the best way to infuse drugs. Most will allow you to select different modes and can provide great flexibility with adjunctive CRIs or medications. (Courtesy of Jennifer Sager, BS, CVT, VTS [Anesthesia], VTS [Emergency & Critical Care].)

addition, enterally administered drugs need to be dissolved before they can pass through capillary membranes. This makes dissolution the major limiting factor in the absorption of orally administered drugs. The physical action of "churning" facilitates the dissolution of drugs. Hypomotility, or delayed gastric emptying, will allow a drug to reside in a certain part of the GI tract for a longer period of time. In contrast, hypermotility may reduce a drug's effect as well. The quicker a drug passes across the intestinal lumen, the less of the drug may be absorbed.

An additional barrier to enteral drug absorption is the "first pass effect." A drug must pass through the hepatic portal system, before it is distributed to the body. Thus, drugs may be partially metabolized before they reach systemic circulation. Additionally, ion trapping may prevent drug particles from diffusing through capillary membranes. Drugs are typically weak acids or bases, and thus have charge. Their pH affects the degree to which a particular drug is ionized or not. The more ionized a drug, the more it will dissociate in water, thus resisting transfer across a lipophilic membrane. Because the pH varies greatly from the lining of the stomach, to within the cellular membrane (pH 2, to pH 7.4, respectively), molecules may diffuse into the cell but then be unable to pass out. This can result in drug accumulation within cells. Ion trapping can not only result in accumulation of drugs within a specific body tissue, but also can assist in drug removal, if the ions are trapped within the renal tubules, for example (Bill 2006).

Rectal drug administration remains an effective way to administer drugs with regard to certain patients. Intrarectal administration of diazepam during status epilepticus represents an example of use of this route. The rectum has a large blood supply with little tissue separating blood vessels from the lumen. Thus, drugs can be readily absorbed into the systemic circulation, and 50% of the drug bypasses the hepatic portal system, allowing for increased drug uptake (Bill 2006).

Drug Uptake

Once a drug is ready to pass through the capillary membrane, entering the intravascular space, it must pass through small windows, or gaps, if unable to diffuse through capillary endothelial cells. Thus, both hydrophobic and lipophobic molecules may enter circulation. However, larger hydrophilic molecules that cannot fit through these gaps and cannot diffuse through endothelial cells remain unable to enter systemic circulation. An exception to this resides in the "blood–brain barrier." The capillaries in the brain lack these gaps; their endothelial cells are tightly conjoined. In addition, there are cells surrounding the capillaries, providing an additional barrier to drug absorption. This makes it almost impossible for hydrophilic drugs to perfuse into the brain.

Perfusion is an important factor in drug absorption and distribution. When placed within the body, drugs require vasculature to move them to their desired location of effect; however, if the vasculature is smaller than normal, in essence "farther away from where the drug was injected," its uptake time will be greater (Bill 2006). If the perfusion is entirely compromised, the drug may stay in the interstitial space and never enter the vasculature. Thus hypovolemic or dehydrated patients may not benefit from SC or IM injections. In hypovolemic states, as vasoconstriction occurs to shunt blood to the core organs, perfusion in less vital areas (adipose tissue, skeletal and muscle tissue) will greatly affect drug transit time.

Another important factor in drug distribution is plasma protein concentration. Drugs are often found bound to albumin (acidic) or α-1 glycoprotein (basic) drugs. Drugs bound to these proteins are considered functionally inactive. Lack of these proteins results in increased levels of free drug in circulation. Drug effects may be enhanced, potentially to the point of toxicity. Thus, drug dosages should be reduced in hypoproteinemic states. Hypoperfusion and hypoproteinemia will be covered in more depth later in the chapter.

Pharmcodynamics

Pharmcodynamics are what a given drug does to the body. Receptor dynamics, such as agonism/antagonism, govern a large portion of pharmacologic interactions. Other types of interactions include chelation, or non-receptor-mediated drug reactions.

Agonist–Antagonist Interactions

The agonist–antagonist relationship functions on some basic principles. First, there is a receptor to which drugs bind. Second, a drug is classified as either an agonist, eliciting action from the receptor, or an antagonist, blocking action at the receptor. Furthermore, agonist/antagonists can be classified as competitive or noncompetitive, whereby the competitive drugs clash over attachment to the receptor, indicating drugs that have stronger affinity for a receptor. And finally, agonist/antagonists can be classified as either full or partial. Full agonists/antagonists elicit the complete response from the receptor, whether it is to perform the receptor function, or block it. Partial agonist/antagonists elicit a partial response from the receptor, often binding more tightly to the receptor.

Non-Receptor-Mediated Drug Interactions

Chelation

Chelation involves the combination of a drug introduced into the body and a substance within the body, usually an ion. It typically is used to remove harmful substances from the body via elimination in a nontoxic form. For example, penicillamine binds to lead and effectively excretes it, bypassing potential heavy metal induced toxicity. Also, ethylenediaminetetraacetic acid (EDTA) binds with calcium in blood to prevent clotting in hematologic testing.

Metabolism

After a drug has exerted its effect, it is ready to be biotransformed, or metabolized. This process changes the drug from an active to an inactive form, called a metabolite. This readies the drug for elimination from the body. Metabolism is a complex set of chemical reactions aimed at altering the chemical composition of the drug, usually to be more lipophilic, so that its excretion can be maximized.

Metabolism usually occurs in two steps. Phase I reactions consist of an oxidation, reduction, or hydrolysis reaction to make the drug more polar. Oxidation reactions are the majority of reactions that occur in drug metabolism. These reactions are mitigated by a large family of enzymes in the liver called the Cytochrome P450 enzymes. These enzymes are found in the smooth endoplasmic reticulum of hepatic cells. Another group of enzymes carry out oxidation reactions in the cytosol or mitochondria of liver cells. These enzymes include monoamine oxidase (MAO), which oxidizes dopamine, epinephrine, serotonin, norepinpehrine, and aldehyde dehydrogenase, which oxidize alcohols, ethylene glycol, and acetaldehyde.

Phase II involves the conjugation of a drug metabolite with glucuronic acid, glutathione, acetate, or by adding a glycine, sulfate, or methyl group to the drug, making it highly hydrophilic. This allows it to readily pass into the urine for excretion. Felines contain less overall numbers of certain Phase II enzymes, reducing their ability to quickly metabolize drugs and prolonging the drug's effects. In addition, some drugs depress the Cytochrome P450 enzyme system, preventing Phase I metabolism. An example of this type of drug is cimetidine. These drugs are referred to as "enzyme inhibitors."

Excretion

After drugs have been metabolized into less active by-products, they are ready for elimination. Major routes of excretion include renal, fecal, and biliary. The majority of drugs are eliminated via the renal route. Once drugs are more hydrophilic, they are freely filtered by the glomerulus and transferred into the renal tubules. They are then passed into the urine and excreted. This occurs in a passive process. Blood flow via the afferent arteriole passes into the glomerulus and Bowman's capsule. Here, high pressure within the arteriole forces water and small molecules out of the capillaries and into the proximal tubule, through the loop of Henle, into the distal tubule, collecting ducts, and into the ureter. Just as with ion trapping in the GI tract, the same can occur in the kidney if the pH of the urine changes. Some drugs are moved into the proximal tubule via an active transport mechanism, and because of the use of energy, the drugs move without respect to a concentration gradient. Because of this, drugs can be eliminated into the urine in active form, and thus can be carefully selected to work in the tubules, ureter, bladder, or urethra. An example is penicillin, which is transported actively into the tubules, making it a good antimicrobial for urinary tract infections. Drugs can be reabsorbed across the tubule membrane if they are lipophilic because they must be absorbed through endothelial cells that line the renal tubules.

Hepatic excretion occurs when drugs remain in the liver's vasculature and can collect in the sinusoids diffusing into hepatocytes where they can be excreted. They are excreted into the gallbladder either in active or metabolite form. Bile is then injected into the duodenum from gallbladder contraction and the drug may be eliminated in the feces. Drugs can potentially be reabsorbed if they are highly lipophilic and returned to the liver via the enterohepatic circulation.

Clinical Pharmacology

GI Pharmacology

Emesis

The act of vomiting is the active diaphragmatic and abdominal muscle contraction to force out stomach contents. This reflex is coordinated by the vomiting center in the brain. This group of neurons resides in the brainstem and is unaffected by the blood–brain barrier; therefore, it is highly susceptible to blood-borne signals. It is controlled by stimulation from several sources. Direct distension of the various parts of the GI system, including the stomach, esophagus, and small intestine, as well as signals from the peritoneum, kidney, gallbladder, and even uterus, can stimulate vomiting. Stimulation of another group of neurons, dubbed as the chemoreceptor trigger zone (CRTZ), also will stimulate the vomiting reflex. Additional sources of input include direct stimulation of the neurons in the vomiting center, input from the nerves of the inner ear, and input from higher brain centers.

Neurons in the vomiting center are made up of serotonin and α_2 adrenergic receptors. When these receptors are stimulated, they evoke the vomiting reflex. The CRTZ contains specialized neurons that can detect toxins in the blood that pass through it. Thus, vomiting associated with uremia, bacteremia, ketonemia, or the vomiting caused by opioids or poisons, comes from this area. The CRTZ contains a plethora of dopamine receptors, so blockade of these receptors will reduce vomiting input from this center. The CRTZ also contains serotonin (5-HT$_3$) and α_2 adrenergic receptors. It is important to note that cholinergic (M$_1$) and histaminergic (H$_1$) receptors are also present, making anticholinergics and antihistamine drugs potential antiemetics. The vestibular apparatus also provides stimulation to the vomiting center via the histaminergic and cholinergic pathways. Finally, peripheral stimulation comes via 5-HT$_3$ serotonin receptor input.

Emetics

The first class of drugs most commonly used are the emetics. These drugs are used to induce vomiting and are mainly used in the treatment of various poisonings. There are two classes of emetics:central acting and local acting. The central acting emetics are apomorphine and xylazine. Remember that inducing vomiting is always contraindicated with a patient who lacks a gag reflex, caustic ingestion, or risk of aspiration is present.

Central acting emetics. *Apomorphine.* Apomorphine is the emetic of choice in the canine. It is an opioid medication that stimulates dopamine receptors in the CRTZ to induce emesis. Felines have less dopamine receptors in their CRTZ so it is not the first line in feline patients. However, it may possibly be used in felines. Apomorphine has the potential to cause excitement and thus should be used with caution. It will eventually pass through the blood–brain barrier and saturate the emetic center. Because it is a CNS depressant, it can depress the emetic center as well. So, after the initial rise in blood levels triggering the CRTZ, it can eventually depress the emetic center after some time. As an opioid, its main side effect will be respiratory depression and should not be used in patients with a questionable gag reflex to prevent aspiration. Because it is an opioid and agonizes dopamine receptors, its potential respiratory side effects can be reversed with an opioid antagonist (like naloxone) and its vomiting effects reversed with metoclopramide, which is a dopamine antagonist. Apomorphine is available in tablets which can be placed in the conjunctival sac, or compounded into an injection, for IV use.

Xylazine. The emetic of choice in cats is the α_2 drenergic agonist xylazine. It quickly stimulates the CRTZ and the emetic center to induce vomiting. Emesis was induced in 100% of cats studied, when given twice the emetic dose (Hikasa et al. 1989). It is less effective in dogs. The dose used to induce emesis is lower than the sedative/anesthetic dose, so the side effects are minimal.

Locally acting emetics. The locally acting emetics include hydrogen peroxide, syrup of ipecac, and salt paste. Hydrogen peroxide will typically irritate oral and gastric mucosa to induce vomiting; however, it has some serious side effects. The peroxide can cause a severe gastritis and the froth places the animal at risk for aspiration. Syrup of ipecac is another locally acting emetic taken off the market in 2004. It had abuse potential and caused fatal cardiac arrhythmias. The final locally acting emetic is the use of a salt paste placed in the pharyngeal area. This practice has largely fallen out of favor due to its risk to cause dehydration, hypernatremia, and variable emetic effects.

Antiemetics

The next class of pharmacologic agents are the antiemetics. There are a variety of methods to approach the reduction of vomiting. Reducing vomiting through pharmacological intervention requires selecting an agent that will either increase gastric transit time, suppress vomiting signals, or lower gastric acid reducing nausea. Note that antacids are not considered antiemetic medications. The antiemetic classes represent drugs that will perform one or more of those functions.

Phenothiazine drugs. The phenothiazine drugs, such as acepromazine, chlorpromazine, and prochlorperazine reduce emesis through their blockade of dopamine receptors in the CRTZ and emetic centers. These drugs are decent antiemetics but have some severe side effects. Due to α_1 adrenergic antagonism, they can cause hypotension. These agents are discouraged from use in critical patients due to these side effects. An additional adverse reaction with phenothiazine tranquilizer use was its potential to lower the seizure threshold and therefore would be contraindicated in patients with known seizure disorders. A recent retrospective study evaluated acepromazine use in patients either presenting for seizures or with known seizure histories. There was no correlation between seizure activity and acepromazine administration; however, further studies would be needed to evaluate this. However, it appears administering acepromazine to patients with seizures may not be contraindicated (McConnell et al. 2007). Dosage volume is extremely important when working with acepromazine. Overdoses have occurred from improper calculations. Double check the dosage with a fellow technician or the DVM.

Metoclopramide. Metoclopramide is another commonly used antiemetic. It is a dopamine and serotonin antagonist, as well as a cholinergic agonist, stimulating motility of the stomach and small intestine. Metoclopramide reduces vomiting and nausea through its central and peripheral effects. By increasing gastric transit time, nausea is reduced by encouraging gastric emptying, and gastric contents are unavailable for ejection. It also directly suppresses vomiting signals caused by dopamine and/or serotonin in the vomiting center and CRTZ. Major contraindications for use include gastric outflow obstructions, or GI obstruction due to foreign body or intussusceptions, due to its prokinetic properties causing risk of gastric or intestinal perforation.

Serotonin antagonists. Another class of commonly used antiemetics are ondansetron and dolasetron. These two antiemetics block 5-HT_3 serotonin receptors in the CRTZ. They are typically used in chemotherapy-induced emesis but are often used as second-line agents in refractory vomiting. Side effects are rare, and these drugs are appropriate for use in critical patients.

Maropitant. The novel antiemetic, maropitant, was recently introduced into the arena. It works by antagonizing substance P, thus blocking the vomiting reflex in the vomiting center, as well as its antinausea and antimotion sickness properties. Its unique pharmacology makes it an exceptional antiemetic. It can be used as a first-line drug or for use in refractory vomiting (Hsu 2008). It is administered subcutaneously and may sting due to its hyperosmolarity. Anecdotally, refrigerating the drug prior to use may alleviate some symptoms of pain on injection. The package insert labels maropitant for 5-day use for its antiemetic effects. Maropitant's use in cat was investigated in 2008 and was determined to be safe and effective as an antiemetic and antimotion sickness agent in feline patients (Cox et al. 2008). Worth noting is a potential for some analgesic properties of maropitant. Because it is a substance P antagonist, it may alter signals sent to the brain from injured tissue or nerves (Hill 2000).

Acid reducers

Proton pump inhibitors. Acid reduction remains an important cornerstone in the prevention of GI ulcer formation and treatment, as well as treating symptoms of nausea. There are several classes of acid reducers. These include proton pump inhibitors (PPI), and H_2 blockers. The PPIs bind directly to the H^+/K^+-ATPase pump controlling proton deposition into the gastric lumen. This irreversibly inhibits acid secretion, and because they block the pump directly, rather than any chemical signals, making them very potent and able to achieve virtual "anti-acidity" (Hsu 2008). Commonly used PPIs include omeprazole and pantoprazole. Omeprazole is administered orally while the parenteral option is pantoprazole. It is typically given as an IV bolus or constant rate infusion (CRI).

H$_2$ blockers. The H$_2$ blockers bind to the histamine receptor on gastric parietal cells. They effectively block one pathway of input to the H$^+$/K$^+$-ATPase pump. Famotidine is the prototypical drug, with ranitidine and cimetidine having less potent effects, respectively. Ranitidine is a weak prokinetic due to its inhibition of acetylcholinesterase, thereby stiumulating parasympathetic innervations of gastric/intestinal motility. All of the H$_2$ blockers are chemical modulations of histamine and thus, rapid IV injection has the potential to cause severe hypotension from histamine release. In addition, anecdotal reports of hemolytic anemia, associated with famotidine administration to felines intravenously, have been reported. However, a recent retrospective study found no precipitous drop in packed cell volume measurements in cats receiving famotidine intravenously (de Brito Galvao and Trepanier 2008). These drugs are given SQ or IV.

Gastric coating agents. Sucralfate is a sucrose and aluminium hydroxide solution that binds to exposed gastric epithelium and coats exposed ulcerated tissue. The sucrose forms a paste that is activated in the acidic stomach. It inactivates pepsin and bile acids and prevents further damage to gastric mucosa. The aluminium hydroxide helps recruit prostaglandins and local growth factors to help protect the stomach. It is most effective in an acidic environment; therefore, it should be given before other oral antacids. Its use with injectable antacids is variable and unclear.

Prostaglandin analogues. Misoprostol is a prostaglandin analogue that functions to enhance gastric blood flow by mimicking the chemical structure of prostaglandins. This leads to increased mucous production, bicarbonate secretion, and cell turnover. It also binds to the prostaglandin receptor on the gastric parietal cell reducing input from the receptor to the H$^+$/K$^+$-ATPase pump. Misoprostol is given PO and care must be taken when handling the pill. Gloves should be used as it causes spontaneous abortion in humans.

Anti-diarrheals

Diarrhea can be a significant problem in critical patients. Hypermotility can propel contents through the GI tract bypassing normal pauses for electrolyte, water, and nutrient absorption. Hypomotility can also affect resorption by not allowing the longitudinal contractions that help mix food in the lumen of the intestine (Webster 2001). Severe protein loss and hypovolemia can result from fecal losses. Rehydration remains a mainstay of treatment and several antidiarrheal medications exist.

Opiate antidiarrheal medications. Opiate drugs alter intestinal motility to increase water absorption and decrease movement of fecal matter. By doing so, they can both decrease peristaltic motions, through reduced stimulation of acetylcholine, which propel fecal matter along and prevents absorption. They also allow for contractions that mix contents to promote absorption by stimulating mu receptors in the central nervous system (CNS) and gut.

Antisecretory medications. The antisecretory/anti-inflammatory class of drugs, such as bismuth subsalicylate, and sulfasalazine, function to coat inflamed mucosa, reduce GI irritability, and absorb excess water causing hypersecretory diarrhea. Sulfasalazine specifically is cleaved in the small intestine to form mesalamine, also called 5ASA or 5Aminosalicylic acid, which has an antiprostaglandin affect, decreasing inflammatory secretions, and reducing inflammation. Caution should be taken with the salicylate portion of bismuth salicylate in cats.

Metronidazole. Unfortunately, most antidiarrheals are administered enterally, making their use in obtunded or comatose patients contraindicated. Metronidazole is a compound available for both oral and injection that is used for its antidiarrheal properties. It exerts an anti-inflammatory effect on the GI mucosa and also is effective against anaerobic bacterial overgrowth in the small intestine. However, its use is controversial. Anaerobic overgrowth assists with reducing the colony numbers of pathogenic gram-negative bacteria, whicht are mainly considered the perpetrators of sepsis caused by bacterial translocation if the GI barrier is compromised. Therefore, its use in patients with compromised GI perfusion may be at increased risk of pathogenic translocation if anaerobes are killed. Metronidazole is available in oral and parenteral (IV) forms.

Treatment of hepatic encephalopathy

Drugs used for the treatment of hepatic encephalopathy include lactulose and special antimicrobials. Lactulose is a disaccharide sugar that has multiple positive effects to reduce enterohepatic toxin absorption. Lactulose will osmotically attract water into fecal matter diluting toxins and reducing their absorption. It also increases transit time, allowing for less absorption. Lactulose also produces a more acidic colon, which keeps ammonia in its ionized form, preventing its absorption across the luminal barrier. Metronidazole and neomycin are antibiotics that reduce the flora in the intestine, reducing toxic by products produced by bacteria in the gut.

Cardiac Pharmacology

Antiarrhythmics

Antiarrhythmic drugs are the first category of cardiac medications. They are divided into four classes, and the first class has three subgroups.

Class I antiarrhythmics. Class I antiarrhythmics are the membrane stabilizers that block the influx of Na^+ from sodium channels and by this are able to decrease the rate of depolarization (Webster 2001). They are also able to prevent automaticity (spontaneous depolarization) through this method.

Class IA agents include quinidine and procainamide. Procainamide is the more commonly used drug of the two, in small animals, whereas quinidine is used in large animals. Procainamide will be effective against ventricular arrhythmias and is usually used as a second-line agent when dealing with ventricular tachycardias. It has some mild negative inotrope effects, so hypotension is a concern with administration. Procainamide is available orally or parenterally and may be given as a bolus injection or CRI.

Class IB agents include lidocaine and mexiletine. Lidocaine is very effective in reducing the rate of or even converting ventricular arrhythmias to normal rates or sinus complexes. It can be administered via IV bolus or CRI. These drugs are CNS toxicants and thus have the potential to cause CNS excitement or depression. Typically, signs of toxicity begin with CNS excitement (seizures) and progress to depression. Care should be taken to watch for altered mental status, dullness, or seizures. Cats are also very sensitive to lidocaine administration and doses should be reduced with regard to administration. The other Class IB agent is mexiletine which is chemically similar to lidocaine, producing all the same effects, however only available in oral form. Anecdotally, lidocaine may cause nausea/anorexia in hospitalized patients. It may be of benefit to consider discontinuing lidocaine in patients who are anorexic and require nutritional support. Lidocaine is only available in parenteral form and may be given as a bolus injection or CRI. Mexiletine is available as an oral preparation.

The only Class IC agent is flecainide, a rarely used antiarrhythmic drug that causes severe cardiovascular depression.

Class II antiarrhythmics. Class II agents are the beta-blockers, so-called for their ability to be adrenergic blockers at beta receptors. These drugs reduce heart rate (HR), and by doing so reduce myocardial oxygen demand, and increase atrioventricular (AV) conduction time (Hsu 2008). They are used in the treatment of supraventricular and ventricular arrhythmias. They are also used in hypertrophic cardiomyopathy (HCM) to control HR and decrease myocardial oxygen demand. They can also slow the ventricular rate with supraventricular arrhythmias (SVT). They have the potential to cause hypotension from decreased cardiac output; however, they have little negative inotrope activity, and thus only the severely debilitated patients will suffer from these effects. If the beta-blocker is nonselective for the β_1 receptor, it will cause some respiratory side effects, including bronchospasm. Propranolol is the prototypical beta-blocker, but it is nonselective. Esmolol is another injectable beta-blocker with highly selective β_1 activity. Oral agents are also available in the forms of atenolol and metoprolol. The use of parenteral beta-blockers requires diligent monitoring of HR, blood pressure (BP), and electrocardiogram (ECG) rhythms.

Class III antiarrhythmic agents. Class III agents prolong the refractory period. They have some Na^+ channel blocking ability to increase the length of the action potential and block K^+ channels to prolong the refractory period. Sotalol is an oral Class III agent that has Class II properties at higher doses. It can be effective in controlling ventricular arrhythmias. Amiodarone is an injectable Class III agent that shares its properties with all the antiarrhythmic drug classes. It inhibits Na^+, K^+, and Ca^{2+} channels, as well as has alpha and beta blocking properties (Hsu 2008). Amiodarone is indicated for refractory tachyarrhythmias, both atrial and ventricular. There is some indication for its use in refractory ventricular fibrillation.

Class IV antiarrhythmic agents. Class IV agents are the parenteral calcium channel blockers. These agents slow sinoatrial (SA) and AV conduction; however, they have major negative inotropic effects. This is due to their interactions with calcium in smooth muscle. They dilate coronary and systemic arteries, causing vasodilation, and limit the amount of calcium available for cardiac contractility. They are mainly indicated for reducing the rate of arrhythmias that pass through the AV node, such as supraventricular arrhythmias. Verapamil causes significant hypotension and therefore diltiazem has replaced its use. Diltiazem has less of a vasodilitory effect with the same rate-reducing effects. These drugs are used in addition to beta-blockers to treat SVT and is also used in the treatment of HCM in cats to reduce afterload, decrease HR and myocardial oxygen demand, and may decrease wall thickness although this is not proven. Calcium channel blockers, parenteral especially, require monitoring similar to beta-blockers. HR/BP, and ECG rhythms should be monitored carefully in a patient receiving these (Table 18.1).

Table 18.1   Antiarrhythmic class descriptions

Class Number	Class	Drugs in Class	Mechanism of Action	Arrhythmias Indicated
I	Membrane stabilizers/Na^+ channel blockers	Ia: Quinidine, procainamide Ib: Lidocaine, mexiletine Ic: Flecainide	Block influx of sodium via sodium channels and lower rate of depolarization, reduce automaticity	Ventricular arrhythmias (ventricular tachycardia mainly)
II	Beta-blockers	Propranolol, metoprolol, esmolol, atenolol	Antagonize beta adrenergic receptors thus causing reduced heart rate, AV conduction, and myocardial oxygen demand	Supraventricular arrhythmias, ventricular arrhythmias, and HCM
III	Prolong refractory period	Amiodarone, sotalol, bretylium	Posess Na^+, K^+, and Ca^{2+} channel blocking ability	Ventricular arrhythmias, amiodarone = ventricular fibrillation
IV	Calcium-channel blockers	Diltiazem, Verapamil	Block Ca^{2+} channels lowering SA and AV node conduction, vasodilation	Supraventricular arrhythmias

Digoxin

Digoxin competitively binds to the $Na^+/K^+/ATPase$ pump on the mycocyte. This allows Ca^{2+} to enter the cell and causes an increase in contractility. Its use as an antiarrhythmic comes from its slowed AV conduction time from parasympathetic effects. It is used in the treatment of supraventricular arrhythmias by slowing AV node conduction and reduces the ventricular response. It is also a weak positive inotrope and will increase contractility in systolic disease. Digoxin toxicity manifests in three different categories: neurological, GI, and myocardial. Anorexia, lethargy, vomiting, first- and potentially second-degree AV block, ventricular tachyarrythmias, and hyperkalemia are all signs of digoxin toxicity. Treatment involves managing clinical signs and discontinuing digoxin treatment. A very expensive treatment is Digoxin immune Fab(ovine). It is a cardiac glycoside-specific antibody directed at preventing uptake of digoxin from myocytes (Kittleson and Keinle 1998).

Pimobendan

Pimobendan is a positive inotropic and vasodilatory drug for use in congestive heart failure (CHF) from dilated cardiomyopathy or mitral valve disease. This newer type of drug is termed an inodilator. It increases myocardial sensitivity to Ca^{2+} causing increased contractility and inhibits phosphodiesterase III (inhibiting cyclic AMP) causing smooth muscle relaxation and vasodilation. It is not regularly used as an emergency drug, but its pharmacology is important as patients presenting in heart failure may already have been prescribed this drug. Emergent use of pimobendan is being investigated and may have future applications.

Anticholinergics

Anticholinergics, atropine and glycopyrrolate, block parasympathetic stimulation via the vagus nerve and thus may increase HR in vagally mediated bradycardias. Atropine and glycopyrrolate are both available for injection and can be given SQ or IV.

Beta-agonists

Beta-agonists are used as short-term therapy to increase the HR with life-threatening bradyarrhthmias refractory to anticholinergic administration. Isoproterenol may be used in cases of severe bradyarrythmias, such as third-degree AV block, to increase HR if cardiac output is affected causing hypotension. Careful monitoring of ECG rhythms should be done to assess efficacy of treatment.

Diuretics

The next class of drugs used in heart disease are the diuretics. There are several categories, and the ones used in critical care will be mainly focused on. These are the loop diuretics, and the osmotic diuretics, although that class is contraindicated in heart failure due to its ability to cause volume overload. The nonemergent classes are the potassium-sparing diuretics and the thiazide diuretics.

Loop diuretics. The loop diuretic of main interest is furosemide. It works by interacting with the $Na^+/K^+/ATPase$ pump in the thick ascending loop of Henle. By preventing Na^+ resorption, it promotes diuresis by making the filtrate hypertonic and thus encouraging water excretion. Calcium, magnesium, and potassium are lost through the urine as a result of this diuresis. It is extremely effective in decreasing pulmonary edema and ascites related to left- and right-sided heart dysfunction, respectively. It also promotes urine formation in oliguric renal disease and causes a calciuresis in the treatment of emergency hypercalcemia. Furosemide may also have some venodilating ability owing to its effectiveness to reduce pulmonary hydrostatic pressure and shift the fluid balance to the systemic vasculature (Webster 2001). Furosemide is available for parenteral use, and may be given IV or IM. Bolus injection or CRI may be used for the IV route.

Osmotic diuretics. The osmotic diuretc, mannitol, causes fluid shifts from the intracellular/interstitial space to the intravascular space due to its hyperosmolarity. This increases the effective circulating volume, signaling the kidneys to exrete water. This increase in circulating volume makes it contraindicated for use in patients with heart disease but is effective in patients with oliguric renal failure, cerebral edema, and increased intraocular pressure in glaucoma. Mannitol is given as a slow IV injection. Typically, the injection is given over 20–30 minutes, while other fluids are stopped, maximizing its diuretic effects. Mannitol very easily crystallizes at room temperature, so it should be kept in an incubator, and given with an injection filter. Filter needles are another option, if in-line filters are unavailable.

Thiazide diuretics. The thiazide diuretics, such as hydrochlorothiazide, are used in the chronic management of CHF since they are only available in oral form, and are considered weak diuretics since they block Na^+ resorption in the distal tubule, where most of the Na^+ has already been resorbed.

Potassium sparing diuretics. Potassium-sparing diuretics, such as spironolactone, are aldosterone antagonists that block the effects of alodsterone on the kidneys. By competing for aldosterone receptors, they block the resorption of sodium and create a diuresis. They are only available in oral form and take may take several days to reach peak effects.

Vasodilators/antihypertensive medications

The vasodilating or antihypertensive drugs are another class of cardiac medications. These include the angiotensin-converting enzyme (ACE) inhibitors, the calcium channel blockers, nitrates, hydralazine, and alpha-blockers.

ACE inhibitors. The ACE inhibitors are a very commonly used class of drugs used in the treatment of cardiac disease. They are not indicated for emergency use. These drugs block the enzyme that converts angiotensin I to angiotensin II. The vasodilating properties reduce afterload and reduce fluid accumulation caused by aldosterone-mediated angiotensin effects. Commonly used ACE inhibitors in veterinary medicine include enalapril and benazepril.

Calcium channel blockers. Oral calcium channel blockers, amlodipine and nifedipine, dilate smooth muscle through blocking of calcium channels. They are not routinely used in critical care. More often, the parenteral calcium channel blocker, diltiazem, would be utilized for its antiarrhythmic properties. However, development of hypertension in hospital may prompt use of an oral calcium channel blocker.

Nitrates. The nitrate drugs, sodium nitroprusside, and nitroglycerin, are metabolized in the body to form nitric oxide compounds. Their production and subsequent diffusion into vascular smooth muscle cells mediate relaxation and thus vasodilation. Nitroprusside has an extremely short half-life, and must be administered via CRI. It immediately produces a decrease in systemic vascular resistance causing a decrease in arterial BP. Reductions in afterload reduce left ventricular filling pressures. It is used in the treatment of acute hypertensive crises or fulminant pulmonary edema in CHF. It should only be administered when IV rates and BP can be continuously monitored. It is metabolized to cyano-compounds so toxicity can occur. Cyanide toxicosis presents as dyspnea and hypoxemia due to the inability of cells to utilize oxygen. This will not change despite oxygen supplementation. Constant BP monitoring is essential with nitroprusside administration. Direct arterial monitoring is the gold standard, but should not be used on patients who are active around their cage (not usually the case in this patient category). Doppler or oscillometric monitoring should be as frequent as possible if direct pressures are not available (Fig. 18.2).

Nitroglycerin is primarily a venodilator that decreases pulmonary edema in CHF when administered transcutaneously. It can cause hypotension as well, so monitoring of BP is recommended. Nitroglycerin is typically supplied in a paste form. It is applied to epidermal tissue, usually with a decent blood supply. Transdermal application is usually done on the pinna, and this area covered with a piece of tape, labeled with the drug and time

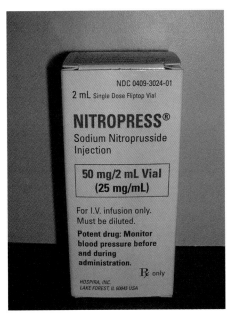

Figure 18.2   Sodium nitroprusside, sometimes known as the "silver bullet" in human medicine because it has an extremely short half-life and comes with a silver cover for the syringe and line, is extremely light-sensitive and therefore must be shieled from light during administration. Additionally, it is always given via CRI. (Courtesy of Thomas Walker, DVM, DACVECC.)

applied. However, as peripheral tissue may be vascocontricted during decreased perfusion states, core locations such as the thorax are likely a better suited administration site. Nitroglycerin must be applied with gloves, and care must be taken when manipulating the patient's ear, as it can cause vasodilation in humans as well.

Hydralazine. Hydralazine is a potent arterio-dilator that reduces afterload. This reduces regurgitant volume and pulmonary venous pressures, reducing congestion. It also helps improve forward blood flow (Hsu 2008). It can be utilized in an emergent situation because it is rapidly absorbed orally.

Alpha-blockers. Alpha-blockers, such as prazosin and phenoxybenzamine, are vasodilators used in the treatment of hypertension, often associated with pheochromocytoma. These agents also relax urethral muscle tone and therefore can be used to treat urethral spasm associated with many lower urinary tract conditions.

Anticoagulants/antithrombotic agents

Antiplatelet drugs. Aspirin blocks the cyclooxygenase (COX) pathway that forms prostaglandins and thromboxane A_2. This prevents platelet aggregation and is used in the prevention of thrombus formation. Salicylates are not metbolized well by felines and so dosing is greatly reduced in this species. Clopidogrel is a newer antiplatelet drug which reduces aggregation by blocking adenosine diphosphate (ADP) binding sites on the platelet surface, thus causing platelet inhibition.

CHAPTER 18

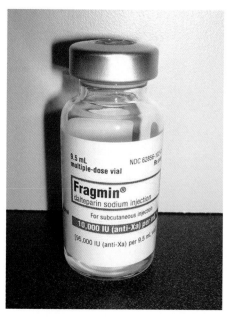

Figure 18.3 Dalteparin is a low molecular weight heparin product commonly used in many critical care departments for the the treatment of hypercoagulability and prevention of thrombus formation. (Courtesy of Thomas Walker, DVM, DACVECC.)

Anticoagulants. The anticoagulant medications consist of heparin, and the low molecular weight heparin (LMWH) drugs enoxaparin and dalteparin. These drugs bind to antithrombin III and inhibit thrombin, and factors IX, X, XI, and XII. Heparin can cause bleeding through its inhibition of thrombin. LMWHs are smaller molecular size and minimally inhibit thrombin and thus cause less bleeding. These do not markedly alter coagulation times (partial thromboplastin time), thus monitoring is usually unnecessary (Hsu 2008). Investigation into anti-Factor Xa levels is underway for LMWH monitoring. Heparin overdose is rarely seen, but protamine zinc serves as an antidote to heparin toxicity. Heparin and LMWH preparations are available for parenteral use. Heparin may be given SQ or IV and enoxaparin and dalteparin is given SQ. A major limitation to enoxaparin and dalteparin is that they are expensive, especially in larger patients (Fig. 18.3).

Vasoactive drugs/inotropes

Dopamine. Dopamine is a precursor to norepinephrine and stimulates its release from adrenergic neurons. Low concentrations of dopamine (1–5 µg/kg/min stimulate dopaminergic receptors in the renal, mesenteric, and coronary vasculature. Administration of dopamine causes dilation of these vascular beds. An increase in glomerular filtration rate (GFR) will result as renal blood flow increases. Dopamine has been traditionally used as an adjunctive therapy to stimulate urine production in oliguric or anuric acute renal failure. Human intensivists have no longer recommended use of dopamine as studies have shown no affect on mortality. Its use in veterinary medicine requires more investigation but may also show improvement in GFR and urine output initially, but no change in mortality overall (Sigrist 2007) (Fig. 18.4).

CHAPTER 18

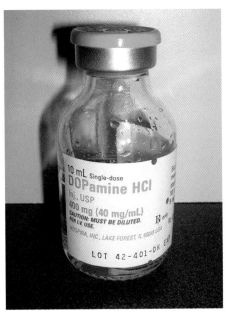

Figure 18.4   Dopamine is a positive inotrope and vasopressor used most commonly for the treatment of hypotension. It can increase systemic vascular resistance (SVR) and contractility depending on what dose range is used. It must be diluted before administration and is always given via CRI due to its very short duration of action. (Courtesy of Thomas Walker, DVM, DACVECC.)

Medium range doses (5–10 µg/kg/min) stimulate beta-adrenergic receptors, causing a positive inotropic, or increased contractility, effect on the heart. High doses of dopamine (10–20 µg/kg/min) stimulate alpha receptors causing peripheral vasoconstriction. Dopamine is arrhythmogenic, and ECG monitoring is advised with its use. Arrythmias are usually ventricular in origin and often respond to reduction of dose or switching inotropic medications. It is rapidly metabolized and must be given via CRI. Perivascular injection may cause tissue necrosis, and careful monitoring of IV sites and BPs is necessary for patients on pressors.

Epinephrine. Epinephrine is a potent adrenergic agonist catecholamine which will stimulate all receptors (α and β). It produces vasoconstriction, positive inotropic and chronotropic effects, and is also quite arrythmogenic. It is used to treat anaphylaxis and hypersensitivity reactions due to its bronchodilation and antihypotensive effects. Epinephrine is also used extensively in CPCR for its vasoconstricting and α/β stimulating properties. Epinephrine may be given intravenously, intracardiac, subcutaneously, or intratracheally. Intracardiac injection has fallen out of favor in part due to its risk to cause iatrogenic cardiac trauma and hemorrage. If the intratracheal route is to be used, a sterile red rubber catheter, or tom cat catheter should be passed down the ET tube and the drug administered, followed by a plain saline flush. Twice the drug dosage should be used in the intratracheal route.

Norepinephrine. Norepinephrine is another adrenergic catecholamine with α_1 and β_1 effects. It is used mainly for its vasoconstrictive effects to raise systemic vascular resistance

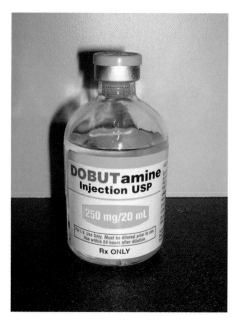

Figure 18.5 Dobutamine is a positive inotrope used to treat hypotension associated with a loss of systolic function. It must be diluted and administered via a CRI due to its very short duration of action. (Courtesy of Thomas Walker, DVM, DACVECC.)

in refractory hypotension. It is rapidly metabolized and must be given via CRI. It carries some risk of ventricular arrhythmia and so ECG monitoring is warranted.

Dobutamine. Dobutamine is a mainly positive inotropic drug, increasing cardiac contractility. It has only β_2 effects. It will increase cardiac output by increasing contractility and stroke volume. Because of this mainly positive inotropic effect, myocardial oxygen demand and work increase drastically. It may be used to treat hypotension associated with systolic heart failure. It is also very rapidly metabolized and must be given via CRI. There are anecdotal reports of dobutamine causing seizures in feline patients, on CRIs greater than 24 hours (Fig. 18.5).

Ephedrine. Ephedrine is a mixed adrenergic agonist with alpha and beta effects. However, it mainly causes vasoconstriction and may resolve hypotension. It is metabolized slowly, and its effects are longer lasting than the above catecholamines. Thus, it is given as a bolus injection. It causes an increase in myocardial work and also may be arrythmogenic.

Phenylephrine. Phenylephrine is a synthetic vasoactive drug with mainly alpha effects causing vasoconstriction. Because it is an alpha-agonist, it will increase only systemic vascular resistance, and thus may spare any negative cardiac effects like increased myocardial work and oxygen demand. It is present in the body for around 20 minutes so one-time dosing may be appropriate for treatment of hypotension (Hsu 2008). Reflex bradycardia, from an increase in afterload, may occur.

Vasopressin (antidiuretic hormone). Vasopressin is a peptide stored in the pituitary gland and released with hyperosmolality or reduction in plasma volume. There are two types of vasopressin receptors, V_1 and V_2. V_1 receptors are located in GI tract and vascular

Table 18.2   Vasopressor/inotrope descriptions

Drug	Route	Primary Receptor(s)	Agonist/ Antagonist	Clinical Effects	Side Effects
Dopamine	Constant rate infusion	Low dose-Dopaminergic Middle dose-beta High dose-alpha	Agonist	↑ renal blood flow, ↑ Inotropy and HR ↑ TPR	Arrhythmias, tachycardia Hypertension
Dobutamine	Constant rate infusion	Beta-1	Agonist	↑ Inotropy +/− HR	Arrhythmias, tachycardia, hypertension, bradycardia,
Norepinephrine	Constant rate infusion	Alpha-1, Beta 1	Agonist	↑ Inotropy & HR ↑ TPR	Tachycardia, hypertension, vasoconstriction
Phenylephrine	Constant rate infusion	Alpha-1	Agonist	↑ TPR	Potent vasoconstrictor
Ephedrine	Bolus injection	Alpha-1 Beta-1	Agonist	↑ TPR, ↑ Inotropy + HR	Arrhythmias Tachyphlaxis (reduced sensitivity after repeated administration)
Vasopressin	Constant rate infusion	V1	Agonist	↑ TPR	Potent vasoconstrictor

smooth muscle. V_2 receptors are found in the kidney and mediate the antidiuretic effects of this hormone (Drobatz et al. 2007).

It is reported, *in vitro*, to be a more potent vasoscontrictor than angiotensin II, or or norepinephrine. Some evidence suggests that patients with shock, especially vasodilatory or distributive, may have decreased levels of vasopressin. Its use in shock is still being investigated. It is also used in cardiac arrest for its epinephrine-like vasoconstrictive effects. Initial studies appear to support its use to increase mean arterial pressure (MAP) in patients with refractory shock; however, further studies are needed to validate these findings (Drobatz et al. 2007) (Table 18.2).

Respiratory Pharmacology

The respiratory system functions to exhange waste gas, CO_2 for fresh gas, O_2 to provide to the circulatory system for delivery to tissues. Its ability to provide adequate gas exchange is dependent on its ability to keep itself intact and functioning. It has many intrinsic safety procedures it goes through, including cough, mucociliary clearance, secretions, and the ability to bronchoconstrict in the face of an allergen. The respiratory drugs work on these pathways, either protecting the system from harm or suppressing unnecessary responses to attack. Respiratory drugs either dilate bronchioles, clear secretions, suppress the cough reflex, combat infection and inflammation, decrease pulmonary hypertension, or increase the production of surfactant (Hsu 2008).

Bronchodilators

Beta-Agonists. Beta-agonists are either specific β_2-agonists or are nonselective adrenergic agonists. All beta-agonists cause rapid bronchodilation, increased bronchial secretions, and enhanced mucuous clearance via the mucociliary system. Nonselective beta-agonists will stimulate B_1 and alpha receptors causing tachycardia, vasoconstriction, and hypertension, such as epinephrine and isoproterenol (Webster 2001). Terbutaline is a β_2-specific agonist that is able to be administered parenterally. Albuterol is a β_2-agonist that can be given via aerosolization through an inhaler. The Aero-kat (Trudell Medical International, Ontario, Canada) (www.trudellmed.com/animal-health/aerokat) is a device made to give metered inhaler doses to animal patients without them fearing the spray of the inhaler. The inhaler is discharged into a chamber and a face mask connected to the chamber is placed over the animal's face while they breathe in the medication.

Methylxanthines. The methylxanthine class of bronchodilators also represents a class for emergency use. They acheive bronchodilation by two methods: First, they reduce phosphodiesterase levels, increasing cyclic AMP levels. Second, they competitively antagonize adenosine. Both of these function to relax smooth muscle. They also interfere with calcium, thereby affecting the bronchioles' ability to constrict. There is some evidence that this class of bronchodilator may help with diaphragmatic contractility, increased CNS sensitivity to P_aCO_2, and prevention of mast cell degranulation. The methylxanthines include aminophylline and theophylline. Aminophylline may be given parenterally.

Anticholinergics. Anticholinergics are also bronchodilators, via the parasympathetic control of the bronchi. Blocking acetylcholine postganglionic muscarinic receptors results in smooth muscle relaxation of the airways and decreased mucous secretion.

Mucolytics

N-acetylcysteine is a commonly used mucolytic to break disulfide bonds in mucous allowing for easier clearance. However, its efficacy has not been proven in veterinary patients and may cause airway irritation, and resulting bronchoconstriction. It should thus be used with caution in respiratory disease (Webster 2001). It is given via nebulization for its mucolytic properties.

Isotonic saline is also a mucolytic. It is often used in nebulization treatments or infusation into the trachea during mechanical ventilation. Saline will hydrate and humidify the airway, as well as break down mucuous formation.

Glucocorticoids

Glucocorticoids are of benefit with Type I hypersensitivity reactions of the respiratory system. These drugs help reduce bronchoconstriction and prevent thickening of the airways seen with chronic respiratory diseases. They can be used in the treatment of feline asthma in crisis or other acute allergen reactions.

Anti-Inflammatory Drugs

As the cell membrane is damaged, via trauma or infection, its phospholipid layer is converted to arachidonic acid via an enzyme called phospholipase. Arachidonic acid can enter two pathways, either the COX pathway producing thromboxanes and prostaglandins, or the lipooxygenase pathway producing leukotrienes. These chemicals are able to diffuse out of the cell and can cause local and systemic effects. Prostaglandins inhibit platelet aggregation, cause bronchodilation and at times bronchconstriction, vasodilate in the GI tract, renal, mesentery, and coronary vasculature, and vasoconstrict in the pulomonary vasculature. Thromboxanes cause vasoconstriction and decrease platelet aggregation. The leukotrienes vasoconstrict, bronchoconstrict, increase capillary permeability, and increase the secretion of mucous.

Glucocorticoids

The glucocorticoids, such such as endogenous cortisol, or synthetic prednisone, dexamethasone, or hydrocortisone, have many anti-inflammatory properties. Corticosteroids are produced in the body naturally by response to adrenocorticotropic hormone, or ACTH. To control ACTH, corticotropin-releasing factor (CRF) is released from the hypothalamus. The production of cortisol by the adrenal glands depresses the production of ACTH and CRF in the body, in a negative feedback loop. Administration of exogenous corticosteroids will produce the same effects, depressing production of ACTH and CRF. They are classified by their effects and duration of action, or exerted effects.

Short-acting glucocorticoids produce effects that last less than 12 hours. Hydrocortisone (cortisol) represents the prototype of this class.

Intermediate-acting corticosteroids produce effects for 12–36 hours and encompases the prednisone class, made up of prednisone, prednisolone, and methylprednisolone. Prednisone is converted in the liver to prednisolone to achieve the greatest effects and thus, administration of the biologically active metabolite, prednisolone, may often be warranted.

Any long-acting glucocorticoid has effects for 48 hours or greater. These encompass the "methasones:" dexamethasone and betamethasone.

Glucocorticoids exert a wide number of effects. The anti-inflammatory effects include prevention of phospholipase and COX, prevention of cell aptosis, prevention of capillary leak, and decreasing fibroblast activity, thus preventing scar tissue. Although scars are cosmetically unappealing, inhibition of fibroblasts will affect general wound healing and strength. These drugs also have immunosuppressive actions, at higher doses. By inhibiting leukocyte and macrophage function, they effectively limit the immune response and are indicated in immune-mediated disease processes, such as immune-mediated anemias or polyarthropathies. They inhibit the release of interleukin (IL)-1 from macrophages and IL-2 from T-lymphocytes, and inhibit tumor necrosis factor (TNF) release from macrophages. These drugs also increase gastric acid secretion and decrease mucous production, increasing risk for gastric ulceration and GI bleeding. Thus, patients on steroids must be monitored for GI bleeding, and steroids are entirely contraindicated to be administered with nonsteroidal anti-inflammatory drugs (NSAIDs). Steroids should also not be used in shock states, as GI perfusion is often first to go in shock, and thus cannot deal with damage to the mucosa. Glucocorticoids are catabolic and break down proteins for amino acid use for glucose production via gluconeogenesis in the liver. Over time, skeletal muscle can be broken down, resulting in a pot-bellied appearance (from abdominal muscle consumption) and generalized muscle wasting. Glucocorticoid medications are contraindicated with ocular ulceration, as they will prevent healing and deepen the ulcer.

Increased or decreased bodily production of steroids manifest as clinical disease. Hyperadrenocorticism, or Cushing's diease, and hypoadrenocorticism, or Addison's disease, can be caused by an increase or lack of endogenous steroids, respectively. Iatrogenic causes of these diseases can also be caused by medical professionals. Overuse of steroids can result in iatrogenic Cushing's disease, and abruptly stopping exogenous steroids can result in iatrogenic Addison's disease. As iatrogenic Addison's disease can be life-threatening, gradual tapering of exogenous steroids is required to stimulate the production of CRF and ACTH and to maintain cellular integrity.

The current use of corticosteroids includes physiologic replacement, anti-inflammatory, and immunosuppressive therapy. Glucocorticoids are not recommended to be administered to hypovolemic or dehydrated patients, nor at increased ("shock") doses during the aforementioned physiologic states, excluding septic shock, where the purpose is replacement, and doses are physiologic.

In patients that lack endogenous steroids, such as hypoadrenocorticism, physiologic replacement is necessary. These patients are administered enough steroid to maintain cellular functions. Septic patients with hypotension refractory to vasoactive agents may benefit from endogenous steroid administration. The anti-inflammatory use of steroids can decrease clinical signs associated with inflammation. These include swelling/edema, caused by capillary leak, relief of acute life-threatening clinical signs such as bronchoconstriction, and assist with analgesia (Fig. 18.6).

NSAIDs

The NSAIDs represent another class of anti-inflammatory agents commonly used in the veterinary hospital. These agents differ from corticosteroids in that they block the COX

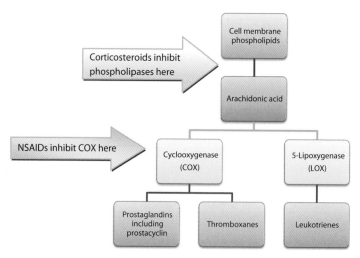

Figure 18.6   Generation of arachidonic acid metabolites and their role in inflammation.

or lipooxygenase pathways resulting in alleviation of clinical signs from inflammation. The two types of COX enzymes exist as COX-1 and COX-2. COX-1 is found in platelets, stomach, kidneys, and is responsible for inducing platelet aggregation, maintaining GI blood flow, bicarbonate and mucous secretion, and regulating renal blood flow. Prostaglandins protect the GI mucosa from the dangerous environment of the stomach. In addition to mucous and bicarbonate production, they enhance perfusion of the GI tract and thus provide the rapidly dividing epithelial cells with much needed nutrients. They also help regulate renal blood flow during hypotensive states. When the body vasoconstricts to maintain core BP, perfusion may be compromised to the kidney. Prostaglandins help vasodilate local arterioles to augment renal blood flow. Blockade of prostaglandin production not only inhibits deleterious side effects of inflammation but also inhibits the body's normal defense mechanisms. Specific targeting of the COX-2 form of the enzyme seems to result in fewer side effects. There are many classes of NSAIDs.

The nonselective COX inhibitors include aspirin, flunxin meglumine, ibuprofen, naproxen, ketoprofen, and phenylbutazone. The prototypical drug is aspirin or acetylsalicylic acid. This drug irreversibly inhibits COX. This drug is metabolized into salicylic acid and is eliminated via glucuronic acid conjugation in the liver. It is used as an analgesic, anti-inflammatory, and antipyretic; however, due to its numerous side effects, and development of COX-2 specifc NSAIDs, its use has declined. It is still used in thromboembolic disease to prevent platelet aggregation and thus incitation of the clotting cascade. Phenylbutazone has many side effects including blood dyscrasias, bone marrow suppression, and interactions with drugs metabolized through the liver. Flunixin is an effective analgesic and has antiprostaglandin effects; however, dogs are reported to be very sensitive to it. Ketoprofen, ibuprofen, and naproxen are all chemically similar but carry the same risks for GI effects. These drugs block both isoforms of the COX enzyme and thus come with many side effects in small animal patients. The newer COX-2 preferential drugs reduce the side effects seen with NSAID administration. However, the COX-2 isoform produces the prostaglandins that augment renal blood flow, making them just as potentially harmful if used during hypotensive states, such as under anesthesia, or in shock. Thus all NSAIDs are contraindicated if any hypovolemia or hypotension has occurred.

The COX-2 selective NSAIDs include carprofen, etodolac, deracoxib, meloxicam, and firocoxib. Tepoxalin is another COX-2 selective drug with lipooxygenase blocking effects as well. These drugs have less GI side effects; however, all have the potential to induce GI ulceration, bleeding, or renal ischemia if used improperly. Meloxicam is the only FDA-approved NSAID approved for use in cats (KuKanich 2008; Lascelles et al. 2005). NSAIDs are available in parenteral and enteral forms. The parenteral options used currently include carprofen, meloxicam, and flunixin (Table 18.3).

Antimicrobials

Antimicrobials are medications intended to kill invading microbes such as bacteria, viruses, protozoa, and fungi. The term "antibiotic" has fallen out of favor because its scope is limited, and antimicrobial encompasses the wide range of micoorganisms, and their respective treatments. Antimicrobials are classified as either -cidal, or -static, and also by the type of organism they affect. For example, a bactericidal antimicrobial will kill bacterial colonies. Drugs that will inhibit the life cycle of the pathogen are called

Table 18.3   Various NSAIDs and their COX-selectivity

Drug Name	COX-Selectivity
Carprofen	COX-2 selective
Firoxoxib	COX-2 selective
Deracoxib	COX-2 selective
Meloxicam	COX-2 selective
Etodolac	COX-2 selective
Tepoxalin	COX-2 selective/lipooxygenase inhibitor
Phenylbutazone	Nonselective
Flunixin megllumine	Nonselective
Over the counter: aspirin, ibuprofen, acetominophen, naproxen	Nonselective

-static drugs and will inhibit future growth, but not necessarily kill that organism outright. Thus, -static drugs can be given to patients with the ability to fight off some infection.

Criteria for use

Antimicrobials are potentially harmful drugs; therefore, criteria must be established for their use. Several requirements exist for antimicrobial therapy to be successful. First, the pathogen must be susceptible to the drug. This requires the knowledge that a particular drug will kill that agent. Second, the drug must be able to reach the concentration required to do its damage. Third, the patient must be able to tolerate the drug, in its forms, and dosages.

The first step in the three step process involves establishing susceptibility. This involves the measurement of the minimum inhibitory concentration (MIC). The MIC refers to the least amount of drug that can prevent growth on an agar plate, after incubation. Most antimicrobials kill all pathogens, but their concentrations may be so high that it would cause detriment to the host. Organisms that are inhibited with minimum concentrations are sensitive, and those that require higher doses are resistant. However, just because an organism is sensitive to a particular antimicrobial does not mean it is the most efficacious one. The second guideline states the drug must reach maximum concentration in the tissues where the infection is. For example, a pneumonia-causing bacterium may be sensitive to a certain type of antimicrobial, but unless this drug can be effectively absorbed, bypass first pass effect, and reach effective concentrations in the lung parenchyma, it should not be chosen.

For this reason, antimicrobial therapy can be seen to fail, if organisms cannot be killed or inhibited. Specific concerns with regard to tissue penetration involve drugs that bypass the blood–brain barrier in CNS infections, blood–retinal and blood–aqueous barriers of the eye. Once the antimicrobial arrives at the site, it still may not be able to work. Sulfa antimicrobials are inactivated in the presence of pus, and aminoglycoside antimicrobials are inactive in necrotic tissue. Also, with -static drugs, these drugs may fail if the host cannot remove some of the offending organisms, since they do not kill the organisms outright, and one generation will still be active. It is recommended that antimicrobial therapy continue for 72 hours before considering failure (Boothe 2009).

Resistance development

Resistance to antimicrobials is becoming an ever-increasing problem in the medical field. The development of "super bugs" has brought to light the concerns regarding antimicrobial therapy. To be responsible "stewards" of antimicrobials, veterinary professionals should be aware of certain recommendations regarding antimicrobial use. A nidus of infection, or clinical signs of an immune response, should guide the practitioner toward antimicrobial therapy. Empirical therapy is being regarded as unnecessary, unless there is appropriate evidence to support their use. Fever is not regarded as a factor for antimicrobial drug use, in the absence of overwhelming evidence of infection. Leukocytosis alone is also another inadequate determinant for antimicrobial use. Additionally, it is recommended that fever with toxic neutrophil changes suggest an infection, and a source should be sought out, yet empirical antimicrobial therapy need not be instituted immediately. However, purulent exudate (with cytology) necessitates antimicrobial use, as will glaring signs of infection, even if a source is not located, such as fever with neutropenia. To avoid overuse of antibiotics, studies indicate that the following are not necessarily conditions that antimicrobials will be of use in:

- Lower urinary tract signs in feline patients otherwise healthy (<5% incidence);
- Upper respiratory tract infections as most are caused by viral infections, and recovery rates typically do not change;
- Acute diarrheas are usually not caused by pathogenic bacteria (salmonella <2%, clostridium <5%, campylobacter <10%) and thus empirical antimicrobial therapy is not indicated, unless the GI mucosal barrier is compromised. Thus hematochezia, or melena are indications for empiric antimicrobial therapy (Trepanier 2009).

Once the need for antimicrobial therapy has been established, its use can be entirely justified. However, the frightening resistance patterns of some organisms require culturing and sensitivity testing to ensure the appropriate drug or drug combinations has been chosen. Choosing to use an antimicrobial on a patient with a resistant infection could be disastrous.

Resistance in organisms develops in many ways. Acquired resistance, via transfer of genetic material, seems to predominate. Chromosomal mutations are also possible, but are considered rare (Webster 2001). Organisms are often able to acquire the instructions for resistance by surviving after antimicrobial therapy and thus retaining that knowledge. This knowledge is then passed, as genetic information, both to subsequent generations of organisms, through vertical transfer, and to other organisms through horizontal transfer. Vertical transfer is accomplished through reproduction, where a copy of the genetic information is given to offspring, and horizontal transfer for information is achieved through plasmids, or small portions of genetic code. Plasmids are able to be taken up by other organisms and encoded in their DNA. This can achieve resistance in entire colonies of bacteria, before the need for reproduction. Another method of resistance transfer involves the use of bacterial viruses, or bacteriophages, who can infect bacteria with the genetic information of previously attacked bacteria.

Organisms, once resistant, will manifest that resistance in different ways. Antimicrobial receptor binding can be altered so that the drugs cannot bind. The organism may begin to produce enzymes that temporarily alter the makeup of the organism, or outright neutralize the antimicrobial. Finally, the organism may develop alternate genetic or metabolic pathways, decreasing the antimicrobial's effectiveness to cause harm via that route (Hsu 2008).

Many classes of antimicrobials exist. They all typically work in five different manners. Antimicrobials either attack the cell wall, cell membrane, ribosomes, enzymes, or nucleic acids. This either kills the organism outright or alters its genetic information to prevent further generations of the pathogen. The classes of antibiotic include the penicillins, cephalosporins, aminoglycosides, quinolones, tetracyclines, sulfonamides, lincosamides, macrolides, and miscellaneous antibiotics such as metronidazole and chloramphenicol. The common classes of antifungals are amphotericin B and the azoles.

Beta-lactam antimicrobials

Penicillins. The first group of antimicrobials are the beta-lactam drugs, which encompass the natural penicillins, the beta-lactamase-resistant penicillins, the extended spectrum penicillins, the carbapenems, the cephalosporins, and vancomycins. The beta-lactam antimicrobials exert their effects by inhibiting the formation of the peptidoglycan polymers that form the bacterial cell wall. These are bactericidal antimicrobials. The gram-positive bacteria are more susceptible to beta-lactam antimicrobials since they have more peptidoglycan polymers, whereas the gram-negative bacteria have a lipophilic coating over their cell wall. They are only effective on cells that are in the growth phase.

Natural pencillins. The natural penicillins are penicillin G and penicillin V. These are both highly effective against gram-positive, but not beta-lactamase-positive, aerobes, some gram-negative bacteria, and anerobes. They are also excreted unchanged in the urine, making their effectiveness in urinary tract infections highly valuable.

Beta-lactamase-resistant penicillins. The beta-lactamase-resistant penicillins are cloxacillin and oxacillin. These drugs are effective against the gram-postitive, beta-lactamase positive organisms and anaerobes. They were developed to counteract resistance among the natural penicillins. Bacteria developed an enzyme to break apart the beta-lactam ring found in the structure of the drugs. This enzyme can be neutralized with the beta-lactamase-resistant drugs.

Aminopenicillins. The aminopenicillins, amoxicillin and ampicillin, have an increased gram-negative spectrum. They are, however, not able to kill beta-lactamase-positive organisms. They also kill enteric flora, and can cause vomiting and diarrhea, as GI upset ensues.

Extended spectrum penicillins. The extended spectrum penicillins, ticarcillin, carbencillin, and piperacillin, have greater gram-negative spectrum and also some anaerobic coverage. They are effective against *Pseudomonas* sp. and *Bacteroides* sp.

Potentiated penicillins. The potentiated penicillins represent a class of penicillin drugs with a beta-lactamase inhibitor attached. Clavulanic acid and sulbactam both have minimal antimicrobial activity by themselves but inhibit the beta-lactamase enzymes used to counteract the pencillin mode of action.

Carbapenems. Carbapenems are highly effective drugs against beta-lactamase-resistant pathogens and anaerobes. In addition to this bactericidal activity, they can penetrate the bacterial cell wall, differing from most other antimicrobial classes. Imipenem is metabolized in great extent by the kidneys, so cilastin is added to reduce the amount of renal metabolism. They are targeted to kill resistant *Staphylococcus* sp. and *Enterococcus* sp.

Cephalosporins. Cephalosporins inhibit bacterial wall synthesis by the same method as penicillins. These drugs are classified by generation.

First-generation cephalosporins are effective against gram-positive organisms and anerobes. They penetrate tissues quite well and are used interchangeably with penicillins to treat gram-positive organisms. This generation includes cefazolin, cephalexin, and cefadroxil.

Second-generation cephalosporins have enhanced gram-positive coverage, and contain some gram-negative coverage as well, in addition to anaerobic coverage. These include cefoxitin and cefuroxime.

The third-generation cephalosporins have enhanced gram-negative coverage, anaerobic coverage, beta-lactamase coverage, and cross the blood–brain barrier. These include cefpodoxime, cefotaxime, ceftriaxone, and ceftiofur.

Fourth-generation cephalosporins have increased activity against gram-positive and negative spectrums with bacteria that developed resistance, as well as anaerobic coverage. An example of a fourth-generation cephalosporin is cefepime.

Vancomycin. Vancomycin is another beta-lactam antimicrobial that inhibits cell wall synthesis by binding to subunits preventing cross-link formation in the peptidoglycan cell wall. It remained effective against *Staphylococcus* sp. and *Enterococcus* sp. without resistance formation until recently when vancomycin-resistant *Staphylococcus aureus*, or VRSA, have been cultured, which poses a serious threat to patients, as this species seems to be resistant to carbapenems as well.

Penicillins, cephalosporins, and vancomycin all have the potential to cause anaphylactic reactions. Allergic signs, such as hives, injected mucous membranes (MMs), hypotension, airway difficulty, and vomiting, should be monitored in these patients. They also have the potential to induce diarrhea due to killing of commensal GI flora.

Cephalosporins anecdotally cause vomiting if given too fast. Recommendations are to give these antimicrobials slowly IV to avoid emesis.

Penicillin and cephalosporin antimicrobials can also induce immune-mediated disease, including immune-mediated hemolytic anemia (IMHA). Sudden, acute hemolytic anemia in a patient on these drugs should prompt the clinician/technician to potentially stop therapy if possible.

Aminoglycosides

Aminoglycoside antimicrobials have a reserved place in critical care due to their serious side effects. They have a unique mechanism of action by binding to the 30S subunit of the ribosome. By altering ribosomal function, essential protein formation is damaged, resuling in fragmented or abnormal proteins, causing immediate short-circuiting in the cell's machinery. Their spectrum includes gram-negative coverage, and they also are synergistic with beta-lactams in killing gram-positive organisms. They are inactivated in an anaerobic environment, due to their need for oxygen in the chemical reaction. Gentamicin and amikacin are the aminoglycosides available for parenteral use. Aminoglycosides are not made for oral use. Aminoglycosides are highly effective against *Pseudomonas* sp. and *Staphylococcus* sp. in addition to their gram-negative aerobic coverage. They tend to accumulate in the ear and kidneys, making patients susceptible to deafness, ataxia, and acute renal failure. Monitoring of renal function, including tubular function, should be performed in patients on aminoglycoside therapy. If clinical signs develop, treatment should be stopped.

Macrolide antibiotics

Macrolide antimicrobials are the first bacteriostatic class to be mentioned thus far. These drugs bind to the 50S subunit preventing the addition of amino acids to protein chains, resulting in defective bacterial protein synthesis. The macrolides of interest in critical care consist of erythromycin, azithromycin, and clarithromycin. These drugs are mainly effective against gram-positive bacteria with aerobic and anaerobic coverage. Erythromycin is a penicillin-alternate drug, with use as a novel prokinetic drug in low doses. Azithromycin is another macolide effective against *Staphylococcus* sp., *Streptococcus* sp., and *Mycoplasma* sp. Clarithromycin is also used for mycoplasma infections.

Lincosamides

Lincosamide antimicrobials have a similar method of action as macrolide antimicrobials, by binding to the 50S subunit on the bacterial ribosome. They are mainly used for gram-positive infections, both aerobe, and anaerobe. They also are effective against *Toxoplasma* sp, *Neospora canis*, and *Mycoplasma* sp (Hsu 2008). Clindamycin is the most common lincosamide and penetrates bone and soft tissue very well. It has good CNS activity but potentially only in cases of CNS inflammation.

Chloramphenicol

Chloramphenicol is a bacteriostatic antimicrobial class unto itself. It also attaches to the 50S subunit of the ribosome, being highly effective against anaerobic bacteria. Chloramphenicol has the potential to cause an aplastic anemia in humans, and should be handled carefully (typically with gloves) to avoid exposure.

Tetracyclines

Tetracycline antimicrobials are also widely used in critical care. They attach to the 30S subunit of the ribosome inhibiting amino acid addition to proteins being synthesized by microorganisms. Tetracylcine antimicrobials have a wide spectrum, with bacteriostatic effects on gram-positive and gram-negative aerobes and anaerobes. They are also effective against *Rickettsia* sp. *Spirochetes*, *Chlamydia* sp., *Mycoplasma* sp, and some protozoans such as *Anaplasma* sp. and *Haemobartonella* sp.

Fluoroquinolones

Fluoroquinolones are commonly used in veterinary medicine. These antimicrobials inhibit bacterial DNA gyrase, which inhibits bacterial replication. They have a broad spectrum against gram-positive and gram-negative organisms. However, anaerobes are mainly resistant. The fluroquinolones include enrofloxacin, ciprofloxacin, marbofloxacin, danofloxacin, orbifloxacin, and difloxacin. They can be administered parenterally or enterally. These drugs are associated with erosion of articular cartilage in young patients. Mainly dogs and foals are affected. They should not be used in growing patients, sometimes up to 1.5 years, until the growth plates are fused. They may also may cause idiosyncratic retinal degeneration in felines.

Metronidazole

The last class of antimicrobial is metronidazole, which belongs to the nitroimidazole class. It is effective against anaerobes where it is absorbed and metabolized to a cytotoxic metabolite by disrupting the synthesis of DNA. In addition to anaerobic bacteria, metronidazole works effectively against protozoans such as *Giardia* and *Trichomonas* sp. Metronidazole is shown to be a CNS toxicant if administered for long periods of time or in high doses. CNS signs such as ataxia, seizures, and vestibular signs, should be monitored for, and dosing discontinued, if they develop (Table 18.4).

Antifungals

The antifungal medications often seen in extended care facilities are the parenterally or orally administered azoles or amphotericin B. Fungal disease can be challenging cases to manage in critical care departments, often manifested as CNS or pulmonary disease. Infection with *Candida* sp. can be another deleterious development in immunosuppressed critical patients. Treating these patients with antifungal medications can be an important step in their recovery.

Azoles. The azole class consists of ketoconazole, itraconazole, and fluconazole, with the latter available for parenteral use. The method of action of these drugs involves a fungistatic process whereby they inhibit the synthesis of ergosterol, an important steroid in fungal cell membranes. These drugs are used for infections caused by *Blastomyces*, *Coccidioides*, *Cryptococcus*, and *Histoplasma* sp.

Amphotericin B. Amphotericin B is a fungicide that creates pores in the fungal cell membrane, allowing fluid entrance and eventual cell death. It is used for *Aspergillus*, *Blastomyces*, *Coccidioides*, *Cryptococcus*, and *Histoplasma* infections. Amphotericin B is highly nephrotoxic, causing decreased GFR, renal vasoconstriction, and tubular necrosis. If azotemia develops, treatment should be discontinued. Amphotericin B is diluted in 5% dextrose and is administered IV.

Disinfectants

Disnfectants and antiseptics have wide use in emergency and critical care medicine. They are used for preparation of surgical sites, preparation of invasive catheter sites, wound cleaning, and cage cleaning. A brief understanding of their mechanism of action, spectrum, and required contact time is essential for the veterinary technician. Failure to adhere to appropriate contact time or inappropriate agent use in the face of a certain microorganism can lead to incomplete destruction of an organismal colony and the development of resistance. Nosocomial infections are becoming a widely recognized problem in veterinary hospitals. The development of multidrug resistant organisms can be worrisome for

Table 18.4   Antimicrobial class descriptions

Anti-Microbial Class	Mechanism of Action	Bacteriostatic or Bactericidal	Spectrum of Coverage
Penicillins (β-lactams)	Inhibit cell wall synthesis	Bactericidal	Gram-positive and some gram-negative. Extended spectrums have better gram-negative and some anaerobic coverage and β-lactamase coverage
Carbapenems (β-lactams)	Inhibit cell wall synthesis, penetrate cell wall	Bactericidal	Gram-positive, gram-negative, and some anaerobic coverage β-lactamase coverage
Cephalosporins (β-lactams)	Inhibit cell wall synthesis	Bactericidal	First generation: Gram-positive Second generation: Gram-positive and gram-negative Third generation: Gram-positive and gram-negative and β-lactamase coverage Fourth generation: Gram-positive and gram-negative
Vancomycin (β-lactams)	Inhibits cell wall synthesis	Bactericidal	Resistant *Staphylococcus/ Enterococcus* sp.
Aminoglycosides	Bind to 30S subunit of ribosome	Bactericidal	Gram-positive and gram-negative, synergistic with β-lactams
Macrolides	Bind to 50S subunit of ribosome	Bacteriostatic	Gram-positive aerobic/anaerobic
Lincosamides	Bind to 50S subunit of ribosome	Bacteriostatic	Gram-positive aerobic/anaerobic
Chloramphenicol	Bind to 50S subunit of ribosome	Bacteriostatic	Gram-positive anaerobes
Tetracyclines	Bind to 30S subunit of ribosome	Bacteriostatic	Gram-positive/gram-negative aerobes and anaerobies, *Rickettsia*
Metronidazole	Disrupts DNA	Bacteriostatic	Anaerobes, Protozoa

health-care providers. These "super bugs" can cause local and systemic infections and greatly increase mortality of emergency and intensive care unit (ICU) patients.

Choosing the appropriate agent

Choosing an agent involves knowledge of the products available in the market. Disinfectants are agents that kill or inhibit microorganismal growth on nonliving matter, such as inanimate objects, whereas antiseptics are agents used to kill or inhibit growth on living tissue and can be killing (-cidal) or inhibitory (-static) to various microbes.

There are several recommendations for selecting a disinfectant. An accepted agent is one that is broad spectrum, nonirritating to tissues, maintains surfaces or equipment, is stable and does not lose effectiveness easily, and is inexpensive (Bill 2006). The agent's spectrum should ideally include all microorganisms, but should at least be effective against a wide range of bacteria, viruses, and hopefully, fungi. However, most agents are stronger in certain areas than others, and selecting an agent that targets the main offenders should be of high priority. Ensuring the agent is nonirritating to tissues is also important, for causing tissue trauma at the expense of antisepsis is counterproductive. In addition, damaging surfaces is also detrimental as organisms can grow in grooves caused by destruction of the surface. Finally, stability is also important, in that the agent should potentially be left on the surface for as long as required for maximum inhibition of organisms (Bill 2006).

Alcohols

One of the most commonluy used disinfectants is isopropyl or rubbing alcohol. This is a very effective agent against gram-positive and gram-negative bacteria, but must remain on the skin for 15 minutes to be effective. It is not effective against spores or some viruses. It also cannot penetrate organic matter such as feces, so the skin must be cleaned first prior to application. Alcohol should be at least 70% concentration and works by denaturing proteins it comes in contact with. If applied to open wounds, it may react with exudate and cause it to thicken, trapping bacteria underneath. Not to mention it stings, and is therefore contraindicated in open wounds.

Bleach

Bleach or sodium hypochlorite is a member of the chlorine compound class. This agent is effective against most bacteria, viruses, and fungi. Bleach has many drawbacks, including corrosiveness and foul odor. It also should be used only when the organic debris has been cleaned. It should be dilute prior to use. There are various dilutions described but 1 cup bleach to 1 gallon water is an acceptable dilution. Another acceptable dilution is 1 part bleach to 40 parts water.

Iodines

Iodine compounds are also common in the veterinary hospital. Iodine is used as a surgical scrub and at times, for wound cleaning. However, it is cytotoxic and should not be used on open wounds. The iodine class is bactericidal, virucidal, protozoacidal, and fungicidal (Bill 2006). These compounds also require the cleaning of organic debris prior to application and require 15 minutes of contact time. Dilution is required with these agents. They should be diluted 1 part iodine to 9 parts water before use.

Quaternary ammonium compounds

Quaternary ammonium compounds, such as benzalkonium chloride, represent another commonly used veterinary disinfectant. These agents have a weaker spectrum, including only gram-positive bacteria and some viruses. They are not effective against gram-negative bacteria. They are generally considered nonirritating; however, large amounts for extended periods of time have the potential to cause dermal or respiratory irritation. As with the above agents, they require a clean surface to work.

Chlorhexidine

Chlorhexidine is another commonly used disinfectant with good bacterial, viral, and fungal coverage. It is also more active in the presence of organic debris; however, it will still lose some efficacy. Chlorhexidine has powerful staying power, often still working after 24 hours of contact. Chlorhexidine is known to be toxic to fibroblasts, which help wound healing, so treatment in open wounds is contraindicated. However, if carefully applied to intact skin, it can be highly effective, and is considered nonirritating. It should be diluted 1 part chlorhexidine and 40 parts water before use on skin.

Hydrogen peroxide

Hydrogen peroxide is the last commonly used disinfectant. It is considered a weak bacteriocide but is not effective against other microorganisms. It is damaging to healthy tissue, and only works in the presence of necrosis, providing some chemical debridement properties. It is not recommended as a common antiseptic. It is used as a sterilization technique for surgical instruments.

Endocrine/Reproductive Pharmacology

Much endocrine/reproductive physiology is noncritical in nature. But several drugs are routinely utilized in the emergent patient. The critical emergencies in the endocrine system are Addisonian crisis, diabetic ketoacidosis, dystocia, hypocalcemia, and hypercalcemia. The drugs of note are glucocorticoids, insulin, oxytocin, and calcium gluconate. Since glucocorticoids were discussed earlier, only the remaining three need exploration.

Insulin

Insulin is the mainstay of treatment in insulin-dependent diabetes mellitus. Insulin is a hormone secreted by beta cells of the pancreas, and is regulated by many factors. Secretion of insulin is controlled by glucose levels, cholecystokinin (CCK), glucagon, among others. Inhibition of insulin is controlled by somatostatin and catecholamines. Porcine, human, and canine insulin are quite similar, whereas bovine and feline insulins are similar in chemical structure. Insulin decreases blood glucose levels by inhibiting glycogen synthesis from absorbed carbohydrates, and reduces hepatic production of glucose via gluconeogenesis and glycogenolysis. It also activates glucose transporters into skeletal muscle cells and adipocytes, allowing glucose to be transported into the cell. Insulin increases the creation of lipids and decreases their metabolism for energy use. Insulin also moves potassium into the cells via the N/K/ATPase pump.

Short-acting insulin. Regular insulin, also called crystalline zinc, is a short-acting human insulin, that peaks at 2–4 hours and lasts 5–7 hours. Because of its rapid onset, it is useful in diabetic ketoacidosis but not appropriate for long-term management. It can be given IV or IM, making it useful for volume-depleted patients, of which diabetic patients presenting for emergencies are often.

Intermediate-acting insulins. NPH insulin, or isophane insulin, is an intermediate acting insulin that contains protamine, a protein that slows insulin absorption. It peaks in 8–12 hours and lasts 24 hours.

Lente insulin is another intermediate-acting insulin with a zinc buffer causing a slowed absorption. It can be subclassified as either semilente, ultralente, or lente. Semilente insulin peaks in 4–6 hours and lasts 12–16 hours. Lente insulin, and the newer porcine Vetsulin (Intervet, Merck, Whitehouse Station, NJ), is similar to NPH in its peak and duration, 8- to 12-hour peak and 24-hour lasting time.

Long-acting insulins. Ultralente insulin is a long-acting insulin that peaks in 16–18 hours and lasts up to 36 hours.

Protamine zinc insulins (PZIs) are long acting due to the protamine and zinc buffers creating extremely slow absorption. PZI peaks in 16–18 hours and can last up to 36 hours. It is often used in feline diabetics. Its long duration makes it quite variable, and tight glycemic control is hard to achieve.

Insulin glargine, or Lantus (Sanofi-Aventis, Bridgewater, NJ), is a recombinant human insulin that forms microprecipitates at the injection site that last for 24 hours. The result is no-peak insulin blood level, but a steady state, creating stable lowered blood glucose levels.

Complications of insulin therapy are hypoglycemia and insulin resistance. The insulins other than regular are usually in suspension and are *only* to be given SQ.

Oxytocin

Oxytocin is a pituitary hormone responsible for uterine contractions. Its primary use is to induce labor and increase uterine contraction strength. However, it is contraindicated in breech births, and can potentially damage the fetus if the cervix is closed, as contractions against a closed gate could be detrimental. It is given parenterally, usually IM or SQ.

Calcium

Calcium, available parenterally in the form of calcium gluconate, is indicated for hypocalcemia, potentially caused by puerperal tetany, or hyperkalemia-induced arrhythmias. It provides ionized calcium for uptake by skeletal muscles and stabilizes the threshold potential of cardiac myocytes to prevent prearrest arrythmias in hyperkalemia. Parenteral calcium is usually given as calcium gluconate. It is given IV slowly, as it may cause bradycardia. ECG/HR monitoring are essential.

Antineoplastic Drugs Used in Critical Care

The main antineoplastic drug of note in critical care medicine is vincristine for its use in immune-mediated thrombocytopenia. Vincristine is a vinca alkaloid which binds to tubulin, a protein that assists with microtubule formation, and arrests microtubular polymerization. It thus prevents cell division. It is used to increase blood levels of platelets from platelet precursors, by an unknown mechanism. It is a neoplastic drug, potentially causing tissue necrosis, and thus must be handled by appropriately trained personnel. Clean, swift venipuncture is necessary, and any chance to dislodge the needle should be avoided to ensure no extravasation occurs.

CHAPTER 18

Immunosuppressive Medications

Immunosuppression is a hallmark treatment of many diseases seen by the critical care service. Immune-mediated anemias and thrombocytopenias represent a critical patient population benefitting from immunosuppression. In addition, complications of immunosuppression, such as infections, can present to the emergency and critical care service. Drugs of note are azathioprine, cyclosporine, corticosteroids, and human intravenous immunoglobulin therapy (IVIG). For the oral medications azathioprine and cyclosporine, because these are toxic to tissue, gloves should be worn when handling these medications.

Azothioprine

Azothrioprine is an immunosuppressive drug with a complicated mechanism of action. It essentially inhibits DNA and RNA synthesis and can target lymphocyte populations responsible for immune interactions. It has a greater effect on the T-lymphocyte than the B-lymphocyte. It is administered orally and takes several weeks to exert effects. Side effects include reversible bone marrow suppression of all cell lines.

Cyclosporine

Cyclosporine is a hydrophobic peptide that enters T-lymphocytes and prevents IL-2 formation, which halts the deleterious effects of T-lymphocytes. It also halts the formation of macrophages. Side effects include GI signs, weight loss, and potential hepatotoxicity, reported in humans.

Human IVIG

Human IVIG is an intravenous infusion that contains IgG. Exact mechanism of action is unkown, but it primarily binds to Fc receptors on macrophages and prevents B-lymphocytes from producing autoantibodies. This limits cell destruction in IMHA and ITP. Because it is a human product, the biggest side effect is a Type 1 hypersensitivty (IgE-mediated) reaction to it. Thus, it should be administered with strict monitoring protocols and infusion stopped at any signs of reaction.

Special Pharmacologic Concerns of Critical Patients

Critical care patients present a particular patient population receiving many drugs for many different problems, and are themselves physiologically compromised. Some conditions affecting drug absorption, distribution, metabolism, and excretion are hypoproteinemia, hypoperfusion, acidosis/alkalosis, age, and species.

Hypoalbuminemia

Hypoalbuminemia is of particular concern with many patients that enter the emergency unit or ICU. Protein-losing diseases, such as protein-losing nephropathy/enteropathy, blood loss, and hepatic dysfunction can all affect levels of blood proteins involved in binding to drugs. Acidic drugs bind mainly to albumin and basic drugs to α-1 glycoprotein. Binding to these proteins affects drug pharmacology in many ways, including reduced renal excretion due to inability of proteins to be filtered across the glomerulus, slowed delivery to site of action, lowered amount of free drug in the plasma, competitive agonism for binding sites on respective protein. Patients with low levels of plasma proteins can be at risk for increased amounts of free drug in circulation, enahancing pharmacological effects. Drug dosages of protein-bound drugs should be lowered in patients with low blood protein levels.

Acidemia/Alkalemia

Acid–base abnormalitles include acidemia and alkalemia. These changes in blood pH levels affect many aspects of pharmacology. Blood pH directly affects how much drug is dissociated in a given environment. An ionized drug that is lipophilic and is able to traverse cell membranes easily. An ionized drug that is hydrophilic cannot cross cell membranes as easily. Depending on the pH of the environment, it may be beneficial to have the drug be lipophilic or hydrophilic.

Hypovolemia/Hypoperfusion

Hypoperfused patients have reduced ability to uptake drugs from sites other than with a strong blood supply. The IV route will be preferred in these patients. Reduced perfusion to organs involved in metabolism and excretion, such as the liver or kidney, can alter the amount of drug that would undergo these processes. Reduced perfusion to the liver means less available enzymes for metabolism, and reduced renal perfusion means a reduced GFR and excretion of active or inactive metabolites. Along with this, renal and hepatic disease or dysfunction can alter the metabolism and excretion of drugs due to cell damage. Drug dosages should be reduced in these cases as well.

Pediatric/Geriatric patients

Another category of critical patient involves those who are young and old. Pediatric and geriatric patients represent a particular category of critical patient, those which face natural impediments to pharmcokinetics, as opposed to pathologic ones. It is of great importance in pediatric patients to ensure adequate drug clearance, as potential side effects may greatly affect the paient's quality of life. Geriatric patients need to have their already frail physiology stabilized rather than destroyed with the use of pharmaceuticals. As these patients both represent a fragile physiology, they are often spoken of together, although each presents its own challenges.

Pediatric patients

Pediatric patients have immature renal and hepatic function. Therefore, drug metabolism and excretion are impaired. Specifically, pediatric patients possess increased GI

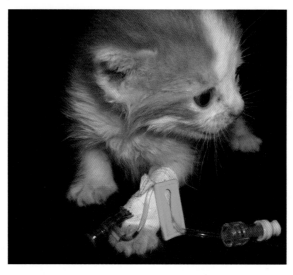

Figure 18.7   This kitten has an IV line with a T-connector attached. The T-connector allows for drug/fluid administration and a separate port for injections. (Courtesy of Thomas Walker, DVM, DACVECC.)

permeability in the first 24 hours of life. High plasma levels of oral drugs may be achieved by the breaching of the gut barrier. They have relatively basic gastric pH (>3.0) up to 5 weeks of age, making drugs absorbed in acidic environments of little efficacy, nor do antacid medications have much of an effect. Milk residue in the GI tract also can chelate drugs and make them ineffective. And finally, motility of the GI tract is "relatively imma- ture" making use of prokinetic efficacy unknown (Gelens 2003). Drug distribution in the pediatric patient is also altered due to increased body water, decreased fat stores, and hypoproteinemia. Protein-bound drugs and hydrophilic drugs may exert greater effects at dosages based on current weight.

Metabolism of drugs is also affected by youth. Pediatric patients contain less CP450 enzymes, making drug metabolism prolonged as there is less available enzyme to catalyze the reaction. Glucuronidation metabolism is also reduced in pediatric patients (Fig. 18.7).

The pediatric renal system is also not fully developed until around 8 weeks of age. Thus, some drug metabolism and drug excretion can be stunted due to low amount of nephrons and reduced GFR. In addition, the pediatric patient has an increased permeabil- ity with regard to the blood–brain barrier, allowing CNS toxicants to exert an increased effect.

Geriatric patients

As with pediatric patients, geriatric patients present concerns regarding pharmacology. With regard to the renal system, geriatric patients are at increased risk of chronic renal failure, making drug clearance reduced. Age-related changes lead to reduced GFR and potential drug mobilization in the kidneys.

Hepatic metabolism and clearance of drugs seems to be somewhat well preserved in the elderly due to the adequate amount of CP450 enzyme conserved in geriatric patients. Reduced blood flow to the liver, however, may cause concern when administering "flow- limited" drugs such as beta-blockers, and fentanyl (reported in humans). These drugs should be reduced 50% in their doses (Trepanier 2007). Geriatric patients may also be

CHAPTER 18

overweight, having increased fat stores, and should be dosed on lean body weight, to prevent drug accumulation in adipocytes.

Most anesthetic doses should be reduced for both pediatric and geriatric patients. Propofol, as an anesthetic induction agent, was examined for its viability in geriatric patients. Propofol's clearance was markedly reduced, and the effects were seen at doses of 5 mg/kg (Nolan and Reid 1996).

Feline Patients

Feline patients are of a unique challenge with regard to pharmacology. Cats tend to be very sensitive to many pharmaceuticals, due in part to their inability to effectively perform Phase II metabolism, specifically glucuronidation. Cats cannot synthesize glucuronic acid to the extent needed to metabolize some drugs, causing an accumulation of the active form. Certain pharmaceuticals are also known to inhibit the cytochrome system of enzymes preventing Phase I metabolism. Feline patients are higly susceptible to any inhibition of this system. For example, ketoconazole, cimetidine, and erythromycin were found to be potent inhibitors of Cytochrome CYP_{3A} activities (Shah et al. 2009). Steroids and NSAIDs are also of particular concern in feline patients. Felines carry a high risk for adverse events with steroid for NSAID use. Currently, meloxicam is the only NSAID approved for use in cats. Also, when determining corticosteroid choices, prednisolone may be a better choice according to a 2009 study. Prednisolone was found to be less diabetogenic in cats than its counterpart dexamethasone (Campbell et al. 2009).

Medical Calculations

Basic Calculations

1. A patient needs 0.5 mg of metoclopramide given SQ. Metoclopramide is 5 mg/mL. How many milliliters do you need?

   Step 1: Divide amount of ordered drug by concentration:

   $$0.5 \text{ mg} / 5 \text{ mg per mL} = 0.1 \text{ mL}$$

2. A patient needs 187.5 mg of Clavamox. You only have 62.5 tablets. How many does this patient need?

   Step 1: What you want by what you have:

   $$187.5 / 62.5 = 3 \text{ tablets}$$

3. A patient needs 0.5 mg/kg of famotidine IV. The patient weighs 12 lb. How many milligrams will you give?

   Step 1: Convert pounds to kilograms:

   $$12 \text{ lb} / 2.2 \text{ kg} = 5.45 \text{ kg}$$

Step 2: Calculate how many milligrams you need:

$$0.5 \text{ mg/kg} \times 5.45 \text{ kg} = 2.7 \text{ mg of famotidine}$$

4. A patient that weighs 4.5 lb needs 22 mg/kg of cefazolin IV. Cefazolin comes in 100 mg/mL concentration. How many milliliters will you give?

Step 1: Convert pounds to kilograms:

$$4.5 \text{ lb} / 2.2 = 2.05 \text{ kg}$$

Step 2: Calculate how many milligrams you need:

$$2.05 \text{ kg} \times 22 \text{ mg/kg} = 45 \text{ mg}$$

Step 3: Calculate how many milliliters you need:

$$45 \text{ mg} / 100 \text{ mg/mL} = 0.45 \text{ mL}$$

Percent Solutions and Dilutions

1. A patient is hypoglycemic and needs 5 g of 50% dextrose diluted 1:5 with a crystalloid solution. How many milliliters of 50% dextrose and crystalloid will you draw up? What will your final solution volume be?

Step 1: Break the question into three parts: How much dextrose, how much crystalloid, how much final volume.

Step 2: Start with part one. You need 5 g of 50% dextrose. Fifty percent dextrose means 50 g/100 mL or 500 mg/mL. Set up equivalent fractions:

$$5 \text{ g} / X\text{mL} = 50 \text{ g} / 100 \text{ mL}$$

Step 3: Cross multiply and solve for x:

$$50x = 500$$

$$x = 10 \text{ mL}$$

Step 4: Calculate your dilution; 1:5 means 1 part dextrose 5 parts crystalloid. If the 1 part dextrose is 10 mL then 5 × 10 = 50 mL crystalloid:

Step 5: Calculate your total volume:

$$50 \text{ mL crystalloid} + 10 \text{ mL dextrose} = 60 \text{ mL total solution}$$

2. A patient needs 10 g of mannitol given slowly IV. Mannitol is 20%. How many milliliters will you draw up?

Step 1: Calculate how many grams per 100 mL in solution:

$$\text{Mannitol } 20\% = 20 \text{ g} / 100 \text{ mL}$$

Step 2: Use an equivalent fraction to find how many milliliters to draw up:

$$10 \text{ g} / x \text{ mL} = 20 \text{ g} / 100 \text{ mL}$$

Step 3: Solve for x:

$$20x = 1000$$

$$x = 50 \text{ mL Mannitol to administer}$$

3. What percent is a 1:40 dilution?

   Step 1: Divide 1 by 40:

   $$1 / 40 = 0.025$$

   Step 2: Multiply by 100:

   $$0.025 \times 100 = 2.5\%$$

4. What dilution is a 5% solution?

   Step 1: Divide 5 by 100:

   $$5 / 100 = 0.05$$

   Step 2: Divide 1 by 0.05:

   $$1 / 0.05 = 20$$

   $$1 : 20 \text{ dilution}$$

Adding Fluids to IV Bags (Fig. 18.8)

1. You need to add 20 mEq KCL/L of fluids to a patient. The patient is on 25 mL/h and has been on IV fluids for 12 h. How many milliequivalent do you add?

   Step 1: Calculate how much fluid is left in the IV bag:

   $$25 \text{ mL/h} \times 12 \text{ h} = 300 \text{ mL}$$

   $$1000 \text{ mL} \times 300 \text{ mL} = 700 \text{ mL}$$

   Step 2: Calculate how much KCL to add to 700 mL:

   $$\text{If you add 20 mEq KCL/L, you add 2 mEq/100 mL}$$

   $$2 \times 7 = 14 \text{ mEq}$$

Alternate way

Setup fractional relationship:

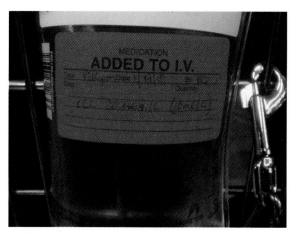

Figure 18.8   All fluids with additives should be labeled as such. These bright red stickers alert the technician to additives and allow for time, date, and initials to be marked as well. (Courtesy of David Liss, BA, RVT, VTS [ECC].)

$$20 \text{ mEq}/1000 \text{ mL} = x \text{mEq}/700 \text{ mL}$$

Solve algebraically by cross multiplying and solving for x:

$$1000x = 14,000$$

$$x = 14$$

2. You have a hypophosphatemic, hypokalemic patient. His potassium level is 2.2 mmol/L. He needs 60 mEq KCL according to the sliding replacement scale. You decide to replace half of his potassium via KCL and half vi KPO4. KCL is 2 mEq/mL and KPO4 is 4.4 mEq/mL. You want to add this to a buretrol with 82 mL left in it. How many milliliters of each drug do you add?

Step 1: Calculate how much of *each* drug to add:

$$60 \text{ mEq total divided by two drugs} = 30 \text{ mEq of each}$$

Step 2: Calculate how many mL/L of each drug:

$$\text{KCL: } 30 \text{ mEq}/2 \text{ mEq/mL} = 15 \text{ mL/L}$$

$$\text{KPO4: } 30 \text{ mEq}/4.4 \text{ mEq/mL} = 6.8 \text{ mL/L}$$

Step 3: Calculate how many milliliters to add to 82 mL:

$$\text{KCL: } 15 \text{ mL}/1000 \text{ mL} \times x \text{mL}/82 \text{ mL} = 1000x = 1230$$

$$X = 1.23 \text{ mL KCL}/82 \text{ mL}$$

$$\text{KPO4: } 6.8 \text{ mL}/1000 \text{ mL} \times x \text{mL}/82 \text{ mL} = 1000x = 557.6$$

$$x = 0.56 \text{ mL}/82 \text{ mL}$$

Continuous Rate Infusion Problems

1. You want to administer metoclopramide at 2 mg/kg/day in a patient's IV bag. The patient weighs 12 kg, metoclopramide is 5 mg/mL, the IVF are running at 12 mL/h, and there are 750 mL left in the bag. How many milliliters of metoclopramide will you add to the patient's bag?

    Step 1: Calculate how many milligrams of Reglan to administer per day:

    $$2 \text{ mg/kg/day} \times 12 \text{ kg} = 24 \text{ mg Reglan/day}$$

    Step 2: Calculate how many milligrams of Reglan to administer per hour:

    $$24 \text{ mg Reglan/day} / 24 \text{ h} = 1 \text{ mg/h}$$

    Step 3: Calculate how many hours the patient's IV fluids will last:

    $$750 \text{ mL} / 12 \text{ mL/h} = 62.5 \text{ h}$$

    Step 4: Calculate how much Reglan to add to the IV bag:

    $$1 \text{ mg/h} \times 62.5 \text{ h} = 62.5 \text{ mg Reglan to add}$$

    Step 5: Calculate how many milliliters to add to the bag:

    $$62.5 \text{ mg} / 5 \text{ mg/mL} = 12.5 \text{ mL}$$

2. A patient needs dobutamine administered at 5 µg/kg/min in a separate 250 mL D5W fluid bag. The patient weighs 2 kg and dobutamine is 5 mg/mL. The patient is not on IV fluids due to volume overload so you want to administer this at a slow rate, 1 mL/h. How many milliliters dobutamine do you add to the 250 mL of D5W?

    Step 1: Calculate how many µg/kg/min to administer to the patient:

    $$2 \text{ kg} \times 5 \text{ µg/kg/min} = 10 \text{ µg/min}$$

    Step 2: Calculate how many µg/h to administer:

    $$10 \text{ µg/min} \times 60 \text{ min/h} = 600 \text{ µg/h}$$

    Step 3: Calculate how many mg/h to run to administer:

    $$600 \text{ µg/h} / 1 \text{ mg} / 1000 \text{ µg} = 0.6 \text{ mg/h}$$

    Step 4: Calculate how many hours the fluid bag will last:

    $$250 \text{ mL} / 1 \text{ mL/h} = 250 \text{ h}$$

    Step 5: Calculate how many mg to add to D5W bag:

    $$0.6 \text{ mg/h} \times 250 \text{ h} = 150 \text{ mg dobutamine to 250 mL D5W bag}$$

    Step 6: Calculate how many milliliters to add to D5W bag:

    $$150 \text{ mg} / 5 \text{ mg} / \text{mL} = 30 \text{ mL dobutamine to bag (Remember to remove 30 mL D5W)}$$

CHAPTER 18

3. A patient needs a furosemide CRI at 1 mg/kg/h. The patient is in fulminant CFH and needs little to no IV fluids. You pick a rate of 1 mL/h and to add it to 150 mL of D5W in a buretrol. Furosemide is 50 mg/mL. How many milliliters will you add to the buretrol if the patient weighs 9.6 kg?

Step 1: Calculate how many milligrams/hour to administer of furosemide:

$$1 \text{ mg/kg/h} \times 9.6 \text{ kg} = 9.6 \text{ mg/h}$$

Step 2: Calculate how many hours the fluid will last:

$$100 \text{ mL} / 1 \text{ mL} / \text{h} = 100 \text{ h}$$

Step 3: Calculate how many milligrams to add to 100 mL D5W:

$$100 \text{ h} \times 9.6 \text{ mg/h} = 960 \text{ mg of furosemide}$$

Step 4: Calculate how many milliliters to add to D5W bag:

$$960 \text{ mg} / 50 \text{ mg/mL} = 19.2 \text{ mL furosemide to } 80.8 \text{ mL D5W}$$

4. A critical patient is going to be undergoing anesthesia. They will need 0.5 mg/kg diazepam, 5 mg/kg ketamine, 2 mg/kg lidocaine and a 50 μg/kg/min CRI, glycopyrrolate at 0.01 mg/kg, dopamine at 5 μg/kg/min, and a fentanyl CRI at 5 μg/kg/h. The patient weighs 28 kg. How much of each will you administer to the patient? Dopamine will be put in 250 mL of D5W at 1 mL/h. The lidocaine is administered in the surgical rates of fluids, which are running at 280 mL/h and is a full liter. The fentanyl will be administered by itself in a 12 mL syringe. The drug concentrations are listed below:

Diazepam: 5 mg/mL
Ketamine: 100 mg/mL
Lidocaine: 20 mg/mL
Glycopyrrolate: 0.2 mg/mL
Dopamine: 40 mg/mL
Fentanyl: 50 μg/mL

Answers:

Diazepam: 2.8 mL
Ketamine: 1.4 mL
Lidocaine bolus: 2.8 mL
Lidocaine CRI: 15 mL to liter of fluids
Glycopyrrolate: 1.2 mL
Dopamine CRI: 52.5 mL dopamine to the 250 mL D5W
Fentanyl CRI: 2.8 mL/h

References

Bill, RL. 2006. *Clinical Pharmacology and Therapeutics for the Veterinary Technician*, 3rd ed. St. Louis, MO: Mosby Elsevier.

Boothe, DM. 2009. *Antimicrobial Resistance: Decreasing the Risk.* Western Veterinary Conference 2009 Conference Proceedings.

Campbell, K, et al. 2009. A pilot study comparing diabetogenic effect of dexamethasone and prednisolone in cats. *Journal of the American Animal Hospital Association* 45(5): 215–224.

Cox, SR, et al. 2008. Safety, pharmcokinetics and use of the novel NK-1 receptor antagonist maropitant (Cerenia) for the prevention of emesis and motion sickness in cats. *Journal of Veterinary Pharmacological and Therapeutics* 31(3):220–229.

de Brito Galvao, JF, Trepanier, LA. 2008. Risk of haemolytic anemia with intravenous famotidine administration to hospitalized cats. *Journal of Veterinary Internal Medicine* 22:325–329.

Drobatz, K, et al. 2007. Vasopressin therapy in dogs with dopamine-resistant hypotension and vasodilatory shock. *Journal of Veterinary Emergency and Critical Care* 17(4): 399–408.

Gelens, H. 2003. *Drug Therapy in Pediatric Practice.* Western Veterinary Conference 2003 Conference proceedings.

Shah, SS, et al. 2009. Inhibitory effects of ketoconazole, cimetidine, and erythromycin on hepatic CYP3A activities in cats. *Journal of Veterinary Medical Science* 71(9): 1151–1159.

Hikasa, K, et al. 1989. Evidence of involvement of alpha 2-adrenoceptors in emetic action of xylazine in cats. *American Journal of Veterinary Research* 50(8):1348–1351.

Hill, R. 2000. NK1 (Substance P) receptor antagonist—why are they not analgesics in humans? *Trends in Pharmacological Sciences* (21)12:461–462.

Hsu, WH. 2008. *Handbook of Veterinary Pharmacology.* Ames, IA: Wiley-Blackwell.

Kittleson, MD, Keinle, RD. 1998. Management of heart failure—digitalis glycosides. In *Small Animal Cardiovascular Medicine*, edited by Kittleson, MD, Kienle, RD, St. Louis. MO: Mosby.

McConnell, J, et al. 2007. Administration of acepromazine maleate to 31 dogs with a history of seizures. *Journal of Veterinary Emergency and Critical Care* 17(3): 262–267.

Nolan, AM, Reid, J. 1996. Pharmcokinetics of propofol as an induction agent in geriatric dogs. *Research in Veterinary Science* 61(2):169–171.

Sigrist, NE. 2007. Use of dopamine in acute renal failure. *Journal of Veterinary Emergency and Critical Care* 17(2):117–126.

Trepanier, LA. 2007. *Neonatal and Geriatric Pharmacology.* International Veterinary and Critical Care Symposium 2007 Conference Proceedings.

Trepanier, L. 2009. *Appropriate Empirical Antimicrobial Therapy: Making Decisions without a Culture.* ACVIM 2009 Conference Proceedings.

Webster, CRL. 2001. *Quick Look Series in Veterinary Medicine Clinical Pharmacology.* Jackson Hole, WY: Teton NewMedia.

Fluid Therapy, Electrolyte, and Acid–Base Disorders

David Liss

Introduction

Fluid therapy is one of the most important modalities in treatment of emergent patients. It serves vital functions including enhancing perfusion, affording maintenance fluid requirements, and replenishing dehydrated cells. The veterinary technician is essential in assisting the veterinarian with a fluid plan and monitoring a patient receiving fluid therapy. This chapter serves to provide a basis for any veterinary technician working in the emergency and critical care setting on the topics of fluid therapy, electrolyte disorders, and acid–base disturbances.

Fluid Therapy in Critical Care

Fluid Compartments

The body is composed of 60% water (DiBartola 2006). Water comprises almost all bodily fluids and is readily distributed to all bodily compartments. These compartments consist of intracellular and extracellular sections. Extracellular fluids (ECFs) can be further categorized into the intravascular, interstitial, and transcellular sub-compartments. The intracellular fluid (ICF) compartment represents the fluid contained within bodily cells. This gives them shape and form, and the ability to function. Of the 60% total body water, two-thirds is contained within bodily cells (DiBartola 2006).

Any fluid not contained by a cellular membrane represents ECF. The ECF represents one-third of total body water, and is further distributed into the intravascular, interstitial, and transcellular compartments. The intravascular compartment represents the body of fluid inhabiting the space within blood vessels. This fluid is mainly composed of plasma and represents one-fourth of the ECF. Interstitial fluid is the fluid in the spaces surrounding cells (in tissues) and makes up three-fourths of the ECF. Finally, the transcellular fluids are those fluids requiring their own subcategory. Examples of these fluids are bile, cerebral spinal fluid (CSF), synovial fluid, glandular secretions, and respiratory secretions. These make up a small amount, around 1% of the ECF (Fig. 19.1).

Electrolyte Distribution

Water and solutes are in equilibrium within all of these compartments. Water flows freely between all compartments. However, electrolytes (or solutes) are either freely permeable across membranes, or selectively permeable depending on the electrolyte. Vascular endothelium (tissue lining blood vessels) is freely permeable to ionic solutes, but relatively impermeable to large plasma proteins and blood cells. Thus, the interstitial and intravascular fluid compartments have relatively similar ionic concentrations but different protein levels. In contrast, intracellular and ECF compartments have vastly different electrolyte concentrations. Cells maintain specific intracellular and extracellular ions with cellular

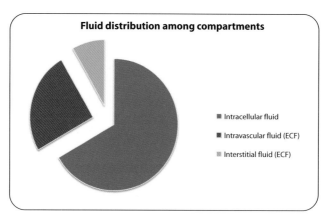

Figure 19.1   The main fluid compartments in the body are the intracellular and extracellular compartments. The extracellular compartment contains the intravascular and the interstitial compartments.

CHAPTER 19

pumps. This keeps a very tight equilibrium on cations (positively charged ions) and anions (negatively charged ions).

The main extracellular cation is sodium. This means that a large majority of the sodium (Na^+) concentration is kept outside the cell. The cell membrane is freely permeable to sodium, but the Na^+-K^+-ATPase pump removes most sodium that diffuses across the membrane. There is thus a steep concentration gradient with regards to sodium (DiBartola 2006). The extracellular space also contains a small amount of potassium (K^+). Although the numbers are small (roughly 4 mEq/L of potassium compared to roughly 140 mEq/L), this meager amount of potassium is physiologically required for proper muscular function.

The major extracellular anions are chloride (Cl^-) and bicarbonate ($HCO3^-$). Bicarbonate is formed as a result of the reaction between CO_2 (carbon dioxide) and water (H_2O) in the presence of the enzyme carbonic anhydrase. Its highly important job is to serve as a buffer so the body remains in a very tight pH range. Chloride is highly important in maintaining acid–base status as well as osmolality of fluid.

Intracellular cations are composed of potassium (K^+) and magnesium (Mg^{2+}). Cell membranes are permeable to potassium. However, any potassium that leaks out is typically replaced via the Na^+-K^+-ATPase pump. Magnesium is responsible for muscle function and is an important co-factor in ATP production, making it required for any cellular function. Potassium is responsible for cellular function and needs to be available for proper cardiac muscle function extracellularly.

Intracellular anions represent phosphorus and proteins (which are mainly negatively charged). An additionally important ion is Calcium (Ca^{2+}). It has a slightly increased extracellular concentration and is responsible for nerve, muscle, and cardiac function. It also is instrumental in blood clotting and skeletal bone function (Fig. 19.2).

Osmolarity, Osmolality, and Tonicity

Understanding solutions and effects of solutes on water concentrations across gradients and membranes is essential in formulating a fluid plan. Solutions can be spoken of in

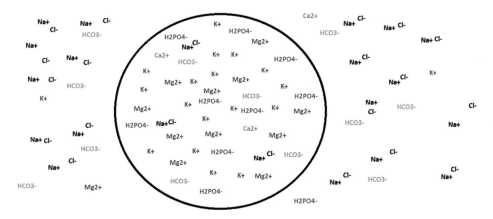

Intra/extracellular distribution of electrolytes

Figure 19.2   Electrolytes, such as Na^+ and Mg^{2+}, have very different intracellular and extracellular concentrations. The numbers above are simply proportional.

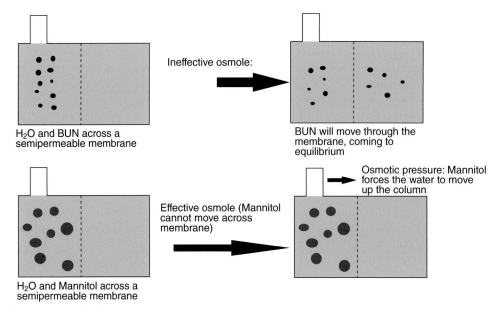

Ineffective osmole:

H₂O and BUN across a
semipermeable membrane

BUN will move through the
membrane, coming to
equilibrium

Osmotic pressure: Mannitol
forces the water to move
up the column

Effective osmole (Mannitol
cannot move across
membrane)

H₂O and Mannitol across a
semipermeable membrane

Ineffective versus Effective Osmolality

Figure 19.3   When effective osmoles are present in solution across a membrane, they increase the osmotic pressure, as displayed here.

regard to their tonicity, and solutes can be described in terms of their osmolality/osmolarity. Osmolarity is the number of osmoles per kilogram of solution. An osmole is a determined number of molecules of a particular solute. Thinking of osmoles as solutes is appropriate, as only the number of molecules in solution changes, but the main function of an osmole stays the same regardless of the number of molecules. Tonicity is how effective the osmoles are at creating osmotic pressure. Isotonic solutions do not cause changes in water movement. Hypotonic solutions have a tonicity less than plasma and cause fluid to move into cells. Hypertonic fluid has a tonicity higher than plasma and fluid will move out of cells to balance the tonicity (Fig. 19.3).

$$\text{Calculated Osmolality: } 2 \times (Na^+ + K^+) + \text{Glucose}/18 + \text{BUN}/2.8$$

Fluid Dynamics and the Starling Equation

Fluids move in and out of vascular structures, into the interstitial spaces, based on various pressures found within each of those compartments. The relationship is explained in a monumental equation pioneered by Frank Starling. He identified four forces that work in concert to guide fluid distribution among the major ECF compartments. The four forces are as follows: capillary hydrostatic pressure, capillary oncotic pressure, interstitial hydrostatic pressure, and interstitial oncotic pressure. Oncotic pressure is the pressure generated by plasma proteins in the vascular space. Hydrostatic pressure is the pressure generated as a result of increased water volume. The equation is as follows:

$$\text{Net filtration} = Kf\,[(Pcap\text{-}Pif) - (\pi p - \pi if)] \text{ (Dibartola 2006)}.$$

Kf   = Filtration coefficient
Pcap   = Capillary hydrostatic pressure (generated by the heart/blood pressure)
Pif   = Intestitial hydrostatic pressure (generated by tissues)
πp   = Capillary oncotic pressure (determined by plasma proteins)
πif   = Hydrostatic oncotic pressure (determined by mucopolysaccharides in tissues)

So what does this overbearing equation mean for us clinically as technicians? First, increased capillary hydrostatic pressure will favor fluid movement into the interstitium. Second, decreased capillary oncotic pressure will also favor fluid movement into the interstitum (because the lack of plasma proteins decreases the their draw of water into the intravascular space).

If a patient suffers from heart failure and is administered fluid boluses, their hydrostatic pressure increases. Because the fluid will now be redistributed, the patient may develop tissue edema (such as peripheral edema or pulmonary edema). As another example, if a patient has hypoalbuminemia and lacks adequate capillary colloid oncotic pressure, the lack of proteins that cause fluid retention within the vascular space will be altered and peripheral edema may form.

Anion Gap

The solute-rich fluids in the body are usually a mix of cations and anions. The sum of cations and anions are always equal. This means that there is no net electric charge of plasma. If all cations plus all anions must equal each other, then the major cations + unmeasured cations and the major anions + unmeasured anions must also equal each other. Thus, if we add the major cations (Na^+ and K^+) and subtract that from the major anions sum (Cl^- + HCO_3^-), we are left with the measurement of the unmeasured anions and cations. Because there are more unmeasured anions that cations, changes in the "anion gap" represent changes in unmeasured anions. Increases in the anion gap represent an increase in the number of unmeasured anions and can hint at problems clinically without actual electrolyte measurements. For example, lactate is an anion, and a patient with a metabolic acidosis and an elevated anion gap may have a lactic acidosis. In addition, patients that are acidemic and diabetic may have ketosis if they have an elevated anion gap. Other causes of an increased anion gap besides lactate and ketones include urea, ethylene glycol, ethyl alcohol, and aspirin.

Fluids Used in Veterinary Medicine

There are two general categories of fluids used in veterinary medicine for resuscitation, dehydration replacement, and maintenance: crystalloids and colloids. These fluid types can further be broken down into various categories. They can be organized by their osmolality (hypertonic saline), whether they are maintenance or replacement solutions (Normosol-M® vs. Normosol-R® [Hospira, Inc., Lake Forest, IL]), whether they are blood products (fresh frozen plasma [FFP]), their synthetic nature (Hetastarch), whether they are balanced or unbalanced (Lactated Ringer's solution [LRS] vs. 0.9% NaCl) or their purpose (electrolyte replacement, colloidal properties).

Crystalloids

Crystalloids are solutions that contain electrolytes, non-electrolytes, and free water (DiBartola 2006). These solutions may contain a variety of electrolytes such as Na^+, Cl^-, K^+, Mg^{2+}, Ca^{2+}, PO_4^{3-}, and non-electrolytes such as amino acids or buffers (acetate, lactate, bicarbonate, or gluconate) to balance acid–base status. The various crystalloids commonly used in North America include Lactated Ringer's solution, Normosol-R and Normosol-M (Hospira, Lake Forest, IL), Plasmalyte® (Baxter Healthcare Corporation, Deerfield, IL), 0.9% sodium chloride, 5% dextrose in water, 0.45% saline and 2.5% dextrose, and hypertonic saline. These solutions are able to diffuse into the intravascular, interstitial, and ICF compartments. They can also diffuse into some transcellular spaces as well. Crystalloid solutions may be used to expand the intravascular space, but they rapidly redistribute to the interstitial spaces. Around 75%–85% of crystalloids are lost to the interstitial space and intracellular space within 1 hour of infusion (Tonozzi et al. 2009). This makes them effective at rapid volume restoration in hypovolemic states, but you may need large volumes, and repeated boluses to restore effective circulating volume. In contrast, they are highly effective at interstitial rehydration.

Replacement solutions. The replacement solutions consist of Lactated Ringer's, Normosol-R, and Plasmalyte-148® (Baxter Healthcare Corporation). These solutions approximate the ECF and are thus isotonic and friendly to the body's environment when infused.

Normosol-R®. Normosol-R is an isotonic replacement crystalloid with acetate as its buffer. It contains 140 mEq/L of Na^+, 98 mEq/L of Cl^-, 5 mEq/L of K^+, 3 mEq/L of Mg^{2+}, 27 mEq/L of acetate, and 23 mEq/L of gluconate. It is a buffered solution and because it contains some magnesium, may be a good choice for critical patients who may be magnesium deficient. There are some anecdotal reports of hypotension associated with Normosol-R boluses. This is reasoned to be from the acetate buffer causing vasodilation; however, no literature currently supports its occurrence.

LRS. LRS is an isotonic buffered replacement crystalloid. It contains 130 mEq/L of Na^+, 109 mEq/L of Cl^-, 4 mEq/L of K^+, 3 mEq/L of Ca^{2+}, and 28 mEq/L of lactate. It has a slightly lower sodium level than that of the ECF, which may make it a good choice in hypernatremic patients. It does not contain magnesium, but does contain some calcium. However, LRS is not recommended to give with blood products, owing to calcium's large role in the clotting cascade.

Plasmalyte-148. Plasmalyte-148 is another isotonic buffered crystalloid. It is very similar to Normosol-R. It contains 140 mEq/L of Na^+, 103 mEq/L of Cl^-, 10 mEq/L of K^+, 5 mEq/L of Ca^{2+}, 3 mEq/L of Mg^{2+}, 47 mEq/L of acetate, and 8 mEq/L of lactate. Plasmalyte contains Ca^{2+} and Mg^{2+} which may make it a great choice for critical patients, who may be hypocalcemic and hypomagnesemic.

Maintenance solutions. Maintenance solutions such as Normosol-M and Plasmalyte-56® are not commonly used in veterinary medicine. This is probably due in part to stocking issues and limited product availability. They contain less sodium and more potassium than replacement fluids.

Normosol-M. Normosol-M contains 40 mEq/L of Na^+, 40 mEq/L of Cl^-, 13 mEq/L of K^+, 3 mEq/L of Mg^{2+}, and 16 mEq/L of acetate. Because of the high potassium levels, this fluid would not be appropriate for hyperkalemic patients or those with the tendency to develop hyperkalemia.

Plasmalyte 56. Plasmalyte 56 contains 40 mEq/L of Na^+, 40 mEq/L of Cl^-, 16 mEq/L of K^+, 5 mEq/L of Ca^{2+}, 3 mEq/L of Mg^{2+}, 12 mEq/L of acetate, and 12 mEq/L of lactate. The same restrictions apply with Normosol-M.

Other crystalloids. *0.9% Sodium chloride.* "Normal saline" contains only 154 mEq/L of Na^+ and 154 mEq/L of Cl^-. It contains no other electrolytes, making it a weak replacement solution, and definitely not a maintenance solution. It is also very acidic with a pH of 5.0. This solution is most appropriate in cases of hyponatremia or hypochloremia, hypercalcemia, and potentially hyperkalemia. However, hyperkalemic patients are often acidemic from translocation and concurrent disease processes, so a buffered solution such as LRS may be preferred. This will be discussed later in the chapter. Patients with gastric emesis, such as with pyloric obstructions, will lose Cl^-, H^+, and Na^+ ions. They may be profoundly hyponatremic and hypochloremic. These patients will benefit from replacement with 0.9% NaCl. They should have potassium levels added to their fluids based on the degree of potassium levels they have (see potassium supplementation, later in the chapter).

5% dextrose in water. This solution contains 50 g/L of dextrose and the no other electrolytes. This solution contains relatively no caloric content, and thus is used in free water replacement. The dextrose is rapidly metabolized into carbon dioxide and H_2O. The patient will breathe off the carbon dioxide and the free water will serve to translocate depending on the water and sodium contents of the intravascular, interstitial, or intracellular compartments. This will be discussed later in the chapter.

0.45% sodium chloride + 2.5% dextrose. This solution, called "half and half" contains 77 mEq/L of Na^+, 77 mEq/L of Cl^-, 25 g/L of dextrose, and no other electrolytes. This fluid is still considered isotonic because the addition of dextrose makes it so. It is used to replace fluids in patients that are hypernatremic, as a lower sodium solution will cause favorable shifts in lowering sodium content. Again, K^+ should be added if the patient is hypokalemic, or simply to add maintenance potassium during diuresis.

Hypertonic saline. Hypertonic saline represents a crystalloid solution with a concentration of either 7.5% NaCl or 26.5% NaCl. This fluid typically has a specific use. It will expand the intravascular compartment effectively and rapidly in hypovolemic shock states. Because of its hypertonicity, water will rush into the ECF from the ICF and interstitial compartments. This will result in an increase in effective circulating volume, and thus, perfusion. It should not be given to patients who are interstitially dehydrated or hypernatremic. It is also advocated for use in head trauma patients with hypovolemia, as it will decrease cerebral edema, and increase intravascular volume (Table 19.1).

Buffers. Buffers are added to crystalloid solutions because acetate, gluconate, and lactate are all metabolized to bicarbonate. Lactate is found in Lactated Ringer's and acetate and gluconate are found in Normosol and Plasmalyte solutions. Lactated products should be avoided in patients with hepatic failure, as they cannot readily metabolize the lactate in

Table 19.1   Comparison of the composition of various crystalloid solutions

Name	Na^+ (mEq/L)	Cl^- (mEq/L)	K^+ (mEq/L)	Ca^{2+} (mEq/L)	Mg^{2+} (mEq/L)	Dextrose (g/L)	Buffer (mEq/L)
Replacement							
Normosol-R®	140	98	5	0	3	0	Acetate (27) Gluconate (23)
Lactated Ringer's	130	109	4	3	0	0	Lactate (28)
Plasma-Lyte 148	140	103	10	5	3	0	Acetate (47) Lactate (8)
0.9% NaCL	145	145	0	0	0	0	None
Maintenance							
Normosol-M®	40	40	13	0	3	0	Acetate (16)
Plasma-Lyte 56®	40	40	16	5	3	0	Acetate (12) Lactate (12)
5% Dextrose in Water	0	0	0	0	0	50	None
0.45% NaCL + 2.5% Dextrose	77	77	0	0	0	25	None

the fluids, and increased lactate concentrations (in equilibrium with lactic acid) may exacerbate metabolic acidosis. (Cooper and Webster 2006; DiBartola 2006).

Colloidal solutions

Colloids are solutions that have a large molecular weight. These fluids will stay in the intravascular space (provided that patient does not have a leaky vascular epithelium). Examples of these fluids include: Dextran®, Hetastarch, Plasma, hemoglobin-based oxygen carriers (HBOCs) (Oxyglobin®, OPK biotech, Cambridge, MA), species-specific albumin, and human albumin solutions. Because these have a high molecular weight, they cannot fit between the tight junctions of the vascular epithelium, and due to their high colloid oncotic pressure, serve to hold water within the vasculature. Colloids were described in the past by their M_w or average molecular weight. That, however, falsely represented their oncotic ability as larger molecules would make the M_w falsely elevated. Now the solutions are referred to by their M_n or molecular number. For example: Dextran-70 (sold as Gentran® 70 by Baxter, Macrodex® by Medisan) has a M_w of 70,000 (or 70 kDa) but an M_n of 41,000. Dextran-40 has an M_w of 40 kDa and an M_n of 26 kDa (DiBartola 2006). Standard Hetastarch (Hextend® [Hospira, Lake Forest, IL]/Hespan®

[B. Braun Melsungen, Melsungen, Germany]) has an M_w of 670 kDa. This means the M_n of Hetastarch is lower, but still higher than Dextrans. Newer types of Hetastarch have a lower M_w (Voluven® [Fresenius SE & Co., Bad Homburg, Germany]) which is 130 kDa (Dibartola 2006).

Dextrans. Dextrans are long-chain sugars that are synthesized from bacterial conversion of sucrose. The two Dextran products include Dextran-70 and Dextran-40. Dextran-70, usually prepared as a 6% solution, will hold twice as much water in the intravascular space as albumin, making it an effective solution for volume expansion (Concannon 1993). Both the Dextrans (70 and 40 preparations) have the same plasma volume expansion (20–25 mL of H_2O/g Dextran) (DiBartola 2006).

Hydroxyethylstarch (Hetastarch). In contrast to Dextrans, the Hetastarch family contains several different preparations with widely different sizes and is a chemical modulation of amylopectin. Amylopectin resembles glycogen in structure. Hextend® has an M_w of 670 and a colloidal onconic pressure or colloidal osmotic pressure (COP) of around 31 mmHg. Hetastarch-450 has an M_w of 450 and a COP of 29 mmHg.

Voluven. Voluven is a newer generation synthetic colloid, in the Hetastarch family, with a very low molecular weight. Its average weight is 130 kD, and thus can be administered in larger doses, up to 50 mL/kg/day. It has a minimal, if any, effect on prolongation of clotting times, as seen with other synthetic colloids.

Complications of synthetic colloids. Coagulopathies related to synthetic colloids have been subject of much debate. Most sources recommend not exceeding 20 mL/kg/day with respect to each type of synthetic colloid, with the exception of Voluven. The coagulopathies associated with Dextran preparations come about because of its effects on the reduction of circulating levels of factor VIII, vWF factor, and interference with platelet function. Dextrans should not be used prior to surgical procedures (DiBartola 2006). Dextrans potentially can coat platelet membranes, cause hemodilution, and decrease vWF activity. Reports of coagulopathy development occurred in dogs receiving 20 mL/kg of Dextran in 30–60 minutes; however, no dog bled spontaneously. (Concannon 1993).

Hetastarch-related coagulopathies are associated with decreased platelet adhesion due to alterations in circulating vWF and Factor VIII (Jandrey 2010), similar to Dextrans. HES does alter platelet function, *in vivo*, significantly more than dilutional coagulopathies (Jandrey 2010).

The risk of coagulopathy is directly related to the size of the molecules. Thus, Voluven, with its lower average molecular weight, may not affect the coagulation system in the same way as other synthetic colloids. Voluven is able to be administered up to 50 mL/kg/day with minimal effect on hemostasis (Jandrey 2010).

Allergic reactions, such as Type I hypersensitivity reactions, seem to also have the potential to occur with synthetic colloids. However, there are no studies in animals to evaluate this. Reports in human medicine include skin erythema, hypotension, respiratory distress, and cardiac arrest. However, prevalence of these with HES is listed as 0.007% and 0.03%–4.7% with Dextrans (Concannon 1993).

Plasma products. Plasma products, in the form of FFP, and frozen plasma, contain colloidal properties as they contain large molecules, including some albumin. These products may be used as volume expanders in a critical emergency, and have the benefit of being isotonic and also contain coagulation factors and circulating anticoagulants. They are not routinely used for this purpose, and are more often used as a transfusion product, discussed in Chapter 21, "Transfusion Medicine."

HBOCs. HBOCs (Oxyglobin®) are purified solutions of bovine hemoglobin. They are used to increase oxygen delivery to tissues and have a significant COP. They have the advantage of delivering oxygen to tissues where red blood cells may not travel. In addition to their colloidal properties, they exhibit a significant vasoconstriction by blocking nitric oxide, which could be helpful or harmful depending to different patient populations. Hemoglobin contains no surface antigens, so transfusion reactions are unlikely to occur because of incompatibility (Tonozzi et al 2009).

Albumin products. There are currently two albumin products available for transfusion in the veterinary market. Human serum albumin represents a human product and risks incompatibility reactions, and canine albumin has just been released and offers no efficacy data as of yet. Human serum albumin carries real risk of anaphylactoid reactions that can cause severe detriment. Two studies published in 2010 and 2005 observed infusions of 5% human serum albumin (has) and 25% has, respectively. They both found that HSA can be safely administered to critically ill patients (Mathews and Barry 2005; Vigano et al. 2010). However, there is still a high risk of anaphylactic, and Type IV (delayed) hypersensitivity reactions as evident by a 2007 study that found in 4 out of 9 dogs administered 5% HSA suffered either a delayed HS reaction or anaphylactic reaction (Cohn et al. 2007).

Indications for colloidal therapy. There are several indications for colloids in the fluid therapy plan. The first involves rapid volume expansion by augmenting plasma COP. Administering any colloid into the vasculature will retain the fluid currently there, and draw fluid from the interstitium into the vascular space to help with perfusion. In addition, colloids will "last longer" in the IV space because they mostly do not fit between epithelial tight junctions. In disease states where proteins are lost (protein losing enteropathy/nephropathy), plasma COP is reduced, allowing fluid to leech into the intersitium creating edema. This edema can overwhelm the lymphatics and cause a relative hypovolemia as the fluid in the intersititum does not contribute to effective circulating volume. Thus, products with a high COP will assist in fluid retention in the intravascular space. These represent the two main indications for colloidal therapy in regards to a fluid therapy plan.

Several other indications exist for specific products, such as clotting factor replacement via FFP in coagulopathies. Take note that albumin is only effectively replaced with an albumin transfusion. It would take 22/kg of FFP to raise a patient's albumin by 0.5 g/dL (Hopper and Silverstein 2009). Those volumes are not usually cost-effective or available to the veterinary clinician. In addition, the high COP and volume required may potentially cause fluid intolerance or overload.

Fluid therapy principles

Fluid therapy has many different important tasks including replacing ongoing fluid losses, enhancing perfusion, maintaining some level of cellular energy, affording maintenance fluid requirements, and replenishing dehydrated cells, as well as a medium for administering medications and electrolytes.

The benefits of fluid therapy are best described in reference to the depleted fluid compartment. The compartments requiring rehydration are the intravascular compartment, interstitial compartment, and intracellular compartments.

Intravascular deficits. Intravascular fluid deficits represent drastic and life-threatening problems which require immediate intervention. If a patient has an intravascular deficit, they will have derangements in their perfusion parameters, such as mentation, heart rate (HR), arterial blood pressure, mucous membrane(MM)/capillary refill time (CRT), extremity temperature, lactate, pH, urine output, and central venous pressure (CVP). Addressing perfusion deficits involves one of three types of approaches. Either large volume resuscitation, limited volume resuscitation (end point resuscitation), or hypotensive resuscitation may be used. Large volume resuscitation involves use of the blood volume formulas for a dog and cat, (approximately 90 mL/kg and 45 mL/kg, respectively) and administering that volume in a large bolus administered as quickly as possible. This technique has moved now toward the use of limited volume fluid resuscitation techniques. This type, also known as endpoint resuscitation, involves using some aliquots of fluid to resuscitate a patient to acceptable endpoints (Hammond and Holm 2009). Research has shown that there is an increased survival rate using this technique (Hammond and Holm 2009). Patients receive smaller "test" doses of crystalloids and colloids, and their perfusion parameters are monitored after each dose.

Once the parameters have normalized, then the volume resuscitation stops and hydration replacement and maintenance fluids are instituted. Hypotensive resuscitation involves fluid resuscitation to a mean arterial pressure (MAP) of no greater than 60 mmHg, or if the patient is already there, not administering fluid (Hammond and Holm 2009). This technique is typically only used in patients with acute, life-threatening hemorrhage where administering fluids will exacerbate blood loss. An MAP of 60 mmHg will allow organ perfusion but cannot be tolerated for long. These patients need to have the hemorrhage controlled immediately, and fluid resuscitation instituted once hemostasis has been achieved (Table 19.2).

Interstitial deficits. Interstitial fluid deficits and dehydration can be harder to objectively quantify. These patients have fluid loss from their vasculature, most commonly from vomiting, diarrhea, polyuria, adipsia, exudative skin lesions, and third spacing. The intravascular hydrostatic pressure drops, and fluid moves from the interstitium to the intravascular space. These patients are not necessarily in danger of death immediately, unless dehydration is combined with hypoperfusion and hypovolemia. The hydration parameters include skin turgor, body weight, MM/CRT, and packed cell volume (PCV)/total solid (TS). Patients with moderate to severe dehydration may also have enophthalmos. With fluid loss from the interstitium, the skin collagen no longer is elastic and thus takes longer to rebound after being stretched. This parameter can be misleading, as older cats, and some systemic diseases can cause altered skin turgor. Body weight is thought to be a sensitive parameter of hydration in human medicine. However, a study performed in 2002 at a veterinary teaching hospital found no correlation between levels of hydration and weight gain after admission (Hansen and DeFrancesco 2002). Enophthalmos and skin turgor can also be altered with chronic weight loss (with normal hydration) which will result in eye fat pad metabolism, giving the look of sunken eyes and prolonged skin turgor (Tonozzi et al. 2009). MM "wetness" can be a subjective indicator of dehydration. As the interstitial fluid crosses to the intravascular space, membranal tissue such as the MMs, conjunctiva, and so on will become "sticker" or "tacky." The CRT should be

Table 19.2   Perfusion parameters

Parameter	Signs of Hypoperfusion
HR	Elevated or decreased
ABP	Normotensive with tachycardia or hypotension
MM	Pale, white, muddy
CRT	Rapid in hyperdynamic shock Prolonged in hypovolemia/vasoconstriction
UOP	Decreased (<1 mL/kg/h) in hypovolemia
CVP	Lower than baseline (typically <5 cm H_2O)
Pulse quality	Weak/thready, absent distal pulses
Extremities	Cool indicating peripheral vasoconstriction
Mentation	Stuporous/obtunded/dull/depressed/comatose

Table 19.3   Physical assessment of dehydration

Percent Dehydrated	Physical Signs Associated
<5%	Assumed based on history of fluid loss (vomiting). No physical signs
5%–7%	Dry MMs/slightly prolonged CRT
7%–9%	Slight increase in skin tenting, tacky/dry MMs, prolonged CRT, increased PCV/TS
9%–11%	Significant skin tenting, sunken eyes, dry MMs, increased PCV/TS
12% or >	All of the above with signs of perfusion deficits (shock)

somewhat prolonged as hemoconcentration will cause "sludgier" blood. The PCV/TS should both be elevated with significant dehydration. The PCV will increase with hemoconcentration, and the TS will if there is only a loss of fluid without protein. Dehydration associated with protein loss will manifest as hemoconcentration with a low or normal TS. For now, the most sensitive indicator of hydration is the PCV/TS (Table 19.3).

Intracellular deficits. Intracellular deficits have started to become known as deficits worth mentioning. These are not measurable by any clinical or laboratory parameter. If intravascular deficits are solute poor, hypotonic or free water loss, the increase in tonicity of the intravascular fluid (such as with hypernatremia) will result in fluid movement across the cell membrane and into the intravascular space to equilibrate the osmolality. Dehydrated cells can result in organ dysfunction, and notably affect the brain, which responds poorly to acute changes in plasma osmolality and result in cerebral edema.

Ongoing losses. Ongoing losses must also be calculated when putting together a fluid plan. These are made up of sensible and insensible losses. Sensible losses are those which can be calculated, such as vomiting, diarrhea, or polyuria. Insensible losses are those which cannot be measured, such as respiratory losses like excessive panting. Typically only sensible losses are added into the fluid plan with an estimation of the volume using a variety of techniques. Estimating fluid loss can be achieved via "eye-balling" the amount lost, metabolic cages that contain catch pans and measure loss, urinary catheters and measurement of urine output, using "pee pads" that can be weighed empty and full, and "free catching" urine. Typically, the methods used for vomitus and diarrhea are "eye-balling" and using measurable pads. Measuring urinary losses can be more objective. However, 1 g of water is equal to 1 mL, based on its density (www.onlineconversion.com).

Maintenance. Finally, a maintenance rate must be added in to meet the normal metabolic requirements of the body. This is typically achieved using one of several equations: (BW [kg] × 30) + 70 = mL/day for patients 2–50 kg. For patients <2 kg or >50 kg, $BW(kg)^{0.75} \times 70 = mL/day$ can be used. Alternatively, 40–60 mL/kg/day can be used for cats and dogs, respectively (Hopper and Silverstein 2009); 90 mL/kg/day is typically used for pediatric puppies and kittens. There are no validated studies on this range, however; it is extrapolated from metabolic requirements.

The Fluid Plan

The typical approach to a patient and its fluid requirements involves a series of questions. Does the patient have a perfusion or intravascular deficit? If they have derangements in their perfusion deficits, then yes they do. Thus, these patients will benefit from "test" boluses of 15–20 mL/kg of crystalloids or 2.5–5 mL/kg of colloids to restore perfusion. After restoration of perfusion, is the patient interstitially dehydrated? If yes, then estimate the percentage of dehydration and calculate the dehydration deficit by using the following formula: % dehydration × BW (kg) × 1000 = mL to replace. If the dehydration is acute, it can be replaced rapidly in 4–6 hours, while chronic losses are replaced slowly over 24–48 hours (Tonozzi et al. 2009). If ongoing losses are present then additional volume must be added in. Finally, the patient's maintenance rate is calculated and administered. All of these components together constitute the fluid plan. See the following example:

7y MN DSH presents with a history of urinating excessively, then anorexia and lethargy. Acute renal failure is diagnosed via blood work and exposure to Lillies is confirmed. The patient is tachycardic at 220 bpm and hypotensive with a Doppler of 40 mmHg. He has marked decreased skin turgor, his PCV is 63%, and TS is 9.0 g/dL. He weighs 4.2 kg.

Step 1

Does he have a perfusion deficit?: Yes—Perfusion parameters indicate hypovolemic shock.

Replace with 10 mL/kg of crystalloids. HR and BP normalize.

Step 2

Does he have an interstitial fluid loss?: Yes, estimated at 10%–12% (due to perfusion abnormalities).

% dehydration × BW (kg) × 1000 = mL to replace.

Replace with 0.1 × 4.2 × 1000 = 420 mL over 12 hours.

Step 3

Does he have ongoing losses?—Yes, polyuric.

Urination on a pee pad in hospital measures 6 mL of urine. Estimate 6 mL loss per 4 hours.

Step 4

Maintenance: BW (kg) × 30 + 70= 4.2 × 30 + 70 = 196 mL of fluid over 24 hours.

So the fluid plan becomes (after perfusion replacement)

196/24 = 8.2 mL/h for maintenance.

1.5 mL/h for polyuria.

35 mL/h for dehydration replacement over 12 hours.

This means a fluid rate of 45 mL/hour.

Monitoring fluid therapy

Monitoring a patient on fluid therapy involves a dedicated and knowledgeable veterinary technician. Veterinarians will tell you, that we (the technicians) are crucial in this process, because we will notice changes associated with fluid intolerance or overload much quicker than the veterinarians who are not constantly with their patient.

The ultimate consequence of fluid therapy is fluid overload/intolerance. The term intolerance has come into favor, because overload signifies: (1) fault on behalf of the clinician for giving too much, (2) an overloading of a patient, who seemed to need that volume of fluids. Using intolerance means that the clinician made no error, and the patient needed that volume of fluids, but could not tolerate it. Fluid intolerance can take many shapes and forms, but will often manifest as congestive type symptoms. Tachypnea can result from pulmonary edema, as well as interstitial/alveolar/bronchial patterns on radiographs. According to experience, the respiratory rate will most often be the first thing to elevate in a patient on IV fluids experiencing some fluid intolerance. Thus, instituting careful respiratory watches on these patients is essential. Harsh lung sounds can also indicate pulmonary edema, caused by high hydrostatic pressures within the pulmonary vasculature. Peripheral edema can result from excessive interstitial hydration, and chemosis (swollen conjunctiva) can also be appreciated. Clear nasal discharge can also be common, as fluid weeps in the sinus spaces, and a wet cough can also occur from fluid in the lower airways. Although fluid intolerance is iatrogenic, it is not often anyone's fault. Cats are extremely susceptible to fluid overload. A prevailing thought is that because the lung parenchyma is adversely affected in feline shock, they have excessively permeable lung tissue, thus resulting in parenchymal edema and intolerance.

Electrolyte Disorders

Electrolyte disturbances can be life-threatening and challenging to interpret, and treat in small animal patients. A basic understanding of their pathophysiology, and a thorough understanding of their treatment is highly important for the veterinary technician to know. This section will briefly review electrolyte regulation and pathophysiology, and focus heavily on the treatment of each disorder.

Disorders of Sodium

Sodium disorders are far more often derangements in water balance as opposed to total body sodium concentration. If a patient has a loss of free water or solute poor fluid, the sodium concentration in the plasma will increase. Conversely, the same is true. Sodium is a huge component of plasma osmolality and osmolality factors into assessing sodium disorders. Recall Osmolality $= 2\,(Na^+ + K^+) + (BUN\,(mg/dL)/2.8) + (Glu\,(mg/dL)/18)$.

Sodium regulation is more aptly discussed in terms of regulation of osmolality. There are two major regulators of osmolality: thirst and antidiuretic hormone (ADH) concentrations. Small changes in osmolality are sensed by the hypothalamus and alterations in thirst and ADH concentrations ensue. When an increase in plasma osmolality is sensed, the hypothalamus releases ADH. ADH causes water retention in the kidneys via V_2

receptor modulation of Aquaporin-2 channels in the basement membrane. Water is resorbed and osmolality decreases. The converse is true when hypoosmolality is present. Thirst also is stimulated when osmolality increases, and free water can be consumed (Hopper and Silverstein 2009).

Hypernatremia

Hypernatremia typically results from either a free water deficit, a sodium excess, or loss of hypotonic fluids.

A free water deficit is the loss of solute-free water from the intravascular space. This results in a high sodium concentration, but not an increase in total body sodium. This condition is somewhat uncommon, but can occur due to diabetes insipidus (central or nephrogenic), lack of access to water, fever, or high environmental temperature (Hopper and Silverstein 2009).

Sodium excess can also lead to hypernatremia. This refers to an increase in total body sodium from administration of salt containing products. Typical cases of sodium intoxication result from salt poisoning, play-dough or paintball ingestion, hypertonic saline administration, sodium bicarbonate or phosphate administration, and more rarely hyperaldrenocorticism.

Hypotonic fluid loses may result in hypernatremia and refers to fluids with solute concentrations less that of plasma, but still some solutes are contained within the fluid. The typical fluids lost are through the gastrointestinal (GI) tract (vomiting, diarrhea), renal system (diuresis post urethral unblocking, osmotic diuretics, mannitol, hyperglycemia, or chronic renal failure), or potentially third spacing of fluids such as with burns, pancreatitis, or peritonitis (DiBartola 2006).

Determining volume status and acute/chronic development of hypernatremia is very important its treatment. Patients with hypovolemia and hypoperfusion require rapid intravascular volume expansion to counteract shock. Typically a balanced isotonic crystalloid is appropriate for this initial phase. Hypoperfusion typically occurs with loss of hypotonic fluid loss type of hypernatremia. If the volume status of the patient is normal, they may or may not be clinically dehydrated and fluid therapy will focus on replacement of dehydration deficits plus potential free water deficits. In patients that are acutely hypernatremic, restoration of intravascular and interstitial fluid can take place quickly, as there has been no equilibration of the subsequent hyperosmolality. Hypernatremia causes cellular dehydration due to ICF shifts moving from the ICF to the ECF to compensate for the hyperosmolar ECF. This results in cellular shrinkage. A few hours after this occurs, the body begins to make intracellular osmolytes ("idiogenic osmoles") that help restore the osmolality of the intracellular space. Full compensation takes 24 hours. Once the full compensation occurs, osmolalities of the ECF and ICF are matched to prevent any further cellular shrinkage.

Rapid correction of chronic hypernatremia will result in a diluted ECF with a reduced osmolality. The increase in water concentration will begin to flow intracellularly, which is now hyperosmolar compared to the ECF. This will result in cellular swelling and bursting and can result in life-threatening cellular swelling and potentially neurologic dysfunction and edema. Thus, sodium concentration should be decreased slowly to prevent this. Recommendations include that mild to moderate hypernatremia ($Na^+ < 180\,mEq/L$) have their sodium concentration reduced by no more than $1\,mEq/L/h$. Patients with severe hypernatremia ($Na^+ > 180\,mEq/L$) should have their sodium levels reduced even slower, $0.5\,mEq/L/h$ (Hopper and Silverstein 2009).

Fluids used to replace the free water deficit are typically 5% dextrose in water, because the dextrose is rapidly metabolized and only free water is left in the intravascular space. Dehydration fluids (isotonic replacement crystalloids) can also be administered simultaneously to replace electrolytes and hydrate the interstitium. The free water deficit formula helps identify the volume of fluid needed to correct the patient's sodium:

$$\text{Free Water Deficit (FWD)} = ([\text{Current Na}^+]/[\text{Normal Na}^+] - 1) \times 0.6 \times \text{BW(kg)}.$$

Thus, a patient with a Na^+ concentration of 181 mEq/L that is 10 kg has an FWD of 240 mL if we assume normal Na^+ is 140 mEq/L.

They should have their Na^+ concentration lowered by 0.5 mEq/L/h; therefore, they need around 80 hours for replacement of the 240 mL. If patients are drinking and not vomiting, oral water may be used as well.

Na^+ concentrations should be assessed every 4 hours to ensure a slow drop in Na^+ concentration. Patients being treated for hypernatremia should be monitored for any change in mentation or pupil size, as rough estimates of increasing brain swelling. In extreme cases, the Cushing's reflex (hypertension and bradycardia) with mental dullness may indicate an acute brain swelling, increasing intracranial pressure (ICP), and require the use of osmotic diuretics.

Hyponatremia

Understanding hyponatremia is typically described in terms of plasma osmolality, and this should be calculated or measured in a patient with hyponatremia. There are three types of hyponatremia: normal plasma osmolality, hyperosmolality, hypoosmolality.

Normo-osmolar patients typically have a pseudohyponatremia caused by lab error due to the patient's hyperlipidemia or hyperproteinemia. This has been corrected with advanced lab testing machines that are available. Patients with hyperosmolar hyponatremia have an increase in plasma osmolality (increase in an effective osmole concentration) and thus, free water has been pulled into the vasculature. Hyperglycemia and mannitol will cause an increase in plasma osmolality and thus cause free water to migrate from the ICF and interstitial spaces into the ECF. These patients must have their sodium levels corrected, especially in the case of hyperglycemia. Na^+ concentration will decrease 1.6–2.4 mEq/L for every 100 mg/dL increase in glucose concentration above normal. Patients may actually be hypernatremic when the actual sodium is corrected.

Hypo-osmolar hyponatremia is the most complicated in terms reasoning. It has three subcategories: hypo-osmolar hyponatremia with hypervolemia represents a dilutional effect additional fluid has on the sodium concentration. Examples of this include congestive heart failure (CHF), liver disease, nephrotic disease, and advanced renal failure. Hypoosmolar hyponatremia with normovolemia represents a retention of water such as with inappropriate ADH secretion, where a patient's ADH levels soar, and free water is retained. The sodium level drops from water retention, but the patient is not hypervolemic. Lastly, hypovolemic hypo-osmolar hyponatremia represents fluid losses such as GI fluids (vomiting, diarrhea), third space losses (effusions, uroabdomen, pancreatitis/peritonitis, burns), hypoadrenocorticism (from lack of aldosterone), and diuretic administration (DiBartola 2006).

Hyponatremia can be as life-threatning as hypernatremia. Na^+ concentrations less than 120 mEq/L can cause neurological signs as the hypertonic ICF receives fluid that will move from the hypotonic ECF. Cells attempt to protect themselves from hyponatremia by expelling solutes to make the ECF more hyperosmolar and thus influencing free water to leave the intracellular space. Rapid correction of sodium levels to normal can result in dehydration of cells, called myelinolysis, and can result in neurologic damage. If the sodium level rises too fast, treatment is to administer free water to reduce it and halt the cellular shrinkage (Hopper and Silverstein 2009). Sodium levels should not be increased greater than 0.5–1 mEq/L/h. If the patient's Na$^+$ level is <120 mEq/L, rapid increase in the sodium level to 120 mEq/L can be performed.

Standard electrolyte replacement solutions can be given for hydration, and the sodium level monitored. To increase free water excretion, furosemide (0.5–1 mg/kg) and mannitol (0.5–1 g/kg) can be given to ensure solute-free water is excreted (Hopper and Silverstein 2009). In the patient that is hypovolemic, the patient should receive volume expansion, and it should be roughly equivalent to the patient so rapid water shifts will not take place. Hypovolemic hyponatremic patients can be resuscitated with a replacement solution not more than 6 mEq/L above the patient's sodium.

Disorders of chloride

Chloride is absorbed from the small intestine (namely, the jejunum and colon) from the diet. The magnitude of chloride absorption follows the amount of sodium ions absorbed to maintain electroneutrality. The kidneys reabsorb filtered Cl$^-$ as well. The same is true with regards to Cl$^-$ reabsorption in the kidneys; they reabsorb the same magnitude of Cl$^-$ as Na$^+$. Chloride has a strong role in acid–base. Chloride is a strong factor in the anion gap measurement, which will be discussed later. The chloride value must be "corrected" when the patients Na$^+$ level is abnormal (DiBartola 2006). Chloride levels will change, along with Na$^+$, during body water disturbances. However, this may not accurately reflect the Cl$^-$ status in the body. Thus, the following equation is used:

$$Cl^- \text{ (corrected)} = Cl^- \text{ (patient)} \times [Na^+ \text{ (patient)} / Na^+ \text{ (normal)}].$$

Hyperchloremia

If the patient is hyperchloremic, and the corrected Cl$^-$ is normal, then they have an artifactual hyperchloremia. This is most often associated with dehydration, and the Na$^+$ levels should be elevated as well. If their corrected Cl$^-$ is also high, then they have a true hyperchloremia. Hyperchloremia is relatively uncommon. Some causes include excessive gain of Cl$^-$ (NaCl fluid therapy, salt poisoning), lipemic samples (falsely elevate Cl$^-$), and renal chloride retention (renal failure, renal tubular acidosis, hypoadrenocorticism). Highly increased Cl$^-$ levels will reduce the HCO3$^-$ levels, resulting in a hyperchloremic metabolic acidosis.

The treatment of corrected hyperchloremia is usually aimed at resolving the underlying issues. Corrected hyperchloremia, by itself, does not seem to cause life-threatening clinical signs. However, because of the anion gap adjustments, hyperchloremic patients may be acidotic and should have therapy instituted as soon as possible to correct this.

Hypochloremia

Low levels of Cl$^-$ can result from either excessive loss of chloride ions relative to Na$^+$, or administration of a high Na$^+$ fluid without subsequent Cl$^-$. The most important causes in veterinary medicine are vomiting of upper GI contents (mainly HCl) and diuretic therapy (loop and thiazides). The loss of Cl⁻ ions will cause a proportional increase in HCO_3^- concentration resulting in a hypochloremic metabolic alkalosis.

Typically, the patient will require fluid administration. Thus, the infusion of 0.9% NaCL is appropriate. This will typically resolve the hypochloremia. Normal saline contains no other electrolytes, so addition of maintenance or replacement K^+ levels may be necessary.

Disorders of potassium. Potassium is the body's largely intracellular cation. Potassium is 99% intracellular with extracellular concentrations roughly around 4 meEq/L. Potassium levels that are high represent *hyperkalemia*, and those that are low represent *hypokalemia*. Potassium is absorbed in the small intestine, and excreted in the kidneys and the colon. Acid–base status affects the potassium concentration, as H^+ ions are moved into the ICF in place of K^+ ions in the case of metabolic acidosis. Thus, hyperkalemia and acidosis go hand in hand. Finally, potassium plays a role in the membrane potentials of tissues that can contract. A cell can perpetuate a depolarization wave when it has reached its threshold/action potentials. This happens in part due to Na^+ flowing into the cell and potassium flowing out.

If there is less potassium available for exchange (hypokalemia), the cell is less excitable because less Na^+ will flow in. If there is an abundance of potassium ions (hyperkalemia), the resting potential moves closer to the threshold potential because more Na^+ can move intracellularly. As the resting potential comes closer to the threshold potential, the cell becomes more excitable. If the resting potential exceeds the threshold potential, the cell cannot repolarize and cannot subsequently continue to depolarize. Calcium also has a role in this as well. Calcium affects the threshold potential as opposed to the resting potential. Addition of calcium ions to the ECF raises the threshold potential away from the resting potential. Hypocalcemia will lower the threshold potential toward the resting potential making cells hyperexcitable (DiBartola 2006). This will be explained further.

Hyperkalemia

Hyperkalemia can occur for a variety of reasons. The major ones include: translocation, decreased urinary excretion, and increased intake. With translocation, potassium ions flow from the ICF into the ECF due to acidosis, lack of insulin (which drives potassium intracellularly), reperfusion syndrome, acute tumor lysis syndrome, and drug therapy such as B-blockers and digoxin. Decreased urinary excretion results from conditions such as a ruptured urinary bladder, urethral obstruction, acute kidney injury, anuria, hypoadrenocorticism, and hypoaldosteronism, and drug therapy such as angiotensin-converting enzyme (ACE) inhibitors, nonsteroidal anti-inflammatory drugs (NSAIDs), potassium-sparing diuretics (e.g., spironolactone) can also potentially cause hyperkalemia (DiBartola 2006). Increased intake is quite rare, but iatrogenic oversupplementation could occur. It is important to note that Akita dogs have a normal hyperkalemia (DiBartola 2006).

There are two mainstays of treatment for hyperkalemia: drive the potassium back into the ICF and promote diuresis. An ECG should immediately be obtained in a patient with hyperkalemia, as the most life-threatening effects are cardiac arrhythmias. Drug treatment of hyperkalemia includes the use of insulin to promote cellular uptake of potassium, infusion of dextrose to promote insulin release and counteract hypoglycemia, and infusion of 10% calcium gluconate as a cardioprotective measure. Calcium will raise the threshold potential away from the resting potential. This will stabilize the membranes somewhat, but will do nothing to correct the actual potassium level. Intravenous fluid containing none, or minimal potassium can be used to promote diuresis. Then, 0.5–1 mL/kg of 10% calcium gluconate can be given for cardioprotection. Finally, 0.5 U/kg of regular insulin with 0.5–1 g/kg of 50% dextrose (diluted 1:2 or 1:4) can be administered IV. ECG changes with hyperkalemia include bradycardia, tall, peaked T waves, prolonged QRS complex, atrial standstill, and ventricular arrhythmias such as ventricular premature complexes (VPCs) or ventricular tachycardia. In the worst of cases, ventricular fibrillation can result. If the hyperkalemia is due to acute renal failure (ARF), peritoneal or hemodialysis may be necessary to lower potassium levels (Hopper and Silverstein 2009) (Fig. 19.4).

Hypokalemia

Low levels of potassium typically result from either redistribution or relocation to the ICF or urinary loss and inadequate intake. ICF relocation can happen as a result of insulin therapy, metabolic alkalosis, refeeding syndrome, and B-agonist therapy. Urinary loss occurs most commonly from osmotic, or postobstructive diuresis, diuretic therapy, chronic kidney disease, hyperaldosteronism, diabetes, renal tubular acidosis, and severe diarrhea. Inadequate intake or anorexia can result in hypokalemia as well.

Typically, hypokalemia causes skeletal muscle weaknesses, potentially to the point of hypoventilation, from a hyperexcitable cell membrane. Typical clinical signs include recumbency, ventroflexion of the neck, and possibly a plantigrade stance. Although ECG signs are not as predictable with hyperkalemia, life-threatening arrhythmias such as atrioventricular (AV) dissociation, and wide Q-T bradycardia can occur (Hopper and Silverstein 2009). Treatment includes replacing lost potassium and treating underlying disorders. Potassium can be supplemented enterally but is most often supplemented parenterally. The following sliding scale indicates published replacement doses for potassium chloride supplementation. Be careful that the rate of potassium infusion does not exceed 0.5 mEq/kg/h. For severely affected patients (serum potassium <2 mEq/L), infusion of KCL can take place in a separate IV line during the rehydration (high IV rate) period. A separate line can be dedicated to the potassium infusion and given at a rate not to exceed 0.5 mEq/kg/h (Hopper and Silverstein 2009) (Table 19.4).

CHAPTER 19

K+ level >6.0meq/L = Tall, peaked T-waves

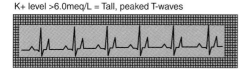

K+ level 7–8meq/L = Wide QRS, P-R interval prolongation

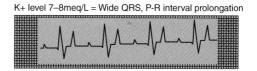

K+ level 8–9 meq/L = Absent p-waves (atrial standstill)

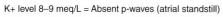
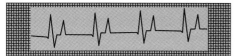

K+ level >9meq/L = Risk for V-tach/V-fib, Bradyarrhythmias

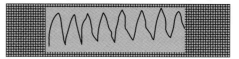

Figure 19.4   Hyperkalemia has characteristic, although not predictable, ECG changes. The four major changes are: tall, peaked T waves; wide QRS; P-R interval prolongation; and atrial standstill.

Table 19.4   Potassium administration chart

Serum Potassium Level (mEq/L)	Amount (mEq) to Add to 1 L of Crystalloid Fluids
<2	80
2.0–2.4	60
2.5–3.0	40
3.1–3.5	30
3.5–4.0	20
>4.0	None

Note: Do not exceed 0.5 mEq/kg/h.

Disorders of calcium

Calcium regulation is a highly complex process. Ninety-nine percent of calcium is contained within bone. Less than 1% of total body calcium is available for cellular or biological processes. Calcium that is found in the ECF has three forms: ionized (metabolically active), complexed, and bound (typically to albumin). Ionized calcium is the only form that is truly of interest clinically (DiBartola 2006). Parathyroid hormone regulates the daily, hourly, and minute-to-minute calcium changes. Calcitriol (vitamin D_3) regulates bigger picture calcium concentrations. Parathyroid hormones (PTH) will signal the kidneys and bones to mobilize more calcium as the body requires it. Intestinal reabsorption is controlled by calcitriol, which is synthesized in the kidneys. Calcitonin is a hormone secreted by the thyroid gland, in response to hypercalcemia, which limits calcium resorption in the bone.

Measurement methods of calcium typically measure total or ionized calcium. Total calcium levels reflect a total body picture of calcium, and do not accurately reflect the metabolically active portions of calcium. Thus, a machine that measures iCa is highly recommended. There is not a good way to extrapolate ionized calcium from total calcium (Silverstein).

Hypercalcemia

Hypercalcemia can result from hyperparathyroidism, hypercalcemia of malignancy (e.g., lymphoma, adenocarcinoma, multiple myeloma), osteomyelitis, acute kidney injury, hypervitaminosis D (typically from rodenticide toxicity), hypoadrenalcorticism, lab error, or be idiopathic in cats.

Hypercalcemia typically is not life-threatening. However, it can cause arrhythmias and renal failure due to mineralization of those tissues. Q-T interval shortening and P-R interval elongation, resulting in bradyarrhythmias and possibly ventricular fibrillation can occur, however rare (DiBartola 2006). Clinical signs of hypercalcemia include polyuria and polydipsia, anorexia, weakness, lethargy, and seizures (Dibartola 2006).

Treatment of hypercalcemia involves inducing diuresis, administering diuretics, glucocorticoids (which increase renal excretion and reduce skeletal reabsorption), and potentially calcitonin, or pamidronate. Normal saline causes competition for calcium ion reabsorption and contains no calcium, making it ideal to induce calciuresis (Hopper and Silverstein 2009). Calcitonin can be given parenterally (4–6 IU/kg SQ) to control hypervitaminosis D intoxication. Pamidronate is a biphosphonate that prevents osteoclast reabsorption of calcium.

Hypocalcemia

Typical causes of hypocalcemia include hypoalbuminemia (loss of bound calcium), chronic kidney disease, acute kidney injury, eclampsia (calcium utilized by neonates), hypoparathyroidism, ethylene glycol toxicity, protein-losing enteropathy, massive blood transfusion with citrate, hypomagnesemia, acute tumor lysis syndrome (Hopper and Silverstein 2009). In addition, ionized hypocalcemia may be a biomarker of sepsis, but more research is needed (Holowaychuk and Martin 2007). A recent study of 58 cases of sepsis admitted to a veterinary ICU found that 24% of them had ionized hypocalcemia (Luschini et al. 2010).

Clinical signs associated with hypocalcemia involve muscle tremors and fasciculations, muscle cramping, facial rubbing, panting, pyrexia, polyuria, polydipsia, and rarely hypotension and death (Dibartola 2006). The most common presentation for hypocalcemia is the bitch who recently whelped and is twitching. An ionized calcium level should be measured immediately and treatment instituted.

Treatment involves immediate calcium administration, monitoring ECG changes, and continuing supplementation in a CRI if necessary. For parenteral use, calcium gluconate is preferred because it does not cause problems if it accidentally extravasates (Hopper and Silverstein 2009). Doses include 0.5–1.5 mL/kg of the 10% solution, slow (over 10–30 minutes) IV. An ECG should be monitored during calcium infusion. Any bradycardia, P-R interval prolongation, or Q-T interval shortening should prompt the technician to stop the infusion and recheck an ionized calcium (Hopper and Silverstein 2009). A CRI of 1–3 mg/kg/h IV can be used if boluses are not sufficient at keeping levels normal (Hopper and Silverstein 2009).

Disorders of phosphorus

Phosphorus represents the body's major intracellular anion. It typically is absorbed and excreted in contrast with calcium concentrations. It is passively absorbed in the small intestine. The kidneys also serve to regulate phosphorus balance as well. PTH stimulation will cause an increase in phosphorus excretion.

Hyperphosphatemia

Increases in phosphorus will normally lower the serum calcium concentration, so the Ca × Pi product is relatively constant. Increases in this product (>60) risk soft tissue mineralization of Ca phosphate salts. Therefore, hyperphosphatemia can cause hypocalcemia by default (DiBartola 2006). Causes of hyperphosphatemia include tumor lysis syndrome (rupture of tumor cells release PO_4^{3-}), tissue trauma, rhabdomyolysis, and metabolic acidosis. In addition, cholecalciferol rodenticides, hypoparathyroidism, acute kidney injury, chronic kidney disease, uroabdomen/urethral obstruction, and physiology (growing animals) can cause hyperphosphatemia.

Typically, hyperphosphatemia involves treatment of the underlying problem, fluid diuresis, and phosphorus binders. Saline diuresis will prevent phosphorus reabsorption by the kidney, as well as treat volume deficits. Dietary phosphorus restriction should commence and phosphate binders (aluminum hydroxide, carbonate) should be administered enterally, if possible. Phosphate binders are much more effective if given with food and thus should be administered only if the patient is able to take enteral nutrition (DiBartola 2006).

Hypophosphatemia

Hypophosphatemia can occur as the result of translocation, increased urinary loss, or decreased absorption/reduced intake. Translocation is a common cause of hypophosphatemia and occurs in the treatment of diabetes (insulin therapy moves PO4 3- intracellularly), or rapid administration of parenteral or enteral nutrition, as insulin release causes the same problems. Hyperparathyroidism will stimulate renal loss of phosphate, and renal tubular disorders (e.g., Fanconi's syndrome) can cause phosphate wasting. Rarely does decreased intake cause hypophosphatemia (DiBartola 2006).

Typically, hypophosphatemia involves phosphorus supplementation parenterally. There is a somewhat wide dose range for potassium phosphate supplementation. Listed as 0.03–0.12 mmol/kg/h in some texts and 0.01–0.06 mmol/kg/h in others (DiBartola 2006; Hopper and Silverstein 2009). Potassium supplementation should not exceed 0.5 mEq/kg/h. Since most of these patients are hypokalemic as well, potassium supplementation may be worthwhile. Some clinicians will decide on potassium supplementation and administer half as KCL and half as KPO_4.

Disorders of magnesium

Magnesium is a co-factor in ATP production, making it vital for all cellular functions. It serves to help support the Na^+-K^+-ATPase pump, which regulates Na^+ and K^+ levels in the ECF and ICF. Magnesium also blocks calcium channels, preventing calcium movement intracellularly (Cortes and Moses 2007). Magnesium is found mainly intracellularly, being the second cation after potassium (Cortes and Moses 2007). Magnesium is found in the serum as ionized, or bioavailable, complexed, and bound, similar to calcium. As with calcium, only ionized Mg^{2+} is able to be utilized in biologic processes. Magnesium is absorbed in the small intestine and regulated further in the kidneys. No one hormone has been found to control magnesium levels within the body (Cortes and Moses 2007). In contrast to the availability of ionized calcium analyzers, we are only able to routinely test for total magnesium, at this time. However, like with calcium, derangements in iMg can present with normal total magnesium levels.

Hypermagnesemia

Hypermagnesemia is quite rare in veterinary literature, but has been documented. One study found that 13% of dogs admitted to a veterinary ICU were hypermagnesemic (Martin et al. 1994) article). Renal failure and iatrogenic overdose are the only two listed causes of hypermagnesemia (Cortes and Moses 2007). Clinical signs are typically weakness, depression, and hypotension. Hypotension can occur as high levels of magnesium will block calcium intracellular influx, contributing to a loss of vasomotor tone and vasodilation (Cortes and Moses 2007).

Treatment involves discontinuing supplementation, administering calcium to antago-nize Mg^{2+} at the neuromuscular junction (NMJ), and administering loop diuretics as needed (Cortes and Moses 2007).

Hypomagnesemia

Causes of hypomagnesemia reflect those of other electrolytes. Renal loss from diuretic therapy, osmotic diuresis, or tubular disease can contribute to hypomagnesemia. Inade-quate intake is rare but possible. Pancreatitis, sepsis, and endocrine disease have also been implicated in hypomagnesemia. Clinical signs include twitching and fasciculations, hyper-excitability, cardiac arrhythmias including ventricular tachycardia, ventricular fibrillation, VPCs, atrial fibrillation, and supraventricular tachycardia (SVT). A special arrhythmia, termed Torsades de Pointes, occurs in human medicine in response to low magnesium. It is a special kind of ventricular tachycardia. There are no reports of it occurring in veteri-nary medicine (Cortes and Moses 2007). Hypomagnesemia can be associated with elec-trolyte derangements, namely refractory hypocalcemia and hypokalemia, based on magnesium's role in cellular transport of these ions. However, to correct these problems, the Mg^{2+} levels must be corrected as well. However, since many hospitals do not run magnesium levels, these problems may not be corrected and abnormal magnesium levels not ever detected (Cortes and Moses 2007).

Treatment involves enteral or parenteral supplementation. Fluid therapy with a mag-nesium containing fluid can provide some support (Normosol-R, Plasmalyte). Parenteral options include magnesium sulfate or magnesium chloride. Magnesium is typically given at 0.7–1 mEq/kg/day IV, diluted in IV fluids (Cortes and Moses 2007). Recommendations for monitoring include rechecking electrolytes, Mg^{2+}, and Ca^{2+} levels every 12 hours. Enteral supplementation can be given as magnesium carbonate, oxide, or gluconate, typi-cally supplied as a powder. The canine reported dose is 1–2mEq/kg/day (Cortes and Moses 2007).

Acid–Base Disturbances

Acid–base measurement and interpretation is a very important part of the workup in a critical patient. Blood gas analysis has many benefits, including identifying underlying disease processes, assessing ventilatory function, and guiding treatment in treating acido-sis and alkalosis. The body works very hard to keep the pH within a very narrow range. Many derangements can alter this pH and cause disastrous consequences with regard to cellular function and cardiac integrity.

Regulation

Acid–base status in the body depends on several factors. The H^+ (or "acid") load is pro-duced as a net result of metabolic processes. One that is notable is the combination of CO_2 and H_2O in the presence of carbonic anhydrase, which forms carbonic acid or H_2CO_3. The carbonic acid equation is $CO_2 + H_2O \text{-} > H_2CO_3 \rightarrow H^+ + HCO^{3-}$.

In addition, the levels of HCO_3 are also regulated to match the amounts of acid being produced. A normal blood pH is generally between 7.35 and 7.45 (DiBartola 2006). H^+

ions and HCO_3 ions are regulated via excretion and resorption in the kidneys. Amounts of CO_2, which effectively means carbonic acid levels, are regulated via minute ventilation by the respiratory center in the brain. Thus, we think of CO_2 having an acidic effect. Too much CO_2 will cause an acidemia. The work horses of acid–base balance in the body are the kidneys and the lungs. The lungs can retain and excrete CO_2 (converted into acid) quite quickly. The kidneys can reabsorb or excrete HCO_3 (base) over a slower period.

An *acidosis* is the clinical syndrome associated with too much acid in the body. An *acidemia* is the presence of too much acid in the blood (pH < 7.35). Acidoses can occur from either too much CO_2, loss of HCO_3 (loss of buffer will increase acid levels), or intake or production of exogenous (outside of the body) or endogenous (inside the body) acids. An *alkalosis* represents too much base in the body and can manifest in the opposite ways. *Alkalemia* is the presence of too much alkaline in the blood (pH > 7.45). Typically, gain of too much bicarbonate or loss of too much CO_2 are the common causes of an alkalosis.

Regulation of the acid–base status of the body is achieved mainly through the quick actions of the lungs, the already present bicarbonate, and the slower resorption of bicarbonate by the kidneys. If an acidosis occurs, the acid will be neutralized by circulating bicarbonate. As the pH drops, the brain stimulates alveolar ventilation to increase, and the CO_2 levels will drop to less than normal (DiBartola 2006). Finally, the kidneys will start to resorb bicarbonate, a process that takes 2–5 days. The reverse process will happen with an alkalosis. Minute ventilation will decrease so that CO_2 levels will rise, and HCO_3^- excretion from the kidneys will commence. These processes, called compensation, help to keep the body's pH normal.

Buffering

Buffering is another important concept to cover. Buffers are weak acids and their accompanying salts that, in the presence of strong acid or base, can receive or donate protons to effectively reduce the change in pH (Dibartola 2006). Essentially, in a hostile environment like the body, strong acids are being created and the way to minimize the changes in pH that may occur, the body has buffering systems to "neutralize" the strong acids. The buffers in the body are bicarbonate, in the ECF, and proteins and phosphates, in the ICF (DiBartola 2006).

Anion gap

Lastly, the anion gap is an important component of acid–base interpretation. As discussed earlier in the chaper, the anion gap represents the amount of unmeasured anions (mostly acids) that may be present in the blood. An elevated anion gap acidosis indicates the presence of unmeasured acids which are titrating and lowering the bicarbonate levels, without chloride changes. This is called a normochloremic metabolic acidosis. A normal anion gap in the face of an acidosis means that bicarbonate levels have dropped and chloride levels have increased as compensation. This is called a hyperchloremic metabolic acidosis.

Parts of the blood gas report

pH = Inverse of the H^+ concentration. An increased pH means an alkalosis (low levels of acid) and a decreased pH indicates an acidosis (high levels of acid). An acidemia and/

or alkalemia refer to the H^+ concentration in the ECF, and acidosis/alkalosis refer to the condition of having a blood pH alteration.

PCO_2 = Concentration of dissolved CO_2 molecules in the blood. It can be arterial, venous, or mixed.

HCO_3 = Concentration of bicarbonate ions in the blood.

AG = Anion gap.

BE = Base excess refers to the amount of strong acid or base required to bring the blood pH back to 7.4. Typically, a negative value (base deficit) means a metabolic acidosis, meaning more base, is needed to normalize blood pH. If the base excess is high, then base needs to be taken away to normalize blood pH, indicating an alkalosis (Table 19.5).

Stepwise approach to blood gas analysis

Approaching blood gas reports systematically will help make analyzing and interpreting the data more efficient in a critical situation. The following steps should be followed every time you read a blood gas analysis.

1. Consideration is first given to pH. Is the patient normal, acidemic (pH < 7.35), or alkalemic (pH > 7.45)?

Table 19.5 Arterial and venous blood gas normals

	Dog	Cat	Elevation?	Decrease?	Normal
Arterial					
pH	7.35–7.45	7.35–7.45	Alkalosis	Acidosis	NA
pCO_2 (mmHg)	35–45	35–45	Respiratory acidosis	Respiratory alkalosis	NA
HCO_3 (mEq/L)	19–23	17–21	Metaolic alkalosis	Metabolic acidosis	NA
AG (mEq/L)	12–24	13–27	*Normo*chloremic metabolic acidosis		*Hyper*chloremic metabolic acidosis
Venous					
pH	7.35–7.45	7.35–7.45	Alkalosis	Acidosis	NA
pCO_2 (mmHg)	35–45	35–45	Respiratory acidosis	Respiratory alkalosis	NA
HCO_3 (mEq/L)	19–23	17–21	Metaolic alkalosis	Metabolic acidosis	NA
AG (mEq/L)	12–24	13–27	*Normo*chloremic metabolic acidosis		*Hyper*chloremic metabolic acidosis

2. Next, evaluate the respiratory component! Is the respiratory component normal or does that patient have a respiratory alkalosis and hypocapnia ($PaCO_2 < 35\,mmHg$) or a respiratory acidosis and hypercapnia ($PCO_2 > 45\,mmHg$)?

3. Evaluate the metabolic component. Is the metabolic component normal or does that patient have a metabolic acidosis ($HCO_3 < 18\,mmol/L$ or base deficit $<-4\,mEq/L$), or metabolic alkalosis ($HCO_3 > 24\,mmol/L$ or base deficit $>+4\,mEq/L$)?

4. If possible, we need to determine which component (respiratory or metabolic) is the primary contributor. Generally, the pH will vary in the direction of the primary disorder. The other component is the secondary or compensatory component attempting to restore pH to normal.

5. Examine the PaO_2; does the PaO_2 show hypoxemia ($PaO_2 < 80\,mmHg$, assuming breathing room air)?

6. Consider clinical picture and history (Wingfield and Raffe 2002).

Metabolic acidosis

Metabolic acidosis is defined as a low blood pH, decreased HCO_3 concentration, and a compensatory drop in PCO_2. There are two different ways to classify metabolic acidosis; either by the anion gap/chloride levels, or by their relationship to loss of bicarbonate or addition of acid. The chloride/anion gap classification is more commonly used. Let us discuss the loss of HCO_3/addition of acid classification briefly. A titrational acidosis refers to an increase in exogenous or endogenous acids, such as lactate, ketones, or uremic acids, which cause titration and loss of free HCO_3 in the plasma. A secretional acidosis refers to loss of HCO_3-rich fluid, such as in diarrhea, or proximal renal tubular acidosis (DiBartola 2006). The chloride/anion gap relationship is more commonly used.

A metabolic acidosis either has an increased anion gap, a decrease in HCO_3^- without compensatory increase in Cl^- concentrations, or a normal anion gap, where bicarbonate ions are lost but chloride ions increase to keep the AG normal. The former is called a normochloremic metabolic acidosis, and the latter is called a hyperchloremic metabolic acidosis. In this case, the Cl^- value is added to the information on a blood gas report to give information about chloride status. The increased AG metabolic acidosis results from the addition of endogenous or exogenous acids. Causes include ethylene glycol intoxication, salicylate intoxication, ketoacidosis, uremic acidosis, lactic acidosis. The normochloremic metabolic acidosis results from loss of HCO_3-rich fluid. The causes are more obscure but include diarrhea, proximal and distal renal tubular acidosis, and hypoadrenocorticism (DiBartola 2006).

Patients with metabolic acidosis will compensate by increasing their minute ventilation, and potentially exhibiting a classic respiratory pattern of deep regular breaths, called Kussmaul's respirations. Metabolic acidosis in itself can cause cardiovascular dysfunction by decreasing cardiac output, hypotension, reduced contractility, and down-regulation of B-adrenergic receptors (DiBartola 2006). Acidosis can also cause venous vasoconstriction, with a shift in the oxyhemoglobin dissociation curve to the right, causing increased oxygen unloading to tissues. In addition, acidosis causes insulin resistance, and hyperkalemia, caused by intracellular exchange of H^+ ions for K^+ ions (DiBartola 2006).

Treatment of metabolic acidosis is typically achieved with treatment of the underlying cause. Many acidoses will normalize with fluid therapy (especially lactic acidosis). In diabetic ketoacidosis (DKA), reduction in ketone levels will normalize the blood pH.

The use of bicarbonate therapy has fallen out of favor, but there are still guidelines for its use. Most sources advocate using sodium bicarbonate only when blood pH is less than 7.1 and/or bicarbonate levels <10 mEq/L several hours after fluid therapy (Holowaychuk and Martin 2006). However, most acidotic patients do not require bicarbonate therapy. If the decision is made to administer bicarbonate, several approaches exist. Calculation of the amount of bicarbonate needed is usually carried out by using the following formula:

$$0.3 \times BW \ (kg) \times base \ excess = mEq \ of \ bicarbonate \ needed.$$

Typically, that amount can be given in small aliquots in a slow bolus, and the rest added to the IV fluids while the pH is constantly monitored (Hopper and Silverstein 2009). Complications with bicarbonate administration include induction of metabolic alkalosis, hypernatremia, hypocalcemia, respiratory acidosis, and hypokalemia or worsening of hypokalemia (Hopper and Silverstein 2009).

In addition, hypoventilation can worsen acidosis tremendously as CO_2 is retained. Thus, in critical patients, where metabolic acidosis is common, hypoventilation should be avoided at all costs. As acidosis can have detrimental side effects, controlling ventilation may be necessary in the hypoventilating, severely acidotic patient.

Metabolic alkalosis

A metabolic alkalosis is defined as an increased blood pH, an increased HCO_3 concentration, and a compensatory increased pCO_2 level (DiBartola 2006). Metabolic alkalosis is typically described by either a loss of chloride-rich fluid or administration of exogenous base. Loss of Cl^- ions can occur with vomition of gastric contents (loss of HCl), diuretic therapy (causing Cl^- loss), and hyperaldosteronism and hyperadrenorcorticism (hypernatremic metabolic alkalosis) (DiBartola 2006; Hopper and Silverstein 2009). Administration of base is rare and can follow chronic administration of sodium bicarbonate or phosphorus binders (DiBartola 2006). A common cause of hypochloremic metabolic alkalosis are patients with a pyloric foreign body, as their vomition is mainly stomach contents.

Treatment of hypochloremic metabolic alkalosis often consists of replacing the chloride levels via 0.9% NaCl fluids. The other types of metabolic alkalosis (those that would not respond to chloride administration such as hyperadrenocorticism) typically will not resolve until the underlying disease process is treated or resolved.

Respiratory acidosis

Laboratory features. Respiratory acidosis is defined as a decreased blood pH, elevated pCO_2 level, and low HCO_3 levels. It is usually always a sign of ventilatory failure (DiBartola 2006). There are numerous causes of respiratory acidosis, and they can be generalized into different categories. Extrapulmonary causes include neuromuscular disease (myasthenia gravis, botulism, polyradiculoneuritis, tick paralysis, tetanus, hypokalemia) and respiratory depression (head trauma, intracranial disease, drug-induced) causes (DiBartola 2006). The pulmonary causes include airway obstructions (e.g., laryngeal paralysis, brachycephalic syndrome, feline allergic airway disease, mass, or tracheal collapse) and small airway diseases (e.g., acute respiratory distress syndrome (ARDS), chronic obstructive pulmonary disease (COPD), pulmonary edema, pneumonia, pulmonary fibrosis, pulmonary thromboembolism) (DiBartola 2006). Finally, chest wall trauma, pleural space disease, and diaphragmatic hernia can cause respiratory acidosis. Respiratory acidosis can be acute or chronic. Most causes of this type of acidosis are acute (trauma, pulmonary disease). However, certainly bracycephalic breeds can have a chronic respiratory acidosis, as well as patients with COPD or Pulmonary fibrosis.

Patients with a respiratory acidosis will typically exhibit a reduced respiratory rate, or shallow, ineffective respirations. Hypoxemia is caused by hypoventilation, and this is the most serious consequence. Hypercapnia will cause tachycardia, hypoxemia, vasodilation, shifting of the oxyhemoglobin dissociation curve to the right, and an increase in cerebral blood flow and ICP (DiBartola 2006).

Treatment includes treatment of underlying disease (removing pleural obstructions, airway obstructions) and removal of CO_2, for which mechanical ventilation is often required. In this situation, increasing tidal volume, respiration rate, or minute volume will help clear CO_2 faster. Supplying oxygen will invariably help with the hypoxemia but not necessarily resolve the hypercapnia.

Respiratory alkalosis

Respiratory alkalosis is defined as an elevated blood pH, subnormal pCO_2 concentrations, and decreased HCO_3 levels. Hyperventilation is the most common category and can have pulmonary and non-pulmonary causes. Pulmonary causes usually induce hyperventilation as a result of hypoxemia. These include ARDS, pulmonary thromboemboli (PTE), pulmonary edema, and pneumonia. Causes of hyperventilation as a result of hypoxemia can also include anemia, CHF, and right to left shunts. Non-hypoxemia-related hyperventilation causes include exercise, pain, fear, anxiety, heatstroke, steroid administration, CNS disease, liver disease, and iatrogenic overventilation (DiBartola 2006). Respiratory alkalosis is an uncommon primary problem. One can often see this condition in a patient that has certainly been hyperventilating in response to some underlying condition but it is not a common acid–base abnormality.

Treatment is aimed at resolving underlying issues and providing oxygen, controlling respiration rate, or administering oxygen carrying capacity support (Table 19.6).

Mixed disorders

Mixed disorders contain a derangement from the typical presentations of each disorder. Some will have a normal pH in the face of an acid–base alteration, indicating a "normalizing" effect. Mixed acid–base disorders can bring pH to normal if you combine an acidosis and an alkalosis. They can be numerous and can take on just about any form you can think of. There can be respiratory-metabolic acidosis, respiratory-metabolic alkalosis, respiratory-metabolic acidosis/alkalosis, and vice versa, normal plus high anion gap metabolic acidosis, mixed high or mixed normal anion gap metabolic acidosis, or even triple disorders.

The key is understanding the physiological response to each disorder. For example, if patients have pneumonia and hypotension, they may have a respiratory acidosis and a metabolic acidosis (lactic acidosis). If their pH is quite low, and the HCO_3 is low, they have, by definition, a metabolic acidosis. If the pCO_2 is high, they have, by definition, a respiratory acidosis. Therefore, such patients have a mixed disorder. If patients have low HCO_3 level, indicating a metabolic acidosis, and low pCO_2 level from panting, they may have a normal pH, indicating a mixed respiratory alkalosis and metabolic

Table 19.6   Compensation in acid-base disturbances

	Primary disorder	Expected change	Compensatory change
Metabolic			
Metabolic acidosis	*Decrease in HCO$_3$*	PCO$_2$ will decrease by 0.7 mmHg for every 1 mEq/L increase in HCO$_3$	
Metabolic alkalosis	*Increase in HCO$_3$*	PCO$_2$ will increase by 0.7 mmHg for every 1 mEq/L increase in HCO$_3$	
Respiratory			
Respiratory acidosis (acute)	*Increase in pCO$_2$*	HCO$_3$ will increase by 0.15 mEq/L for every 1 mmHg increase in pCO$_2$	
Respiratory acidosis (chronic)	*Increase in pCO$_2$*	HCO$_3$ will increase by 0.35 mEq/L for every 1 mmHg increase in pCO$_2$	
Respiratory alkalosis (acute)	*Decrease in pCO$_2$*	HCO$_3$ will decrease by 0.25 mEq/L for every 1 mmHg decrease in pCO$_2$	
Respiratory alkalosis (chronic)	*Decrease in pCO$_2$*	HCO$_3$ will decrease by 0.55 mEq/L for every 1 mmHg decrease in pCO$_2$	

acidosis. Formulas can also be used to identify the expected compensation based on a given disorder. If the compensatory mechanism is not met, there is a mixed disorder. The presence of a normal pH with non-normal pCO$_2$ or HCO$_3$ indicates the suspicion for a mixed disorder.

Acid–Base Case Examples

1. A 6-year-old obese (7.2 kg) FS Chihuahua presents with PU/PD, lethargy, anorexia, and vomiting. Her rectal temperature is 99.8 F, HR 180 bpm, RR 60 bpm, and MM/CRT very tacky, pink, and CRT 3 seconds. The patient has a blood glucose of 600 mg/dL, positive urine ketones, is 7% dehydrated with a decreased skin turgor, has a Doppler blood pressure of 75 mmHg, and has the following blood gas results:

   pH: 7.21 (7.35–7.45)
   pCO$_2$: 24 mmHg (35–45)
   HCO$_3$-: 12 mEq/L (18–24)

   Identify the acid–base abnormality, its cause, and compensation.

   Answers: This patient has a metabolic acidosis, most likely the result of both ketoacids and lactic acids, and has a decreased pCO$_2$ (hyperventilation) as compensation.

2. Analyze the following blood gas abnormalities:

    a. pH: 7.31, pCO_2: 50 mmHg, HCO_3: 24 mEq/L
    b. pH: 7.5, pCO_2: 22 mmHg, HCO_3: 19 mEq/L
    c. pH: 7.2, pCO_2: 20 mmHg, HCO_3: 12 mEq/L
    d. pH: 7.55, pCO_2: 60 mmHg, HCO_3: 25 mEq/L

Answers:

    a. Primary reparatory acidosis with secondary metabolic alkalosis.
    b. Primary respiratory alkalosis with with no compensation.
    c. Primary metabolic acidosis with secondary respiratory alkalosis.
    d. Primary metabolic alkalosis with secondary respiratory acidosis.

References

Cohn, L. et al. 2007. Response of healthy dogs to infusions of human serum albumin. *American Journal of Veterinary Research* 68(6):657–663.

Concannon, KT. 1993. Colloid oncotic pressure and the clinical use of colloidal solutions. *Journal of Veterinary Emergency Critical Care* 3(2):49–62.

Cooper, J, Webster, CRL. 2006. Acute liver failure. *Compendium on Continuing Education for the Practicing Veterinarian* 28(7):498–515.

Cortes, YE, Moses, L. 2007. Magnesium disturbances in critically ill patients. *Compendium on Continuing Education for the Practicing Veterinarian* 29(7):420–427.

DiBartola, SP. 2006. *Fluid, Electrolyte, and Acid-Base Disorders in Small Animal Practice*, 3rd ed. St. Louis, MO: Elsevier Saunders.

Hammond, TN, Holm, JL. 2009. Limited fluid volume resuscitation. *Compendium on Continuing Education for the Practicing Veterinarian* 31(7):309–318.

Hansen, B, DeFrancesco, T. 2002. Relationship between hydration estimate and body weight change after fluid therapy in critically ill dogs and cats. *Journal of Veterinary Emergency Critical Care* 12(4):235–243.

Holowaychuk, MK, Martin, LG. 2006. Misconceptions about emergency and critical care: metabolic disease and intensive care medicine. *Compendium on Continuing Education for the Practicing Veterinarian* 28(6):434–448.

Holowaychuk, MK, Martin, LG. 2007. Review of hypocalcemia in septic patients. *Journal of Veterinary Emergency Critical Care* 17(4):348–358.

Hopper, K, Silverstein, D. (eds) 2009. *Small Animal Critical Care Medicine*. St. Louis, MO: Elsevier Saunders.

Jandrey, KE. 2010. *Colloids and Coagulopathies: Is Hydroxyethylstarch a Cause?* ACVIM 2010 Conference Proceedings.

Luschini, MA. et al. 2010. Incidence of ionized hypocalcemia in septic dogs and its association with morbidity and mortality: 58 cases (2006–2007). *Journal of Veterinary Emergency Critical Care* 20(4):406–412.

Martin, LG et al. 1994. Abnormalities of serum magnesium in critically ill dogs: incidence and implications. *Journal of Veterinary Emergency and Critical Care* 4(1):15–20.

Mathews, KA, Barry, M. 2005. The use of 25% human serum albumin: the outcome and efficacy in raising serum albumin and systemic blood pressure in critically ill dogs and cats. *Journal of Veterinary Emergency Critical Care* 15(2):110–118.

Tonozzi, CC. et al. 2009. Perfusion versus hydration impact on the fluid therapy plan. *Compendium on Continuing Education for the Practicing Veterinarian* 31(12): E1–E14.

Vigano, F. et al. 2010. Administration of 5% human serum albumin in critically ill small animal patients with hypoalbuminemia: 418 dogs and 170 cats (1994–2008). *Journal of Veterinary Emergency Critical Care* 20(2):237–243.

Wingfield, WE, Raffe, M. (eds) 2002. *The Veterinary ICU Book*. Jackson,WY: Teton NewMedia.

Anesthesia and Analgesia

Jennifer K. Sager

Introduction

Patients presented to the emergency room face a variety of physiological and psychological issues relating to their systemic health. The consideration for anesthesia, tranquilization, and pain management should take into account not only the basic fundamentals of general anesthesia, but also an understanding of the current disease or metabolic state that could alter the effectiveness of a chosen anesthetic protocol.

Table 20.1   ASA classification status (*Source*: Tranquilli et al. 2007)

ASA class	Definition
I	Normal, healthy
II	Mild systemic disease—no functional limitations
III	Moderate to severe systemic disease—some functional limitations
IV	Severe systemic disease—incapacitating or threat to life
V	Moribund—not expected to survive with or without surgery

Preanesthetic Preparation

Preanesthetic preparation for the emergent or critical patient may be limited to a few minutes, or a few hours, depending on the stabilization of the systemic disease or injury. The common goals during this period are to evaluate the patient's physical status, maximize hemodynamic stability, choose an appropriate drug plan, and assess the patient's need for analgesia. The American Society of Anesthesiologists (ASA) Physical Status Classification System is helpful in determining the overall status of the patient and potential risk involving anesthesia (Carroll 2008) (Table 20.1).

A thorough physical examination should be performed, with a focus on the patient's cardiovascular, respiratory, and neurologic status. All anesthetic drugs will have an effect on a patient's cardiac output (CO), ventilation, or central nervous system (CNS); therefore, any abnormalities in heart rate (HR), blood pressure (BP), respiratory rate, respiratory effort, and level of consciousness should be immediately identified. Once the above primary systems have been assessed and stabilized, secondary evaluations of the other body systems, involving liver and kidneys, should be performed. This will aid in fluid and electrolyte resuscitation, and will help to determine the severity of any underlying metabolic disease (Tranquilli et al. 2007). Preanesthetic laboratory tests should include a complete blood count (CBC), serum chemistry (including electrolytes), and activated clotting time (ACT) at a minimum. In addition, to adequately assess a patient's acid–base status, a venous or arterial blood gas, including lactate, should be performed. More extensive diagnostic tests may include prothrombin time (PT), partial thromboplastin time (PTT), and blood type/blood crossmatch, as well as thoracic and abdominal radiographs or ultrasound.

In addition to a complete physiological evaluation, the patient's behavior should be considered for adjunctive preoperative sedation or analgesia. Changes in behavior can be indicative of severe systemic disease or a response to pain. An anxious patient can be hard to restrain and appropriately evaluated for therapy (Dyson 2000). The increase in stress level, even if it is due to restraint for such benign procedures as catheter placement, can lead to an influx of catecholamine from the adrenal glands, effectively increasing the chances of cardiac arrhythmias, myocardial oxygen demand, and intraoperative morbidity (Macintire et al. 2005).

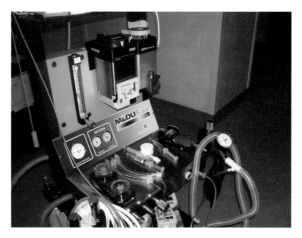

Figure 20.1 A typical anesthesia machine used at a veterinary practice with a non-rebreathing circuit.

Equipment and Monitoring

An anesthetic machine is made of several components vital to the distribution of mixed gases to the patient necessary for general anesthesia (Fig. 20.1). Prior to the invention of this machine, and its components, anesthesia was delivered via liquid drops over a face-mask. Thankfully, we can utilize equipment necessary to stabilize our patient's depth or response to anesthesia and monitor vital body systems.

Simplistically, the typical anesthesia machine contains gas cylinders providing the patient with 100% oxygen, and flowmeters to determine the amount of gas delivered to the patient in liters/minute, and a precision vaporizer (isoflurane, sevoflurane, or desflurane) to turn liquid anesthetic into a gas state (McKelvey and Hollingshead 2000). Breathing systems are chosen dependent on patient weight, with <10 kg animal often placed on a non-rebreathing system, and >10 kg on rebreathing or circle system. Other equipment necessary would include a laryngoscope to facilitate intubation, a face mask for pre-oxygenation of 100% oxygen beneficial in some systemic disease, and endotracheal tubes to maintain a patent airway.

Intraoperative patient monitoring should include electrocardiogram (ECG) to observe cardiac rate and rhythm. An ultrasonic Doppler can be placed along the carpus or tarsus to hear the HR, and aid in indirect BP measurements, with use of a sphygmomanometer and BP cuff. Capnography is beneficial to assess respiratory rate and indirectly determine ventilation status via end-tidal carbon dioxide pressure ($ETCO_2$). Pulse oximetry can be used to determine oxygen saturation, and more invasive monitors can be used such as arterial catheters and central venous pressure (CVP) measurements. Please refer to chapter on patient monitoring for more information (Fig. 20.2).

Mechanical Ventilation

Due to systemic disease, trauma, or pharmacologic influence, an anesthetized patient may require assistance to maintain adequate ventilation and perfusion. The act of ventilation consists of two phases, active and passive, more commonly expressed as inhalation and

CHAPTER 20

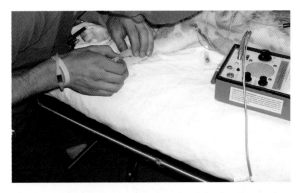

Figure 20.2   An anesthetist places a 20g catheter in the dorsal pedal artery for continuous direct blood pressure monitoring of a canine patient during splenectomy.

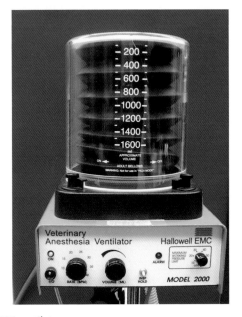

Figure 20.3   A Hallowell 2000 ventilator.

exhalation, respectively. An increase in arterial carbon dioxide levels ($PaCO_2$) triggers the expansion of the thorax via stimulation of the intercostal muscles and diaphragm, creating a negative pressure, resulting in air moving into the airway passages (inhalation). Once the lungs have reached capacity, the CNS system triggers the relaxation of the intercostals muscles and diaphragm, causing the lungs to deflate (exhalation). Most patients will hypoventilate under general anesthesia, due to the respiratory depressant effects of injectable and inhalation agents. In order to maintain adequate $PaCO_2$ levels of 35–45 mmHg, and avoid hypoxemia (PaO_2 levels below 60 mmHg), manual ventilation or intermittent positive pressure ventilation (IPPV) through the use of a mechanical ventilator may be required (Fig. 20.3).

There are several types of small animal ventilators that can be used in conjunction with the anesthesia machine to control the patient's breathing. The type of ventilator can

Table 20.2   Common veterinary ventilators

Ventilator	Power source	Drive Mechanism	Cycling Mechanism	Bellows	Type of Ventilation	Special Features
Drager SAV	Pneumatic	Pneumatic	Time-fluidic	Ascend	Control	Not currently being manufactured; constantly maintains positive-end expiratory pressure (PEEP) pf 2 cm H2O
Hallowell EMC 2000	Pneumatic; electronic	Pneumatic	Time-electronic	Ascend	Control	Three sizes of bellow attachments; use with anesthesia machine
Ohmeda 7000 (7800)	Pneumatic; electronic	Pneumatic	Time-electronic	Ascend	Control	Two bellow assembly; 7000-set by minute ventilation, 7800-set by tidal volume
Mallard 2400V	Pneumatic; electronic	Pneumatic	Time-electronic	Ascend	Control	Controlled by microprocessor
Bird Mark-7	Pneumatic	Pneumatic	Time-electronic	None	Control	Single circuit ventilator; vary inspiratory pressure to 60 mmH20 and inspiratory sensitivity
ADS 1000 Critical Care Ventilator	Pneumatic; electronic	Pneumatic	Time-electronic	None	Control	No bellows, not intended for connection to anesthesia breathing system. Microprocessor determines levels depending on patient's body weight

be classified depending on power source, drive mechanism, and cycling mechanism (pressure, timed, or volume). Most ventilators have a power source that employs electricity, compressed gas, or both. The drive mechanism is most often described as a double circuit, with two gases used to compress the bellows and deliver the oxygen and gas to the patient inside the bellows. The bellows within a ventilator can be ascending or descending, with most current models utilizing ascending bellows.

A *pressure cycled ventilator* will supply air during inspiration until the pressure reaches a predetermined level. A disadvantage of this type of ventilator is that tidal volume delivered may decrease due to a decrease in lung compliance. A *timed cycle ventilator* is set according to a set inspiratory time, and the volume cycle typed delivers a volume regardless of the inspiratory pressure.

Most ventilators can be set with a maximum inspiratory pressure to ensure safety of the patient, as well as controls for tidal volume, I:E ratio, and respiratory rate. An initial setting for these controls include a tidal volume of 10–20 mL/kg, an I:E ratio of 1:2–1:3, and a respiratory rate of 8–10 bpm. Adjustments can then be made from there by monitoring $PaCO_2$, PaO_2, $ETCO_2$, and pH perioperatively.

All ventilators should be attached to a scavenge system, and hooked to the driving gas, oxygen supply, before hooking to the patient. The most common types of ventilators found in small animal veterinary practices include the Drager SAV Small Animal ventilator, Hallowell EMC Model 2000 (Hallowell EMC, Pittsfield, MA), Ohmeda 7000 Electronic Anesthesia Ventilator (Teollisuuskatu, Helsinki, Finland), and Mallard 2400 V Small Animal Anesthesia Ventilator (Mallard Medical, Inc., Redding, CA) and the Bird Mark-7 Ventilator (Carefusion, San Diego, CA). The ADS 1000 Veterinary Anesthesia Delivery System (Engler Engineering Corp., Hialeah, FL) is a single circuit ventilator that functions as a nonrebreathing circuit for critical patients (Table 20.2).

Pain Management

Oftentimes, animals are presented to the emergency room experiencing some level of pain (Fig. 20.4). According to the International Association for the Study of Pain, the definition of pain is an unpleasant sensory and emotional experience associated with actual or potential tissue damage (Lamont et al. 2000). In order to provide appropriate therapeutics, it is necessary to understand pain physiology, its subsequent nociceptive response, and to be able to appropriately assess pain.

Pain can be categorized as physiologic or pathologic. Physiologic pain is the body's initial recognition of pain produced by a noxious stimulus resulting in minimal tissue damage (Carroll 2008). This type of pain acts as defense mechanism to alter behavior between the body and environment, and is usually not evident in a clinical setting. Pathologic pain, or clinical pain, occurs with chronic activation or alteration of nociceptors, peripheral nerve endings that initially signal pain following tissue injury (Lamont et al. 2000). Pathologic pain can be acute (recently occurring) or chronic (long-lasting), and can occur without the presence of a noxious stimulus (idiopathic or spontaneous pain),

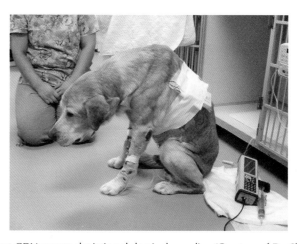

Figure 20.4   A dog post GDV surgery depicting abdominal guarding (Courtesy of Dr. Sheilah Robertson).

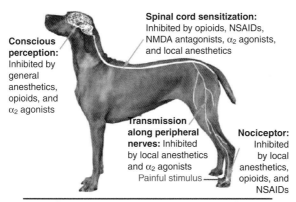

Conscious perception: Inhibited by general anesthetics, opioids, and α_2 agonists

Spinal cord sensitization: Inhibited by opioids, NSAIDs, NMDA antagonists, α_2 agonists, and local anesthetics

Transmission along peripheral nerves: Inhibited by local anesthetics and α_2 agonists

Painful stimulus

Nociceptor: Inhibited by local anesthetics, opioids, and NSAIDs

▲ The different classes of analgesic drugs work at different locations in the pain pathway. With multimodal analgesia, a synergistic response can be achieved by targeting these different locations.

Figure 20.5   Line drawing of the components of the nocioceptive pathway.

in an exaggerated response to a noxious stimulus (*hyperalgesia*), or as a response to a benign stimulus (*allodynia*) (Tranquilli et al. 2007).

The transmission of pain begins with specialized sensory nerve endings called *nociceptors*. In response to an external stimulus, these nociceptors will begin the process of transduction, transmission, and modulation of the neural signal, resulting in the perception of pain (Lamont et al. 2000) (Fig. 20.5).

To simplify a complex neurologic pathway, pain is processed in three steps. The first step, referred to as first-order neuron, involves the *transduction* of mechanical, thermal, or chemical energy by nociceptors into electrical impulses. These impulses are *transmitted* along primary afferent A (fast, myelinated, sharp pain) and C (slow, unmyelinated, dull pain) fibers to the dorsal horns of the spinal cord. Within the dorsal horn neurons, the signal is modulated and divided into three separate populations: inhibitory or excitatory neurons, propriospinal neurons, or projection neurons. These signals form the second-order neurons, following several ascending tracts, with synapses in various regions of the midbrain, medulla, pons, and thalamus. Here the transmission is *modulated* into three separate populations, and transmitted along a third path (third-order neuron) to a high somatosensory area of the brain, resulting in the *perception* of pain (Matthews 2000).

Pain assessment is subjective. Various physiological and behavioral responses occur with the perception of pain (Robertson and Hellyer 2004). Increases in HR, BP, vasoconstriction, myocardial oxygen demand, and respiratory rate can be observed as a stress response in the cardiopulmonary system (Lamont et al. 2000). Other observable changes may include a decrease in gastrointestinal (GI) tone, increase in pupil size, hyperglycemia, and increases in catecholamine and cortisol production (Lamont et al. 2000). However, some of these physiological changes can be affected by the patient's response to a strange environment and administration of drugs (e.g., opioids can cause mydriasis in cats), and should not be the sole indicator of pain (Robertson and Hellyer 2004). It may be beneficial to observe the patient's behavior and utilize a pain scoring system that can include a visual analog scale and a numerical rating scale (Tranquilli et al. 2007). These tools can be used to quantify certain behaviors, such as wound sensitivity, to determine the severity of a patient's pain, but can also be subjective according to the observer. Therefore, the pain scale must be appropriate for the patient, designed to meet their specific needs. Two of the most popular pain assessment tools are the Glasgow Composite Measures Pain Scale and the University of Melbourne Pain Scale, which utilize a descriptive set of phrases and categories to determine a patient's pain score (Robertson and Hellyer 2004). An alternative model of pain assessment is the Colorado State University Pain Scale. This scale can be used for both canine and feline patients, whereas the Glasgow model is only used in pain assessment for dogs (Robertson and Hellyer 2004). The Colorado State University Pain Scale is a combination of pictures and phrases used to evaluate the patient's psychological and behavioral attitude, as well as response to touch and body tension.

Once the pathologic pain has been assessed, several therapeutic agents are available, dependent on the patient's systemic health. *Preemptive analgesia*, or applicable premedicant therapy administered before exposure to a noxious stimulus, is helpful in minimizing postoperative pain. Balanced or *multimodal anesthesia* is the use of different therapeutic agents to modulate the transmission of pain along different points of the physiologic pain pathway (Tranquilli et al. 2007). This can be achieved by using different local and regional techniques such as local infiltrative blocks, epidurals, constant rate infusions (CRIs) or combining the effects of the aforementioned techniques, or in using different drugs with different mechanisms of action (Fig. 20.6).

Opioids, local anesthetics, nonsteroidal anti-inflammatory drugs (NSAIDs), N-methyl-D-aspartate (NMDA) antagonists, and alpha-2 agonists are the most commonly used drugs in pain management therapy (Muir et al. 2000). Opioids (e.g., morphine, methadone, hydromorphone, oxymorphone, butorphanol, fentanyl, remifentanil, buprenorphine) act on receptors located in the peripheral and CNS, inhibiting the release of excitatory neurotransmitters. The three opioid receptors known as mu, kappa, and delta

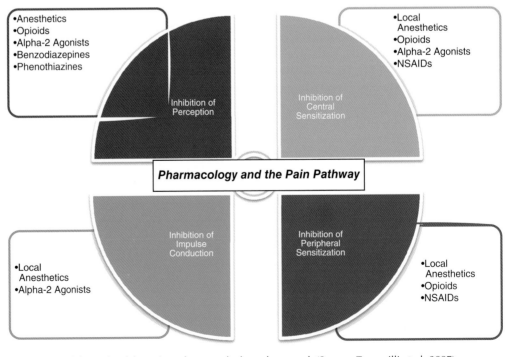

Figure 20.6   Schematic of the pain pathway and where drugs work (Source: Tranquilli et al. 2007).

are primarily responsible for analgesia (Carroll 2008) (see sections on "Opioids" and "Alpha-2 Agonists" for more specific information).

Alpha-2 agonists receptors are located peripherally and centrally along the physiologic pain pathway. These drugs (e.g., dexmedetomidine, medetomidine, xylazine) act to hyperpolarize the cell due to activated g-proteins, causing the cell to become less responsive to sensory input (Tranquilli et al. 2007).

Local anesthetics (e.g., lidocaine, mepivicaine, bupivacaine, ropivicaine) act by decreasing the membrane permeability of sodium ions, preventing conduction of nerve impulses. Their uses include topical anesthesia, infiltrative anesthesia, peripheral nerve blockade, and epidural injection. Because these drugs are typically weak bases, their effectiveness changes based on the pH of the environment. If more acid is present, then more ionized drug is made, and the effectiveness decreases. Conversely, if they are injected into an alkaline environment, their effectiveness increases. This is why adding sodium bicarbonate to lidocaine allows for increased onset time and reduced pain on injection. It can usually be diluted 1:9 sodium bicarbonate to lidocaine.

NSAIDs (carprofen, firocoxib, meloxicam) act by blocking prostaglandin synthesis, through inhibition of COX-1 and COX-2 enzymes, those responsible for the production of inflammatory cells used in the nociceptive transduction of pain (Tranquilli et al. 2007). COX-1 enzymes aide in homeostatic functions, such as platelet aggregation and renal autoregulation, whereas COX-2 enzymes are associated more with the inflammatory process (Robertson and Hellyer 2004). Short-term use is variable among species and specific target enzyme, and deemed relatively safe; long-term therapy can attribute to GI toxicity (Robertson and Hellyer 2004). NSAID toxicity has been a fear in cats due to differences in the glucuronidation pathway, which can lead to a slower metabolism of the drug, prolonged side effects, and drug accumulation (Matthews 2000).

Anesthestic Drug Pharmacology

"There are no safe anesthetic agents...only safe anesthetists." Robert Smith

Premedicants

Most anesthetic plans begin with a premedication to help sedate or calm the anxious patient, prevent pain, aid in muscle relaxation, and decrease the amount of intravenous and inhalant anesthetics needed to maintain general anesthesia. The most common categories of premedicants are anticholinergics, phenothiazines, benzodiazepines, opioids and alpha-2 agonists. Response to any drug used can be unpredictable, especially when a patient is critically ill. However, administration of these drugs in combination with each other can facilitate a less stressful environment for a patient.

Anticholinergics

Anticholinergic or parasympatholytic drugs act on various muscarinic receptors found in the parasympathetic system. Muscarinic receptors can be found in the CNS, sinoatrial (SA), and atrioventricular (AV) node of the myocardium and in the smooth muscle of the GI tract. These drugs act to prevent acetylcholine from binding to the various receptor sites, thereby reducing the effects of the parasympathetic system (Tranquilli et al. 2007). Two of the most commonly used anticholinergic drugs in practice are atropine and glycopyrrolate.

Anticholinergics can be used as part of a preoperative anesthetic plan to manage bradycardia associated with an increase in vagal tone due to surgical manipulation, preexisting bradycardia, or reflexive bradycardia associated with administration of other anesthetic drugs such as opioids. However arrhythmias and subsequent sinus tachycardia can occur, leading to an increase in myocardial oxygen demand and an increase in workload of the heart (not beneficial in some cardiac disease). Anticholinergics also decrease intestinal motility and lowers esophageal sphincter tone, leading to potential postoperative GI complications, such as gastroesophoageal reflux (Tranquilli et al. 2007). Anticholinergics can also be used preoperatively to help dry secretions, acting on the muscarinic receptors found in the salivary glands and respiratory tract. This can aid in intubation of smaller animals, such as cats, or those prone to airway obstructions, such as brachycephalic breeds. Anticholinergics are typically recommended in brachycephalic breeds who may be have higher resting vagal tone as well as pediatric patients (12 weeks of age and under) who are highly dependent on HR to maintain CO and BP.

Atropine can be given SQ, IM, or IV (see Table 20.2), and has a quicker onset of action than glycopyrrolate (Carroll 2008). Atropine is the drug of choice in an emergent bradycardia because it is rapidly absorbed after both IM and IV administration. The peak effects of atropine can be seen within 1–5 minutes and the duration of action about 60 minutes. At a dose range of 0.02–0.04 mg/kg, atropine will increase the conduction of nerve transmissions through the AV node, increasing HR (Tranquilli et al. 2007). However, at subtherapeutic doses, <0.02 mg/kg IV, atropine can delay transmission through the AV node, causing a transient second degree AV block or worsening bradycardia. Atropine has been noted to produce a mild sedation, but has little effect in the CNS. Atropine affects the muscles surrounding the eye, causing a persistent mydriasis; therefore, caution is warranted in glaucoma patients. Atropine does affect the GI system, by acting on specific muscarinic receptors in the smooth muscle, causing a decrease in motility; therefore, it is not widely used in large animals, as colic may result. Atropine crosses the blood brain and placental barriers (Muir et al. 2000).

Glycopyrrolate has similar pharmacokinetic properties as atropine (see Table 20.2 for dosages). It is rapidly absorbed, and has the same affinity for the muscarinic receptors in the cardiovascular, GI, and respiratory systems (Tranquilli et al. 2007). Glycopyrrolate has a longer onset of action, with peak effects between 5–7 minutes if administered IV and has a longer duration of action (60–90 minutes). Unlike atropine, glycopyrrolate does not produce a sedative effect within the CNS, is less likely to produce a tachycardia, and does not cross the blood–brain or placental barrier (Muir et al. 2000). Similarly to atropine, subtherapeutic doses may cause a transient second-degree AV block or worsening bradycardia (Table 20.3).

Phenothiazines

One of the most commonly used drugs in practice is acepromazine, a phenothiazine derivative that acts as a tranquilizer and can produce some mild sedation, muscle relaxation, but does not contain any analgesic properties. 2-acetyl-10-phenothiazine or acepromazine maleate is water soluble and has alpha-1 antagonist, beta-1 antagonist, and dopamine antagonist properties, whose primary mode of action is suppression of the reticular activating system in the CNS. This leads to a period of sedation that typically

Table 20.3 Typical dose ranges for various anesthetic agents (Adapted from Tranquilli et al. 2007; Carroll 2008; Bryant 2010)

Drug	Classification	Route	Bolus Dose	Constant Rate Infusion (CRI) Dose
Acepromazine	Phenothiazine	SQ, IM, IV	0.01–0.05 mg/kg	–
Atropine	Anticholinergic	SQ, IM, IV	0.02–0.04 mg/kg	–
Glycopyrrolate	Anticholinergic	SQ, IM, IV	0.01–0.02 mg/kg	–
Diazepam	Benzodiazepine	IV	0.2–0.5 mg/kg	0.2–0.5 mcg/kg/h
Midazolam	Benzodiazepine	SQ, IM, IV	0.2–0.5 mg/kg	0.2–0.5 mcg/kg/h
Morphine	Pure mu-opioid agonist	IM, SQ	0.1–1 mg/kg (canine) 0.05–0.2 mg/kg (feline)	0.05–0.1 mg/kg/h
Oxymorphone	Pure mu-opioid agonist	IM, SQ, IV	0.05–0.2 mg/kg	
Hydromorphone	Pure mu-opioid agonist	IM, SQ, IV	0.05–0.2 mg/kg	
Methadone	Pure mu-opioid agonist	IM, SQ, IV	0.1–0.5 mg/kg	0.05–0.1 mg/kg/h
Fentanyl	Pure mu-opioid agonist	IM, SQ, IV	2–5 mcg/kg	0.03–1 mcg/kg/min
Remifentanil	Pure mu-opioid agonist	IV	Do not bolus	0.03–1 mcg/kg/min
Bupenorphine	Partial mu-opioid agonist	IM, SQ, IV	0.01–0.03 mg/kg	0.04 mg/kg/day
Butorphanol	Agonist/antagonist	IV, IM, SQ	0.1–0.4 mg/kg	0.1 mg/kg/h
Nalbuphine	Agonist/antagonist	IV, IM, SQ	0.1–0.4 mg/kg	
Dexmedetomidine	Alpha-2 agonist	IM, IV	1–5 mcg/kg	1–5 mcg/kg/h
Atipamazole	Alpha-2 antagonist	IM	Equal volume of dexmedetomidine	
Propofol	Injectable anesthetic	IV	2–10 mg/kg slow	100–400 mcg/kg/min
Etomidate	Injectable anesthetic	IV	0.5–2 mg/kg	

(*Continued*)

Table 20.3   (*Continued*)

Drug	Classification	Route	Bolus Dose	Constant Rate Infusion (CRI) Dose
Thiopental	Injectable anesthetic	IV	2–20 mg/kg	–
Ketamine	Injectable anesthetic	IM-cats only, IV	5 mg/kg	2–10 mcg/kg/min
Tiletamine/ zolazepam (telazol)	Injectable anesthetic	IM, IV	5–10 mg/kg	–
Alphaxalone	Injectable anesthetic	IV, IM	2 mg/kg slowly	4–11 mg/kg/h

lasts a duration of 1–2 hours, longer if combined with an opioid (Tranquilli et al. 2007). Drug duration is unpredictable, varying from patient to patient; however, and in some cardiovascular compromised or pediatric patients, the effects can last up to 24 hours post administration (see Table 20.2 for common dosages and routes of administration). There is no antagonist for acepromazine; therefore, it is not a reversible drug and should be used with caution.

The cardiopulmonary effects of acepromazine have been studied extensively in small animals. The most common side effect noted is vasodilation, due to alpha-adrenergic blockade, resulting in a decrease in arterial blood pressure (ABP). At 0.1 mg/kg IV, it has been noted in conscious animals that a 20%–25% drop in CO and stroke volume, resulting in a reduction of mean arterial pressure (MAP) of 20%–30% (Shih et al. 2010). In anesthetized patients (primarily cats and dogs), the effects of the administration of acepromazine can be influenced by the type of inhalant anesthetic used. Studies have shown that a dose of 0.1 mg/kg IV of acepromazine in combination with halothane causes a reduction in MAP between 10% and 16% (Tranquilli et al. 2007). However, when combined with the use of isoflurane, the administration of acepromazine produces a more dramatic effect on the cardiovascular system, with a reduction in MAP between 20% and 30%.

Therefore, lower doses and close monitoring of the anesthetized patient after receiving acepromazine is warranted, and should be avoided in hypovolemic and hypothermic patients or those not able to tolerate its cardiovascular effects. Acepromazine does not have a notable effect on a patient's HR and antagonizes the effect of epinephrine-induced arrhythmias (Tranquilli et al. 2007). No direct changes have been noted in the pulmonary system, such as a decrease in respiratory rate, or change in the acid–base status of small animals, when given acepromazine.

Acepromazine has been noted to reduce the incidence of vomiting when given 15–20 minutes prior to an administration of an opioid such as morphine, hydromorphone, or oxymorphone (Carroll 2008). However, acepromazine can have an effect on the hematologic status of patients by causing splenic engorgement and a subsequent drop in packed cell volume, or PCV. For this reason, the drug is typically a poor choice for the splenectomy patient. Previous thoughts that acepromainze may inhibit platelet aggregation have recently been called into question.

Metabolism of phenothiazines occurs in the liver, and it has been noted that the sedative effects of acepromazine can be present for up to 48 hours in patients with compromised liver function (Muir et al. 2000). For this reason, acepromazine is typically avoided in patients with immature hepatic function (pediatrics) and those with liver failure. There are some reports of a lowering in seizure threshold after the administration of acepromazine, but there is not conclusive evidence supporting or refuting this theory (Carroll 2008).

Use of acepromazine is beneficial in healthy animals with ample cardiac reserves requiring sedation for routine, elective procedures. It is labeled for small and large animals, and can be given SC, IM, or IV. The administration of acepromazine in a critically ill, geriatric, or neonate patient should be avoided due primarily to its alpha-antagonistic vasodilatory effects.

Benzodiazepines

Benzodiazepines (midazolam and diazepam) are commonly used as a premedicants in compromised or critically ill patients. These drugs do not act as a sedative, instead as a tranquilizer, causing central muscle relaxation with little decompensation of the cardiopulmonary system. Benzodiazepines act primarily in the CNS by influencing the effects of the inhibitory neurotransmitter gamma aminobutyric acid (GABA) (Tranquilli et al. 2007). The influence of agonism at the GABA receptor result in not only a mild calming effect and muscle relaxation, but also acts as an anticonvulsant. However, benzodiazepines do not contain any analgesic properties, and therefore should not be used as a treatment for pain.

Benzodiazepines, as well as many other drugs used in anesthesia, are listed as controlled substances, regulated by the federal government, and logs of use must be maintained by the anesthetist. Controlled substances are categorized or scheduled, according to abuse potential, on a scale of C1–C5. Drugs listed as a CI (marijuana, heroin) are at high risk for abuse potential and those with a CV (codeine) are least likely to merit abuse.

Diazepam (CIV) is a non-water-soluble formulation of propylene glycol and ethanol. Because of the propylene glycol, the drug can be irritating upon IM injection, can cause phlebitis and pain upon IV administration, and should not be mixed in the same syringe with other agents as a precipitate will form (e.g., butorphanol). Additionally absorption of diazepam via IM or SQ routes is poor and unpredictable and therefore is typically avoided. Diazepam does not produce a sedative effect in young or healthy animals; however, it can produce a calming effect in geriatric, neonate/pediatric, or critically ill patients. It has been noted that at higher doses, 0.5 mg/kg IV, excitement and dysphoria can result, as well as aggressive behavior in cats (Tranquilli et al. 2007). Therefore, diazepam is rarely used alone, but in combination with another injectable anesthetic, such as ketamine or propofol, or in combination with an opioid for neuroleptic anesthesia to ensure a smooth induction of anesthesia (see Table 20.2 for common dosages).

Diazepam is rapidly distributed throughout the body, with a half-life noted to be between 2 and 5 hours, depending on a dose range of 0.2–0.50 mg/kg IV (Tranquilli et al. 2007). Diazepam reduces the amount of inhalant anesthetic requirements upward of 20%–30% in dogs, and has been known to synergistically enhance the effects of other general anesthetics such as barbiturates or propofol (Tranquilli et al. 2007). Diazepam does not alter HR or CO, and does not have a marked effect on MAP. However, studies have shown rapid intravenous administration of diazepam can cause an initial bradycardia and hypotension (Muir et al. 2000). Diazepam does not have an effect on the respiratory rate or tidal of the patient. It increases the seizure threshold, therefore making it popular as an anticonvulsant, and has not been noted to have an effect on ICP. Diazepam, along with the other benzodiazepines, is metabolized by the liver and should be used with caution in patients with liver dysfunction and carefully in those with immature hepatic function (e.g., neonates) (McKelvey and Hollingshead 2000). Due to its insolubility with water, diazepam cannot be mixed with other medications, otherwise, a precipitate will result; the exception to this is ketamine. The propylene glycol base can also interfere with certain laboratory tests, such as those used to detect ethylene glycol poisoning (Wingfield 1997).

Midazolam (CIV) and diazepam differ slightly in its characteristics and properties; therefore, the same caution should be exercised when using alone in healthy animals, as excitement may result. Midazolam is water-soluble; therefore, IM injection is less painful than diazepam and has a greater absorption rate than diazepam. Midazolam is distributed quickly throughout the body, and can be mixed with other medications other than ketamine, such as opioids, without fear of precipitation (Muir et al. 2000). Midazolam has similar side effects as diazepam, with little influence on the cardiopulmonary system, and does not have any analgesic properties. It has a greater sedative effect than diazepam and can solely be administered IM or IV at a wide range of 0.1–0.3 mg/kg, or in combination with an opioid as a premedicant or ketamine to induce general anesthesia (see Table 20.2).

Zolazepam (CIV) is also a water-soluble benzodiazepine similar to midazolam, but it is found in combination with a dissociative anesthetic, tiletamine, to produce Telazol (see section on "Induction Agents/Injectable Anesthetics").

Benzodiazepines are antagonized by the drug flumazenil, 0.04 mg/kg IV (Muir et al. 2000). This can be appropriate with patients who have severe hepatic disease, as reversal of the benzodiazepines can alter a patient's level of consciousness, returning them to a more normal state of function (Carroll 2008). Caution should be exercised when reversing the effects of a benzodiazepine, if it has been administered in conjunction with other drugs, such as ketamine. If the effects, such as muscle relaxation, of diazepam are antagonized, the patient may experience severe muscle rigidity and dysphoria upon emergency from anesthesia (Carroll 2008)

Opioids

Drugs that contain a formulation of the naturally occurring compound opium are known as opioids. These compounds are synthetically manufactured in various forms and are controlled via federal regulations due to potential abuse. The schedule of opioids ranges from CII (morphine and similar synthetic derivatives) to CIV (butorphanol).

Opioids are used primarily for pain management and can contain some sedative qualities as well (Tranquilli et al. 2007). There are three main receptor classifications for opioids: mu, delta, and kappa. Interactions with drugs at these specifics sites are responsible for central and peripheral analgesia, with the mu receptor the main site for analgesia for small animals such as dogs and cats. Opioids can be categorized according to the mu receptor, in which they primarily agonize or antagonize, and they are termed mu-agonists (morphine, hydromorphone, oxymorphone, methadone, fentanyl, remifentanil, and meperidine), partial mu-agonists (buprenorphine), and mu-agonist/antagonists (butorphanol, nalbuphine).

Tramadol, a non-opioid, mu-agonist is increasing in popularity for use in chronic pain management therapy. It acts by inhibiting norepinephrine uptake, similar to an antidepressant, but does exhibit side effects similar to mu-agonist opioids (Carroll 2008). Tapentadol is another newer centrally acting analgesic with a dual mode of action as an agonist at the μ-opioid receptor and as a norepinephrine reuptake inhibitor that may become useful in dogs and cats in future years. Clinical experience with the agent is currently lacking.

Although their primary function is to relieve pain, opioids have several side effects that could affect a patient's overall systemic health. In addition to pain relief, opioids can cause varying degrees of behavioral changes, miosis or mydriasis, histamine release, vomiting and regurgitation, and changes to nociceptive stimulation (Tranquilli et al. 2007). A recently published study about opioids addressed the concern about immunosuppressive effects on a variety of patients, including cats, dogs, birds, and humans (Odunayo et al. 2010), the results of which indicated that in a laboratory setting, chronic administration of opioids, such as morphine, interfered with the function of T cells, bone marrow, and other inflammatory mediators, and in some cases caused an increase in infection (Odunayo et al. 2010). Therefore, caution should be exercised in use with patients that are immunocompromised, such as diabetics, septic, and those undergoing chemotherapy treatments. Further research into this subject is underway.

Routes of administration for opioids can vary from SQ, IM, and IV, and some preservative-free formulations of opioids, more specifically morphine, can be administered in epidurals. Some opioids can also be used as a CRI for long-term effects. Buprenorphine has excellent bioavailability when given via the transmucosal route in cats and perhaps dogs as well. Bradycardia can result from the administration of some opioids, but significant changes in stroke volume, CO, and BP typically do not occur, making them good choices for the critically ill. Opioids can depress the respiratory system at higher doses or pediatric patients, resulting in hypoventilation and hypercapnia (Wingfield 1997).

There are species-dependent changes in the CNS system, ranging from CNS depression in dogs and potential CNS excitement in cats. Opioids can also interfere with the body's homeostatic regulation by influencing receptors in the medulla, causing both hyperthermia and hypothermia. Hyperthermic changes in cats have been increasingly linked to the CNS excitement caused by opioids, most commonly with hydromorphone. This phenomenon does not appear to occur with oxymorphone. Opioids can also affect the GI system, with the most common side effect being salivation, regurgitation, emesis, and defecation. The urinary system is also not left unaffected, as some opioids can cause urine retention, oliguria, or dieresis, depending on which opioid receptor has been targeted. Opioids will cross the placental barrier, and therefore should be used with caution in cesarean sections, but most effect can be reversed with the administration of antagonist such as naloxone or butorphanol.

Naloxone and naltrexone are pure mu-antagonists used to antagonize the effects of specific opioids. However, antagonism of the mu receptor will not only reverse the potential undesirable side effects of the opioid, such as bradycardia and respiratory depression, but also the analgesia as well. If a patient is experiencing cardiopulmonary depression, a titration of naloxone at a dose of 1–5 mcg/kg IV can be used until the patient begins to arouse, usually within 2–10 minutes (Carroll 2008). Supplemental analgesia is recommended for painful patients in these cases, as the analgesic effects of the opioids will also be removed. Butorphanol, a mixed kappa agonist/mu-antagonist, can be used to reverse the effects of pure mu-agonists such as morphine and hydromorphone, keeping some of the analgesic effects intact via maintained activity at the kappa receptor site.

CHAPTER 20

Alpha-2 agonists

Alpha-2 adrenergic agonists are a group of agents used to decrease sympathetic outflow in the CNS, by agonizing the alpha-2 receptors peripherally and in the CNS; this results in a decrease of catecholamine release, muscle relaxation, and oftentimes profound sedation. It can also afford potent analgesic effects through the stimulation of the alpha-2 receptors in the CNS, and can produce synergistic effects when combined with other drugs such as opioids (Carroll 2008). Alpha-2 agonists such as dexmedetomidine, medetomidine, and xylazine are similar in function, but vary in duration of action. Xylaine, however, is uncommonly used in dogs and cats at this point because of excessive side effects. Alpha-2 agonists can be given SQ, IM, IV, or epidurally to provide regional analgesia.

Stimulation of the alpha-2 adrenergic receptors can cause profound effects on the cardiopulmonary system. The decrease in sympathetic outflow can cause a sinus bradycardia, commonly with an HR of 20–40 bpm, with an occasional atrioventricular blockade (Tranquilli et al. 2007). Stimulation of the peripheral receptors can cause an increase in peripheral vascular resistance, leading to an initial increase in MAP, and pale mucus membranes. The combination of bradycardia and increased peripheral vascular resistance decreases the patient's overall CO (CO = HR × SV) by nearly 50%. Some have questioned whether the decreases in CO seen by alpha-2 agonists may impair delivery of oxygen to tissue (DO_2). Therefore, its use in cardiac compromised patients, or those in cardiogenic shock, is strongly discouraged. Extremely small doses of dexmedetomidine (e.g., 0.5–2 mcg/kg), however, may have slightly less profound cardiovascular effects and may have a growing role in the critical care setting when used as an intravenous bolus or CRI.

Depression of the respiratory center with alpha-2 agonists is also observed, with a decrease in overall tidal volume and respiratory rate. Some patients can experience stridor or an increase in effort after administration; therefore, proceed with caution in a brachycephalic breed. Alpha-2 agonists can affect the GI system by suppressing gastric motility, inducing vomiting, and reducing esophageal reflexes or the ability to swallow (Muir et al. 2000). Alpha-2 receptors in the pancreas, when stimulated, can suppress insulin release, resulting in an increase in blood glucose levels; therefore, itsuse in diabetic patients is contraindicated. Alpha-2 agonists cross the placental barrier, and xylazine has been associated with oxytocin-like activity or premature birth in some large animal (Tranquilli et al. 2007).

Antagonism of alpha-2 adrenergic receptors can be achieved with the administration of yohimbine or atipamazole. These alpha-2 antagonists are receptor-specific (α-1 or α-2), and can be used to reverse undesired side effects of these drugs. Yohimbine will antagonize xylazine, and atipamazole can be used to reverse dexmedetomidine and medetomidine. Although alpha-2 antagonists can be given IV, atipamazole or yohimbine should typically be given IM to avoid profound cardiovascular effects.

Induction Agents/Injectable Anesthetics

Propofol/Propofol 28

Propofol is a common drug in practice for rapid intravenous induction and maintenance of general anesthesia. Propofol is classified as a nonbarbiturate, and acts upon the GABA neurotransmitter causing sedation, slight hypnosis, and unconsciousness. It does not deliver any analgesic properties, and patients can often be aroused easily by nociceptive stimulation (Tranquilli et al. 2007). Propofol is formulated as an aqueous emulsion, and can promote bacterial growth if left opened and unused after 6 hours; therefore, it is recommended to discard unused portions daily (Carroll 2008). A new formulation of propofol (Propofol 28 by Abbott Laboratories, North Chicago, IL) has recently been released that includes antimicrobial preservatives that provide the drug with a shelf-life of 28 days. Presently, it appears the drug's clinical profile is identical to previous propofol formulation, but further experience with the drug is needed. The drug also appears to be safe for anesthesia induction in cats; however, as the product contains benzyl alcohol, it should not be given repeatedly or used for total intravenous anesthesia (TIVA).

Single boluses of propofol can be given IV at a range of 2–10 mg/kg and used as a short-term CRI to maintain general anesthesia at 200–400 mcg/kg/min. Recovery from a single bolus injection can occur within 20–30 minutes. Propofol does not change the HR, nor is it highly arrhythmogenic, but can cause significant vasodilation and decreases in cardiac inotropy. Vasodilation commonly leads to a decrease in MAPs, resulting in hypotension. Propofol can cause apnea upon rapid injection and more severe respiratory depression can occur at higher doses (Muir et al. 2000). To mitigate these side effects, the drug is generally administered slowly over 60–90 seconds. It is important to understand that because of these cardiovascular and respiratory side effects, propofol may be a poor choice or even unsuitable in many critical patients. The drug should be selected wisely with the understanding that speed of a drug does not necessarily equate to increased safety.

Propofol does decrease cerebral blood flow and cerebral metabolic rate of oxygen consumption ($CMRO_2$); therefore, it does not significantly increase intracranial pressure (ICP) (Tranquilli et al. 2007). Propofol is not only metabolized by the liver, but also undergoes extraheptic metabolism via the lungs and kidneys, and is rapidly distributed throughout the body. Propofol is beneficial for cesarean sections because of this rapid distribution, leading to minimal fetal depression. The agent is typically considered safe for use in patients with hepatic or renal dysfunction and in pediatrics. Other side effects include pain upon injection and myclonus, which can be minimized by the use of premedicants. Research studies have shown long-term infusions may lead to Heinz body formation in cats (Tranquilli et al. 2007).

Etomidate

Etomidate is a propylene glycol-based, imidazole derivative, which is used to induce general anesthesia. It primarily acts through enhancement of the inhibitory neurotransmitter GABA, and depresses the reticular formation of the brain stem, causing hypnosis and unconsciousness (Allen et al. 1998). It is classified as a rapid-acting, noncumulative, nonbarbiturate intravenous anesthetic agent, and does not provide analgesic properties (Muir et al. 2000). Typical dose range is from 1 to 2 mg/kg IV titrated to effect following benzodiazepine administration. Etomidate does not exhibit any changes in CO, stroke volume, or myocardial contractility; nor is there any appreciable change in HR or MAP. Etomidate does not sensitize the heart to catecholamine-induced arrhythmias, and unlike some opioids, does not produce a histamine release (Wingfield 1997). Administration does not have an effect on the patient's respiratory drive, although it has been noted that a brief period of apnea can occur directly after induction. Patients will often maintain a gag reflex or cough upon intubation. Patients induced with etomidate can experience a brief period of myoclonus; however, administration of an intravenous benzodiazepine as part of the induction can greatly reduce the skeletal muscle excitement.

Etomidate is a popular drug of choice in neurological patients because it can decrease the $CMRO_2$, and likely has some anticonvulsant properties due to its interaction with the GABA complex (Tranquilli et al. 2007). Etomidate is rapidly metabolized and distributed by the liver, heart, kidneys, and spleen. Etomidate does cross the placental barrier, but is rapidly cleared, so side effects are often minimal (Muir et al. 2000). Other side effects of etomidate include pain upon injection, due to propylene glycol, inhibition of natural adrenocorticoid production, and long-term infusions that can cause hemolysis of the red cells. The inhibition of adrenal function has raised concern in past years about the drug's use in septic and critically ill patients. More recent human literature suggests that this concern is likely overstated. Carboetomidate and other etomidate derivatives are being developed which do not inhibit adrenal function. These agents may allow for long-term infusions of etomidate-like drugs in the future.

Dissociatives

An NMDA antagonist, classified as a dissociative agent, is another form of injectable anesthesia; two most commonly utilized in practices are ketamine and tiletamine (Carroll 2008). Dissociative drugs, rather than depress neurologic function, produce an anesthetic state by interrupting the transmission of signals along the pathways relating to consciousness. Activation of NMDA receptors has been linked with hyperalgesic responses to pathologic pain (Tranquilli et al. 2007). Subsequently, antagonism of these sites by ketamine and, to a lesser extent, tiletamine, offers a degree of somatic analgesia (Tranquilli et al. 2007). Dissociative agents can have a profound effect in the cardiovascular and neurological system of the body. Dissociatives can mimic sympathomimetic effects such as increased HR, vascular smooth muscle dilation, increased myocardial oxygen demand, and inhibition of catecholamine uptake. Vasodilation can also lead to an increase in cerebral blood flow, increasing ICP, and cerebral metabolic rates (Tranquilli et al. 2007).

Ketamine, the most common of the dissociative drugs, is a highly controlled substance (CIII) due to abuse potential. It is a rapid onset nonbarbiturate, which lasts 15–20 minutes when given in a single IV bolus at 5–7 mg/kg, and can be useful for maintenance anesthesia for short procedures. It can be given IM or IV in cats, and can be painful upon injection due to a low PH (Carroll 2008). It is not recommended for IM administration in dogs. Ketamine is extensively metabolized by the liver in dogs; however, in cats, it is excreted unchanged by the kidneys (Carroll 2008). Patients with urinary obstructions or in the stages of renal failure should probably avoid ketamine, due to the decrease in glomerular filtration rate (GFR) and longer recovery time. Ketamine can cause skeletal excitement when administered alone, leading to a poor recovery period; therefore, it is recommended to combine ketamine 5 mg/kg with another drug, such as a benzodiazepine, or α-2 agonist, such as dexmedetomidine, to facilitate muscle relaxation (Allen et al. 1998). Ketamine can be administered as a CRI for adjunctive analgesia at 2–10 mcg/kg/min. Ketamine increases CO by increasing HR, MAP, and myocardial contractility, and should be used with caution in patients with cardiovascular disease such as hypertrophic cardiomyopathy (HCM) or dilated cardiomyopathy (DCM). Furthermore, ketamine can lead to an increase in ICP due to an increase in cerebral blood flow, and is contraindicated in patients with or at risk for increased ICP due to neurologic disease. Ketamine does not depress the respiratory drive but can lead to apnea or apneustic breathing at high doses (>8 mg/kg IV) (Carroll 2008).

Tiletamine (CIII) is found in combination (1:1) with zolazepam to create the solution telazol. Tiletamine, as compared with ketamine has a longer duration of action (half-life of 1–3 hours, species dependent) and is more analgesic for painful procedures. Combined with zolazepam, tiletamine provides the patient with a smoother induction and recovery, than solely using tiletamine (Muir et al. 2000). Telazol can be given IV or IM to both cats and dogs, with a dose range of 1–6 mg/kg as a premedicant or induction agent, and is useful when dealing with aggressive cats and dogs (Carroll 2008). Human studies have reported psychosomatic effects such as hallucinations and agitation. Telazol causes profound catalepsy, amnesia, and analgesia, but the patient is hyperresponsive to noxious stimulus. Therefore, when using to aide in restraint of an aggressive animal, caution should be taken when causing a potential pain stimulus, as the patient can be aroused briefly (Tranquilli et al. 2007). Similar to ketamine, telazol can be combined with an opioid to reduce the amount needed for induction. Tiletamine also increases CO, similar to ketamine, but is more respiratory depressive than ketamine at doses greater than 15 mg/kg IV. Oftentimes, excessive salivation is noted as a side effect of telazol; therefore, caution should be used in respiratory compromised or brachycephalic breeds. Due to prolonged recovery, repeated doses of telazol are not recommended (Tranquilli et al. 2007). Telazol, more specifically only the zolazepam portion of the telazol, can be reversed using flumazenil. However, without the muscle relaxant qualities of the benzodiazepines, the patient can often arouse from anesthesia experiencing muscle contraction, dysphoria, and agitation (Muir et al. 2000).

Barbiturates

Although currently the availability is limited due to manufacture shortages, short-acting barbiturates such as thiopental (CIII), methohexital (CIV), and pentobarbital (CII) can be beneficial for patients with neurologic disease, as no increase in ICP or $CMRO_2$ has been noted with administration. Barbiturates act primarily by inhibiting GABA transmission in the nervous system, similar to propofol or etomidate, causing depression of the CNS in a dose-dependant manner (Carroll 2008).

Thiopental (2–10 mg/kg IV bolus) has a rapid onset of action and duration, and does not provide analgesia. It is metabolized by the liver, but is redistributed through fat and muscles after initial uptake in the CNS (Carroll 2008). Therefore, accumulation in these body systems can occur, prolonging recovery and exacerbating CNS effects. Caution is indicated in animals with severe liver disease, as reduced hepatic blood flow, or the reduction in P450 enzyme in sighthounds, can result in slower metabolism of thiopental (Tranquilli et al. 2007). If administered perivascularly, thiopental can cause sloughing of the skin and tissue necrosis. Thiopental can also lead to a reduction in myocardial contractility, leading to a reduction in stroke volume, and increase the incidence of cardiac arrhythmias, such as ventricular bigeminy and tachycardia (Carroll 2008). It is also contraindicated in hypovolemic patients, due to a systemic hypotension that can result from a decrease in CO, coupled with volume depletion.

Methohexital and pentobarbital are not commonly used in practice as an anesthetic agent, as the short duration of action, and lack of analgesia can lead to dysphoric recoveries. However, pentobarbital is used for humane euthanasia. The lethal dose of this drug is 20–25 mg/lb IV, and acts as an anesthetic overdose, depressing cardiovascular and pulmonary function (Muir et al. 2000).

Alphaxalone

Alphaxalone is a newer neurosteroid injectable anesthetic agent that is not yet at the time of writing available in the United States but is widely used throughout the rest of the

CHAPTER 20

world. The agent works by modulation of neuronal cell membrane chloride ion transport, induced by binding of alphaxalone to GABA-A cell surface receptors. Alphaxalone has minimal cardiovascular and respiratory depressing effects, a short duration of action, and can be administered by bolus for induction or via CRI for maintenance of anesthesia. The agent also appears safe for use in patients with renal, liver, and brain disease. Its use within the veterinary critical care setting has many applications and will hopefully be available within the United States for use in future years.

Maintenance Anesthetic Agents

Inhalant anesthetics (sevoflurane, isoflurane)

Maintenance of general anesthesia can be achieved through the use of inhalant agents in the form of a gas (nitrous oxide) or volatile liquid (isoflurane, sevoflurane, desflurane) (Tranquilli et al. 2007). The redistribution of these agents is dependent on specific pharmacokinetics of alveolar partial pressure gradients and blood-gas solubility, while the *minimum alveolar concentration*, or MAC, is a determination of the potency of an inhalation anesthetic (Carroll 2008). The lower the blood-gas solubility coefficient of an agent, the longer the agent will remain in the alveoli before entering into circulation. As a result, when the concentration of the inhalation anesthetic is high in the alveoli of the lungs, the diffusion into the blood is minimal, with the biotransformation occurring rapidly in the brain; this in turn leads to a rapid induction and recovery (isoflurane, sevoflurane, desflurane—in order of high to low blood-gas solubility coefficients). This factor may be ideal for mask or chamber inductions. Agents with a high blood-gas solubility coefficient will distribute throughout the body into various tissues, resulting in a slower onset of general anesthesia and prolonged recovery (e.g., methoxyflurane). The MAC of an anesthetic agent is the lowest concentration of drug needed to not produce a gross motor response in 50% of patients when a painful stimulus is administered; the more potent a volatile liquid, the lower the MAC.

Inhalation anesthetics have varied effects on different systems throughout the body. CO, through direct myocardial depression and reduced sympathetic activity, is influenced by the dose of the agent, concurrent drugs that may depress CO, and the duration of the anesthesia. HR is not usually affected, but vasodilation and decreases in MAP are observed regularly, especially with higher concentrations of inhalation agents (Tranquilli et al. 2007). As a result, it is critical to minimize inhalant anesthetics in both the critically ill and healthy patient alike. Some older inhalant agents (e.g., halothane) can predispose the myocardium to arrhythmias, sensitizing the heart to catecholamine release. This may be contraindicated in some surgical procedures such as an adrenalectomy; therefore, it is ideal to use lowest possible setting while maintaining an appropriate anesthetic depth or use newer inhalant agents (Carroll 2008). Besides depressing the cardiovascular system, all inhalation anesthetics depress the respiratory system in a dose-dependant manner.

Both sevoflurane and isoflurane can be used with essentially all commercially available tranquilizers, sedatives, analgesics, and injectable anesthetics (Norkus 2006). Both sevoflurane and isoflurane produce dose-dependent increases in cerebral blood flow and ICP. Clinically, however, the increased ICP observed with either drug can be effectively counteracted by minimizing hypercapnia and employing an induction technique that reduces or does not increase ICP. Both drugs have some anticonvulsant effect (Norkus 2006).

Renal blood flow (RBF) and GFRs are also reduced through the use of inhalation agents, albeit in a dose-dependant manner, and influenced by the patient's hemodynamic status throughout anesthesia. Other systemic changes linked to use of inhalation anesthetics includes liver damage, diffusion hypoxia, and skeletal muscle hyperthermia (Tranquilli et al. 2007). The administration of inhalational anesthetic agents is a precise process that utilizes specific equipment (precision vaporizers, anesthetic machine, O_2 and due diligence from personnel to lessen the risk of morbidity under anesthesia.

Neuromuscular Blocking Agents

Neuromuscular blocking agents, depolarizing and nondepolarizing, are not used routinely in emergency settings, but may be of use in patients undergoing long-term ventilation. The neuromuscular junction is the locus where nerves and muscles attach to create contraction. When a neuronal signal reaches an end terminus of a neuron, calcium channels open, allowing the free influx of calcium ions; this opening stimulates the neurotransmitter acetylcholine to travel across the synaptic cleft. Acetylcholine will bind with postsynaptic nicotinic receptors, forcing Na^+ and K^+ channels open. The influx of Na^+ ions in, and K^+ ions moving out, propagate an action potential. Acetylcholine is then rapidly hydrolyzed by acethycholinesterase, terminating the effects of acetylcholine in the postsynaptic receptor shortly after integrating with the nicotinic receptors. This protects the nerve muscle innervations from accumulation of acetylcholine leading to constant depolarization. They do not cross the blood–brain or placental barriers, and have been used in some cesarean sections as an alternative for general anesthesia. Neuromuscular blocking agents must be used with caution, since apnea can result from paralysis of intercostal muscles, requiring mechanical ventilation, as well as vigilant monitoring of the cardiopulmonary system. A peripheral nerve stimulator to evaluate the "train of four" twitch response to stimulation is helpful in determining the level of muscle paralysis.

Succinylcholine is a depolarizing neuromuscular blocking agent that mimics the effects of acetylcholine. This agent binds to nicotinic receptors, generating depolarization of the nerve-muscle fiber, but is not degraded by acetylcholinesterase, rather butyrylcholinesterase. Degredation, rather than antagonism, of succinylcholine occurs more slowly than acetylcholine; therefore, an accumulation of the agent in the neuromuscular junction will lead to constant depolarization of the muscle fiber, resulting in paralysis. Some side effects encountered with the administration of succinylcholine include hyperkalemia, malignant hyperthermia, and increased ICP.

Non-depolarizing agents, such as atracurium, pancuronium, and vecuronium competitively agonize nicotinic receptors on both pre- and postsynaptic sites. These agents will bind to Ach receptors, and unlike achethylcholine, there is propogation of the action potential, resulting in muscle relaxation. They also have many side effects including blockade of muscarinic receptors, causing sympathomimetic effects such as tachycardia, hypertension, and histamine release causing ereythema, pruritus, hypotension, and bronchoconstriction. Thus, these drugs can be antagonized by synthetic acetylcholinesterase drugs such as neostigmine and edrophonium.

Anesthetic Considerations for the Critically Ill

Cardiovascular Emergencies and Shock

Most anesthetic agents, injectable or inhalant, will have an effect on the HR, stroke volume, myocardial contractility, or vascular tone, which can significantly alter CO and BP. Patients with a preexisting cardiac disease can have either anatomical or physiologic changes to the heart, also affecting CO. The subsequent changes to the cardiovascular system can alter the delivery of oxygen to tissues vital in sustaining life. Care must be taken to determine the best combination of agents that will have minimal effect on the patient's HR, preload, afterload and contractility, all determinants in CO (Carroll 2008). Additional effort is made to minimize myocardial oxygen demand, improve diastolic filling and myocardial perfusion, and minimize patient stress resulting in catecholamine release and arrhythmias.

A thorough physical exam should be performed including ascultation for murmurs, gallop rhythms, arrhythmias, HR, lung sounds, and evaluation of pulse strength and jugular vein distension. If a patient is suspected of having cardiovascular disease, thoracic radiographs and echocardiography are beneficial in determining the severity of the disease, including the presence of congestive heart failure, risk for volume overload, and cardiac contractility. Patients without true underlining heart disease but rather in shock states should have their perfusion status maximized (e.g., volume resuscitation, pharmacological agents) before undergoing general anesthesia. Intraoperatively, both those cases with cardiac disease or shock states should be monitored closely with a direct ABP catheter, ECG, capnography, and CVP to evaluate appropriate fluid administration.

Patients with preexisiting cardiovascular disease or shock states should receive pre-oxygenation prior to anesthesia induction. Patients with concurrent cardiovascular disease typically should receive lower rates of intraoperative fluids (e.g., 2.5–5 mL/kg/h). However, patients with hemodynamic collapse (e.g., hypovolemic shock) should be aggressively fluid-resuscitated prior to anesthesia and may require increased fluid therapy perioperatively (e.g., >10 mk/kg/h) (Fig. 20.7).

Premedicants could include an opioid for pain management, with or without a benzodiazepine, for increased sedation and muscle relaxation. Acepromazine is cautioned due

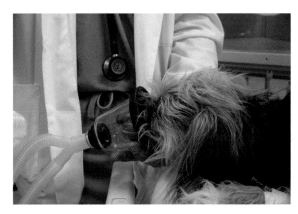

Figure 20.7   Preoxygenation of a canine patient prior to receiving propofol induction (Courtesy of Luisito Pablo, DVM, MS, DACVA, University of Florida).

to its profound vasodilatory effects, but can be beneficial in small doses in some select patients requiring a decrease in afterload (e.g., mild well-compensated heart disease). Alpha-2 agonists and anticholinergics are not routinely recommended. Induction agents can include etomidate, as this is an excellent choice with cardiovascular disease, offering no change in HR, vascular tone, stroke volume, or contractility.

Other induction options would be using a neuroleptic agent (e.g., a benzodiazepine) and an analgesic (e.g., opioid) together as a neurolepanalgesic induction to minimize hemodynamic changes in a patient. An example of this would be using intravenous fentanyl and intravenous midazolam to accomplish intubation in a critically ill patient.

Propofol can cause cardiac depression due to vasodilation, but may be appropriate in low doses for some cases with less severe heart disease. In some cases of heart disease, reduction of afterload with propofol may actually be beneficial (e.g., mild to moderate disease states that are well compensated). Propofol should be avoided in cases of shock or dehydration. Alphaxalone, where available, may also be an appropriate induction agent for patients with heart disease.

Ketamine increases HR and contractility, but can cause myocardial depression in critically ill patients who have exhausted their sympathetic reserves. The drug is not recommended in hypertrophic or hypertensive disease states and should be used selectively in shock states. Some dogs with mild heart disease that is well compensated may be able to tolerate the effects of ketamine.

Inhalants such as sevoflurane and isoflurane cause cardiovascular depression in a dose-dependant manner; therefore, it is recommended to lower the amount of inhalant, by providing injectable drugs in a multimodal approach. An opioid CRI, such as fentanyl up to 48 mcg/kg/h with or without midazolam up to 0.48 mg/kg/h is a popular choice with cardiac-compromised patients (Carroll 2008).

Generally, inadequate tissue perfusion, sometimes accompanied by hypotension, can be classified as shock; this can be related to blood loss (hemorrhagic shock), decreased cardiac function (cardiogenic shock), sepsis (septic shock), or related to changes in vascular integrity (anaphylactic, neurologic shock). For hemorrhagic shock during anesthesia, administration of colloids such as hetastarch (max 20 mL/kg/day) or whole blood at a rate of 5 mL/kg/h is beneficial for patients experiencing acute blood loss due to surgery. IV hypertonic saline at 4–6 mL/kg IV bolus has been proven beneficial by increasing plasma volume concentrations, thereby increasing MAP and CO. It is also useful in head trauma patients to reduce the risk of cerebral edema (Tranquilli et al. 2007). The use of inotropic or vasopressor support such as ephedrine (0.01–0.05 mg/kg IV bolus) or phenylephrine (0.15 mg/kg IV bolus, 0.5–1.0 mcg/kg/min CRI) can be indicated to increase peripheral vasoconstriction, shunting blood to the body's major organs. Caution should be used with inotropic therapy (e.g., dopamine, dobutamine) in patients with underlying cardiovascular disease, as stimulation of the b-adrenergic receptors can directly affect myocardial contractility, HR, and function (Tranquilli et al. 2007).

Respiratory Emergencies

The function of the pulmonary system is to oxygenate the blood via the exchange of oxygen and carbon dioxide in the alveoli of the lungs. This complex feedback ventilation control system is influenced by many factors and alterations in such things as oxygen and carbon dioxide tension, rate, sensory input, and thermoregulation. To adequately assess a patient's ventilation and subsequent perfusion, an arterial blood gas can be evaluated

CHAPTER 20

to examine the arterial carbon dioxide partial pressure ($PACO_2$), arterial oxygen partial pressure (PAO_2), and pH levels.

Most anesthetic drugs will depress respiratory rates and rhythms, further declining the patient's pulmonary function. Patients with respiratory disease should be stabilized with oxygen support via nasal cannulas or oxygen cages. Thoracic radiographs should be performed to assess severity and type of disease. Alpha-2 agonists, barbiturates, opioids, and inhalant anesthetics are respiratory depressants in a dose-dependant manner. Phenothiazines and benzodiazepines have minimal effect on respiratory function. Preoxygenation via face mask with 100% oxygen, rapid sequence induction (RSI), and rapid intubation is necessary to stabilize the airway and begin ventilation.

Drugs used for RSI include ketamine/benzodiazepine combinations, propofol, thiopental, alphaxalone, and etomidate. Neuroleptic analgesic inductions and inhalant mask inductions are contraindicated for these patients. Controlled or mechanical ventilation is safe, but should be kept at a low peak inspiratory pressure to avoid postexpansion pulmonary edema. Pulse oximetry to measure oxygen hemoglobin saturation, and end-tidal CO_2 to indirectly measure $PaCO_2$ levels, are more tools designed to aid in evaluation of the patient's ventilation during anesthesia. Patients with respiratory emergencies should also be monitored via direct ABP catheter and ECG.

Neurological Emergencies

Neurological disease can elicit a variety of signs, depending on the location of the lesion within the nervous system. Cerebellar disease can result in seizures, behavioral changes, and sensory deficits (Carroll 2008). Cerebellar disease can lead to ataxia, tremors, and vestibular signs. Brainstem lesions can cause changes to mentation, behavior, cranial nerve, and postural deficits. Spinal cord lesions can cause upper and lower motor neuron signs depending on the location of the lesion, whereas peripheral nerve disease causes lower motor neuron signs.

Determining the origin of the lesion is done by performing diagnostic imaging (e.g., magnetic resonance imaging [MRI]) of the brain and or spinal tract. Keeping $CMRO_2$ low and minimizing ICP will hopefully minimize the chance of cerebral ischemia or brain herniation (Tranquilli et al. 2007). To minimize increases in ICP, excitement, coughing, and vomiting should be avoided. Patients should be evaluated primarily to determine changes in cardiovascular or respiratory function, as a result of a lesion in the brain or increase in intracranial hemorrhage causing pressure within the tissues. Patients should be restrained with care, as pressure on the jugular veins can increase ICP.

Acepromazine is cautioned due to controversy of whether or not acepromazine will decrease the seizure threshold or alter BP. Additionally, the agent is not reversible. Benzodiazepines are routinely used as anticonvulsants, and would be beneficial to patients experiencing seizures or skeletal muscle rigidity, due to its ability to increase the seizure threshold, and cause minimal changes in ICP (Carroll 2008). Opioids can be used for pain management, but vomiting can increase ICP; therefore, the use of butorphanol (0.1–0.3 mg/kg IV) or methadone (0.1–0.5 mg/kg IV), instead of morphine or hydromorphone, which commonly cause vomiting, may be warranted (Muir et al. 2000).

Induction agents can include barbiturates such as thiopental (4–10 mg/kg IV bolus), offering no change in $CMRO_2$ or ICP, etomidate 1–2 mg/kg IV after benzodiazepine administration, alphaxalone, or propofol (4–6 mg/kg IV bolus) because it, too, has minimal changes in ICP (Tranquilli et al. 2007). Ketamine increases HR and contractility, and can lead to an increase in ICP through direct increase in MAP as well as lower the seizure threshold; therefore, it is not recommended in most neurologically compromised patients. Small doses of lidocaine (e.g., 1 mg/kg) are sometimes included as part of the induction technique in dogs to reduce the chance of coughing. The effectiveness of this technique in dogs and cats is debatable.

Both sevoflurane and isoflurane can contribute to increased ICP and therefore, a balanced anesthesia technique including a propofol CRI at 200–500 mcg/kg/min with or without a fentanyl CRI may be used in place of or in conjunction with inhalational anesthetics, especially as maintenance for general anesthesia in MRI cases with suspected brain injury (Carroll 2008). When used, inhalants should be kept to the lowest amount possible (below MAC), and careful attention should be paid to ventilation. Hypercapnia and hypocapnia must be avoided. Hypertonic saline is optimal for fluid support during resuscitation to decrease the chance of cerebral edema. Mannitol, a diuretic, at 0.5–1 gm/kg IV over 20 minutes and methylprednisolone sodium succinate (MPSS) can also be administered if cerebral edema is suspected.

GI Diseases

The most common GI emergencies requiring anesthesia are gastrointestinal dilation volvulus (GDV) and foreign body obstruction. These patients typically have some degree of hypovolemia, electrolyte/acid–base abnormalities, and pain.

A GDV patient should immediately undergo decompression of the stomach via orogastric tube placement and external trocarization (gastrocentesis) of the stomach through a large bore needle. Oftentimes, these patients present in distress, are laterally recumbent, and in shock. Cardiac dysrhythmias, such as ventricular premature depolarizations or ventricular tachycardia, are noted due to an increase in catecholamine release, myocardial ischemia, and splenic contraction. The engorged stomach can also displace the diaphragm, causing a decrease in pulmonary reserve capacity. Electrolyte imbalances, such as hypokalemia, are often reported as a result of lactic acid metabolism. Patients should be stabilized aggressively before anesthesia is performed.

Rapid access to the airway is important to maintain ventilation of a patient; therefore, propofol to effect IV after 0.2 mg/kg IV diazepam is one option in very stable GDV cases. Etomidate IV to effect after a benzodiazepine can be used in cardiovascular-compromised patients. Alphaxalone, where available, may also be an appropriate induction agent. Lidocaine at 2 mg/kg IV bolus followed by a 40–75 mcg/kg/min CRI can be used to treat ventricular tachycardia. Ketamine IV to effect after 0.2 mg/kg IV diazepam or midazolam is another acceptable induction for the stable and sick GDV alike. Preoperative administration of pure mu-agonists such as morphine 0.3–0.5 mg/kg or hydromorphone 0.05–0.1 mg/kg can be given IV, rather than IM, to reduce the incidence of vomiting. Opioids can be used intraoperatively for analgesia, and as part of a balanced technique to reduce the level of inhalants necessary to maintain anesthetic depth; fentanyl up to 48 mcg/kg/h with or without midazolam up to 0.48 mg/kg/h can be considered (Carroll 2008). NSAIDs are typically withheld for analgesia in the postoperative period to not potentially alter a damaged GI tract.

Reproductive

Anesthetic management for a cesarean section must take into account the altered metabolic and physiologic state of the dam and the effect of drugs across the placental barrier

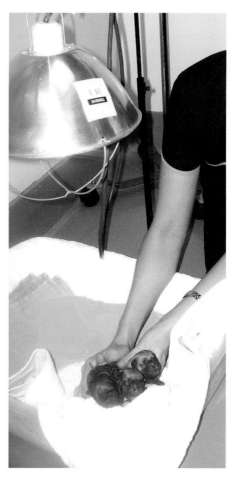

Figure 20.8   French bulldog puppies delivered via emergency cesarean section due to prolonged dystocia.

(Fig. 20.8). During gestation, CO is increased due to increases in HR and stroke volume (CO = HR × SV) (Tranquilli et al. 2007). MAP is oftentimes unchanged due to a decrease in vascular resistance from the circulating hormone, estrogen, and total blood volume increases by 40%, attributing to the increase in CO. Changes in cardiac reserve are further exacerbated by an additional increase in CO during labor due to compression of the vena cava and extrusion of blood from the uterus.

Other body systems influenced by gestation and parturition include the pulmonary, hepatic, and GI system, to name a few. Increases in respiratory rates and oxygen consumption rates have been noted in the pregnant dam. However, functional residual capacity (FRC) of the lungs is decreased during pregnancy due to the displacement of the diaphragm. If during anesthesia the patient experiences hypoventilation, hypoxemia can result due to this decrease in FRC; therefore, drugs that depress the pulmonary system or respiration rate should be avoided (Tranquilli et al. 2007). Hepatic function is varied slightly by a slight decrease in plasma protein concentrations. GFRs and RBFs are increased, resulting in a decrease in blood urea nitrogen (BUN) and creatinine (CRE) concentrations. Pregnant patients are at a high risk of aspiration due to a decrease in gastric motility from physical displacement of the stomach by the uterus.

Anesthetic drugs should be chosen to compensate for the maternal physiological changes and to avoid fetal depression. Phenothiazines, benzodiazepines, alpha-2 agonists, and barbiturates readily cross the placental barrier, causing decreases in cardiac and respiratory function, as well as a decrease in physical activity during labor and post parturition (see section "Premedicants"). Propofol can lead to respiratory depression at high concentrations but is rapidly redistributed and metabolized. Inhalants cross placental barriers, causing dose-dependent cardiac and respiratory depression. Local anesthetics are used with caution due to absorption via fetal blood flow, which can cause neonatal depression. An anticholinergic, such as glycopyrrolate (atropine crosses the placental barrier), can be used to decrease salivary secretions and inhibit increases in vagal tone due to uterine contractions (Tranquilli et al. 2007).

In an ideal cesarean section, the patient should be pre-oxygenated with 100% oxygen via face mask. A fluid bolus of crystalloid fluids at 10–20/kg IV can be administered as needed to reduce hypovolemia associated with fluid loss. The patient should be pre-clipped prior to induction of anesthesia to reduce anesthetic and surgical time to facilitate delivery of puppies. Premedicants are controversial because most will cross the placental barrier causing fetal depression, but will aid in reducing maternal anxiety and aid in analgesia. Rapid induction and stabilization of an airway is important due to the risk of regurgitation and aspiration. Propofol at 4–6 mg/kg IV bolus is ideal, but if the dam is cardiovascular-compromised, this can profoundly depress the cardiovascular system. Etomidate at 1–2 mg/kg IV after benzodiazepine administration is an alternative to a propofol or barbiturate induction, which will include cardiovascular support and rapid induction. Alphaxalone, where available, may also be an appropriate induction agent for such cases. Opioids provide analgesia, and if cardiovascular or respiratory depression is of concern, can be antagonized. Bradycardia associated with opioid administration can be reduced through the use of an anticholinergic (glycopyrrolate 0.01 mg/kg IM, IV). Methadone (0.3–0.5 mg/kg IV), butorphanol (0.1–0.3 mg/kg IV), or buprenorphine (0.01–0.03 mg/kg IV) do not cause vomiting and still provide adequate pain relief. Oftentimes, adjunctive analgesia can be administered after fetal delivery to provide maternal analgesia and avoid the potential fetal depression (Tranquilli et al. 2007). Alpha-2 agonists have been linked to an increase in fetal mortality and should be avoided. Intraoperative fluid support is necessary to lower maternal hypotension due to blood loss. Prior to delivery, inotrope support with ephedrine 0.04–0.1 mg/kg IV can be used if necessary, with minimal reduction in uterine blood flow.

Pain Management in Trauma

Effective pain management in trauma is beneficial in reducing pain and patient anxiety but should be balanced with cardiopulmonary resuscitation and support (Matthews 2000). Alpha-2 agonists, opioids, NMDA antagonists, NSAIDs, and local anesthetics are primarily used in pain management protocols (see section on pathophysiology of pain).

Alpha-2 agonists have significant cardiovascular and pulmonary effects, including profound bradycardia, peripheral vasoconstriction, and hypoventilation, and increase the incidence of cardiac dysrhythmias. They are generally not selected in the acute care setting for these reasons. NSAIDs should be used with caution in renal-compromised, dehydrated, and hypovolemic patients, as decreases in RBF are a major side effect of the drug and potentially result in acute kidney injury. Gastric ulceration can also occur with prolonged exposure to NSAID therapy. NSAIDs are more beneficial in chronic pain management and should be used when the animal is stabilized, ruling out renal and GI disease.

In general, within the acute care setting, opioids are typically the safest and most effective agents for analgesia. However, it should be remembered that they may cause vomiting, regurgitation, bradycardia, respiratory depression, and hypoventilation that can potentially cause increased ICP (Wingfield 1997).

Later during the critical care setting, CRIs of opioids (e.g., morphine, fentanyl, buprenorphine) can be selected to provide continued drug without peaks and valleys of analgesia. Ketamine and/or lidocaine can also be added via CRI for additional multimodal analgesia if needed. NSAIDs can be introduced in select patients as can oral gabapentin to control neuropathic or chronic pain. Nondrug adjunctive pain control techniques such as adequate bedding, ice packing inflamed tissue, acupuncture, and tender love and care should also not be overlooked.

After analgesia, addressing anxiety in the emergency and critical care setting can be a common issue. Benzodiazepines are most appropriate to treat older and sicker patients alike. Very low doses (e.g., 0.01 mg/kg) of acepromazine may be excellent in appropriate patient populations (e.g., patients who have the cardiac reserves to tolerate the drug). Micro doses of dexmedetomidine (e.g., 0.05–1 mcg/kg) can also provide profound sedation and added analgesia in select stable patients. CRIs of dexmedetomidine at 0.05–5 mcg/kg/h can also be administered for extended effects. It is important to remember that even a low dose of alpha-2 agonists may have profound cardiovascular effects (Carter et al. 2010). When selected, they should be used with great care.

References

Allen, D, Pringle, J, Smith, D, et al. 1998. *Handbook of Veterinary Drugs*, 2nd ed. Philadelphia: Lippincott-Raven.

Bryant S. (ed.) 2010. *Anesthesia for Veterinary Technicians*, 1st ed. Hoboken, NJ: Wiley-Blackwell.

Carroll, G. 2008. *Small Animal Anesthesia and Analgesia*. Ames, IA: Blackwell.

Carter, JE, Campbell, NB, Posner, LP, et al. 2010. The hemodynamic effects of medetomidine continous rate infusions in the dog. *Veterinary Anaesthesia Analgesia* 37(3):197–206.

Dyson, D. 2000. Chemical restraint and analgesia for diagnostic and emergency procedures. In *The Veterinary Clinics of North America Small Animal Practice Managementof Pain*, Vol. 30, 4th ed., edited by Matthews, K. pp. 703–723. Philadelphia: W.B. Saunders.

Lamont, L, Tranquilli, W, Grimm, K. 2000. Physiology of pain. In *The Veterinary Clinics of North America Small Animal Practice Management of Pain*, Vol. 30, 4th ed., edited by Matthews, K. pp. 703–723. Philadelphia: W.B. Saunders.

Macintire, D, Drobatz, K, Haskins, S et al. 2005. *Manual of Small Animal Emergency and Critical Care Medicine*. Baltimore, MD: Lippincott Williams & Williams.

Matthews, K. 2000. *The Veterinary Clinics of North America Small Animal Practice Management of Pain*. Philadelphia: W.B. Saunders.

McKelvey, D, Hollingshead, KW. 2000. *Small Animal Anesthesia& Analgesia*, 2nd ed. St. Louis, MO: Mosby.

Muir, W, Hubbell, H, Skarda, R et al. 2000. *Handbook of Veterinary Anesthesia*, 3rd ed. St. Louis, MO: Mosby.

Norkus, C. 2006. Balacing act: combining inhalant anesthetics and injectable drugs. *Veterinary Technician* 12:770–780.

Odunayo, A, Dodman, J, Kerl, M et al. 2010. State-of-the-art-review: immunomodulatory effects of opioids. *Journal of Veterinary Emergency and Critical Care* 20(4):376–385.

Robertson, S, Hellyer, P. 2004. How do we know they hurt? In *Symposium on Managing Medical, Surgical, Chronic and Traumatic Pain*, edited by Pfizer. Wilmington, DE: The Gloyd Group. p. 13. abstract 1.

Shih, A, Robertson, S, Vigani, A et al. 2010. Evaluation of an indirect oscillometric blood pressure monitor in normotensive and hypotensive anesthetized dogs. *Journal Veterinary Emergency Critical Care* 20(3):313–318.

Tranquilli, W, Thurmon, J, Grimm, K. 2007. *Lumb & Jones' Veterinary Anesthesia and Analgesia*, 4th ed. Ames, IA: Blackwell.

Wingfield, W. 1997. *Veterinary Emergency Medicine Secrets*. Philadelphia: Hanley & Belfus.

Transfusion Medicine

Lindan Spromberg

Introduction

Over the past decade, increasing interest and availability of blood products has helped to make transfusion medicine a common practice at almost every veterinary clinic. The veterinary industry, especially veterinary emergency and critical care, has seen a drastic increase in value placed on pets and their importance within the family. This positive move has helped blood banks increase the number of these essential blood products produced, allowed for technical advances in specialized blood products and storage methods, and enabled veterinarians to provide life-saving treatments to their patients. Advances in component therapy has allowed for multiple patients to benefit from one transfusion while also reducing transfusion-related reactions from unnecessary components that previously were unable to be separated. Because of these advances, it is crucial that veterinary support staff understand the basics of transfusion medicine, component therapy, and the administration and monitoring of blood products. This chapter will serve as an introduction to the foundations of transfusion medicine and the principles behind donor selection, product collection, transfusion administration, and recognition and treatment of transfusion-related reactions.

Blood Cell Physiology and Blood Types

Erythrocytes, otherwise known as red blood cells (RBCs) are vital for our existence in that they contain hemoglobin, the carrier of oxygen that our cells depend upon for survivability and function. The process in which these cells develop from hemopoietic progenitor cells into erythrocytes is called erythropoiesis (Car 2006). Oxygenation levels within our tissues are determined by the concentration of erythrocytes in the blood. As oxygenation decreases, receptors within the interstitial cells of the renal inner cortex and, to a lesser extent, receptors in the liver excrete a hormone called *erythropoietin* (Epo) (Car 2006). This substance is the primary hormone responsible for red cell production and regulation within the bone marrow. The release of this hormone begins the chemical cascade that results in erythropoiesis and the production of new RBCs that enter into the bloodstream and increase oxygenation levels back to normal.

All mammals are born with a specific inherited blood type. This blood type is determined by the presence or absence of antigens on the RBC surface. These antigens are composed of a combination of polysaccharides and proteins, and each antigen is unique in its composition and shape. Blood typing is therefore a two-part description in which you note the antigen site and then note if there is an antigen found at that site. If a site contains that specific antigen, it is said to be positive (+), and conversely, if the site does not contain an antigen it is said to be negative (−).

Opposite to the antigen is the antibody, which is either naturally occurring within the body or formed after a sensitization to a foreign antigen. The severity of an antibody/antigen reaction depends on the levels of the antibody in the recipient's body; the higher the level of antibodies the more severe the reaction. In addition, antibody reactions that are mediated by immunoglobulin M (IgM) are more severe in nature compared with immunoglobulin G-mediated reactions (IgG) (Abrams-Ogg 2000).

Canine Blood Types

Canine blood typing is classified using the *Dog Erythrocyte Antigen* (DEA) system. Currently within the DEA system there are six recognized antigen sites defined by the availability of international standardized antisera. These antigen sites are known as DEA's 1.1, 1.2, 3, 4, 5, and 7. Although not fully defined or recognized, there are said to be upward of 18 or more antigen specificities described. DEA 6 and DEA 8 are two examples of antigens that have been identified, yet typing sera is unavailable at this time for these sites. Donors are said to be universal negative if they are negative for the above 6 antigen sites with the exception of DEA 4 as 99% of dogs are positive at that site. Therefore, universal donors can be DEA 4 positive or negative and still referred to as universal negative donors.

The first antigen is the "DEA 1 Group" and is considered the most antigenic group. This group is composed of DEA 1.1 and DEA 1.2 which are actually alleles, meaning that the patient can be negative for both, but can only be positive for one of them. In recent years, a third allele has been described at the DEA 1 site, DEA 1.3. Dogs can therefore be negative for DEA 1.1 and 1.2, but positive for 1.3. Because conventional antisera testing only tests for the 1.1 and 1.2 sites, it is possible that the donor will turn up "negative" even if it is DEA 1.3 positive, and consequently, a production of antibodies could be formed within the recipient at the DEA 1. site due to the DEA 1.3 antigens present within the donor blood.

Dogs lack naturally occurring alloantibodies to the DEA 1.1 and 1.2 sites. Thus, no antigenic reaction will occur within the patient's first transfusion. However, if the patient is negative for DEA 1.1 and is given DEA 1.1 positive blood on the first transfusion, likely, a delayed transfusion reaction will occur as the body is sensitized to the donor's DEA 1.1 positive antigens and the patient's immune response would be to create anti-DEA 1.1 antibodies. This reaction would be delayed, likely occurring 1–2 weeks out from the original transfusion when enough antibodies have been formed within the patient to start attacking the foreign DEA 1.1 antigens still circulating in the vascular system.

This is where the common phrase of "it does not matter in dogs what type of blood is used with the first transfusion" comes from. However, this misconception should be abandoned as it does matter, and delayed hemolytic reactions can and will occur. This is additional significance when blood typing and crossmatching products are inexpensive and readily available.

If the patient has a chronic or nonimproving illness, any destruction to the transfused cells decreases their RBC numbers and may lead to the requirement of an additional transfusion, increasing the risk of transfusion-related reaction. If that same patient is later given another transfusion of DEA 1.1 positive blood, it will have a severe acute hemolytic reaction as the immune system has had ample time to create anti-DEA 1.1 antibodies. If this transfusion occurred, the recipient's immune system and antibodies would immediately recognize the DEA 1.1 positive antigens as foreign, and rapid RBC destruction would occur (Abrams-Ogg 2000). It is estimated that an acute hemolytic reaction could wipe out the transfused RBCs within 12–16 hours (Table 21.1).

DEA 1.2 sensitization does occur as well to a lesser extent, but total RBC destruction will take place over a longer period of time, 24–36 hours. However, the overall end result is the same; the transfusion of DEA 1.1 or 1.2 positive blood to a DEA 1.1 negative patient who has already been sensitized prior to the DEA 1. positive antigens will lead to complete hemolysis of the transfused unit within a few days. Therefore, it is recommended that if full DEA 1. typing is not available that the patient receive universal negative blood, typed fully out to DEA 7, to prevent sensitization and future mismatch transfusion reactions. In addition, crossmatching should be performed on every subsequent transfusion due to the possible presence of the DEA 1.3 antigen which is not currently tested in commercially available antisera test kits.

Outside of the DEA 1. site there are four additional sites that have varying degrees of naturally occurring antibodies. DEA sites 3 and 5 do have naturally occurring alloantibodies, and a sensitization reaction could be seen on the first transfusion if the levels of antibodies are high enough in the recipient. DEA site 4 is unique in that approximately 99% of dogs are positive for DEA 4. Therefore, the vast majority of dogs could receive DEA 4 positive or DEA 4 negative blood and show no antibody reaction. DEA 7 has been a topic of recent discussions on whether or not dogs carry naturally antibodies to this antigen site. Some references document that despite the controversy we know that approximately 15%–50% of dogs have naturally occurring antibodies to the DEA 7 site (Abrams-Ogg 2000). Although not currently recognized in the DEA system due to lack of typing sera, DEA 6 is very similar to DEA 4 in that the DEA 6 antigen site is present in approximately 99% of dogs. The last of the antigen sites, DEA 8, is estimated to be found in approximately 40% of the canine population. Again, this site is currently unable for typing due to lack of typing sera (Wardrop 2006).

CHAPTER 21

Table 21.1   Canine blood groups

DEA Antigen	Incidence (Positive)	Reaction Seen with Mismatch
1.1	45%–50%	Acute hemolytic immunologic reaction
1.2	20%–25%	Acute or delayed hemolytic reaction
1.3	Unknown	Delayed hemolytic immunologic reaction
3	6%–10%	Naturally occurring anti-DEA 3 in approx. 15%–20% of DEA 3 negative dogs. Acute hemolytic reaction or RBC removal within 5 days of use
4	97%–99%	No naturally occurring antibodies reported
5	10%–15%	Naturally occurring anti-DEA 5 in approx. 8%–10% of DEA 5 negative dogs. Acute or delayed red cell removal
6*	99%–100%	Typing sera no longer available, anti-DEA 6 not reported (prevalence at ~100%)
7	40%–55%	Naturally occurring anti-DEA 7 in approx. 35%–45% of DEA 7 negative dogs. Acute or delayed hemolytic reaction (RBC removal)
8*	40%–45%	Typing sera no longer available, anti-DEA 8 unknown reaction

*Typing sera no longer available.
Created using average numbers of multiple sources (Abrams-Ogg 2000; Feldman and Sink 2006).

One phenomenon that has been documented regarding DEA 1.1 positive sensitization is *Neonatal Isoerythrolysis (NI)*. Although very uncommon, this unfortunate situation occurs when a DEA 1.1 negative female that has had DEA 1.1 sensitization is bred to a DEA 1.1 positive male. The pups that are born DEA 1.1 positive will likely have a hemolytic reaction occur when they nurse from the bitch as her colostrums is full of DEA 1.1 positive antibodies. This hemolytic reaction begins as general lethargy and failure to thrive soon followed by death, and may be a component of fading puppy syndrome.

Feline Blood Types

Unlike the canine, felines currently only have one recognized blood group known as the AB system. Cats can be either Type A, Type B, or Type AB. Of these three types, Type A is by far the most common blood type in the United States with approximately 95% of the domestic short and long-hair cats having this blood type (Wardrop 2006). Of the remaining 5%, the majority is Type B with less than 1% of the population typing as AB. Although Type A is the predominant type in domestic short- and long-haired cats, certain exotic and rare breeds, such as the Devon and Cornish rex, are not predominately Type A and actually have almost 50% of their population as Type B blood.

Type A cats do have natural antibodies to Type B blood but these anti-B alloantibodies are fairly weak and may cause a delayed hemolytic reaction leading to transfused red cell destruction. Type B cats, however, have very strong anti-A alloantibodies and Type B cats transfused with Type A blood will have a severe hemolytic reaction often leading to death within the recipient. Type AB cats do not have any alloantibodies as they have both the A and B antigens present on their red cells. NI is a concern with felines as well, and Type B queens have shown the highest rate of NI fatalities due to severe hemolysis of Type A or Type AB kittens.

Blood Typing

Commercially available blood typing kits have made it possible for in-house rapid blood type determination in both dogs and cats. The readily available and easy-to-use typing kit is the Rapid Vet-H typing cards produced by DMS Laboratories, Inc. (Farmington, NJ). These kits include a card that has wells containing lyophilized antisera. A drop of diluent (supplied with the kits) is used to reconstitute the antisera and once reconstituted, a drop of the patient's blood is added to the patient well. The user is instructed to slowly rotate and rock the card for two minutes and then read and record the results. In canine cards, agglutination in the patient well means a positive result; the patient is DEA 1.1 positive, while lack of agglutination means the patient is DEA 1.1 negative. In feline cards, the blood type of the patient is determined by which control well the patient well matches, either the Type A well or the Type B well. The card kits contain control vials of typed blood to assist with type determination and help eliminate false positive or negative results. These kits are easy to use and are inexpensive compared to blood typing using an outside laboratory. One reported disadvantage is frequently seen false-positive reactions which can be problematic if the patient is actually DEA 1.1 negative and is given DEA 1.1 positive blood (sensitizing it to DEA 1.1 antigens) (Wardrop 2006).

False-negative reactions have also been reported but are less harmful as the patient is assumed to be DEA 1.1 negative and is therefore given universal negative blood. This is another reason crossmatching should be performed before all transfusions. Another disadvantage to the typing cards is seen with patients that are auto-agglutinating. Due to red cell agglutination, the patient well will contain agglutinants regardless of actual blood type, and an accurate blood type cannot be determined.

A newer blood typing kit has been introduced by Alveda marketed as DME typing kits. This blood typing kit employs using a strip kit that contains all the necessary parts for each test in individual packages. An antisera embedded strip is placed in a well containing the patient's blood and a drop of diluent at an angle close to 90°. Via capillary action, the blood flows up the strip over an embedded control line and then over the positive and negative antisera sites. Once the proper time has elapsed, the strip is removed and replaced back into its original horizontal position within the kit. The patient's blood type is determined by the presence or absence of lines at the DEA 1.1 positive and DEA 1.1 negative antisera marker sites, or for felines, the presence or absence of lines at the A, B, or both A and B marker sites.

Tests are not considered accurate unless a line occurs at the control marker site. If the patient is DEA 1.1 negative you will only see a line at the control marker site (as no antibodies were present to react to the antisera), but if the patient is DEA 1.1 positive, you will see a line develop at both the control marker site and the DEA 1.1 positive marker site. The benefit of these kits over the card kits is that they are marketed as being effective in typing patients who are experiencing auto-agglutination because the agglutinants remain at the bottom of the well, unable to travel up the strip via the capillary action. In addition, animals who are anemic make it harder to accurately see agglutination on the card kits (due to the low RBC count), leading to false-negative results. The makers of the DME strip kits state their typing kits are still effective in typing anemic animals because only a small amount of red cells need to travel over the antisera to cause a reaction and subsequent line formation to occur.

If you are in need of blood typing outside of your hospital, or are looking to fully type your donors or recipients, there are numerous outside laboratories that provide typing services for cats and dogs. Two of the most well-known facilities include

1. Animal Blood Resources International
   1-800-243-5759 or www.ABRInt.net located in California and Michigan
2. Stormont Laboratories
   1-530-661-3078 located in California

Crossmatching

The crossmatch is performed to determine incompatibility between the donor and recipient. More specifically, blood typing identifies certain known RBC antigens in the patient and donor, but it does not identify antibodies in the patient or donor. The crossmatch procedure is done to determine if there is an antibody reaction to either known or unknown antigens within the donor and the recipient, making it a crucial part in transfusion medicine. As we learn more about antigen sites on both canine and feline red cells, our blood typing technology becomes more specific and less transfusion reactions occur due to proper product selection. However, there are still many antigen specificities that have not yet been fully described and determined. Due to the likelihood of unknown antigens and/or antibodies, a crossmatch procedure should be performed to ensure the blood product's compatibility with the recipient's blood.

Crossmatching does not indicate if the donor and the recipient have the same blood type, it only indicates that the no antibody/antigen reaction was detected. It is recommended that crossmatching be done even if the patient has been typed (Wardrop 2006). In addition, crossmatching should always be done in the following circumstances:

1. The patient had a previous transfusion more than 4 days prior. If the patient was sensitized to foreign antigens, it is likely the immune system has developed antibodies and a crossmatch should be performed to ensure compatibility and prevention of a hemolytic transfusion reaction.
2. The patient is a feline. As discussed above, there is no universal feline donor and Type B blood has strong anti-A alloantibodies which can lead to an acute hemolytic reaction which may be fatal. Due to the possibility of inaccurate typing and the potential for unknown antigens, it is highly suggested that a crossmatch be performed before all feline transfusions.
3. The patient is a breeding animal. Crossmatching would be performed to avoid sensitization to foreign antigens which would increase the risk of NI.
4. A crossmatch is strongly recommended if the patient has been pregnant.
5. If the patient's transfusion history is unknown (Abrams-Ogg 2000).

Crossmatching Procedure

Crossmatching can be done within the hospital using a centrifuge, saline, and blood from both the potential donor and recipient. In addition to in-hospital saline procedure, recent crossmatching kits have been introduced by DMS Laboratories Inc. marketed as Rapid Vet-H Companion Animal Crossmatch. This crossmatch involves a fully pre-packaged set of positive, negative, and patient controls and uses gel technology to determine compatibility. This test can be used on both dogs and cats; it is a universal crossmatch kit (Table 21.2).

Table 21.2   Crossmatch procedure

1. Obtain an anticoagulated (EDTA) blood sample from both patient and donor.
2. Centrifuge both tubes and separate plasma from RBCs at standard blood speed.
3. Remove the plasma from each tube and place each plasma sample in a labeled red top serum separating tube. Be sure to note which tube has the donor serum and which tube has the recipient serum.
4. Remove remaining packed red cells from the bottom of each tube and place them into individual red top serum separating tubes. Be clear to label both tubes are containing RBCs from the donor versus the recipient.
5. Fill the tube three-fourths full with sterile saline. Mix gently and centrifuge for 1 minute. Be clear to state here fill the tube containing the red blood cells with sterile saline *not* the serum tube.
6. Decant the saline and repeat Step 5 three more times. This is known as cell washing and helps to remove proteinaceous debris.
7. After the last wash, decant supernatant.
8. Resuspend the cells with saline to give a 2%–4% suspension of RBCs. It should look like "weak" tomato juice.
9. Make the following mixtures by adding the RBC suspension and plasma to new red top tubes.

	Major Crossmatch	Minor Crossmatch	Control
Patient	2 drops plasma	1 drop 2%–4% RBC Suspension	1 drop patient 2%–4% RBC suspension with 2 drops patient
Donor	1 drop 2%–4% RBC Suspension	2 drops plasma	Plasma

10. Incubate tubes for 20–30 minutes at 37°C.
11. Centrifuge for 15 seconds at standard blood speed.

Interpreting the Results

Macroscopic—Examine tubes for hemolysis. This is done by gently rolling the tubes between fingers and observing cells for hemagglutination as they come off the "button" in the bottom of the tube.

Microscopic—Place a drop on a slide with a cover slip and look under the microscope at 10× and 40×. Look for presence of agglutination. Agglutination measured as 0 (none), +1 (rare), +2 (few), +3 (many). If agglutination is present on the major crossmatch, the units are not compatible. If agglutination is 0 or +1 on minor crossmatch, the unit may be accepted; however,, a transfusion reaction to the donor plasma may occur.

Source: Modified from Abrams-Ogg (2000 and Wardrop (2006).

Blood Donors

Transfusion medicine wouldn't exist without the presence of our blood donors. There are numerous facilities and hospitals across the United States that have in-house and community blood donor programs that supply veterinary hospitals with an array of blood products. Although blood banking and component separation requires the addition of specialized blood separation equipment, most hospitals can have a small in-hospital blood donor program for emergency whole blood transfusions (WBTs). Donors should be in good health, be an appropriate age and size, and be screened and typed prior to admittance into a blood donor program. Donors in the program should get yearly blood work, physical exams, and be up to date on vaccinations, heartworm prevention, and flea and tick medications for the safety of the donor and the blood product recipient.

Canine Donors

Canine donors should be young and in good overall health and behavioral standing determined by clinical history and physical exam. It is extremely helpful to have a thorough travel history to alert you of possible exposure to regional transmissible diseases. Ideal donors would be between the ages of 1 and 7 years old. Although there is no specific medical condition or event that occurs at 7 years of age, we do know that as canines age (especially larger breeds), they run a higher risk of having underlying undiagnosed conditions such as heart, renal, or hepatic disease, and run a higher risk of complications from blood donations. In addition, some facilities have their donors in the donor program for a minimum amount of time to balance out the costs associated with initial testing and screening.

If this is the case, then 7 years of age is likely the oldest age accepted for a canine donor who is expected to donate for 24–36 months. Donors should be 25 kg or larger; however, smaller dogs can be donors when smaller volume transfusions are required. Most veterinary clinics do not have small dogs as donors because it is not as cost-effective as the larger dog donors. The same testing and screening must be done but the total volume of blood and blood products over time is significantly less than that of the larger donors.

Donors should be free of parasites and infectious disease. In 2002, the American College of Veterinary Internal Medicine (ACVIM) developed a blood donor consensus statement on canine and feline blood donor screening, and an updated consensus statement was published in 2005. Because different viruses and infections are found in different regions in the United States and around the world, there is not one universal screening recommendation. However, the ACVIM consensus statement does give us a minimum screening recommendation for canine donors with additional testing being recommended and suggested for specific regions and specific breeds of dogs. The minimum screening for canine donors should include the following: complete blood count (CBC) and chemistry panel, *Babesia canis* and *Babesia gibsoni* via serology testing and/or polymerase chain reaction (PCR) assay, *Ehrlichia canis* via IFA or point-of-care test for *E. canis* and *Brucellosis* (if breeding dogs are accepted into the blood donor program). Canine donors should also be tested for canine heartworm.

This recommendation is not for the recipient, as heartworm is not transmitted via transfusion, but rather for the donor as underlying heartworm disease could severely affect the blood donor's health. It is highly recommended that the ACVIM consensus statement on canine and feline blood donor screening for infectious disease be reviewed and the recommendations followed for donor screening. Accepted donors should have chemistry and hematologic screening (CBC/chemistry) every 12–18 months and have subsequent disease testing if repeated exposure to risk factors occur; this is especially important if the donor is involved in travel.

Canine donor blood collection

Canines can safely donate approximately 15 to 20% of their overall blood volume every 3–4 weeks, equating to approximately 15–18 mL/kg (Abrams-Ogg 2000). Donors should be fasted if possible prior to the donation to minimize lipemia within the plasma, and in case the donor requires sedation or anesthesia for blood collection. In general dogs do not require any chemical restraint and lie still for the collection process. New dogs to the program may be more nervous and potentially need sedation, but over time and exposure the donor becomes adjusted to the procedure. If sedation is needed there are a variety of medications that may be used to help calm the patient including: opioids such as butorphanol (0.05 mg–0.2 mg/kg IV), tranquilizers such as diazepam (0.2–0.4 mg/kg IV), and/or low doses of acepromazine (0.01–0.2 mg/kg IV or IM) (Abrams-Ogg 2000). If general anesthesia is required for a canine donation it is recommended that this donor be removed from the donor program.

The collection processes includes at least two staff members; one to restrain and one to perform the blood draw. A closed collection system that is designated for the collection and processing of blood products should be used. These bags are readily available through multiple vendors and help reduce the risk of bacterial contamination. Collection bags are usually polyvinyl chloride (PVC), a type of plastic which is inexpensive to make, readily available, and allows gas exchange to occur which is necessary for the release of carbon dioxide and consumption of oxygen by the red cells within the unit. During the collection process, blood flows into the bag using gravity or can be expedited along using a blood-approved vacuum system that gently pulls the blood into the bag. A standard single 450 mL bag is available and contains citrate-phosphate-dextrose-adenine (CPDA), an anticoagulant and nutrient solution for the preservation of RBCs and prevention of coagulation. Satellite bags are also available for collection and storage of blood components. The satellite bags are generally three or four bag systems that contain the standard single 450 mL CPDA bag, one or two satellite bags for plama, and a red blood nutrient source for the red cells (such as Optisol [Terumo Corporation, Tokyo, Japan]) so the lifespan of the product can be extended. RBC units preserved with Optisol have a storage life of around 5–6 weeks in the refrigerator.

Sterile technique should be used when obtaining blood from a donor. The area over the jugular vein should be shaved and the area cleaned prior to venipuncture. The person drawing the blood would gently hold off the jugular vein and upon visual confirmation, the needle should be advanced into the vein in one steady motion. The restrainer's job is to assure the patient is doing well during the procedure and to prevent any movement from occurring so the collection is smooth and the needle does not travel outside of the vein. As blood flows into the bag, a staff member should gently rock the bag to ensure the blood has come in contact with the CPDA solution (Fig. 21.1).

The use of a gram scale is helpful to determine when a unit is filled. Each milliliter of blood weighs 1 g. Therefore, after zeroing the gram scale, a 450 mL unit of blood should weigh 450 g once filled. Once finished, the restrainer uses gauze to apply pressure over

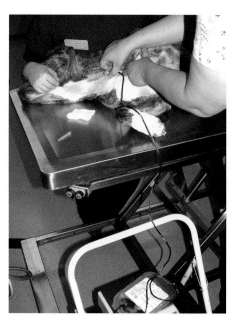

Figure 21.1 Most dogs do not require sedation to donate blood; however, a tolerant patient and adequate restraint is mandatory. Cats, however, are routinely given chemical restraint to when they donate blood.

the venipuncture site to prevent hematoma formation while the phlebotomist prepares the now full collection bag for sealing (Abrams-Ogg 2000). If the donor is in good health and does well during the procedure it can be returned to its cage, given a small amount of food and water, and monitored for 15–30 minutes post transfusion. Subcutaneous fluids are not necessary in canine donors unless general anesthesia was used or if complications such as hypotension arise during or after the collection. Should volume replacement be required, SQ or IV crystalloid solutions should be given at two to three times the blood loss.

The bag should be labeled with the date, type, and volume of blood product, donor information including blood type, and expiration date. Each canine donor should have a donation file in which donation information is recorded in the event problems arise within the donor or within the donated blood.

Feline Donors

Much like canine donors, feline donors should be in good overall health and have a good temperament. Ideal donors would be between the ages of 1 and 8 years old. Donors should be at least 5 kg in weight and in good physical condition. If the donor is overweight the blood collection volume should be based on the ideal body weight as additional fat does not equate to additional RBCs.

Feline donors should be able to lie still for blood collection, but will most likely require some form of anesthesia or sedation for the collection of the unit. It is highly recommended that donor cats are indoor cats and that they remain indoors to eliminate possible exposure to parasites and disease.

As discussed with canine donors, it is recommended to follow the ACVIM consensus regarding feline screening for infectious disease. The minimum screening for felines includes the following: CBC and Chemistry Panel, feline leukemia virus (FeLV)/feline immunodeficiency virus (FIV) testing, *Mycoplasma haemofelis* preferably by PCR, and *Bartonella*. The ACVIM have other conditional and regional recommended testing for feline donors including cytauxzoonosis, ehrlichiosis, anaplasmosis, and neorickettsiosis (Wardrop et al. 2005). Feline donors should be tested for the above during the pre-donor screening period and have subsequent testing done if repeated exposure to risk factors occur, this includes if the pet is allowed to start going outdoors. Repeat chemistry and hematologic testing should be performed every 12–18 months.

Feline blood donor collection

Feline donors can safely donate 10%–15% of body weight every 3–4 weeks, equating to approximately 11–13 mL/kg (Abrams-Ogg 2000). Unlike canines, most feline donors require general anesthesia or neuroleptanalgesia to remain still enough through the entire blood draw procedure. This does pose a higher risk of anesthetic complications and possible death to donor. Care should be taken to give the minimum anesthetic volume required to keep the patient from moving during the donation. Analgesics and anesthetic agents are chosen based on the patient, the comfort level of the veterinarian with the medications and blood collection, and the time required for unit collection. To avoid excessive time under anesthesia, the staff member responsible for the blood collection should have all the necessary supplies out ahead of time and be ready to draw as soon as the patient is unconscious and/or sedated. Common drugs used during feline donations are neuroleptanalgesia combinations such as:

- Butorphanol (0.2–0.4 mg/kg) and midazolam (0.2–0.5 mg/kg) IV or IM
- Butorphanol (0.2–0.4 mg/kg) and acepromazine (0.04–0.10 mg/kg) IV or IM
- Oxymorphone (0.05–0.1 mg/kg) and acepromazine (0.04–0.10 mg/kg)IV or IM (Abrams-Ogg 2000)

These combinations allow the patient to remain awake and in a state of profound sedation without the need for general anesthesia. The use of acepromazine as a sedative agent or part of a neuroleptanalgesic combination has the potential to cause hypotension and is not only dose-dependent but also dependent on the donor's metabolism of this agent. If hypotension is a concern or if the patient is very relaxed and calm to begin with, the administration of a solo opioid drug can be used for the donation.

If general anesthesia is required, many facilities use the combination of ketamine and a sedative or tranquilizer as their anesthetic agent of choice. Ketamine causes excitement within the CNS, often leading to tachycardia and hypertension which is dose-dependent and may facilitate the visualization and collection of blood. In contrast, other injectable anesthetics such as propofol and gas anesthetic like isoflurane can cause hypotension and potential respiratory depression and are avoided by some in blood collection. Since the donor will be undergoing blood loss, it has been recommended that hypotensive agents (e.g., propofol) be avoided as the primary anesthetic agent so the patient does not become both hypovolemic and hypotensive. Some general anesthesia protocols include:

- Ketamine (100 mg/mL) mixed with diazepam (5 mg/mL) at a 1:1 ratio or 1:2 ratio and given at 0.1–0.2 mL/kg IV to effect.

■   Ketamine 2 mg/kg and midazolam 0.1–0.2 mg/kg mixed and given IV to effect (Abrams-Ogg 2000)

Once the donor is safely sedated or anesthetized, care should be taken to ensure that the airway is secure and, if necessary, endotracheal intubation performed. The eyes should be lubricated with an artificial tear formula to prevent drying of the cornea during the procedure. As soon as the patient is ready, the blood collection can begin and vitals should be monitored through the procedure. The restrainer places the cat in lateral recumbency with the neck region exposed for the staff member to visualize the jugular vein for blood collection. The area over the jugular vein is shaved and the area cleaned prior to venipuncture. For whole blood donations that are going to be used right away, the blood can be collected directly into syringes containing CPDA. CPDA is used at a ratio of 1 mL per 7–8 mL of blood drawn. One large 60-cc syringe can be used but often, staff find the suction to be too strong and leads to vein collapse.

An alternative to one 60-cc syringe is to use two 35-cc syringes (each with half of the calculated CPDA) and attach them to a 3-way stopcock. A 19-g butterfly catheter is attached to the 3-way stopcock system and is inserted into the jugular vein in one fluid motion. As the jugular vein is held off, slow and steady suction is used to collect the blood into the first syringe. Once that syringe is full, the stopcock is turned and the second syringe is filled to the appropriate amount. The butterfly catheter is then removed and pressure is placed over the vein for 10–15 minutes to ensure clot formation and to prevent a hematoma (Fig. 21.2).

Because of the need for sedation and/or anesthesia, cat donors are routinely given subcutaneous fluids at a volume of two to three times the blood volume removed. The syringe(s) should be labeled with the date, type, and volume of blood product, donor information including blood type, and expiration date. Each feline donor should have a donation file in which donation information is recorded in the event problems arise within the donor or within the donated blood. If the blood is being collected for separation and storage, a special feline collection bag should be used as syringes do not allow for adequate gas exchange to occur for the viability of the RBCs. Closed collection systems are available with one or two small bags that allow for both single bag collection and satellite

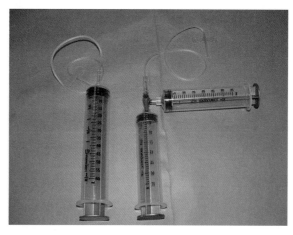

Figure 21.2   Feline blood donation is commonly collected via a butterfly catheter and a 35- or 60-cc syringe containing an anticoagulant.

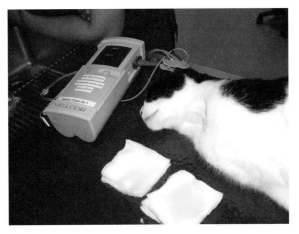

Figure 21.3   Here a sedated cat prepares to donate blood. A combination of intravenous ketamine and midazolam or diazepam is an excellent combination frequently selected for cats donating blood.

bag component collection. These systems may or may not contain CPDA and/or a nutrient solution such as Optisol. For these systems, sterile technique should be used to add the anticoagulant and/or the nutrient solution to the bags to prevent coagulation and to extend the life of the RBC unit (Fig. 21.3).

Blood Products and Component Therapy

Blood is composed of a variety of cells and components that each has their own unique jobs and function with the patient. Whole blood is composed of RBCs, platelets, white blood cells (WBCs), and plasma. Within the plasma, we see the presence of coagulation factors, plasma proteins, antibodies, and immunoglobulins. Most blood contains approximately 38%–50% RBCs and 45%–58% plasma, with the remaining 1%–2% owing to WBCs and platelets. With advancements in technology and availability of specialized equipment for blood products, we not only can collect whole blood for immediate use, but we can collect blood, separate components from each other, and store them for later use. Care is taken to ensure that stored blood products are collected in closed collection systems and as sterilely as possible to minimize the potential for bacterial growth within the product (Abrams-Ogg 2000).

Whole Blood Transfusion (WBT)

Fresh whole blood is defined as blood that is taken directly from the donor into a closed collection system and, with the proper administration sets and filter, is then given directly to the recipient. Whole blood, therefore, contains RBCs, functional platelets, coagulation factors, and plasma proteins (Callan 2006). WBTs are utilized for a variety of reasons within veterinary medicine, including replacement therapy in patients who have a decrease in oxygen-carrying capacity with hypovolemia to a significant degree (Bergeron 2005). Examples of this are patients experiencing massive hemorrhage and blood loss from

CHAPTER 21

trauma, shock, disseminated intravascular coagulation (DIC), or other serious illness/injury.

Additionally, whole blood is utilized in patients requiring various types of blood components where it is more economical and practical to do one large transfusion from a single donor than components from possibly multiple donors. An example of this can be seen with canine patients who have ingested anticoagulant-type rodenticides who are suffering both from anemia and decreased clotting factors.

Finally, whole blood is often used over components simply because it is the only blood product available to the patient at the time (Callan 2006). Blood product backorders occur on some level within every blood bank facility due to low supply and high demand. Patients might only require one particular component, but due to limitations they are given a WBT. This is a safe and accepted practice if the patient can handle the increase in vascular volume seen with whole blood administration. Fresh whole blood should be used within 4 hours of collection.

To determine the amount of blood needed or how much the recipient's packed cell volume (PCV) will increase, you can use the following equation:

$$\text{(Desire PCV of patient—actual PCV of patient)\% PCV of donor.}$$

This number is then multiplied by the blood volume of the patient. Dogs have approximately 90 mL/kg of blood while cats have approximately 70 mL/kg (Feldman and Sink 2006). Another simple method is the "rule of 1's". The "rule of 1's" states that 1 mL of whole blood per 1 lb of body weight will increase the PCV of the reciepient by 1%.

Stored Whole Blood (SWB)

SWB is similar to fresh whole blood except that instead of immediate administration into the patient, these units are stored under refrigeration at 1–6°C until use. Stored blood hemostatic properties vary from those found in fresh blood. Stored red cells have been documented to have changes to the RBC shape and various biochemical alterations which can affect red cell function and viability. Due to these changes, the addition of nutrient and preservative solutions is imperative to help increase red cell viability (Callan 2006).

Platelets almost immediately begin to lose viability and function when refrigerated, with a 50% decrease occurring within the first 12–18 hours. Approximately 72 hours after storage, there are no longer any viable platelets found within the stored unit (Abrams-Ogg 2000). Labile clotting factors such as factors V, VIII, and von Willebrand factor (vWf) also lose function under refrigeration. The loss of labile clotting factors is at a much slower rate than that of platelets. At the 24-hour mark, approximately 85% of factor VIII, 75% of vWf, and 90% of factor V is still present within the unit. These percentages will continue to decline the longer the unit is left under refrigeration. There is very little loss of the non-labile clotting factors and antithrombin III, and they are thought to be viable through the entire storage process (Abrams-Ogg 2000; Bergeron 2005).

SWB can be used for patients requiring replacement of blood volume and oxygen carrying capacity as RBC viability is high. SWB can also be used in circumstances where fresh whole blood is not available or in situations where plasma components are unavailable and the patient needs a source of non-labile clotting factors, albumin, and/or plasma proteins.

Packed Red Blood Cells (PRBC)

PRBCs are the result of centrifugation (or sedimentation) of a unit of whole blood. These units provide only RBCs and do not contain any plasma components. Once the donor unit has been centrifuged and the red cells separated from the plasma, a nutrient solution such as Optisol is added, and the units are stored in the fridge at 1–6°C. The storage time of PRBCs can vary from 3–6 weeks depending on the type of anticoagulant and nutrient solution used (Abrams-Ogg 2000; Schneider 2006). Packed red cell units should be stored in either a specialized blood bank fridge, a designated blood product fridge, or in a lab fridge that has a separate area only for the placement of blood products.

The units should be stored away from other medications, chemicals, and with space between the units. Red cells are living cells that require enough space for fresh oxygen and carbon dioxide diffusion in and out of the bags. It is recommended that red cell units either be suspended/hung in the refrigerator or laid flat; not allowing the units to lie on top of each other or be put into bundles (Abrams-Ogg 2000). Red cell units should not be placed in refrigerator drawers as oxygen exchange may be inhibited by drawer moisture/air controls (Fig. 21.4).

Indications for use of packed RBCs include the presence of anemia without concurrent hypovolemia. One example of this is the chronic renal failure patient; in which erythropoietin is poorly produced and subsequently, bone marrow production of red cells into the circulation is decreased, leading to anemia. Another example would be immune-mediated hemolytic anemia (IMHA) cases. Packed RBCs can also be used in patients that require fresh whole blood but no donor is available and the patient requires an immediate source of red cells for oxygen-carrying capacity (Abrams-Ogg 2000).

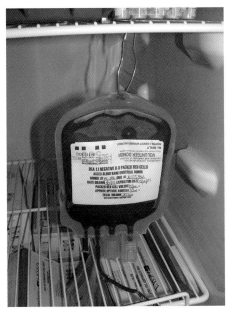

Figure 21.4 Stored units of blood, such as this unit of canine packed red cells, should be stored upright and apart from each other.

CHAPTER 21

Fresh Frozen Plasma (FFP)

FFP is defined as the plasma portion separated from the red cells via centrifugation and subsequently frozen to −18°C within 8 hours of collection. Pending additional studies, FFP expires within 1 year of preparation and collection. Once stored for 1 year, the unit should be pulled and relabeled as frozen plasma (FP) and stored for an additional 4 years (Abrams-Ogg 2000; Schneider 2006).

FFP contains all labile and non-labile clotting factors (hemostatic proteins), plasma proteins, albumin, and globulin. FFP does not contain appreciable amounts of platelets as these remain in the packed RBC units. It is vital that the plasma be completely frozen within the 8 hours to best preserve the amount and viability of the labile clotting factors (V, VIII, vWf) and fibrinogen.

Plasma products require an anticoagulant but do not require the addition of a nutrient solution as there are no living cells within the preparation. Storage of FP products should be in either a specialized blood bank freezer, a designated plasma freezer, or a laboratory freezer as far away from the door as possible. The minimum temperature to maintain the units is −18°C; a freezer that is constantly opened can significantly decrease the temperature possibly leading to thawing of the unit and potentially reduced levels of labile clotting factors such as factor V, VIII, and vWf. The use of a freezer without an automatic defrost cycle is recommended (Abrams-Ogg 2000; Schneider 2006).

FFP is used to treat a variety of inherited or acquired coagulopathies and hemostatic disorders. This includes the treatment of hemophilia A and B, anticoagulant rodenticide toxicities, von Willebrand disease, and other factor deficiencies. FFP is also used to treat help treat shock and hypoproteinemia caused by multiple disease processes such as pancreatitis, protein losing enteropathies (PLE), and protein losing nephropathies (PLN), DIC, sepsis, and hepatic failure (Fig. 21.5).

FFP has also been used in puppies with parvovirus as protein replacement therapy and additionally to provide immunoglobulins. The volume required is specific to the underlying condition and individual patient requirements, but a general range of 6–15 mL/kg is

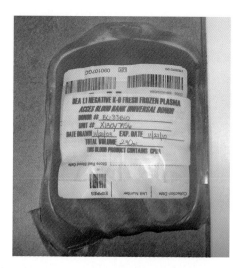

Figure 21.5   Stored units of blood products must be labeled carefully and include information about the donor, when the product was drawn, when the product expires, how much the unit contains, and what anticoagulant is used.

widely accepted for treatment of coagulopathies and/or hypoproteinemic states (Abrams-Ogg 2000; Brooks 2006).

Frozen Plasma (FP)

FP is either the product of the above "expired" FFP with a 4-year shelf-life, or it is plasma that was collected but not completely frozen within the 8-hour time requirement to label it as FFP. FP does not contain labile clotting factors (V, VIII, IX, vWf), but it does contain the non-labile clotting factors (II, VII, and X) and plasma proteins such as albumin and globulin (Abrams-Ogg 2000).

FP is effective in the treatment of acquired deficits of non-labile coagulation factors. Anticoagulant rodenticide toxicity affects production of factor VII, so fresh frozen or FP can be used to treat the coagulopathy. Just like FFP, FP can be used to treat shock and hypoproteinemic states. The dose of FP required follows the recommendations given for FFP and is primarily determinant on the underlying disease and individual patient needs (Abrams-Ogg 2000; Brooks 2006).

Cryoprecipitate

Cryoprecipitate is a precipitate that is specially prepared from existing units of FFP. Cryoprecipitate is made by slowly thawing a unit of FFP at a steady temperature (4°C) until the unit has a slush-like frothy appearance. The unit is then centrifuged at 5000 g for 5–7 minutes. The supernatant is expressed off, and the small amount of precipitate remaining is the cryoprecipitate. This small amount of precipitate (often 15–20 mL) is a concentrate of factor VIII, vWf, and fibrinogen (Brooks 2006). Although these factors can be found in FFP, the factor volume necessary for treatment of the disease may make it impractical to use multiple FFP units, as volume overload would likely occur in the patient.

Cryoprecipitate is the treatment of choice for hemophilia A, von Willebrand disease, and hypofibrinogenemia. In recent years, Animal Blood Resources International, a merger of Animal Blood Bank and Midwest Blood Bank, has introduced a lyophilized cryoprecipitate product for both canines and felines. The cryoprecipitate, marketed as part of their HemaGold line, is collected through Cohn cold ethanol fractionation to get a 98% pure cryoprecipitate product. The cryoprecipitate is then lyophilized, or freeze dried, allowing the product to be stored in the refrigerator for up to 12 months and quickly reconstituted at the time of use.

The benefit of fractionation is that the product is not only pure but multiple bottles can be purchased and given to the patient, reducing the amount of in-hospital FFP units that must be thawed and taken apart. In addition, fractionation means that only factor VIII, fibrinogen, and vWf are present in the cryoprecipitate, eliminating the need for crossmatching or blood typing before use. The cryoprecipitate may be administered at a dosage of 1–2 mL/kg with severe deficits requiring up to 5 mL/kg. Lyophilized cryoprecipitate can also be used as a pretreatment prior to surgery if a potential coagulopathy is of concern. Administration should be within 4 hours of the surgery to be effective. The manufacturers do caution that because this product has been derived from canine donor plasma that the same risk of infectious disease applies as with other plasma products (Hale 2009) (Table 21.3).

CHAPTER 21

Table 21.3   Blood products and their respective components

Blood Product	RBCs	Labile Clotting Factors	Non-Labile Clotting Factors	Plasma Proteins and Immunoglobulins	Functional Platelets	Miscellaneous Components
Fresh whole blood	Yes	Yes	Yes	Yes	Yes	
Stored whole blood	Yes	No	No	Yes	No	
Fresh frozen plasma	No	Yes	Yes	Yes	No	
Frozen plasma	No	No	Yes	Yes	No	
Cryoprecipitate	No	Factor VIII, fibrinogen	No	No	No	Von Willibrand factor (vWf)
Cryo-poor plasma	No	All except VIII, XIII, and fibrinogen	Yes	Yes	No	Lacks vWF
Canine albumin	No	No	No	Albumin only	No	
Feline albumin	No	No	No	Albumin only	No	

Cryoprecipitate Poor Plasma

Cryoprecipitate poor plasma (cryo poor) is the supernatant that was first removed off the cryoprecipitate after thawing and centrifugation (as described above). Cryo poor plasma still contains albumin and non-labile clotting factors, including the vitamin K-dependent clotting factors. Cryo poor plasma can be used for the treatment of anticoagulant rodenticide toxicities, hemophilia B (factor IX deficiency), and albumin deficits or hypoproteinemia. Cryo poor plasma should be stored at −18°C and is good for up to 5 years (Abrams-Ogg 2000; Brooks 2006).

Administration of Blood Products and Patient Monitoring

Although each blood product is unique in how it is collected, stored, and prepared, there are a few universal standards that exist with all transfusions, regardless of the product being delivered. When administering blood products, no other fluids or drugs should be given concurrently in the same line with the exception of 0.9% saline solution. The concurrent administration of Lactated Ringer's solution (LRS) in the same line is contradicted due to the presence of calcium in the fluid as calcium will negatively interact with the anticoagulant in the unit (Abrams-Ogg 2000; Brooks 2006). If possible, all medication administration should be avoided during blood product administration to better distinguish transfusion reactions from medication-related reactions. During the transfusion, the catheter should be inspected to make sure it remains patent (Abrams-Ogg 2000).

Patient monitoring is vital during transfusions to catch potentially serious transfusion reactions and to have documentation of the patient's vitals during the transfusion. One staff member should remain and monitor the patient during the entire transfusion to watch for transfusion reactions. The patient should have vitals such as temperature, heart rate, respiratory rate, mucous membrane color, capillary refill time, and blood pressure assessed throughout the transfusion. Many documented transfusion reactions occur within the first 15–30 minutes of the transfusion, so the rate of assessment is high at first with vitals obtained and recorded every 5 minutes to best obtain early recognition of a reaction (Abrams-Ogg 2000; Callan 2006).

If the patient is tolerating the transfusion well, the assessment time period can be extended out to every 15–45 minutes until the transfusion is complete. In addition to the abovementioned parameters, the patient should also be monitored for any signs of vomiting, hives, dypsnea, swelling, or itching as these can be indicators of an allergic transfusion reaction. Various transfusion forms exist and are a useful tool for documenting information regarding the donor, recipient, and transfusion administration. This form can easily be created in-hospital and kept with the patient's record (Abrams-Ogg 2000; Feldman and Sink 2006).

Administration Rates

Early recognition of transfusion reactions is crucial when performing a blood product transfusion. In addition to diligent monitoring, the rate of administration over the first 15–30 minutes is slowed to help catch potentially serious transfusion reactions. A variety of administration rates have been published and care should be taken to tailor the administration to the patient and their overall condition. In emergency situations where hypovolemia or severe hemorrhage is present, the blood product can be given as fast as the unit can be infused into the patient. Ideally, the unit would be warmed to help prevent hypothermia, but in an emergency situation, the unit of blood can at least be administered with the tubing running through warm water and then warming procedures performed on the patient (Callan 2006). A standard beginning transfusion rate for patients experiencing some form of hypovolemia or diminished oxygen-carrying capacity is 0.5–2 mL/kg/h. This rate is continued for the first 15–30 minutes so early recognition of a transfusion reaction can be monitored and caught. If no signs of a transfusion reaction have occurred, the rate can be increased to a rate of 3–5 mL/kg/h for the next 30 minutes while monitoring is continued (Fig. 21.6).

Pending additional studies, ideally, blood products will be transfused within 4 hours, so the rate of administration may need to be adjusted after the first hour so the unit is fully infused within that timeframe (Abrams-Ogg 2000; Brooks 2006; Callan 2006). In patients with cardiac disease or normovolemic anemia, the maximum administration rate is 10–20 mL/kg/h. Going higher than this rate may lead to volume overload and/or pulmonary edema (Abrams-Ogg 2000; Callan 2006).

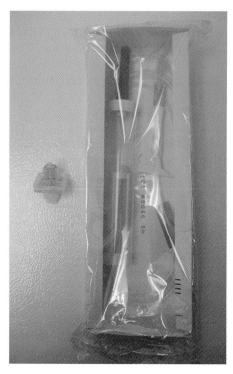

Figure 21.6 Commercial administration sets such as the one seen here on the right are available for blood product administration. Another option is use a standard intravenous fluid administration set and place a commercial filter as seen on the left yourself.

Blood Administration Sets and Filters

A variety of transfusion sets and filters are available for use in veterinary transfusion medicine. Hemo-Nate filters (Gesco International, San Antonio, TX) are recommended for small volume or feline transfusions. The Hemo-Nate filter is a small, square 18–20 μm filter that fits in between the patient and the blood product within the administration line. This small micron filter will filter out some leukocytes, broken down platelets, fibrin, and other microaggregates (Callan 2006). These are small-volume filters; if large volumes are transfused through the filter, you run a higher chance of aggregate clumping, slowed transfusion rates, and eventual filter blockage.

Standard canine blood infusion sets are IV sets with an in-line filter. These filters have a much larger micron size, varying from 170–260 μm, and are ideal for use on canine blood products. These filters are made by multiple manufacturers including Baxter and Abbott. If administering red cell products, care should be taken to completely fill the filter chamber with blood so drops land on RBCs rather than impact onto the filter leading to possible red cell destruction. Lastly, there is a Y-Type filter which allows concurrent administration of saline to dilute RBC solutions that are high in viscosity. The Y-Set is above the filter so both the PRBCs and the saline go into the filter which is an in-line component to the IV line (Abrams-Ogg 2000).

Administration of Fresh Whole Blood/Stored Whole Blood (SWB)

Fresh whole blood should be given immediately after drawing off the donor. Fresh whole blood from cats is most often drawn using syringes, so the blood should be set up on a syringe pump with a Hemo-Nate filter attached and an extension set leading to the patient. If the blood is not given immediately to the patient, it should be labeled and placed into the fridge until the time of administration. Fresh whole blood from dogs is collected into an anticoagulated sealed transfusion bag, so an in-line filter can be attached and the unit administered straight from the collection bag. In the case of SWB from feline donors, the blood can be administered to the cat via an approved blood infusion pump or can be sterilely removed from the bag into a 60-cc syringe and given on a syringe pump as described.

Whenever possible, the blood should be allowed to come to room temperature on its own and never aggressively heated before administration to the patient (Abrams-Ogg 2000; Feldman and Sink 2006). This small and gradual warming prevents accelerated red blood deterioration or bacterial growth in the red cell product. Patients that are already hypothermic or receiving large volumes of red cells should have their units warmed closer to body temperature (37°C) to prevent hypothermia. Blood products can be warmed by laying out at room temperature, in warm-water baths (not to exceed 37°C), or by warming it with approved in-line RBC warmers (Callan 2006).

Packed Red Cell Administration

Packed red cells from felines come in small collection bags and are generally 20–30 mL in volume. Because cats are very small and the transfusion rate is very slow, it is generally recommended that the blood be either transfused through a blood-approved infusion pump or sterilely removed from the bag and given on a syringe pump rather than a gravity drop system (A. Abrams-Ogg 2000). The red cells should be sterilely removed from the bag and placed into an appropriate-sized syringe. The blood should be allowed to come to room temperature as described in the above section.

Because of the viscosity of the unit due to the high PCV of the red cells, it is often recommended that the blood be diluted with saline before administration to facilitate passage through the filter and intravenous catheter. This can be achieved by sterilely adding 8–10 mL of 0.9% saline solution to the syringe. The syringe is then attached to an extension set with a Hemo-Nate filter attached and run on a syringe pump. If the red cells are warmed and drawn up and then no longer needed, they should be replaced back into the refrigerator with the expiration date decreased to 24 hours (A. Abrams-Ogg 2000).

Packed red cells from canines generally come in two volumes: single units which are approximately 125 mL and double units which are approximately 250 mL. The volume will vary depending on the blood bank that created the units. Because most dogs are an appreciable size and the transfusion rates are faster than those used for feline patients, a syringe pump is not required, and gravity administration can be used when appropriate.

As discussed earlier, packed red cell units are often high in viscosity and may require dilution to facilitate administration through the filter and patient. Y-type administration sets can be used on highly viscous canine RBC units. One port of the Y-Set will be attached to the blood unit while the other port is connected to a bag of 0.9% saline solution. The unit only needs to be diluted by 10%–20%; a large amount of dilution is not required and adds additional transfusion volume, potentially leading to volume overload within the patient (Abrams-Ogg 2000).

Red cell transfusions should be completed within 4 hours of administration. Pending additional studies, this time period ensures transfusion of functional and viable red cells while also preventing the growth of bacteria if contamination was present (A. Abrams-Ogg 2000; Callan 2006). As discussed with feline red cell units, if the unit is warmed to room or body temperature, the unit can be placed in the refrigerator and with the expiration decreased to 24 hours (Abrams-Ogg 2000).

Plasma Products

Feline plasma generally comes frozen in small units, 20–30 mL in size and can be fresh frozen or frozen depending on the manufacturing blood bank used. Because hemophilia A is considered rare in cats, many blood banks sell FP, not FFP, for cats. Canine plasma comes in fresh frozen and frozen units in single unit size (125 mL) or double unit size (250 mL). The plasma products should be thawed in a warm water bath not exceeding 37°C until all the frozen crystals have dissolved. Manual manipulation and agitation of the unit will help speed up the thawing process and is not thought to disrupt or damage the plasma proteins.

When thawing the unit you should place it into a freezer or Ziplock® bag (S.C. Johnson & Son, Inc., Racine, WI) to prevent contamination through the collection bag or ports (Abrams-Ogg 2000; Yaxley et al. 2010). Plasma is safe to administer through standard IV infusion pumps as well as syringe pumps. A filter is required for plasma administration so a Hemo-Nate filter should be used in felines and small-volume canine transfusions, while a standard in-line filter should be used for larger canine patients (Abrams-Ogg 2000).

Administration of cryoprecipitate is also monitored for transfusion reactions as it is a blood component product. A Hemo-Nate filter should be attached to the syringe and the above protocol for the first 30 minutes followed to watch for transfusion reactions. Due to the volume size of cryoprecipitate, this rate can be increase or remain the same as the entire volume will likely be administered within 30–90 minutes (Hale 2009).

Occasionally, patients will only require a portion of the plasma unit with the remainder to be transfused at a later time. If this is required, the unit can be thawed by appropriate methods to body temperature (37°C) and the desired amount removed from the bag using sterile technique. The remainder of the unit should be labeled and placed in the fridge until needed. The labile clotting factors and fibrinogen should remain present and viable if the unit is used within 5 days (Abrams-Ogg 2000).

One recent study determined the viability of hemostatic proteins (coagulation factors) when a unit of FFP is thawed to body temperature (37°C) kept refrigerated for 1 hour and then refrozen. Results of the study suggest that FFP units that are thawed to body temperature and then are no longer needed can be refrozen and remain as FFP with no decrease in expiration date if the product is placed back in the freezer within 1 hour of thawing (Yaxley et al. 2010). This is promising as the standard up until this time has been to refreeze the unit but relabel it as FP as it was assumed the labile coagulation factors were significantly reduced after the warming process.

The study did not focus on the potential for bacterial proliferation when warmed to body temperature. If possible contamination is suspected, the unit should be thrown out, or if hospital protocol dictates that thawed units be used within a reduced time frame, then the unit should be placed in the fridge with the expiration decreased to 24 hours (Abrams-Ogg 2000). Pending additional studies, FFP that has been thawed but refrozen within 1 hour of thawing can be kept as FFP for up to 1 year. After that time the unit is relabeled as FP and the expiration period extended by 4 years (Yaxley et al. 2010). If the unit is thawed at body temperature (37°C) but remains at room temperature for greater than 4 hours, it is recommended that the unit either be placed in the fridge as FFP for up to 5 days or refrozen and relabeled as FP with the expiration date changed to reflect that of FP units in case labile clotting factors are significantly decreased (Abrams-Ogg 2000; Brooks 2006).

Transfusion Reactions

There are four categories of transfusion reactions that are described in canine and feline transfusion medicine. Transfusion reactions are either acute immunologic or acute nonimmunologic, or delayed immunologic or delayed nonimmunologic. Acute reactions are said to occur within minutes to hours of the transfusion while delayed reactions occur days to months after the transfusion. It is also possible for animals to have multiple reactions from different categories (Abrams-Ogg 2000; Brooks 2006; Hohenhaus 2006).

In general, pretreatment for transfusion-related reactions is not required unless the patient has a history of fever reactions or previous transfusion reactions. In addition, many of the adverse side effects from the transfusion reaction do not alter with the pretreatment of steroids or antihistamines (Abrams-Ogg 2000; Brooks 2006; Hohenhaus 2006). Pretreatment should be based on the individual patient and attending veterinarian along with the type and amount of blood product used.

Immunologic Reactions

Immunologic reactions are caused by antigen–antibody interactions between the donor and recipient. This category of reactions includes antigen reactions from red cells, white cells, plasma proteins, and/or platelets (Abrams-Ogg 2000; Hohenhaus 2006). This category is further broken down into subtypes listed as follows.

Red blood cell incompatibility reactions (hemolytic reactions)

The mechanism of this reaction is discussed at the beginning of the chapter and involves red cell antigen–antibody incompatibility. More specifically, antibodies present within the recipient plasma recognize the red cell antigens as foreign, and an immunologic response is formed. The interaction triggers an inflammatory response in the recipient resulting in red cell hemolysis and systemic inflammation (Abrams-Ogg 2000; Hohenhaus 2006).

An acute hemolytic reaction usually occurs within the first 30–60 minutes of the transfusion but can occur all the way up to 48 hours after the transfusion administration. In felines, this reaction is severe, likely owing to their strong naturally occurring alloantibodies. Numerous sources site that a Type B feline that is inadvertently transfused with as little as 1 mL of Type A blood can develop a severe acute hemolytic reaction (Abrams-Ogg 2000; Wardrop 2006; Hohenhaus 2006). Clinical symptoms vary based on species, type of blood product, and the volume of transfused product. In a feline hemolytic reaction, such symptoms as recumbency and stretching of the limbs, tachycardia, respiratory distress, and tachypnea occur and if left untreated then can progress to hypotension, bradycardia, pulmonary edema, and potential death (Abrams-Ogg 2000; Hohenhaus 2006). Additional symptoms reported with this type of reaction are cyanosis, seizures, tremors, vomiting, diarrhea, hyper salivation, and weakness (A. Abrams-Ogg 2000).

Canine acute hemolytic reactions often do not show the same symptoms or symptom severity as feline patients; more often, tachycardia, fever, panting (tachypnea), and urination/defecation are the first symptoms displayed along with hemoglobinuria and hemoglobinemia (Abrams-Ogg 2000; Hohenhaus 2006). In dogs, this type of reaction would occur from previous sensitization to foreign red blood antigens. This type of reaction can best be prevented by crossmatching the donor blood to the patient prior to administration; however, future reactions due to sensitization during this transfusion cannot be prevented (Hohenhaus 2006). Treatment for both feline and canine acute immunologic (hemolytic) reaction includes immediate discontinuation of the transfusion and notification of the attending clinician. Pretreatment of antihistamines and/or corticosteroids will not prevent a hemolytic reaction as they do not acutely suppress the production of IgG or IgM antibodies or prevent binding of IgE to mast cells (A. Abrams-Ogg 2000).

Once the transfusion has been stopped, the patient should receive supportive care, which may include IV fluids (shock doses of 60 mL/kg/h in cats and 90 mL/kg/h in dogs), colloids (hetastarch at 5–15 mL/kg/day), diuretics (furosemide at 2–4 mg/kg IV), pressors (dopamine at 2–5 mcg/kg/min as a CRI), and/or oxygen supplementation (Abrams-Ogg 2000; Feldman and Sink 2006; Hohenhaus 2006). In addition, a blood sample should be drawn for a Coombs test and to test for presence of hemoglobinemia and hemolysis. During this time, it is recommended that a urinary catheter be placed to monitor fluid outputs (Feldman and Sink 2006; Hohenhaus 2006).

Delayed RBC immunologic reactions (hemolytic) begin to occur 3–5 days post transfusion. The most common cause of this is antibody production within the recipient as a result of the presence of foreign antigens in the donor cells. Although there are no naturally occurring antibodies to DEA 1.1 and 1.2, if a DEA 1.1 negative dog is transfused (first transfusion) with DEA 1.1 positive blood, antibodies production will begin within the immune system. These antibody levels increase and build up within the recipient and eventually, an anamnestic response will occur, with clinical symptoms often emerging around 5–10 days post transfusion (Abrams-Ogg 2000; Feldman and Sink 2006; Hohenhaus 2006).

Symptoms of a delayed hemolytic reaction include a steady decrease in posttransfusion PCV over a period of 3–5 days, development of jaundice, fever, and anorexia (Abrams-Ogg 2000; Hohenhaus 2006). In general, transfused red cells are expected to remain in the patient for 4–6 weeks. Delayed hemolytic reactions can greatly decrease this as the red cells are slowly being destroyed as the patient builds antibodies. This illustrates another reason why the saying "the first transfusion is always safe" should be abandoned as delayed reactions can be detrimental to animals who have an absent or slower bone marrow response to their anemia.

Although a crossmatch cannot predict a delayed transfusion reaction, typing and crossmatching of the donor and recipient to identify blood types and blood compatibility can help minimize the chances of an acute immunologic reaction (Hohenhaus 2006; Wardrop 2006).

White blood cell and platelet incompatibility reactions (nonhemolytic)

This type of immunologic reaction occurs when antibodies to donor WBC and/or platelet antigens are present in the patient. This type of reaction is nonhemolytic in nature, but it can lead to fever and or/vomiting within the first 1–2 hours of the transfusion. As with immunologic hemolytic reactions, pretreatment with antihistamines will not prevent this type of incompatibility reaction and subsequent fever from occurring, although some authors have suggested that pretreatment with a steroid (dexamethasone sodium phosphate at 0.5–1.0 mg/kg IV 5–15 minutes prior) may help in patients with a transfusion history (Abrams-Ogg 2000; Callan 2006).

Treatment for both feline and canine acute nonhemolytic immunologic reactions includes immediate discontinuation of the transfusion and notification of the attending clinician. Treatment may include administration of steroids, if not given prior to transfusion (dexamethasone sodium phosphate 0.5–2 mg/kg IV), supportive care for the fever including administration of cooled IV fluids (0.9% NaCl or another crystalloid in a separate vein), removing bulky blankets and towels, and other cooling methods (A. Abrams-Ogg 2000; Feldman and Sink 2006; Hohenhaus 2006).

If the transfusion must be continued, it is suggested that the rate be slowed down and monitoring of vitals performed more often. In general, this type of reaction will resolve on its own within 12–24 hours (Abrams-Ogg 2000). One other form of preventative treatment include purchasing WBC filters, which can filter out WBCs from the blood products. They are becoming more available and more affordable, but may not be practical for every transfusion (Abrams-Ogg 2000; Callan 2006).

Acute hypersensitivity reaction (nonhemolytic)

This reaction occurs from an immunologic reaction to gamma globulins found in the plasma. This is a type of allergic reaction, often referred to as a hypersensitivity reaction (IgE-mediated) and is fairly rare, occurring in approximately 1%–2% of transfusions (Abrams-Ogg 2000; Hohenhaus 2006). This type of reaction usually occurs within the first 15–45 minutes, but it can emerge anytime throughout the transfusion. Hypersensitivity reactions are of concern because of the potential for anaphylaxis. Common symptoms of this reaction include pruritis, urticaria (hives), vomiting, and/or diarrhea. If the patient has a severe reaction, anaphylaxis may occur, leading to edema, ascites, and pleural effusion (Abrams-Ogg 2000; Hohenhaus 2006; Feldman and Sink 2006). Treatment includes stopping the transfusion and notifying the attending clinician. This type of reaction can sometimes be affected by the rate of administration, so if the transfusion is continued, it should be performed at a slower rate. Antihistamines should be administered (diphenhydramine at 1–2 mg/kg SQ, IM, or slow IV). Corticosteroids can also be administered (dexamethasone sodium phosphate 0.5–1.0 mg/kg IV, IM). If anaphylaxis is suspected, the transfusion should be stopped completely and supportive care given until the patient is stable (Abrams-Ogg 2000).

Preventative treatment should be considered in any animal who have received prior transfusions greater than 4 days prior. This includes avoiding using blood products from the same donor (donor rotation), pretreatment with antihistamines and/or steroids (15–30 minutes prior to administration), and for patients with documented allergic reactions to a previous transfusions, strict monitoring and reduced administration rates for early reaction detection (Abrams-Ogg 2000; Feldman and Sink 2006; Hohenhaus 2006).

Nonimmunologic Transfusion Reactions

These reactions occur from outside factors and are not reactions that are directly related to red cell, platelet, white cell, or protein antigen–antibody reactions. Most often, these reactions occur from collection, storage, and/or administration errors.

Volume overload

Volume overload is a common nonimmunologic reaction occurring often in cat transfusions. Blood products are potent natural colloids, and blood transfusions often include the administration of large volume of blood products. Volume overload (hypervolemia) can occur from transfusing too much product or transfusing it too quickly. One big contributor to hypervolemia is the inadvertent concurrent administration of crystalloids during the transfusion. Some patients do require both blood product and concurrent crystalloid/colloid administration, but those that are normovolemic or at risk for volume overload (underlying heart disease, renal disease) should have their intravenous fluids discontinued prior to and during the transfusion (Abrams-Ogg 2000; Hohenhaus 2006).

Symptoms of volume overload can include dyspnea, cyanosis, coughing (pulmonary edema), vomiting, and/or ascites formation. Treatment of volume overload includes either decreasing the transfusion rate or stopping the transfusion altogether depending on the severity of hypervolemia and clinical signs (Feldman and Sink 2006; Hohenhaus 2006). For those who are clinical for volume overload, diuretics can be given (furosemide at 2–4 mg/kg IV), oxygen supplementation implemented, and in extreme circumstances, emergency phlebotomy can be done to try to decrease overall volume (Abrams-Ogg 2000; Hohenhaus 2006).

Sepsis

Blood products are an excellent source of nutrients for bacteria, and because of this, contaminated anticoagulants, improper handling, storage, and administration can lead to bacterial growth within the blood product. Some sources of contamination include donor sources (bacteria on skin, improper area prep), transfusion material contamination (donor bags, needles, anticoagulant solutions), and/or mishandling of blood products (thawing, elevated temperatures, contamination during spiking) (Abrams-Ogg 2000).

Severe bacterial contamination can occur in stored blood products as bacterial proliferation easily occurs with the available nutrients in the unit. Newly developed blood banks (in-hospital or commercial) should perform random cultures on their units to make sure bacterial growth is not occurring (Abrams-Ogg 2000). Bacterial contamination can be avoided by using strict sterile technique when collecting and handling blood products, and by following suggested expiration dates (Abrams-Ogg 2000; Feldman and Sink 2006; Hohenhaus 2006).

Sepsis can occur within a few hours of the transfusion, but can take 1–3 days to fully appear in the recipient. Common symptoms of sepsis can include acute vomiting, diarrhea, fever, hypotension, hypoglycemia and, if severe, dyspnea, collapse, DIC, and cardiopulmonary arrest. It should be noted that many of these symptoms are also seen in acute immunologic reactions, so staff must look for other signs to confirm sepsis within the patient.

Blood products should be inspected upon arrival and at regular intervals during refrigeration. Blood products are usually a medium to bright red color, and units that are black or dark red should be set aside and a culture sent out to confirm or rule out contamination

(Abrams-Ogg 2000). If it is suspected that a patient became septic from a blood product, a blood culture of the patient and the unit should be sent off for analysis.

Treatment of sepsis is a complex process and varies depending on the severity, underlying conditions, hospital supplies and medications, and so on. Often, antibiotic therapy is started along with crystalloid and/or colloid therapy to help correct hypotension, electrolyte/glucose support, and general supportive care (Abrams-Ogg 2000; Hohenhaus 2006).

Miscellaneous Reactions

There are many other nonimmunologic transfusion reactions that can occur with transfusion products.

Hyperammonemia

It is crucial to remember that blood products contain red cells and contain living, breathing cells. These red cells require oxygen and nutrients for survival, and during storage, the amount of viable red cells reduces over time. When red cells within the unit become inactive and die, they are broken down and release potassium and ammonia as a by-product (Abrams-Ogg 2000; Feldman and Sink 2006). As units approach their expiration date, the bag contains a higher amount of ammonia and inactive red cells than fresher units. Hyperammonemia can pose a problem for animals with underlying hepatic disease as they are unable to fully filter out ammonia. Ammonia accumulation in the patient can lead to exacerbation of the hepatic disease, CNS symptoms, and hepatic encephalopathy. Patients with underlying hepatic disease that require RBC products should be given the freshest product available to prevent additional hepatic compromise. In addition, because of the loss of viable red cells and the high levels of ammonia and potassium, blood products should never be used past their expiration dates (Abrams-Ogg 2000; Feldman and Sink 2006).

Hypothermia

Hypothermia can occur from transfusing blood products that are below body temperature or from multiple product administration. This is especially dangerous in small and/or young animals (Abrams-Ogg 2000; Feldman and Sink 2006). Blood products should be warmed to at least room temperature, and if required, body temperature (37°C) before administration. This can be achieved by placing the blood product in a warm water bath, using an approved blood warming device, or simply holding the blood product at body temperature until warm. When thawing the unit you should place it into a freezer or Ziploc bag to prevent contamination through the collection bag or ports (Abrams-Ogg 2000; Yaxley et al. 2010).

References

Abrams-Ogg, A. 2000. Practical blood transfusion. In *Manual of Canine and Feline Haematology and Transfusion Medicine*, edited by Day, M, Mackin, A, Littlewood, J. Ontario, Canada: British Small Animal Veterinary Association. pp. 263–302.

Bergeron, DA. 2005. Component preparation. In *Textbook of Blood Banking and Transfusion Medicine*, 2nd ed., edited by Rudmann, SV. Philadelphia: Elsevier Saunders. pp. 232–257.

Brooks, M. 2006. Transfusion of plasma and plasma derivatives. In *Schalm's Veterinary Hematology*, 5th ed., edited by Feldman, BF, Zinkl, JG, Jain, NC. Ithaca, NY: Blackwell. pp. 838–842.

Callan, MB. 2006. Red blood cell transfusions in the dog and cat. In *Schalm's Veterinary Hematology*, 5th ed., edited by Feldman, BF, Zinkl, JG, Jain, NC. Philadelphia: Blackwell. pp. 833–837.

Car, BD. 2006. Erythropoiesis and erythrokinetics. In *Schalm's Veterinary Hematology*, 5th ed., edited by Feldman, BF, Zinkl, JG, Jain, NC. Newark, DE: Blackwell. pp. 105–109.

Feldman, BF, Sink, CA. 2006. *Practical Transfusion Medicine for the Small Animal Practitioner*. Blacksburg, MD: Tenton NewMedia.

Hale, A. 2009. *Animal Blood Resources HemaGold Line*. Retrieved 09 01, 2010, from Animal Blood Resources International: www.abrint.net.

Hohenhaus, A. 2006. Transfusion reactions. In *Schalm's Veterinary Hematology*, 5th ed., edited by Feldman, BF, Zinkl, JG, Jain, NC. New York: Blackwell. pp. 864–868.

Schneider, A. 2006. Principles of blood collection and processing. In *Schalm's Veterinary Hematology*, 5th ed., edited by Feldman, BF, Zinkl, JG, Jain, NC. Annapolis, MD: Blackwell. pp. 827–831.

Wardrop, J. 2006. Clinical blood typing and crossmatching. In *Schalm's Veterinary Hematology*, 5th ed., edited by Feldman, BF, Zinkl, JG, Jain, NC. Pullman, WA: Blackwell. pp. 795–797.

Wardrop, J, Reine, N, Birkenheuer, A, et al. 2005. Canine and feline blood donor screening for infectious disease. *Journal of American College of Veterinary Internal Medicine (JACVIM)* 19(1):135–142.

Yaxley, P, Beal, M, Jutkowitz, L, et al. 2010. Comparative stability of canine and feline hemostatic proteins in freeze-thaw-cycled fresh frozen plasma. *Journal of Veterinary Emergency and Critical Care (JVECC)* 20(5):472–478.

CHAPTER 21

Nutrition for the Critically Ill

Ann Elise Wortinger

Introduction

Inadequate calorie intake in critically ill dogs and cats due to anorexia, inability to eat or tolerate feedings (e.g., vomiting), or decreased absorptive capabilities is a frequent but often overlooked problem (Chan 2005a,b). When looking at veterinary patients, the most common reasons for in-hospital starvation and failure to provide a positive energy balance appear to be poorly written feeding orders, direct orders to withhold food, and refusal by the animal to consume the food offered (Chan 2005a,b). Energy supply, even if modest and close to resting energy requirements (RERs), appears to be positively associated with veterinary hospital discharge (Brunetto et al. 2010).

While withholding food for pretreatment and preanesthetic events is often necessary, when performed repeatedly and for prolonged periods of time, the loss of intake can be significant. The problems include alterations in wound healing, compromised immune function, decreased cardiac and respiratory function, and potentially, a negative impact on overall survival (Chan 2005a,b; Wingfield 1997). Prolonged malnutrition can ultimately lead to organ failure and eventually death (Buffington et al. 2004; Michel 2006a,b). In an effort to help avoid these consequences, improvements in nutritional assessment, nutritional plan formulation and execution is essential. Therefore, once patients are stable, consideration should be made to address the nutritional status of the patient and develop an appropriate and feasible feeding plan (Fig. 22.1).

CHAPTER 22

523

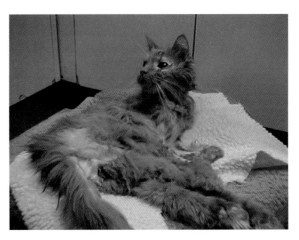

Figure 22.1   A cat with severe weight loss from malnutrition.

Nutrition and the Body

While healthy animals lose primarily fat when they do not receive adequate caloric intake, sick or traumatized patients catabolize lean body mass when they are not provided with sufficient calories (Chan 2005a,b). When subjected to starvation, all body tissue (except the brain and bone) loose cell mass to varying degrees. Neoplasia and tissue injury may act as additional burdens, and can further increase the patient's caloric and nutritional requirements (Donaghue 1989). When the body uses *exogenous stores* (those provided outside of the body) rather than *endogenous stores* (those provided by the animals own body's reserves), the breakdown of lean body mass is minimized and the patient's response to therapy is optimized (Abood 1997).

Nutrition Goals

Overall, the goal of nutritional support is to meet the patient's nutritional requirements and, if possible, prevent further deterioration of the patient's general health status. This can be achieved by providing calories in the form of protein, carbohydrate, and fat, while including other nutrients (vitamins, macrominerals, microminerals) necessary for survival. To achieve this, a formula must be utilized that will be maximally utilized by the body and have minimum adverse effects (Donaghue 1989). Even with initiation of adequate nutritional support, muscle wasting and negative nitrogen balance can occur (Wingfield 1997). The longer the wait before nutritional intervention is started, the more significant the changes that can occur (Table 22.1).

Guidelines for Nutritional Support

Nutrition has gained increased recognition in the management of emergency and critical care cases and as a result, the recommended duration of time that an animal is permitted

Table 22.1 Recommended levels of protein, fat, and carbohydrate in critical care diets expressed as metabolizable energy (ME)

Species	Protein % ME	Fat % ME	Carbohydrate% ME
Dogs	20–30	30–55	15–50
Cats	25–35	40–55	15–25

Source: Tennant (1996).

Table 22.2 Guidelines for initiating nutritional support

Loss or anticipated loss of 10% or more of body weight
Anorexia of >3 days
Trauma
Surgery
Severe systemic infiltrative disease
Diarrhea, vomiting, draining wounds or burns

Source: Wingfield (1997).

to have relative anorexia (insufficient caloric intake to meet the body's requirements) to absolute anorexia (no intake of calories) has decreased from weeks to days. Most veterinary nutritionists agree that no animal should go longer than 5 days without adequate nutrition, and many feel this number is ideally closer to 3 days. It is important to remember that this 3- to 5-day interval is not "hospital days" but rather total days without adequate food intake (Chan 2006). Still the current tendency is to wait too long before instituting nutritional support (Chan 2005a,b).

General guidelines for initiating nutritional support include the loss or anticipated loss of more than 10% of the patient's body weight; anorexia lasting 3 days or longer; trauma; surgery (including elective surgeries); severe systemic infiltrative disease; increased nutrient loss through diarrhea, vomiting, draining wounds, nephropathy, or burns associated with decreased serum albumin (Wingfield 1997) (Table 22.2).

Nutritional Assessment

The cornerstones of nutritional assessment are conducting a complete physical examination, obtaining a detailed patient history (including food intake estimates and diet history), documenting body weight, assessing the patient's body condition using one of the recognized body condition score (BCS) systems, evaluating blood chemistry profiles, and performing a complete blood count (Abood 1997). The specific blood profiles required will depend on the patient's condition and individual clinician's preference.

There are five specific areas of the patient history that need to receive special attention when making a nutritional assessment. These would include

- The presence of any weight loss and over what period of time that weight loss occurred.
- Whether there is voluntary oral dietary intake.
- Presence of gastrointestinal signs such as nausea, vomiting, diarrhea, or gastroesophageal reflux.
- Patient's functional capacity (e.g., exercise intolerance or lack thereof).
- Metabolic demands from any underlying disease state.

It is important to note over what period of time the weight loss has occurred because rapid weight loss involves a greater percent loss of lean body mass than does a gradual weight loss (Michel 2006a,b).

Body Condition Scoring

The BCSs used for healthy animals often do not convert well to sick animals. This is because when an animal is physiologically stressed, lean body mass is its preferred energy source. In contrast, healthy animals use stored body fat for energy. The result is increased catabolism of body protein in the sick animal (Buffington et al. 2004). The catabolism of lean body mass is an adaptive response by the body where endogenous amino acids are prioritized for the synthesis of proteins vital for survival. The problem is that there are no protein stores within the body as all endogenous protein serves some functional purpose; therefore, this breakdown of lean body mass when sick or injured will have a negative effect on the patient (Michel 2006a,b). Decreased lean body mass can be clinically observed with decreased functional reserves in all the organs, decreased muscle activity that can be seen with decreased ventilatory effort, cardiac arrhythmias, and generalized muscle weakness.

A patient may present with increased amounts of body fat but still be at serious risk of malnutrition-associated complications caused by protein catabolism. Careful examination, including palpation of skeletal muscles over bony prominences (e.g., the scapula, vertebrae, hips, and occipital crest) can help identify any muscle wasting consistent with increase protein catabolism. Other physical indicators of poor nutritional status include peripheral edema and ascites, which result in alteration to colloidal osmotic pressure from low serum albumin levels secondary to malnutrition. Poor hair coat and skin condition can also result from inadequate food intake or micronutrient deficiencies (Remillard et al. 2000).

The findings of the historical and physical assessment are used to categorize the patient as well nourished, moderately malnourished, at risk for becoming malnourished, or significantly malnourished. Using this classification scheme in conjunction with the patient's underlying disease and current status will help in deciding whether to initiate nutritional support (Michel 2006a,b).

Calculating Energy Requirements

Caloric requirements are determined by a patient's body weight and function and can be calculated by using the resting energy requirement (RER) formula for healthy adults at rest in environmentally comfortable cages (Donaghue 1989). Most hospitalized patients are not expending more energy than RER since they are usually caged in a thermoneutral environment. Therefore, if a patient's caloric intake is at least RER, it should not lose significant amount of weight (Michel 2006a,b). In the past years, RER was often multiplied by a potential illness factor coefficient. More recently, the application of illness factors to the RER is believed to be a source of increased morbidity rather than improving clinical outcome and is therefore currently discouraged (Chan 2005a,b). Water requirements equal those for energy (1 mL = 1 kcal) (Torrance 1996). Patients that wish to eat more than the calculated RER amounts should not be discouraged from doing so while recovering from surgery, trauma, or chronic disease.

RERs can be calculated by several formulas. The most widely used formula is:

$$RER = (weight\ in\ kilograms \times 30) + 70$$

This formula can be utilized in ill and healthy cats and dogs between 2 kg and 45 kg (Hand et al. 2000). Alternately, for cats, weight in kilograms × 40 + RER.

For animals less than 2 kg or above 45 kg, the formula most commonly used is:

$$RER = (70 \times weight\ in\ kilograms)^{0.75}$$

RER should be calculated for a patient's current weight first to prevent any further deterioration but, most importantly, calculate again using ideal or desired weight. Often one will start feeding a case at the lower RER, and as the patient improves, will gradually increase the caloric intake to the higher RER for the desired weight.

RER is a general guideline or caloric need and may need to be adjusted as necessary for individual patients. The more critically ill the patient is, the less likely it is to tolerate 100% RER. The patient's condition may help dictate the volume of food administered. It is not abnormal to take 5–7 days for the animal to be able to tolerate full RER feeding and sometimes as long as 10–14 days.

For a sick animal that is ambulatory and minimally active, calculating the metabolic energy requirements (MERs) can provide a transition caloric goal. To calculate MER, the calculated RER is multiplied by 1.2–1.3. Numbers higher than these are usually not necessary because MER is dictated by activity level and most ill patients are only minimally active. If nutritional support is to continue after discharge from the hospital, be sure to recalculate your numbers to include enough for activity outside the hospital by figuring out a more accurate MER for the new activity level (Table 22.3).

Overfeeding can result in metabolic and gastrointestinal complications, hepatic dysfunction, increased carbon dioxide production (with subsequent decrease in plasma pH), and weakened respiratory muscles. Of the metabolic complications encountered in critical care nutrition, the development of hyperglycemia is the most common, and possibly the most detrimental (Chan 2006).

Table 22.3   Enteral nutrition worksheet

Client: _____ Patient: _____ Case #_____

Date: _____ Body Condition Score: _____/5

Actual Body Weight (kg): _____ Desired Body Weight (kg): _____

Resting energy requirements (RER) = (wt in kg) 30 + 70 = kcal/day

RER: _____ kcal/day   Product selected_____

Contains: _____ kcal/mL, kcal/can, kcal/cup (circle one)

Feeding Instructions:

For canned food: Feed _____ cans _____ times/day OR

For dry food: Feed _____ cups _____ times/day

Total volume to be administered/day:

kcal required/day

kcal/mL in diet = _____ mL/day

Administration schedule (differs for hepatic lipidosis)

1/3 of total requirement on Day 1 = _____ mL/day

2/3 of total requirement on Day 2 = _____ mL/day

Total requirement on Day 3 = _____ mL/day

Feeding schedule

Divide total daily volume into 4–6 feedings/day (depending on patient needs)

Day 1 = _____feedings/day

Day 2 = _____feedings/day

Day 3 = _____feedings/day

Volume/feeding

Day 1 = _____mL/feeding

Day 2 = _____mL/feeding

Day 3 = _____mL/feeding

Individual Patient Considerations

The gut is generally the safest and most natural route for administering nutrients. This has promoted to school of thought of "If the gut works... then use it!" Maintaining the intestinal mucosa may also help prevent bacterial translocation from the gut to the rest of the body and avoid patient sepsis. This is best accomplished with enteral feeding (Hill 1994). Voluntary oral intake is the preferred route for enteral nutrition; however, patients must be able to consume at least 85% of their calculated RERs for this method of feeding to be effective (Donaghue 1989). Veterinary technicians often need to devise ways to encourage patients to accept oral feedings. Appetite stimulants (e.g., cyproheptadine,

---

Box 22.1   Hints for Increasing Oral Intake of Food

- Hand-feed or pet the patient during feeding.
- Warm the food to slightly below body temperature; if microwaving, be sure food is stirred well before feeding.
- Add warm water to dry food or make slurry from canned foods by adding warm water.
- Use baby food meats as a top dressing; dogs may also like cat food used as a top dressing.
- Try various shapes and types of bowls. Shallow dishes for cats and brachycephalic dog breeds; plastic may have a strange smell to the animals.
- Use foods that have a strong smell or odor.
- Add appetite stimulants to "jump-start" the feeding process (usually ineffective over the long term) (Torrance 1996).

---

mirtazepine, diazepam) are often inappropriately and overconfidently used. In reality, they are inadequate long-term solutions as they do not ensure adequate caloric intake and often have clinically short effectiveness. The better assumption would be that appetite will not improve without supportive care, and nutritional intervention should be attempted (Chan 2005a,b).

If a patient is unwilling or unable to eat voluntarily, tube feeding should be considered. Tube feeding, however, is limited by diet selections. In most instances, only liquid or gruel diets can be fed through the tube due to its small internal diameter. In addition, tubes can become clogged and must be flushed regularly with water to help prevent occlusion (Remillard et al. 2000).

To assess the advisability of enteral nutritional support in a given patient, several considerations should be made, including gastrointestinal tract function, other organ systems that may have an impact on the patient's ability to tolerate specific nutrients, the patient's ability to tolerate the tube and tube placement, and the patient's risk for pulmonary aspiration (Michel 2006a,b).

The gastrointestinal assessment should include evaluation of the patient for nausea and vomiting and indications of gastrointestinal dysfunction such as ileus, malabsorption, or maldigestion. Also take into consideration whether the patient will be receiving any medication that might cause nausea (e.g., antibiotics) or ileus and whether the patient has had any recent alimentary tract surgery or injury that you may wish to bypass.

Hypothermia and hypotension will also decrease gut perfusion and motility and should be evaluated. Enteral nutrition should not be given until the animal is hemodynamically stable with normal body temperature. An animal that is hypothermic and/or hypotensive will likely have compromised gut perfusion and motility and should not receive enteral nutrition until it has been warmed and stabilized (Michel 2006a,b).

Impairment of other organ systems may have an impact on diet selection as they may not be able to tolerate specific nutrients. Renal failure or hepatic encephalopathy may affect protein tolerance. Infiltrative mucosal disease or lymphangiectasia may affect the patient's ability to assimilate dietary fats (Michel 2006a,b).

With the exception of nasoesophageal (NE) tubes, all types of feeding tube placement require some form of anesthesia and analgesia. Feeding tubes requiring some level of anesthesia for placement would include esophagostomy, gastrostomy, and jejunostomy

Table 22.4   Which type of tube to use?

Type of Tube	Cost	Food Used	Length of Time for Use
Nasoesophageal/naosgastric	$	Thinned liquid	3–7 days
Esophagostomy	$$	Undiluted liquid to gruel	1–20 weeks
Gastrostomy	$$$	Undiluted liquid to gruel	1 week to permanent
Jejunostomy	$$$$	Liquid CRI	3–10 days

tubes. Looking at nutritional status at the time of a planned anesthetic event can decrease the number of times the animal is anesthetized as well as decrease the time until nutritional intervention can occur (Michel 2006a,b). Tube placement typically is a short procedure, and can easily be carried out during the recovery phase of anesthesia, as surgical depth of anesthesia is generally not required (Table 22.4).

The most serious complication of enteral feeding is aspiration pneumonia. This can become a fatal consequence in critically ill patients. Patients most at risk include those who have prior history of aspiration pneumonia, depressed mental status from sedatives or analgesics, patients with head trauma, neuropathies, megaesophagus, those with reduced or absent gag or cough reflexes, and patients on mechanical ventilation (Michel 2006a,b).

The availability of nursing care will also influence the choice of feeding tube and feeding route used. Considerations should include whether 24-hour care is available, how long nutritional support is anticipated, whether the patient can be fed via bolus or whether constant rate infusion (CRI) is required, and whether owners are able to manage the tube at home if needed (Michel 2006a,b). CRI of nutrition is often easier and less time-consuming for nursing staff but ties up equipment and requires an initial equipment investment. It would appear, however, that at least as far as nasoenteric feeding tubes go, continuous versus intermittent delivery of nutrition result in no significant difference in gastrointestinal complications (Campbell et al. 2010).

Diet selection will also help to determine tube type and site of placement. With a gruel or blenderized diet, you are limited to a larger bore tube (>12–14 French) such as an esophageal or gastrostomy tube. If you are limited to smaller bore tubes, then liquid diets will be your only option.

Many of the currently available critical care diets are available as either gruel foods, or are easily made into a gruel form. A consideration with gruel or liquid diets is the caloric density of the food. The lower the caloric density (the fewer calories provided/milliliter of diet) the more food will need to be given to the animal to meet the RER or MER. Ideally, feeding a diet with the highest caloric density will provide all the required nutrients while decreasing the volume of food being fed either through voluntary eating or assisted feeding. If an animal has been severely catabolic or anorexic for a prolonged period of time, significant changes may have occurred in the intestinal tract, decreasing the ability of the animal to digest and utilize the nutrients being provided.

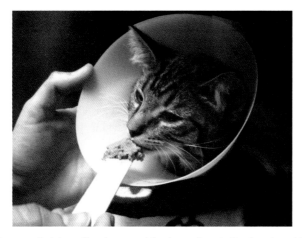

Figure 22.2   A veterinary technician offered warmed food to a hospitalized patient. Many patients will start eating when food is provided warm and they are encouraged. (Courtesy of David Liss, RVT, VTS [Emergency & Critical Care].)

Diets

The selection of food type should be based on several factors including the medical condition and how it affects the patient's tolerance of fat and protein, the preferred route of feeding (oral, feeding tube, intravenous), nutritional requirements for that given patient, access to specific diets, and the cost of use and cost to client (Michel 2006a,b) (Fig. 22.2).

There are three basic types of diets available for use. The least expensive would be commercial diets or, for use in feeding tubes, blenderized commercial diets. These diets tend to be more readily available than some other diets, decreasing the number of diets needed in your inventory. The disadvantage to these diets would be their lack of caloric density when compared with recovery diets (Michel 2006a,b).

There are a number of commercially available recovery diets formulated specifically for cats and dogs. These diets can be fed both orally and through feeding tubes. The size of tubes the individual diet will pass through will vary based on the product. The disadvantage to these diets is they are more expensive than nonrecovery commercial diets and they tend to be high in fat (Michel 2006a,b). Maximum calorie canned diet manufactured by the Iams Company (Dayton, OH), A/D canned diet manufactured by the Hill's Company (Hill's Pet Nutrition, Topeka, KS), and Clinicare liquid diet manufactured by Abbott Laboratories (Worcester, MA) are examples of commercially available recovery diets.

The last category of recovery diets would be commercially available human products. This would include products such as Jevity, Osmolite, and Ensure, all manufactured by Abbott Laboratories. These not only offer the same advantages as the veterinary enteral diets, but also provide a wider range of formulas allowing the clinician a more varied selection to choose from. The primary disadvantage is that they are not balanced for the veterinary patient. Therefore, they need to have protein, taurine, arginine, and B vitamins added in sufficient amounts to meet the unique needs of the veterinary patients (Michel 2006a,b).

CHAPTER 22

Commercial pet foods are specifically designed to meet the dietary requirements of cats and dogs and contain ingredients (e.g., glutamine, taurine, carnitine) not usually found in liquid or parenteral diets. The principal differences between human and animal liquid diets are the extent that ingredients are subject to hydrolysis and the protein contents. For example, most human enteral diets contain 14%–17% protein, which is insufficient for both dogs and cats. In addition, arginine and methionine levels in human enteral diets tend to be too low, especially for cats (Tennant 1996). Unfortunately, after the addition of these nutrients, any perceived savings seen by using the human product is generally lost in the cost of the additions.

Patients with stress starvation can be glucose intolerant and if so, use glucose less efficiently as an energy source. Therefore, protein and fat are important sources of energy. Before evaluating the need for fat, protein, and carbohydrate, however, a good diet strategy should address the animal's requirement for water and correct any preexisting fluid and acid–base deficits. After these needs have been satisfied, sufficient fat, carbohydrate, and protein should be provided to meet the animal's energy requirements and minimize the gluconeogenesis from amino acids (Tennant 1996).

In human medicine, the presence of hyperglycemia is seen as a poor prognostic indicator in all hospitalized patients. Because of this, it has become a target of therapy since reducing the hyperglycemia with insulin improves patient outcome. In dogs, mortality rates dramatically increased when comparing animals that were mildly hyperglycemic to those who were severely hyperglycemic (Chan 2006). When faced with a hyperglycemic animal in a critical care situation, the decision to treat with insulin should not be made lightly, and could well influence the final outcome for the animal. Insulin not only exerts an effect on glucose transportation into the cells, but also effects the transportation of potassium, phosphorus, and magnesium into the cells. This can result in hypoglycemia, as well as a decrease in the intracellular electrolytes as measured in the plasma. A small number of animals may also show an allergic reaction to insulin, as it is a foreign protein (Nelson and Couto 2009).

Pediatric or growth pet diets are often recommended because they are highly digestible, have a high fat and protein contents, and are very palatable (Hill 1994). Meat-based baby foods contain 30%–70% protein and 20%–60% fat. However, because they are deficient in calcium, vitamin A, and thiamine, baby foods should not be used as the sole dietary source (Wingfield 1997). Caution should also be made to avoid baby foods with onion or garlic powder, as such substances may be toxic to veterinary patients.

Enteral Feeding Tubes

The best feeding tubes for prolonged use are made of polyurethane or silicone. For short-term feeding, usually less than 10 days, polyvinylchloride (PVC) tubes can be used. These are not appropriate for long-term feeding because they tend to become stiff with prolonged use, causing additional discomfort for the patient. Silicone, however, is softer and is more flexible than other tube materials, but has a greater tendency to stretch and collapse. Polyurethane is stronger than silicone, allowing for thinner tube walls and a greater internal diameter, despite the same French size. Both the silicone and polyurethane tubes do not disintegrate or become brittle *in situ*, providing a longer tube life.

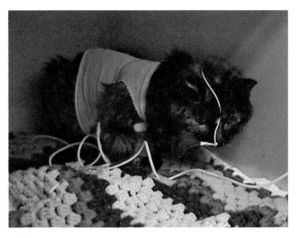

Figure 22.3   A cat being fed via nasoesophageal tube.

Nasoesophageal (NE)/Nasogastric Tube

NE tubes are useful for providing short-term nutritional support, usually less than 10 days. They should be used only in patients with a functional esophagus, stomach, and intestines. NE tubes are contraindicated in patients that are vomiting, comatose, or lack a gag reflex (Willard 1992; Hand et al. 2000). Complications include epistaxis, lack of tolerance of the procedure, inadvertent removal by the patient, and aspiration. These tubes should not be used in vomiting patients or those with respiratory compromise (Guilford et al. 1996; Hand et al. 2000) (Fig. 22.3).

Due to the small internal diameter of these tubes, only liquid enteral diets may be used. Patients with NE tubes can either be fed through a syringe pump as a CRI or bolus fed. If feeding through a syringe pump, completely change the delivery equipment every 24 hours to help prevent bacterial growth within the system. Tube clogging is a common problem, and a syringe pump may help to decrease the incidence of obstruction as will flushing well with warm water before and after bolus feeding. If the tube becomes clogged, replacement may be necessary. Diluting the liquid with water may also help prevent obstruction, though this further decreases the caloric concentration of the diet and therefore increases the volume necessary to meet the caloric needs.

When removing an NE tube, the tube may be simply pulled out after the glue or sutures are removed.

Esophagostomy Tube

Esophagostomy tube ("E tube") placement does require anesthesia to perform, but this generally does not need to be a surgical depth of anesthesia. The patient needs to be deep enough to place a mouth gag to prevent anyone from getting bit.

Complications include tube displacement due to vomiting or removal by the patient, skin infection around the exit site, and biting off of the tube end by the patient after vomiting.

Depending on the technique used and the size of the patient, an 8 Fr–20 Fr catheter is selected. The large bore of these catheters allows for feeding of a gruel recovery diet,

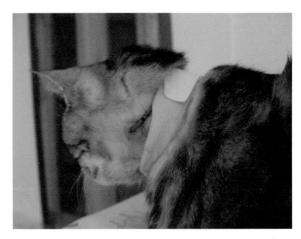

Figure 22.4   A cat with an esophagostomy tube ("E Tube"). These tubes are easy to place and maintain for extended periods of time.

sometimes without dilution with water. These catheters are also easy for clients to use and maintain as long as vomiting is not a problem (Hand et al. 2000). For cats with chronic kidney disease, esophagostomy tube places offers clients another means of fluid administration and may be able to replace uncomfortable and stressful subcutaneous fluid therapy (Fig. 22.4).

When removing, the tube may be simply pulled out after the sutures are removed. The exit hole is allowed to heal by second intension. A light bandage may be applied for the first 12 hours.

Gastrostomy Tube

Gastrostomy tubes ("G tube") can be placed either endoscopically, blindly, or surgically. All three techniques require general anesthesia, but again, this often does not need to be of surgical depth. Percutaneous endoscopic gastrostomy (PEG) tube placement allows for visualization of the esophagus and stomach as well as biopsy collection from the stomach and proximal duodenum and foreign body removal. Blind biopsy allows placement of a gastrostomy tube without the investment in an endoscopic unit. Surgical placement is useful during surgical exploratory or when the scope cannot be passed through the esophagus due to trauma or esophageal strictures (Fig. 22.5).

A minimum of 12 hours is needed for a temporary stoma to form before feeding can begin when a gastrostomy tube is used. The feeding tube should be left in place for a minimum of 7–10 days to allow a permanent stoma to form before removal. The tubes can be left in long term (1–6 months) without replacement. When replaced with another PEG tube, low-profile silicone tube, or Foley-type feeding tube, the stoma can be used for the rest of the patient's life.

Complications associated with PEG tubes include those seen from tube placement such as splenic laceration, gastric hemorrhage, and pneumoperitoneum. Delayed complications can also be seen such as vomiting, aspiration pneumonia, tube removal, tube migration, peritonitis, and stoma infection (Hand et al. 2000).

CHAPTER 22

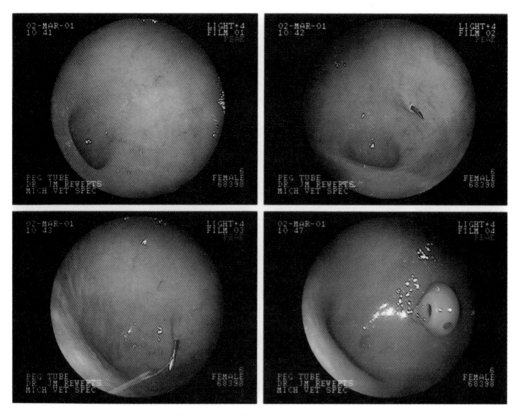

Figure 22.5   An endoscopic view of the stomach during PEG tube placement.

Gastrostomy tube placement is the technique of choice of long-term enteral support. These tubes are well tolerated by the patient, produce minimal discomfort, allow feeding of either gruel recovery diets or blenderized commercial foods, and can be easily managed by owners at home (Willard 1992) (Fig. 22.6).

Patients are able to eat normally with gastrostomy tubes in place and can easily be nutritionally supplemented via the tube until the patient is totally self-feeding. For patients that are difficult to medicate and require long-term medications, many medicines can also be given through the feeding tube. The major disadvantage of gastrostomy tubes is the need for general anesthesia and the risk of peritonitis (Willard 1992).

For animals requiring long-term management, the initial latex Pezzer catheter can be replaced with either low-profile silicone tubes or with Foley-type gastrostomy tubes. Both of these types can be placed through the external stoma site without the endoscope. Sedation or anesthesia may be necessary based on the individual patient (Hand et al. 2000).

For removal, if the tube has been in place 16 weeks or less, the tube may be simply removed. This is best accomplished by placing the patient in right lateral recumbency. The tube is grasped with the right hand close to the body wall, with the left hand holding the animal over the rib cage. Pull firmly and consistently to the right in an upward motion. Some force may be required for this. It is also helpful to ensure that the patient has been fasted and that a towel is placed over the tube site to catch any gastric contents that may be removed with the tube. If the tube has been in longer than 16 weeks, the incidence of

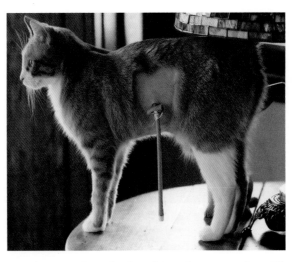

Figure 22.6   PEG tube use at home can be a simple and stress-free means of providing nutrition.

tube breakage is much higher. Depending on where the breakage occurs, the remaining tube pieces may need to be endoscopically retrieved. Larger patients can easily pass retained parts; smaller patients may need to have them endoscopically retrieved.

Upon tube removal, the exit hole is allowed to heal by second intension. A light bandage may be applied for the first 12 hours.

Jejunostomy Tubes

Jejunostomy feeding is indicated when the upper gastrointestinal tract must be rested or when pancreatic stimulation must be decreased. Jejunal tubes can be placed either surgically or threaded through a gastrostomy tube for transpyloric placement. Standard gastojejunal tubes designed for humans are unreliable in dogs due to frequent reflux of the jejunal portion of the tube back into the stomach. Investigation is ongoing involving endoscopic placement of transpyloric jejunal tubes through PEG tubes (Marks 2000) (Fig. 22.7).

Due to the small diameter of these tubes and the location, liquid enteral diets are recommended. Because the jejunum has minimal storage capacity compared with the stomach, continuous rate infusion using a syringe pump is the preferred method of delivery.

Common complications include osmotic diarrhea and vomiting. It is recommended that the jejunal tube be left in place for 7–10 days to allow adhesions to form around the tube site and prevent leakage back into the abdomen (Guilford et al. 1996).Completely changing the delivery equipment every 24 hours will help prevent bacterial growth within the system. Clogging is a common problem; a syringe pump may help to decrease the incidence as will flushing well with warm water every 4 hours.

When removing, the tube may be simply pulled out after the securing sutures are removed. The exit hole is allowed to heal via second intension. A light bandage may be applied for the first 12 hours (Hand et al. 2000).

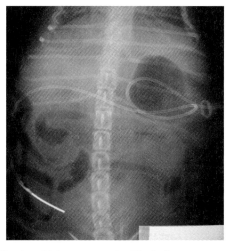

Figure 22.7   An endoscopically placed jejunostomy tube ("J tube").

Parenteral Nutrition

When enteral nutrition is not an option as with gut failure, when enteral nutrition could exacerbate a disease (e.g., necrotizing pancreatitis), or the animal's airway cannot be protected and aspiration pneumonia is a concern, parenteral nutrition is an option (Remillard et al. 2000).

Using parenteral nutrition as the only means of calories (total parenteral nutrition [TPN]) is recommended only for patients that cannot be fed enterally. Due to expense, difficulty in obtaining parenteral nutrition solutions, and ongoing need by the patient, short-term use is usually not justified (Remillard et al. 2000).

Partial parenteral nutrient (PPN) can be used in conjunction with oral or tube feeding to either help meet caloric requirements or when transitioning from TPN back to enteral nutrition. Typically, PPN solutions will have fewer lipids than would TPN solutions, giving them a lower osmolality and allowing peripheral vein infusion. Currently, commercially available PPN solutions do not contain lipids, but if a PPN solution is formulated on-site or by a pharmacist, lipids can be added. An example of a commercially available PPN solution would be ProcalAnime manufactured by B. Braun/McGaw Inc. (B. Braun Medical Inc., Irvine, CA), which is a 3% amino acid 3% glycerin solution with electrolytes.

Parenteral nutrition uses a modified solution with nutrients that can be absorbed by the cells without passing through the gut first. Parenteral solutions can be used alone or as a supplement to enteral feedings when insufficient caloric intake is seen. High lipid TPN diets have been recommended because free fatty acids are the primary energy source in catabolic patients. But the use of this type of diet is not without controversy due to the possible association between hyperlipidemia and pancreatitis. Despite these concerns, lipid emulsions have been used successfully in dogs and humans with pancreatitis when the patient is not hyperlipidemic prior to initiating TPN (Elliott 2004).

Parenteral nutrition has several disadvantages. A dedicated central venous catheter is required, and the special nutrient solution must be properly prepared. Intensive monitoring is necessary; thrombophlebitis and sepsis are serious complications if strict aseptic technique is not followed (Tennant 1996). Lack of nutrients in the intestinal lumen may lead to breakdown of the bacterial barrier in the gut, further increasing the incidence of sepsis. A transitional period is necessary to wean the patient from parenteral to enteral feedings (Donaghue 1989).

As most parenteral solutions have very high osmolality (often greater than 800–1200 mOsm/L), a central venous catheter should be used to help prevent phlebitis and thrombosis from occurring. If a peripheral catheter is used, the solutions must be substantially diluted to <600 mOsm/L to decrease the risk of thrombophlebitis. By diluting the osmolality, you are also diluting the caloric content and increasing the volume infused. Because of this, TPN cannot be administered through a peripheral vein, since a large volume of fluid would be necessary to meet the energy requirements of the patient. TPN administration must carefully be adjusted to prevent fluid overload. Line separation or breakage must be avoided to decrease the incidence of introducing bacteria to the solution (Elliott 2004; Tennant 1996).

Because TPN can also cause refeeding syndrome to occur, the parenteral formula should contain at least 40 mEq/L of potassium to compensate for the insulin-mediated transcellular potassium shift associated with reintroduction of nutrition (Elliott 2004).

Monitoring of the patient receiving TPN is extensive and is best assigned to one individual per shift. This helps in continuity of care as well as decreasing chances of contamination from other patients. Body temperature, heart and respiratory rates, twice daily body weight measurements, assessment of hydration status, and mental attitude should be performed on all patients receiving PPN or TPN. Metabolic complications that may occur include hyperglycemia, glucosuria, hypokalemia or hyperkalemia, hypophosphatemia, and hyperlipidemia. The presence of any of these may necessitate adjusting the nutrient ratios, slowing the rate of infusion, or administering insulin, potassium, or phosphate supplements (Elliott 2004).

Rate of Diet Initiation

Because nutritional support is not an emergency procedure, the general guidelines are to start slowly (Hill 1994). Food intake should be gradually increased over a 2- to 3-day period until the estimated caloric intake is met (Tennant 1996). If the patient shows discomfort, vomits, is nauseous, or becomes distressed, the diet and the route and rate of delivery need to be assessed.

Generally, 30%–50% of the RER, divided into multiple small meals, is offered the first day. If this amount is well tolerated, then 60%–100% of the RER can be fed the second day. By the third day of feeding, the patient should be being fed 100% RER. If the feedings are not well tolerated, the increases should be more gradual over the next 2–3 days. Smaller meals tend to be better tolerated because they do not cause overdistension of the stomach and subsequent delayed gastric emptying or aggravate nausea as can occur with larger meals (Remillard et al. 2000). Sometimes, with patients receiving assisted feedings via NE, esophageal, or gastrostomy tube, delivering the food using a syringe pump for a CRI will allow more food to be fed than if bolus feedings were used, and significantly decrease the incidence of nausea because only small amounts of food are in the stomach at any given time. This also is much easier on the nursing staff than if frequent small bolus feedings are being fed every 2–4 hours (Fig. 22.8).

Refeeding syndrome, an electrolyte disturbance that can occur in patients with depleted intracellular cations (e.g., potassium, phosphorus, magnesium, and calcium), can be seen

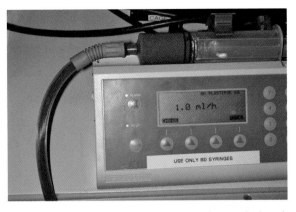

Figure 22.8   A syringe pump set up to administer a constant rate infusion of a liquid gruel diet.

with malnutrition, starvation as with feline hepatic lipidosis, or prolonged diuresis as seen with uncontrolled diabetes or renal failure. Patients at greatest risk are severely malnourished with significant loss of lean body mass. Reintroduction of nutrition results in a rapid shift of these cations from the serum (where levels may be normal prior to feeding) to the intracellular space. Profound hypophosphatemia, hypokalemia and/or hypomagnesemia may result and can lead to muscle weakness, intravascular hemolysis and possible cardiac and respiratory failure. This syndrome can be avoided by monitoring the patient closely, introducing feeding cautiously (CRI of a commercial recovery diet), monitoring electrolytes frequently (every 12–24 hours), and supplementing the diet as needed to correct any deficiencies found (Donaghue 1989).

Implementing Feeding Orders

Technicians responsible for patient treatments should be given instructions listing the type of food to be offered along with how much to give and how often. A flowchart can be used to record the amount eaten, the technique used to feed the patient, and the food that was offered (e.g., one-half can of slightly warmed dog food offered by hand at 3:00 P.M., ate well). The technician can then draw a circle on the flow chart and fill in the amount of food the patient consumed (e.g., filling in one quarter of the circle if the patient ate one-fourth of the amount offered). If the patient refused to eat, the technician should record an R in the circle. The technician should also note whether any food, amount, or technique recorded differs from the instructions. Such recordkeeping provides veterinarians with an accurate measurement of food intake and technicians with feeding methods that succeed on a per-patient basis, which is especially helpful during shift changes and during 24-hour ongoing care.

Diet Transitions

Although diet transitions may occur while the patient is hospitalized, typically, this is carried out 2–6 weeks after discharge from the hospital. Transition depends on the diet being fed, condition of the patient, the patient's response to therapy, and the comfort level of the owner. As with diet initiation, it is best to proceed with diet transitions slowly. For example, when shifting from a support diet to a maintenance diet, each dietary change should represent an additional one quarter of the current diet every 3–4 days. For days 1–4, feed three-fourths of the therapeutic diet and one-fourth of the maintenance diet; days 5–8, feed one-half of the therapeutic diet and one-hald of the maintenance diet; days 9–12, feed one-fourth of the therapeutic diet and three-fourths of the maintenance diet; day 13, feed 100% maintenance diet (i.e., transition phase of 12–16 days). If a problem develops at any stage, the owners should be instructed to return to the last diet combination that worked.

Technicians should supply owners with well-written, concise discharge instructions and reasonable expectation of what the diet being fed can do. Unfortunately, therapeutic diets cannot "cure" inflammatory bowel disease, chronic renal failure, or diabetes, though they are often used to help control the signs of these diseases. It is very important that owners are aware of this.

Conclusion

Being aware of the nutritional aspects of patient care can improve the long-term outcome of the patient's health as well as the client–patient–veterinary team relationship. Technicians can assume a primary role in providing excellent nutritional support to our patients. Even if we are not able to save our patients every time, providing adequate nutrition is an easy step to have a direct impact on each hospitalized individual that truly can effect patient outcome.

References

Abood, SK. 1997. Nutritional assessment of the critical care patient. In *Purina Nutrition Forum*. St. Louis, MO: Ralston Purina, pp. 16–19.

Brunetto, M, Gomes, M, Andre, M, et al. 2010. Effects of nutritional support on hospital outcome in dogs and cats. *Journal of Veterinary Emergency and Critical Care* 20(2):224–2341.

Buffington, CA, Holloway, C, Abood, SK. 2004. *Manual of Veterinary Dietetics*. St. Louis, MO: Elsevier Saunders.

Campbell, JA, Brown, AJ, Santoro, K, Hauptman, JG, Jutkowitz, LA. 2010. Continuous versus intermittent delivery of nutrition via nasoenteric feeding tubes in critically ill canine and feline patients. *Journal of Veterinary Emergency and Critical Care* 20: 232–236.

Chan, DL. 2005a. *In-Hospital Starvation: Inadequate Nutritional Support*. 11th International Veterinary Emergency & Critical Care Symposium Proceedings, pp. 515–518.

Chan, DL. 2005b. Parenteral nutritional support. In *Textbook of Veterinary Internal Medicine*, Vol. 1, 6th ed., edited by Ettinger, SJ, Feldman, EC. Philadelphia: Elsevier Saunders, pp. 596–591.

Chan, DL. 2006. *Controversies in Clinical Nutrition Therapy*. 12th International Veterinary Emergency & Critical Care Symposium Proceedings, pp. 499–502.

Donaghue, S. 1989. Nutritional support of hospitalized patients. *Veterinary Clinics of North America Small Animal Practice* 19(3):475–493.

Elliott, DA. 2004. *Parenteral Nutrition*. 29th World Congress of the World Small Animal Veterinary Association, pp. 1–5.

Guilford, WG, Center, SA, Strombeck, DR. 1996. Nutritional managementof gastrointestinal disease. In *Strombeck's Small Animal Gastroenterology*, 3rd ed., edited by Guilford, WG, Center, SA, Strombeck, DR, Williams, D, Meyer, D. Philadelphia: Elsevier Saunders, pp. 904–908.

Hand, MS, Thatcher, CD, Remillard, RL, Roudebush, P. 2000. Appendix V: assisted feeding techniques. In *Small Animal Clinical Nutrition*, 4th ed. Marceline, MO: Walsworth, pp. 1145–1153.

Hill, RC. 1994. Critical care nutrition. In *The Waltham Book of Clinical Nutrition of the Dog and Cat*, edited by Wills, JM, Simpson, KW. Tarrytown, NY: Pergamon Press, pp. 39–57.

Marks, SL. 2000. Enteral and parenteral nutritional support. In *Textbook of Veterinary Internal Medicine*, Vol. 1, 5th ed., edited by Ettinger, SJ, Feldman, EC. Philadelphia: Elsevier Saunders, pp. 275–282.

Michel, KE. 2006a. *Monitoring the Enterally Fed Patient to Maximize Benefits and Minimize Complications*. 12th International Veterinary Emergency & Critical Care Symposium Proceedings, pp. 495–498.

Michel, KE. 2006b. *Nutritional Clues: Tailoring Nutritional Support to the Patient*. 12th International Veterinary Emergency & Critical Care Symposium Proceedings, pp. 491–493.

Nelson, RW, Couto, CG. 2009. Disorders of the endocrine pancreas. In *Small Animal Internal Medicine*, 4th ed. St. Louis, MO: Mosby. pp. 779–783, 792–795.

Remillard, R, Armstrong, PJ, Davenport, D. 2000. Assisted feeding in hospitalized patients: enteral and parenteral nutrition. In *Small Animal Clinical Nutrition*, 4th ed., edited by Hand, M, Hatcher, C, Remillard, R, Roudebush, P. Marceline, MO: Walsworth, pp. 352–370.

Tennant, B. 1996. Feeding the sick animal. In *Manual of Companion Animal Nutrition and Feeding*, edited by Kelly, NC, Wills, JM. Ames, IA: Iowa State University Press, pp. 171–180.

Torrance, AG. 1996. Intensive care nutritional support. In *Manual of Companion Animal Nutrition and Feeding*, edited by Kelly, NC, Wills, JM. Ames, IA: Iowa State University Press, pp. 171–180.

Willard, M. 1992. The gastrointestinal system. In *Essentials of Small Animal Internal Medicine*, edited by Nelson, RW, Couto, CG. St.Louis, MO: Mosby Year Book, pp. 305–309.

Wingfield, WE. 1997. The essentials of life in critically ill animals. In *Purina Nutrition Forum*. St. Louis, MO: Ralston Purina.

CHAPTER 22

Appendices

To make a 2.5% dextrose solution
Add 50 cc   to 1000 mL
Add 25 cc   to 500 mL
Add 12.5 cc   to 250 mL

To make a 5% dextrose solution
Add 100 cc   to 1000 mL
Add 50 cc   to 500 mL
Add 25 cc   to 250 mL

Appendix B Biochemical Formulas

Equation	Formula	Units	Normal
Anion gap	$(Na + K) - (Cl + HCO_3)$	mEq/L	12–24 mEq/L
Corrected calcium	Measured Ca^{2+} − albumin (g/dL) + 3.5	mg/dL	
Corrected chloride	Cl (patient) × [Na (normal)/Na (patient)]		
Corrected sodium (with hyperglycemia)	Measured Na + [(Glucose − 100)/100 × 1.6]		
Calculated osmolality	$2 \times Na + (BUN/2.8) + (Glucose/18)$	mOsm/L	290–310 (dogs) 290–330 (cats)
Effective osmolality	$2 \times Na + (Glu/18)$	mOsm/L	Non-azotemic: 300–310
Base deficit	Normal HCO_3 − patient HCO_3	mEq/L	0–6
Sodium bicarbonate dose	0.4 × BW (kg) × base deficit	mEq/L	
Free water deficit	BW (kg) × 0.6 × (Na − 140/140)	Liters	N/A
Coronary perfusion	CPP = aortic diastolic pressure − right atrial pressure		
Cerebral perfusion	CPP = MAP − ICP	mmHg	N/A
Arterial oxygen content (CaO$_2$)	$1.34 \times Hb \times SaO_2 + (0.003 \times PaO_2)$	mmHg	N/A
Oxygen delivery	CO × CaO2 × 10	mL 02/100 mL blood	
Arterial blood pressure	CO × SVR	mL/min	
Mean arterial blood pressure	Diastolic + (Systolic − Diastolic)/3	mmHg	
Blood volume (dog)	90 mL/kg		
Blood volume (cat)	60 mL/kg		

Note: CO = cardiac output

Equation	P:F Ratio	PaO_2/FiO_2	Normal:
			400–500
			<300 = ALI
			<200 = ARDS
	A-a gradient	PAO_2 (room air at sea level) $= 150 - (PaCO_2/0.8) - PaO_2$	Normal: <10 mmHg
		Visit: http://www.mdcalc. com/a-a-o2-gradient	
Blood Gas Values			
	Arterial blood gas: pH	Canine: 7.35–7.46	Feline: 7.31–7.46
	Arterial blood gas: $PaCO_2$	Canine: 32–43	Feline: 26–36
	Arterial blood gas: HCO_3	Canine: 18–26	Feline: 14–22
	Arterial blood gas: PaO_2 (at sea level)	Canine: 80–105	Feline: 95–115
	Venous blood gas: pH	Canine: 7.36	N/A
	Venous blood gas: $PvCO_2$	Canine: 40–46	N/A
	Venous blood gas: HCO_3	Canine: 22–24	N/A
	Venous blood gas: PvO_2	Canine: 49–67	N/A

Conversion	Formula
Celsius to Fahrenheit	$(C \times 1.8) + 32$
Fahrenheit to Celsius	$(F - 32) \times 0.555$
% Solution to g/100 mL	x% solution = xg/100 mL
% Solution to mg/mL	x% solution $\times$ 10 = mg/mL
mmHg to cmH_2O	1 mmHg = 1.36 cmH_2O
cmH_2O to mmHg	1 cmH_2O = 0.736 mmHg
inches to centimeters	1 in. = 2.54 cm
centimeters to inches	1 cm = 0.4 in.
pounds to kilograms	1 lb = 2.2 kg
kilograms to pounds	1 kg = 0.45 kg
ounce to gram	1 oz = 28.35 g
1 mL H_2O to grams	1 mL H_2O = 1 g
grams to grains	1 g = 15.43 grains
milligrams to grains	1 mg = 1/65 grain
liters to quarts	1 L = 1.06 quarts
liters to fl oz	1 L = 23.80 fl oz
drams to grams	1 dram = 3.9 g
ounce to grams	1 oz = 31.1 g
fluid ounce to milliliters	1 fl oz = 29.57 mL
pint to milliliters	1 pint = 473.2 mL
quart to milliliters	1 quart = 946.4 mL
tablespoon to milliliters	1 tbsp = 15 mL
teaspoon to milliliters	1 tsp = 5 mL
cm to French	Outside diameter (cm) $\times$ 3

| RER for >2 kg and <30 kg | BW (kg) × 30 + 70 = kcal/day |
| RER for <2 kg and >30 kg | $70 \times BW \ (kg)^{0.75}$ |

TPN formulation	Protein requirements	Nonprotein requirements
Canine	5 g/100 kcal (normal) [2–3 g if decreased requirements]	RER: (grams protein/day × 4) = NPC (nonprotein calories)
Feline	6 g/100 kcal (normal) [3–4 g if decreased requirements]	RER: (grams protein/day × 4) = NPC (nonprotein calories)
Dextrose requirement	NPC × 0.5 = kcal/day dextrose	
	kcal/day dextrose × 1.7 kcal/mL = mL/day dextrose	
Lipid (20%) requirement	NPC × 0.5 = kcal/day lipid	
	kcal/day lipid × 2 kcal/mL = mL/day lipid	
kcal/mL of various diets	Procalamine: 0.25 kcaL/mL	
	Lipid 20% – 2 kcal/mL	
	Hils A/D: 1.15 kcal/mL	
	Eukanuba Max Cal: 2 kcal/mL	
	Abbott Clinicare: 1 kcal/mL	
	Royal Canine Recovery: 2.4 kcal/mL	

Temperature	Canine: 100–102.9 F	
	Feline: 100–102.9 F	
Pulse	Feline: 160–220 bpm	
	Small to medium breed: 100–140 bpm	
	Large breed: 60–100 bpm	
Respiration	15–30 breaths/min	
MM/CRT	Pink, CRT > 1 second < 2.5 seconds	
Systolic blood pressure	90–140 mmHg	
Diastolic blood pressure	60–90 mmHg	
Mean arterial pressure	70–105 mmHg	
Central venous pressure	0–5 cmH$_2$O	*Note*: Trend more important!!
Urine output	1–2 mL/kg/h on maintenance fluids	

When you have	Multiple by	To find ....
Grain	60	Milligram
Milligram	1000	Microgram (mcg) or (µg)
Milligram	0.001	Gram (g)
Gram	0.035	Ounce (oz)
Gram	1000	Milligram (mg)
Gram	0.001	Kilogram (kg)
Kilogram	2.21	Pound (lb)
Kilogram	1000	Gram
Pound	16	Gram
Pound	453.6	Gram
Pound	0.4536	Kilogram
Parts per million (ppm)	0.0001	% (percentage)
Mcal	1000	Kcal
Milliliter (mL)	0.20	Teaspoon (tsp)
Milliliter (mL)	0.06	Tablespoon (tbsp)
Liter	4.23	Cup
Liter	2.12	Pint (pt)
Liter	1.06	Quart (qt)
Drop (gt)	0.06	Milliliter
Milliliter	15	Drop (gt)
Teaspoon	4.93	Milliliter
Tablespoon	14.78	Milliliter
Fluid ounce (fl oz)	29.57	Milliliter
Cup	0.24	Liter
Pint	0.47	Liter
Quart	0.95	Liter
Inch	2.54	Centimeter (cm)
Foot	30.48	Centimeter
Yard (yd)	91.44	Centimeter

Appendix H   Drug Compatibilities

Note: Any drug combinations not listed have not been tested and should therefore be considered "not compatible."

Ampicillin
Famotidine
Furosemide
Magnesium Sulfate
Medetomidine
Morphine
Pantoprazole
Potassium Chloride
Propofol
Insulin-regular

Butorphanol
Diphenhydramine
Medetomidine
Metoclopramide
Propofol

Cefazolin
Clindamycin
Dextrose 5%
Diltiazem
Famotidine
Fluconazole
Heparin
Magnesium Sulfate
Medetomidine
Metronidazole
Midazolam
Morphine
Ondansetron
Propofol
Insulin-regular
Sodium Chloride 0.9%

Cefoxitin
Clindamycin
Dextrose 5%
Diltiazem
Famotidine
Fluconazole
Heparin
Hydromorphone
Lidocaine
Magnesium Sulfate
Medetomidine
Morphine
Ondansetron
Propofol
Insulin-regular
Sodium Bicarbonate
Sodium Chloride 0.9%

Clindamycin
5% Dextrose
Cefazolin
Cefoxitin
Diltiazem
Heparin
Hydromorphone
Medetomidine
Methyprednisolone Sod Succ
Metoclopramide
Midazolam
Morphine
Ondansetron
Propofol
Sodium Bicarbonate

Diazepam
Fentanyl
Morphine

Diltiazem
Cefazolin
Cefoxitin
Clindamycin
Dextrose 5%
Dobutamine
Dopamine
Epinephrine
Fentanyl
Hydromorphone
Lidocaine
Medetomidine
Metoclopramide
Metronidazole
Midazolam
Morphine
Norepinephrine
Sodium Chloride 0.9%
Sodium Nitroprusside
Vasopressin

Dobutamine
Dextrose 5%
Diltiazem
Dopamine
Epinephrine
Famotidine
Fentanyl
Hydrom or phone
Lidocaine
Medetomidine
Meropenem
Morphine
Norepinephrine
Procainamide
Propofol
Sodium Chloride 0.9%
Vasopressin

Dopamine
Dextrose 5%
Diltiazem
Dobutamine
Epinephrine
Famotidine
Fentanyl
Hydromorphone
Lidocaine
Medetomidine
Meropenem
Metronidazole
Midazolam
Morphine
Norepinephrine
Propofol
Sodium Chloride 0.9%
Sodium Nitroprusside
Vasopressin

Famotidine
Ampicillin
Cefazolin
Cefoxitin
Dexamethasone
Dextrose 5%
Dobuatmine
Dopamine
Furosemide
Heparin
Hydromorphone
Lidocaine
Magnesium
Metoclopramide
Midazolam
Morphine
Norepinephrine
Ondansetron
Propofol
Insulin-regular
Sodium bicarbonate
Sodium Chloride 0.9%

Fentanyl
Dexamethasone
Diazepam
Diltiazem
Dobutamine
Dopamine
Epinephrine
Heparin
Hydromorphone
Lidocaine
Medetomidine
Metoclopramide
Midazolam
Morphine
Norepinephrine
Ondansetron
Propofol

Furosemide
Ampicillin
Atropine
Dexamethasone
Fentanyl
Heparin
Hydromorphone
Lidocaine
Medetomidine
Propofol

Heparin
Buprenorphine
Cefazolin
Cefoxitin
Clindamycin
Dexamethasone
Famotidine
Fentanyl
Furosemide
Lidocaine
Magnesium Sulfate
Meropenum
Metoclopramide
Metronidazole
Midazolam
Norepinephrine
Ondansetron
Procainamide
Propofol
Insulin-regular

Imipenem
Diltiazem
Famotidine
Ondansetron
Propofol
Insulin-regular
Vasopressin

Insulin-regular
Ampicillin
Cefazolin
Famotidine
Heparin
Imipenem
Lidocaine
Magnesium Sulfate
Meropenem
Metoclopramide
Midazolam
Morphine
Nitroprusside
Propofol

Compiled by Andrea Steele BSc, RVT, VTS (ECC), Ontario Veterinary College. *Reference: Lawrence Trissel, Pocket Guide to Injectable Drugs: Companion to the Handbook of Injectable Drugs*, 15th ed.

Lidocaine
Calcium Gluconate
Dexamethasone
Dextrose 5%
Diltiazem
Dobutamine
Dopamine
Famotidine
Furosemide
Heparin
Insulin-regular
Procainamide
Sodium Chloride 0.9%

Magnesium Sulfate
Ampicillin
Cefazolin
Cefoxitin
Dextrose 5%
Famotidine
Heparin
Hydromorphone
Medetomidine
Meropenem
Metoclopramide
Metronidazole
Morphine
Ondansetron
Propofol
Sodium Chloride 0.9%

Meropenem
Dopamine
Furosemide
Heparin
Insulin-regular
Magnesium Sulfate
Metoclopramide
Metronidazole

Medetomidine
Dextrose 5%
Ampicillin
Atropine
Butorphanol
Cefazolin
Cefoxitin
Dexamethasone
Diltiazem
Dobutamine
Dopamine
Epinephrine
Famotidine
Fentanyl
Furosemide
Heparin
Hydromorphone
Lidocaine
Magnesium Sulfate
Metoclopramide
Metronidazole
Midazolam
Morphine
Norepinephrine
Ondansetron
Procainamide
Propofol
Sodium Bicarbonate
Sodium Chloride 0.9%

Metronidazole
Cefazolin
Clindamycin
Diltiazem
Heparin
Hydromorphone
Magnesium Sulfate
Medetomidine
Midazolam
Morphine

Metoclopramide
Butorphanol
Clindamycin
Dexamethasone
Dextrose 5%
Diltiazem
Famotidine
Fentanyl
Heparin
Hydromorphone
Insulin-regular
Lidocaine
Magnesium Sulfate
Medetomidine
Meropenem
Midazolam
Morphine
Ondansetron
Sodium Chloride 0.9%

Midazolam
Buprenorphine
Cefazolin
Clindamycin
Dextrose 5%
Diltiazem
Dopamine
Famotidine
Fentanyl
Hydromorphone
Insulin-regular
Metoclopramide
Metronidazole
Morphine
Norepinephrine
Ondansetron
Sodium Chloride 0.9%

Norepinephrine
Dextrose 5%
Diltiazem
Dobutamine
Dopamine
Epinephrine
Famotidine
Fentanyl
Furosemide
Heparin
Hydromorphone
Magnesium Sulfate
Medetomidine
Meropenem
Midazolam
Morphine
Propofol
Sodium Chloride 0.9%
Sodium Nitroprusside

Ondansetron
Cefazolin
Cefoxitin
Clindamycin
Dextrose 5%
Dopamine
Famotidine
Fentanyl
Heparin
Hydromorphone
Imipenem
Magnesium Sulfate
Medetomidine
Midazolam
Morphine
Propofol
Sodium Chloride 0.9%

Pantoprazole
Ampicillin
Dextrose 5%
Procainamide
Sodium Chloride 0.9%

Propofol
Ampicillin
Buprenorphine
Butorphanol
Cefazolin
Cefoxitin
Clindamycin
Dexamethasone
Dextrose 5%
Dobutamine
Dopamine
Epinephrine
Famotidine
Fentanyl
Furosemide
Heparin
Hydromorphone
Imipenem
Insulin-regular
Ketamine
Magnesium Sulfate
Medetomidine
Naloxone
Norepinephrine
Ondansetron
Sodium Nitroprusside

Glossary

Acclimatization: The body's physiological ability to adapt to varying environmental temperatures. Detrimental effects of these temperatures are minimized through this biological process.

Acidemia: Increased amounts of acid concentrations in the extracellular fluid (ECF) and blood.

Acidosis: The clinical condition associated with an increase in acid in the body.

Acute kidney injury (AKI): See acute renal failure.

Acute renal failure (ARF): A potentially reversible syndrome of diverse etiology characterized by an abrupt and sustained decline in renal function producing impaired excretion of metabolic wastes, impaired ability to maintain fluid, electrolyte and acid–base balance, and uremia.

Acute-on-chronic renal failure: An acute decompensation of chronic renal failure.

Afterload: The pressure the heart chambers must overcome to pump blood out of the heart.

Alkalemia: Increased amounts of base in the ECF and blood.

Alkalosis: The clinical condition associated with an increase in base in the body.

Allodynia: Painful response to a stimulus that does not normally elicit pain.

Analgesic: An agent that provides pain relief.

Anamnestic response: An immune response to an antibody in which the body has previously encountered.

Anaphylaxis: A life-threatening hypersensitivity allergic reaction where the immune system responds to a substance.

Anemia: An abnormally low number of erythrocytes.

Angiogenesis: Growth of new blood vessels at the site of tissue.

Anisocoria: Unequal size of the pupils.

Antibody: Unique protein structures found within the immune system that react to foreign antigens.

Anticholinergic: A drug that blocks effects of the parasympathetic nervous system, often summarized into SLUD: salivation, lacrimation, urination, defecation.

Antigen: A substance that can elicit an antibody response. Blood type antigens are polysaccharide/protein complexes found on the red cell.

Antimicrobial drug: Antibacterial, antifungal, antiviral drugs administered to rid the body of pathogens.

Antisera: Serum that contains sensitized antibodies that are capable of prompting an immune response to antigens.

Anuria: the absence of urine production, or <0.08 mL/kg/h.

Arrhythmia: Any variation from the normal rhythm of a heartbeat.

Ataxic: Loss or decrease of the ability to coordinate muscular movement.

Auto-agglutination: An immune response within the patient that causes the antibodies within the plasma to react to the antigens present on its own red cells. The result is clumping of the red blood cells and eventual destruction.

Azotemia: An abnormal concentration of urea, creatinine, and other nitrogenous waste products in the blood.

Beta-lactamase: An enzyme produced by bacteria developing resistance to penicillin and cephalosporin antimicrobials. It destroys the beta-lactam ring both antimicrobials have in their chemical structure.

Blepharospasm: Spasmodic winking from involuntary contraction of the orbicularis muscle of the eyelids.

Borborygmus: A rumbling or gurgling sound caused by the movement of gas moving through the intestines.

Bradycardia: A heart rate that is below normal.

Bradypnea: A decreased respiratory rate.

Bronchodilator: Agent that causes expansion of the lumina (cavity or channel within a tube or tubular organ) of the air passages of the lungs.

Cachexia: General ill health with emaciation.

Capillary refill time (CRT): The amount of time required for empty capillaries to refill.

Capnogram: Continuous measurement of carbon dioxide concentrations in the exhaled air.

Cardiac output: The blood volume pumped from the left heart in one minute.

Cardiogenic: Originating in the heart.

Cardiomegaly: Enlargement of the heart.

Catacholamine: "Fight-or-flight" hormones released by the adrenal glands in times of stress.

Central sensitization: Pain receptors in the central nervous system become used to pain signals and respond with a heightened response. Also called "wind up."

Chronic kidney disease: See chronic renal failure (CRF).

Chronic renal failure (CRF): A gradual and progressive loss of the ability of the kidneys to excrete waste, concentrate urine, and conserve electrolytes.

Chronotrope: Any agent that increases heart rate.

Colloid: A fluid containing large molecules with oncotic pull. These molecules expand the intravascular space and draw water into the intravascular space from the interstitial space.

Conscious proprioception: An awareness of where a body part is in space.

Crossmatch: A procedure for blood products that indicates immune responses and potential compatibility between a donor and recipient.

Crystalloid: A fluid containing water and electrolytes. It has no oncotic pressure and thus large volumes are needed for resuscitation.

Cyanosis: A condition in which the skin and mucous membranes turn a bluish color because there is not enough oxygen in the blood.

Deoxyhemoglobin: Hemoglobin not combined with oxygen, formed when oxyhemoglobin releases its oxygen to the tissues.

Descemetocele: A protrusion of Descemet's membrane through the cornea.

Dialysate: A solution which interfaces directly with the blood when performing hemodialysis or peritoneal dialysis.

Diuretic: An agent that promotes the excretion of urine.

Dysautonomia: A rare neurological condition resulting in abnormal functioning of the autonomic nervous system.

Dyschezia: Inability to defecate without pain or difficulty.

Dyspnea: Difficult or labored breathing

Dysuria: Painful urination

Ecchymosis: A small hemorrhagic spot, larger than a petechia, in the skin or mucous membrane forming a nonelevated, rounded, or irregular, blue or purplish patch.

Echinocytosis: Special red blood cell pathology characterized by multiple projections from the red cell surface. Indicative of rattlesnake envenomation.

Edema: An abnormal excess accumulation of serous fluid in connective tissue or body cavity.

Electroporation: Opening of cellular pores as a result of applied electrical current.

End point resuscitation: Intravenous fluid resuscitation to specific end points to satisfy perfusion parameters (mucous membrane [MM] color, CRT, pulse rate and character, mentation)

Epiphora: Excessive secretion of tears or watering of the eye.

Episclera: The layer of connective tissue between the conjunctiva and sclera of the eye.

Epistaxis: Nosebleed; hemorrhage from the nose.

Epithelialization: Development of a new skin layer over an existing, healing wound.

Erythropoietin: A hormone excreted primarily by the kidneys that regulates red blood cell production in the bone marrow.

Eschar: Blackened, thickened layer of skin that develops after a partial or full thickness burn.

Extravasation: To force the flow (of blood or lymph) from a vessel out into the surrounding tissue.

First-pass effect: The process of a drug entering enterohepatic circulation and being partially metabolized by the liver, before entering systemic circulation.

Fresh frozen plasma (FFP): Plasma that is collected from the donor, separated from the red blood cells, and frozen to −18°C within 6–8 hours of collection. FFP contains both labile and non-labile clotting factors. FFP has a 1-year expiration date.

Frozen plasma (FP): Plasma that is collected from the donor, separated from the red blood cells, and frozen to 18°C where complete freezing occurs >8 hours after collection. Frozen plasma does not contain labile clotting factors but does contain plasma proteins and non-labile clotting factors. This term is also used for FFP that has expired after 1 year but still retains the non-labile clotting factors for an additional 4 years.

Glomerular filtration rate (GFR): The total filtration rate of both kidneys.

Heat shock proteins: Proteins that can continue their enzymatic function, despite abnormally high environmental temperatures.

Hematachezia: Frank blood in stool.

Hematemesis: Bloody vomitus.

Hematuria: Bloody urine.

Hemoptysis: Blood produced from the lower respiratory tract.

Hydration: Adequate interstitial water levels.

Hydrophilic: "Water"-loving. The ability of a drug to dissociate in water.

Hydrostatic pressure: The tissue fluid pressure against which osmosis has to achieve a positive gradient if small molecules are to pass the cell membranes and be absorbed.

Hyperalgesia: A heightened painful response to a stimulus that normally elicits pain.

Hypercalcemia: High blood calcium levels.

Hypercapnia: Excess of carbon dioxide in the blood.

Hypercarbia: See hypercapnia.

Hyperchloremia: High blood chloride levels.

Hyperkalemia: High blood potassium levels.

Hypermagnesemia: High blood magnesium levels.

Hypernatremia: High blood sodium levels.

Hyperphosphatemia: High blood phosphorus levels

Hypertension: Elevated blood pressure.

Hyperventilation: Decreased $PaCO_2$ <35.

Hypocalcemia: Low blood calcium levels.

Hypochloremia: Low blood chloride levels.

Hypoglycemia: Low blood sugar.

Hypokalemia: Low blood potassium levels.

Hypomagnesemia: Low blood magnesium levels.

Hyponatremia: Low blood sodium levels.

Hypoperfusion: Decreased blood flow through an organ.

Hypophosphatemia: Low blood phosphorus levels.

Hypotension: Low blood pressure.

Hypothermia: Decreased body temperature.

Hypoventilation: Elevated $PaC0_2$ >45 mmHg.

Hypovolemia: Abnormally decreased volume of circulating fluid in the body.

Hypoxemia: Deficient oxygenation of the blood.

Hypoxia: Deficient oxygenation of the body.

Iatrogenic: Resulting from the activity of those treating the patient.

Idiopathic: Coming from an unknown cause or etiology.

Inotrope: Any agent that improved myocardial contractability.

Inotropy: Ventricular myocardial contractabiliy.

Interstitial: Fluid that bathes and surrounds cells.

Intravascular: Within blood vessels

Iris bombe: A condition in which the iris is bowed forward by an accumulation of fluid between the iris and the lens.

Ischemia: Local deficiency of blood supply produced by vasoconstriction or local obstacles to the arterial flow.

Labile factors: Referring to unstable or easily altered coagulation factors; specifically factor V, VIII, and von Willebrand factor.

Lipophilic: "Fat"-loving. The ability for a drug to be absorbed by fat.

Lyophilized: Freeze-dried, undergoing the process of dehydration and subsequently changing from a liquid to powder form.

Medial canthus: The meeting of the upper and lower eyelids medially.

Melena: The discharge of black, tarry, or bloody stools, usually a result of hemorrhage in the intestinal tract.

Menace reflex: a reflex that may be tested by gesturing a finger or hand toward the eye.

Miosis: Pinpoint pupils, pupils that are smaller than normal.

Mydriasis: Dilated pupils, pupils that are larger than normal.

Neonatal isoerythrolysis (NI): A hemolytic reaction that occurs when the mother contains blood cell antibodies to the blood cells present within one of her offspring. The reaction leads to severe red blood cell destruction in the offspring.

Neurogenic pulmonary edema: Pulmonary edema (fluid in interstitial/alveolar/bronchial) spaces as a result of massive catecholamine from central nervous system damage. Characterized by increased afterload and decreased left ventricular stroke volume.

Neuroleptanalgesia: A profound state of analgesia and sedation from the combination of an opioid and either a sedative or tranquilizing agent.

Nystagmus: A periodic, rhythmic, involuntary movement of both eyeballs in unison.

Odynophagia: Pain produced when swallowing.

Oliguria: An abnormally small production of urine with resultant output ranging from <0.27 mL/kg/h to <1–2 mL/kg/h.

Oxyhemoglobin: Hemoglobin combined with molecular oxygen, the form in which oxygen is transported in the blood.

Parasympathetic: Pertaining to the parasympathetic aspect of the autonomic nervous system.

Perfusion: The passage and delivery of fluid/nutrients through the vessels of an organ and tissues.

Periobit: Related to tissues surrounding the orbit of the eye.

Petechia: A pinpoint, nonraised, perfectly round, purplish red spot caused by intradermal or subcutaneous hemorrhage.

Pharmacokinetics: How a drug is administered, absorbed, metabolized, and excreted.

Pleural effusion: Accumulation of fluid in the space between the membrane encasing the lung and lining of the thoracic cavity.

Pneumomediastinum: An abnormal state characterized by the presence of air in the mediastinum.

Polydipsia: Increased water intake.

Polymyositis: Inflammation of several voluntary muscles simultaneously.

Polyphagia: Increased eating.

Polyuria: An abnormally excessive or inappropriate urine production.

Popliteal: Lymph nodes behind the knee.

Postrenal failure: Inability of the body to eliminate urine produced in the kidneys. Most commonly associated with a urethral obstruction, ureteral obstruction, or urine leakage.

Premature ventricular contractions/complexes (PVCs): See ventricular premature depolarizations (VPDs).

Prerenal azotemia: An abnormal concentration of urea, creatinine, and other nitrogenous substances in the blood arising from conditions such as decreased renal blood flow, hypovolemia, or excessive vasoconstriction.

Proptosis: The forward displacement or protrusion of an eyeball.

Ptyalism: Excessive secretion of saliva.

Pyelonephritis: Infection and secondary inflammation of the kidney.

Pyrogen: A substance that induces fever. It can be a toxin, drug, or pathogen. It can be endogenous or exogenous.

Renal disease: A global term relating to disease of the kidney, and may involve any part of the kidney including vasculature, glomeruli, tubules, or interstitial tissues. It is not synonymous with renal failure.

Renal failure: Inability of the kidney to eliminate products of metabolism or concentrate or dilute urine. Failure occurs after 66%–75% of the kidneys' function has been compromised.

Renal insufficiency: A reduced ability of the kidney to eliminate products of metabolism or concentrate or dilute urine. Insufficiency is the early stage of kidney failure, where 66% of the kidneys' function has been compromised.

Rewarming shock: Vasodilation that occurs during rewarming of a hypothermic patient. Causes reduction in blood flow leading to decreased oxygen delivery to tissues.

Rostral: Situated toward the oral or nasal region.

Strabismus: Inability of the eye to attain binocular vision with the other because of imbalance of the muscles of the eyeball.

Stridor: A shrill, harsh sound, especially the respiratory sound heard during inspiration in laryngeal obstruction.

Stroke volume: The blood pumped from the left ventricle in one heart beat.

Stupor: A state of lethargy and immobility with diminished responses to stimulation.

Symbiosis: An association that is beneficial or mutually reinforcing to both.

Synechiae: An adhesion of parts and especially one involving the iris of the eye.

Tachycardia: A heart rate above normal.

Tacypnea: A respiratory rate above normal.

Tamponade: Pathological compression of the heart.

Tarsorrhaphy: The operation of suturing the eyelids together entirely or in part.

Thermoregulation: The ability of the hypothalamus to keep the body within a narrow temperature range.

Tidal volume: The amount of gas passing into and out of the lungs in each respiratory cycle. Typically 10–15 mL/kg for cats and dogs.

Total body surface area (TBSA): Represents the amount of body surface affected by burn injury. Can help predict severity of injury.

Traumatic brain injury (TBI): Sudden and traumatic injury to the brain.

Uremia: When azotemia is associated with metabolic and physiological alterations.

Ventricular premature complexes/contractions (VPCs): See ventricular premature depolarizations (VPDs).

Ventricular premature depolarizations (VPDs): A common arrythmia where the heartbeat is initiated by the heart ventricles rather than by the sinoatrial node, causing the electrocardiogram (ECG) waves to appear wide and bizarre.

Wind up: See central sensitization.

Index